Combatting Antimicrobial Resistance Through Medical Microbiology

Syed Sohail Ahmad
Rehman College of Allied Health Sciences, Pakistan

Aman Ullah
Rehman College of Allied Health Sciences, Pakistan

IGI Global
Scientific Publishing
Publishing Tomorrow's Research Today

Vice President of Editorial	Melissa Wagner
Director of Acquisitions	Mikaela Felty
Director of Book Development	Jocelynn Hessler
Production Manager	Mike Brehm
Cover Design	Jose Rosado

Published in the United States of America by
IGI Global Scientific Publishing
701 East Chocolate Avenue
Hershey, PA, 17033, USA
Tel: 717-533-8845 | Fax: 717-533-7115
Website: https://www.igi-global.com E-mail: cust@igi-global.com

Library of Congress Cataloging-in-Publication Data

LCCN: (CIP Data Pending)
ISBN13: 9798337338255
Isbn13Softcover: 9798337338262
EISBN13: 9798337338279
British Cataloguing in Publication Data
A Cataloguing in Publication record for this book is available from the British Library.

Table of Contents

Detailed Table of Contents

M. Nisha, Department of Microbiology, Sacred Heart College, Tirupattur, India
U. Subhalakshmi, Department of Microbiology, Sacred Heart College, Tirupattur, India
V. Vaishnavi, Department of Microbiology, Sacred Heart College, Tirupattur, India
P. Prakathi, Department of Microbiology, Sacred Heart College, Tirupattur, India
P. Amudhanila, Department of Microbiology, Sacred Heart College, Tirupattur, India

The human microbiome contains a large number of antimicrobial resistance genes. In this introduction, we will discuss how horizontal transmission of antimicrobial resistance might impact microorganisms in the human gut, skin, respiratory system, and mouth. Additionally, antibiotics will be highlighted as a means of controlling bacteria to avoid illnesses or as a means of treating infections. Among the several human infection sites, the gut microbiota is known to be the primary site where AMR enters microorganisms via integrons, transposons, plasmids, and phage-related sequences. A apparently endless number of factors, including dietary changes, illness, hospitalization, treatment, and the host's immune systems, appear to have an impact on the development of AMR. Metagenomics, transcriptomics, and culturomics have made significant strides in measuring bacteria and the resistome. The advent of microbe-targeted approaches including phage therapies, fecal microbiota transplants, prebiotics, and narrow-spectrum antibiotics has made it possible to lower AMR.

Antimicrobial resistance (AMR) represents a major threat to global public health, driven by the overuse and misuse of antibiotics across human and animal health sectors. Its emergence followed the discovery of penicillin, and the rise of multidrug-resistant organisms now significantly complicates treatment, leading to therapeutic failure, increased morbidity and mortality, and substantial economic burdens. This chapter provides a comprehensive overview of contemporary strategies to mitigate AMR. Key approaches include the promotion of antimicrobial stewardship programs, which are essential for optimizing antibiotic use and preserving their efficacy. Complementary tools such as vaccination, antimicrobial peptides, bacteriophage therapy, monoclonal antibodies, and the development of new antibiotics also form a critical part of the response. The chapter concludes that combating AMR requires a multifaceted and system-wide approach, integrating these diverse strategies to address this complex challenge.

Antimicrobial resistance (AMR) is considered to be one of the most significant ongoing crises in global healthcare, as it jeopardizes the effectiveness of contemporary medicine and control of infectious diseases. This chapter is a detailed review of the molecular and mechanistic pathogenesis of AMR in the context of medical microbiology. It explains the mechanisms of adaptations and survival of bacterial populations in antimicrobial pressure. Major molecular mechanisms, including enzymatic inactivation of antibiotics, alteration of target sites, overexpression of efflux pumps, and decreased membrane permeability, are thoroughly explained. The chapter goes on to discuss the resistance occurring within biofilms, and horizontal gene transfer, which provides conjugation, transformation, and transduction, is investigated as a path of utmost importance. New alternative approaches are required to cope with this current issue. Knowledge of these molecular bases is important in creating successful antimicrobial stewardship initiatives.

AMR is a problem of significant global health concern, which threatens to reduce decades of medical advancement by weakening the efficacy of antibiotics, as well as other antimicrobials. The genetic mechanisms of AMR are spontaneous mutations and horizontal gene transfer of plasmids and transposons and phenotypic adaptation, such as biofilm formation, efflux pumps, and persister cell states which increase bacterial survival. Improper use of antibiotics in healthcare and agriculture such as environmental contamination aids the transmission of resistant strains within the ecosystems. Global surveillance should be conducted with advanced diagnostic tools, such as PCR, CRISPR-based, and whole genome sequencing. The fight against AMR needs combined measures, antibiotic stewardship, new therapeutics, alternative solutions, like bacteriophages and the One Health approach, which involves the connection of human, animal, and environmental health to maintain antimicrobial activity across the globe.

Biofilm production is one of the biological modes of bacterial survival, prolonged existence, and resistance to various forms of antimicrobial agents. A biofilm refers to a self-made polymer matrix that encloses a microbial body of organized bacteria, referred to as Exopolysaccharides (EPS), which adheres to both biological or non-biological surfaces. This unique structural organization makes it difficult for antibiotics to work effectively by inhibiting the functioning of this shielded environment. The physical barrier provided by the EPS matrix further enhances the sequestration or deactivation of antimicrobial drugs and limits the penetration of medicines. Due to this fact, biofilm-associated bacteria can express antibiotic resistance several hundred times higher than that of their free-living counterparts, hence biofilms are a major cause of recurring and chronic infections.

Pseudomonas aeruginosa is a rod-shaped, Gram-negative bacterium in the family Pseudomonadaceae that is native to soil and water environments. It is also found in other unlikely places, including surgical equipment and on the hands of hospital personnel. This chapter discusses how multidrug-resistant (MDR) P. aeruginosa plays a significant role in hospital-associated opportunistic infections. MDR P.

aeruginosa strains are primarily responsible for the high global prevalence of opportunistic pneumonia, bloodborne, and surgical wound infections, particularly in immunocompromised patients. Key mechanisms of resistance in MDR P. aeruginosa can be intrinsic, acquired, and genetic. Addressing antimicrobial drug resistance requires stewardship, hygiene practices, and combining antimicrobials due to limited therapeutic options. Future attempts may involve leveraging multidisciplinary techniques in molecular biology, bioinformatics, and machine learning to improve understanding and management of drug resistance. Novel therapies, vaccine development, and global surveillance are also useful.

This chapter addresses the revolution of antimicrobial resistance (AMR) detection and response by microbial genomics and diagnostic innovation. Three diagnostic platforms (PCR, CRISPR-based detection and Whole Genome Sequencing, WGS) were evaluated in terms of accuracy, reproducibility and turnaround time using 100 clinical isolates. WGS had the best detection rate of (97), the best genotype-phenotype correlation ($r = 0.86$), whereas CRISPR is the most rapid. Genome Data + AI analytics allowed foreseeing resistance and mainstream public health surveillance. The results highlight genomics as a foundation of accurate microbiology, which promotes real-time AMR surveillance and evidence-based policy intervention in a One Health context.

Antimicrobial resistance (AMR) is a growing global health crisis that threatens to undermine decades of medical progress. This chapter examines the transformative role of microbial genomics in addressing AMR, emphasizing advancements in

One of the most important global public health issues of the twenty-first century is antimicrobial resistance (AMR), which compromises the efficacy of currently available antibiotics and causes extended illness, higher death, and a substantial financial burden. Both acquired and innate genetic processes that allow microorganisms to withstand antimicrobial exposure by restricting drug absorption, changing drug targets, and enzymatic drug inactivation are responsible for the fast evolution of resistant infections. The abuse and prescribing of antibiotics in healthcare, agriculture, and farming are examples of human activities that greatly accelerate the development of resistance. The emergence of multiple-drug-resistant organisms and insufficient infection control procedures exacerbate the problems related to AMR. Novel scientific strategies are being explored to tackle these issues. The creation of small-molecule antibiotics is being revolutionized by artificial intelligence, which makes it possible to identify new compounds more quickly.

This chapter examines the transformative impact of precision medicine in combating antimicrobial resistance (AMR), emphasizing the potential of advanced diagnostics, targeted therapies, and personalized treatment strategies. With AMR becoming a significant global health threat, the integration of AI, genomics, synthetic biology, and nanotechnology offers innovative solutions for diagnosing and treating resistant

Preface

INTRODUCTION

Antimicrobial resistance (AMR) represents one of the most urgent and complex challenges confronting modern medicine, threatening to erode decades of progress in the prevention and treatment of infectious diseases. Once-curable infections are increasingly becoming difficult, and in some cases impossible, to treat due to the rapid emergence and global spread of resistant pathogens. This crisis is not confined to any single region or discipline; rather, it is a multifaceted problem that intersects human health, animal health, environmental systems, and global public policy. Medical microbiology lies at the heart of this challenge, providing the tools and knowledge necessary to understand, detect, and ultimately combat antimicrobial resistance.

The purpose of this edited volume, *Combatting Antimicrobial Resistance Through Medical Microbiology*, is to bring together contemporary scientific perspectives that illuminate the biological mechanisms, clinical implications, and technological innovations shaping the global AMR landscape. By integrating foundational microbiological principles with emerging genomic, diagnostic, and therapeutic approaches, this book seeks to bridge the gap between basic science and applied clinical practice. The chapters reflect the growing recognition that AMR cannot be addressed through isolated efforts, but instead requires coordinated, interdisciplinary, and evidence-based strategies.

This volume has been developed for a broad readership that includes microbiologists, clinicians, public health professionals, researchers, educators, and advanced students in biomedical and allied health sciences. The contributing authors represent diverse institutions and geographic regions, underscoring the global nature of antimicrobial resistance and the shared responsibility to address it. Collectively, the chapters emphasize not only the severity of the AMR crisis, but also the promising scientific innovations and collaborative frameworks that offer pathways toward sustainable solutions.

CHAPTER OVERVIEW

The book opens with **Chapter 1**, which explores the role of the human microbiome in the emergence and transmission of antimicrobial resistance. This chapter highlights the gut microbiota as a critical reservoir of resistance genes and examines how horizontal gene transfer, antibiotic exposure, and host-related factors contribute to the expansion of the resistome. It also introduces microbiome-targeted interventions as emerging tools to reduce resistance.

Chapter 2 provides a global perspective on AMR, outlining its public health impact, major challenges, and strategic approaches for prevention. Emphasis is placed on antimicrobial stewardship, vaccination, alternative therapies, and the need for coordinated global action to preserve antimicrobial efficacy.

In **Chapter 3**, the focus shifts to the molecular and mechanistic foundations of antimicrobial resistance. This chapter offers an in-depth discussion of bacterial adaptation under antimicrobial pressure, detailing enzymatic inactivation, target modification, efflux mechanisms, biofilm-associated resistance, and horizontal gene transfer.

Chapter 4 expands on genetic and phenotypic dimensions of AMR, addressing mutations, plasmid-mediated resistance, and adaptive survival strategies. The chapter also highlights the importance of surveillance, advanced diagnostics, and the One Health approach in controlling resistance across ecosystems.

The role of biofilms in persistent and recurrent infections is the focus of **Chapter 5**, which examines how biofilm formation dramatically enhances bacterial tolerance to antimicrobial agents and complicates treatment outcomes.

Chapter 6 presents a clinically focused case study on multidrug-resistant *Pseudomonas aeruginosa* in nosocomial infections. It discusses resistance mechanisms, infection control challenges, and future strategies involving molecular biology and data-driven approaches.

Advances in diagnostics and surveillance are addressed in **Chapter 7**, which evaluates PCR, CRISPR-based detection, and whole-genome sequencing as transformative tools for AMR detection and public health response within a One Health framework.

Chapter 8 explores the application of microbial genomics and artificial intelligence in understanding resistance mechanisms and guiding precision-based interventions, emphasizing real-time surveillance and personalized treatment strategies.

Healthcare-centered interventions are examined in **Chapter 9**, highlighting the central role of medical microbiology laboratories in diagnostics, stewardship, infection control, and data integration for sustainable AMR management.

Chapter 10 reviews emerging therapeutic strategies aimed at mitigating antimicrobial resistance, including novel antibiotic discovery, synthetic biology, and AI-assisted drug development, underscoring the importance of multidisciplinary innovation.

Chapter 11 focuses on microbiological innovations in diagnostics, surveillance, and alternative therapeutics, demonstrating how laboratory-driven advances contribute to early detection and effective resistance management.

The convergence of advanced technologies is further explored in **Chapter 12**, which discusses CRISPR-Cas systems and AI-driven approaches as next-generation tools for antibiotic discovery and resistance prediction.

Precision medicine takes center stage in **Chapter 13**, where personalized diagnostics, targeted therapies, and ethical considerations are examined within the context of global AMR strategies and future roadmaps.

The volume concludes its thematic exploration with **Chapter 14**, which integrates microbiome research into AMR solutions, highlighting engineered probiotics, microbiome restoration, and global collaboration as transformative approaches in resistance management.

CONCLUSION

Taken together, the chapters in this volume present a comprehensive and forward-looking examination of antimicrobial resistance through the lens of medical microbiology. The contributions emphasize that AMR is not merely a consequence of microbial evolution, but a reflection of human practices, healthcare systems, and environmental interactions. Understanding resistance mechanisms at molecular, clinical, and population levels is essential for developing effective and sustainable interventions.

A central theme throughout this book is the critical role of innovation—particularly in genomics, diagnostics, artificial intelligence, and precision medicine—in reshaping how antimicrobial resistance is detected, monitored, and managed. Equally important is the reinforcement of antimicrobial stewardship, infection prevention, and global surveillance systems. The integration of these elements within a One Health framework emerges as a recurring and necessary strategy for addressing AMR at scale.

As editors, we hope that this volume will serve not only as a scholarly reference but also as a catalyst for interdisciplinary dialogue and collaborative action. Combatting antimicrobial resistance requires sustained commitment from researchers, clinicians, policymakers, and educators alike. By advancing scientific understanding and promoting evidence-based solutions, this book aims to contribute meaningfully to the global effort to safeguard the effectiveness of antimicrobials for future generations.

Chapter 1
Role of the Human Microbiome in AMR Emergence and Transmission

M. Nisha
https://orcid.org/0009-0000-0862-7631
Department of Microbiology, Sacred Heart College, Tirupattur, India

U. Subhalakshmi
https://orcid.org/0009-0007-8989-5486
Department of Microbiology, Sacred Heart College, Tirupattur, India

V. Vaishnavi
https://orcid.org/0009-0006-8922-5231
Department of Microbiology, Sacred Heart College, Tirupattur, India

P. Prakathi
https://orcid.org/0009-0000-4457-9008
Department of Microbiology, Sacred Heart College, Tirupattur, India

P. Amudhanila
https://orcid.org/0009-0003-1970-6150
Department of Microbiology, Sacred Heart College, Tirupattur, India

ABSTRACT

The human microbiome contains a large number of antimicrobial resistance genes. In this introduction, we will discuss how horizontal transmission of antimicrobial resistance might impact microorganisms in the human gut, skin, respiratory system,

DOI: 10.4018/979-8-3373-3825-5.ch001

and mouth. Additionally, antibiotics will be highlighted as a means of controlling bacteria to avoid illnesses or as a means of treating infections. Among the several human infection sites, the gut microbiota is known to be the primary site where AMR enters microorganisms via integrons, transposons, plasmids, and phage-related sequences. A apparently endless number of factors, including dietary changes, illness, hospitalization, treatment, and the host's immune systems, appear to have an impact on the development of AMR. Metagenomics, transcriptomics, and culturomics have made significant strides in measuring bacteria and the resistome. The advent of microbe-targeted approaches including phage therapies, fecal microbiota transplants, prebiotics, and narrow-spectrum antibiotics has made it possible to lower AMR.

1. INTRODUCTION

Antimicrobial resistance affects both people and animals. In other words, bacteria that are resistant to drugs develop survival mechanisms that allow them to avoid the negative effects of medicines. The rate at which new antibiotics are being developed is slowing down, and new resistance strains of both old and new drugs are still emerging at an accelerating rate, despite the fact that we are killing most harmful bacteria. This fact increases bacteria' resistance to specific drugs. Misuse of antibiotics raises AMR and contributes to the development of drug-resistant diseases like TB/XDR-TB.

Additionally, the atmosphere is crucial. Resistance genes can transfer between bacteria and even between species, according to Berendonk and colleagues. This idea has evolved along with microbiota's nomenclature. Once a broad word for microorganisms found inside or on hosts, it now often refers to the complete population connected with a specific environment or niche, such as human bodies, soil, or mouths, and includes viruses, bacteria, fungi, and archaea. The main question is how their metabolic and genetic processes impact their environments.

One of the biggest advances in medicine is the development of antimicrobials. As a result, the mean lifespan has doubled and diseases that were once lethal have turned chronic. The mean lifespan has actually grown by about 23 years since the first antibiotic was discovered in 1910. The finding by Alexander Fleming of penicillin, a genuinely revolutionary breakthrough in the field, marked the beginning of their so-called golden age.

But resistance happened in a typical way: bacteria developed ways to resist drugs, such penicillinase, which defeated penicillin. Antibiotics like ampicillin and larger groups like carbapenems and cephalosporins were crucial in treating illnesses in both humans and animals. Over 150 antibacterial compounds have been found since then.

2. ANTIMICROBIAL RESISTANCE

2.1 Nature

There are two primary types of antimicrobial resistance: inherent and acquired. The phrase "innate AMR" refers to the inherent resistance that some bacteria have.

Antimicrobial resistance in microorganisms is an inherent process. On the other hand, acquired AMR occurs when some genes are changed or new genes are produced, initiating the process that gives the microbe resistance (Morton et al., 2015). Antibacterial, antifungal, and antiparasitic medication resistance (AMR) is present despite the predominance of antibiotic resistance.

The widespread use of powerful drugs to treat illnesses and encourage cattle growth has prompted concerns about AMR in both natural and artificial contexts (Moossavi, 2014). Microorganisms tend to become resistant to antimicrobials when they are misused (Mathur & Singh, 2005).

Genes that are resistant to disinfectants and antimicrobials are directly linked to the confluence of environmental, animal, and human problems. In light of this, Morio et al. (2017) discuss the relationship between agricultural practices and the emergence of AMR. The use of antibiotics is intimately linked to AMR in both humans and animals, while it is uncertain how the characteristics of present hosts with AMR may alter. Hokken et al. (2019) claim that the prior research offers a narrow foundation for comprehending the premise and potential modifications to the mechanisms in connection with the development of AMR.

Although "tuning" antibiotics has rarely been utilized in human studies, several attempts have been made to see if it could assist regulate AMR in populations of humans and animals.

Second, the concept of "sentinel species," which includes field rats, chickens, rabbits, and insectivorous mammals, has been widely evaluated and acknowledged as being essential to the investigation and management of AMR.

2.2 Mechanisms of AMR

The increased usage of antibiotics in the environment is making bacteria more resistant. This is due to the fact that antimicrobial resistance genes, or ARGs for short, encode certain microorganisms. These bacteria, along with many others, are easily resistant to antibiotics due to their ARGs. These ARGs continuously contribute to the rise in bacterial resistance because of environmental resistance. ARGs and environmental antibiotic use are the two main causes of microorganism antimicrobial resistance. New antibiotics are finding it more difficult to withstand common bacterial infections due to the rising use of pharmaceuticals and the increased transmission of ARGs by mosquitoes and plasmids.

Bacterial resistance affects not only humans but also cockroaches and both domesticated and wild animals, such as rats and pigeons. Other animals kept in similar circumstances are also exhibiting same behavior. These particular microbes have the ability to infect sick people. Mice, for example, prey on other animals that might contain fleas that harbor the fatal bacteria Yersinia pestis.

Body fluids can transmit pneumonic plague, while fleas from wild mice, cats, and other rodents can transmit bubonic plague. Further studies are needed to completely comprehend the importance of wild small animals as important AMR carriers and reservoirs. AMR genes are easily transferred to animals because houseflies carry AMR enterococci on their bodies. Antibiotic resistance mostly contributes to the development of AMR in the following ways: Microbes modify host, plasmid, or chromosomal genes and/or develop new defense mechanisms. Genes found in various hosts are the cause of AMR.

There has also been research on the transmission of AMR resistance between individuals and their environment. The horizontal gene transfer of flexible bacterial genes is what leads to the rapid establishment of AMR. There are three primary methods that bacteria can transfer genes horizontally. They are conjugation, phage-mediated bacterial transformation, and natural transformation..

2.3 Conventional and Emerging Analytical for Antimicrobial Resistance

Bacteria can be removed using conventional techniques, including saline washes, after host rodents or animals, like mice and other fly species, have been collected. Numerous well used techniques can be used to evaluate their antibacterial susceptibility (Kmet et al., 2018). The Minimum Inhibitory Concentration (MIC) of an antibiotic can be used to identify Antibiotic-Resistant Bacteria (ARB) in a sample (Guo et al., 2017). The Minimum Inhibitory Concentration (MIC) is still unknown for many ecological microorganisms that often do not flourish on culture media. These techniques are biased because they focus on specific bacteria that vary depending on the kind of extraction medium, even if other prevalent diseases may also exhibit resistance but go undetected (Saidi et al., 2013). This approach does not pinpoint the ARGs causing the reported resistance and is mainly anecdotal. Standardizing culture-based methods typically provides a useful and affordable means of comparing outcomes, especially in resource-constrained host environments. Cultural viewpoints have a tremendous impact on AMR research. Utilizing state-of-the-art techniques and resources is crucial, such as sequencing the complete genomes of antibiotic-resistant bacterial species.

This could aid in the identification of mobile genetic elements, dominant microbial strains, and drug-vulnerable genes, among other crucial information (Le et al., 2018). By measuring resistance-conferring genes, antimicrobial-resistant organisms, and variations in mobile genes, especially within rodent gastrointestinal tracts, metagenomics may provide a more accurate and comprehensive understanding of the mechanisms or dynamics of antimicrobial resistance relationships (Pai et al., 2005). Evaluating AMR requires knowledge of the advantages and drawbacks of both traditional culture-based and molecular-based methodologies. Only some bacterial and microscopic species that are easily cultivated using synthetic media and require rapid sample preparation can be used with culture-dependent approaches (Pai, 2013). This suggests that the use of functional but uncultivable bacteria, non-target microbes that contain ARG, or carefully cultured environments does not promote development. This could lead to false negative results. The quantitative polymerase chain reaction (qPCR), a widely used molecular technique for identifying ARGs, requires the NAA's growing strength (Nasirian, 2017). It uses DNA from a range of sources, including microbial cells, to produce ARGs with specific, predefined properties. Certain genetic characteristics of bacteria can be identified using predefined primers. Oyeyemi et al. (2016) claim that qPCR is a highly accurate, rapid, and focused technique.

qPCR can be used to determine the total ARG content of any microbial strain, phage, transcribed coefficient, atmospheric DNA, eDNA, and mobile DNA elements, such as integrons and plasmids (Nasirian, 2017). Additionally, by using propidium acetate as the preferred reagent in sample preparation, qPCR can differentiate between DNA from living cells and DNA from phages, non-viable cells, or ambient DNA fragments. A list of potential ARG ABR donors may result from this. To identify particular resistance-generating genes in bacteria or their effects on human health, PCR is insufficient. Furthermore, the approach cannot assess the overall resistance to a particular antimicrobial medication because it is restricted to known DNA sequences.

3. HUMAN HEALTH RISK ASSESSMENT AND MITIGATION

3.1 Health Risk Assessment

In a nutshell, we need to consider how much the sources mentioned above contribute to the decline in human health brought on by the emergence of antibiotic resistance. The framework for the risk evaluation of AMR problems has been identified by Guiyoule et al. (2001). The concerns related to treatment goals and resistance attributed to domestic or pet animals, such as rats and insects, as well as their human interaction and the potential transmission of AMR and ARGs inside domestic mammals, are the main emphasis of the current review.

Despite the fact that animal farming and other animals are known to be AMR reservoirs, it was previously believed that companion animals, such as dogs and cats, supplied the minuscule portion of ARGs that could be accessible to humans. We should conduct additional research to produce data that is essential for assessing the health risk connected with the sap of rats, dogs, and other animals exposed to antibiotics, as the harm to human health still seems to be underestimated. As noted by the European Medicines Agency in Perry & Wright, 2013, if the high prevalence of AMR in the domestic animal rat, for example, and the related risk factors seem ambiguous, determining the specific health risk may appear challenging.

Clearly, further research is needed, especially given the uncertainty surrounding the hazards associated with rodents and insects. These writers (2014) advocate for national surveillance using certain standards. According to the authors, every strategy meant to accelerate the spread of information must include empirical research. It is important to remember that less developed nations do not have supportive policies. According to Warnes et al. (2012), additional study on antibiotic resistance in companion animals and their owners may be sparked by the government's pivotal role in this context and the requirement for international funding.

3.2 Mitigation

This guarantees a degree of flexibility while maintaining the basic idea. In contrast to utilizing antimicrobials, the fourth and fifth steps focus on teaching veterinarians how to manage resistance, with the goal of improving animal immunity. Additionally, educating pet owners about the need of antimicrobial regulations takes effort.

The health of the pets' teeth may be directly impacted by what they eat. Because teeth are made to process hard, chewed food, soft food diets are associated with a higher incidence of oral health issues. When creating a plan to lower MDR/AMR levels, dental health is an important factor to take into account. The usage of antibiotics must be specified in a unified strategy that will aid in lowering the levels of MDR/AMR.

Particularly for domesticated dogs and cats, it is imperative that antimicrobial medications be prescribed exclusively through a veterinary facility. Precautions must be taken to protect both people and pets because the majority of diseases do not require antibiotics. The current approach primarily focuses on lowering the usage of antibiotics in dogs when treatment is administered in a medical facility. Cleaning the surroundings, avoiding direct contact—such as sharing a bed or making direct eye contact—and maintaining a safe distance—particularly when handling antibiotics—are among the recommended precautions.

To avoid contamination from bug, mouse, or other domestic or wild animal urine and feces, it is crucial to handle AMR cases with additional caution and to wear gloves made of rubber, silicone, or vinyl materials. Safety measures can be taken even in the absence of rats, such as shielding pet food from contamination, covering trash cans, and caulking potential entry points such open windows, cracks around building corners, and holes. In temperate climates, this is particularly true.

Table 1. Human Health Risk Assessment and Mitigation for AMR from Pets and Household Pests

Aspect	Challenges	Proposed Actions / Mitigation Strategies	Reference
General Approach	Risk must be routinely assessed. Guidelines exist, but application to pets/pests is less developed.	Follow established frameworks (e.g., Guiyoule et al., 2001) and adapt for domestic settings.	(Guiyoule et al. 2001)
Focus of Assessment	Focus on AMR in pets (dogs, cats) and inadvertent household pests (rodents, insects).	Primary information sources should be: 1. Prevalence of AMR in these animals. 2. Human-animal contact patterns. 3. Transmission pathways of AMR/ ARGs to humans.	(Perry and Wright 2013)
Major Knowledge Gaps	1. **Companion Animals:** Historically seen as minor source; risk data is scarce. 2. **Pets & Pests:** Insufficient data for quantitative risk assessments due to unclear indicators/ pathways. 3. **Surveillance:** Government surveillance is inadequate, especially in developing countries.	1. **More research is urgently needed** to generate risk assessment data. 2. Implement **national surveillance** using standardized techniques. 3. In developing countries, **external funding and support** are required for research and monitoring.	(Zurek and Ghosh 2014)
Overarching Policy	Need for a holistic approach restricting antibiotic use and environmental release from all sources.	Implement **strict limitations** on non-essential antibiotic use across human and animal sectors.	(Warnes et al., 2012)
For Veterinary Practice	Need to optimize antimicrobial use and explore alternatives.	1. **Educate veterinarians** on prudent antimicrobial selection. 2. Base treatment on **official guidelines** and clinical advice. 3. Promote **non-clinical treatments** (e.g., nutrition for oral health).	(Guzman & Vilcinskas, 2020)

continued on following page

Table 1. Continued

Aspect	Challenges	Proposed Actions / Mitigation Strategies	Reference
For Pet Owners	Owners play a critical role in prevention and hygiene.	1. **Educate owners** on following antimicrobial guidelines. 2. Promote **hygiene:** handwashing, avoiding sharing beds/kissing pets. 3. Use **protective gear** (gloves) when cleaning animal waste.	(Dolejska & Literak, 2019).
For Household Management	Inadvertent pests (rodents, insects) pose a contamination risk.	1. **Rodent Control:** Seal trash, secure food, cover entry points, use traps/repellents. 2. **Pet Management:** Keep cats indoors to reduce prey contact. 3. **General Hygiene:** Maintain clean homes, reduce human-animal contact during antibiotic treatments.	(Ahlstrom et al., 2018).
International & National Action	Need for coordinated governance of critical antimicrobials.	Establish **monitoring and regulations** on the use of Critically Important Antimicrobials (CIAs) at national and international levels.	(Mulani et al., 2019)

4 MECHANISMS OF RESISTANCE IN ORAL MICROORGANISMS

4.1 Resistance in Candida and Other Oral Fungi

Candida albicans may form an extremely complex biofilm on almost any surface, including live tissue and hard, inert objects. Because it is a web of many interconnected cells that is very difficult to eradicate, it is a common nemesis in medical settings, inside hosts, and around the surfaces of implanted devices. Its stubbornness is mostly due to the fact that just six of its thirty-three cellular components show significant antifungal resistance. Furthermore, by increasing the cells' environmental endurance, the biofilm's defense against the fungal invaders raises the risk of reinfection.

The problem's worldwide impact is highlighted by the high fatality rate and persistent treatment difficulties associated with Candida infections, especially invasive candidiasis. The ubiquitous presence of Candida albicans has led to the rapid proliferation of its sister species, Candida glabrata and Candida auris, which have developed resistance and undermined previous treatments (Skarzyńska et al., 2020). In addition to the more obvious mechanisms, such as altered drug targets, efflux pumps, and reduced drug permeability, resistance can also develop through more subtle means. Yeast transcription factors such as YRR1 and TAC1 in Candida albicans are important regulators that synchronize the expression of genes linked to biological, thermal, and nutritional stresses. Without antifungal drugs, microbes like fumigatus Aspergillus, Candida species, and Cryptococcus neoformans, among others, can acquire intrinsic resistance.

Understanding the regulation of the resistant phenotypes is important since adaptive resistance may make therapy even more challenging. For example, genetic alterations that alter therapeutic targets by upsetting intracellular sterol pools and rerouting ergosterol synthesis are the cause of polyene resistance. Increased efflux pump activity, overexpression caused by aneuploidy or transcriptional reprogramming, or an enzyme target that is less sensitive to the medication can all account for the azoles decreased pharmacological action. In yeasts and prokaryotes, a variety of transcription factors indicate an efflux pump mechanism that is always in operation. Changes in the genes generating enzymes that are involved in cell wall production result in echinocandin resistance.

Figure 1. Resistance in Candida and Other Oral Fungi

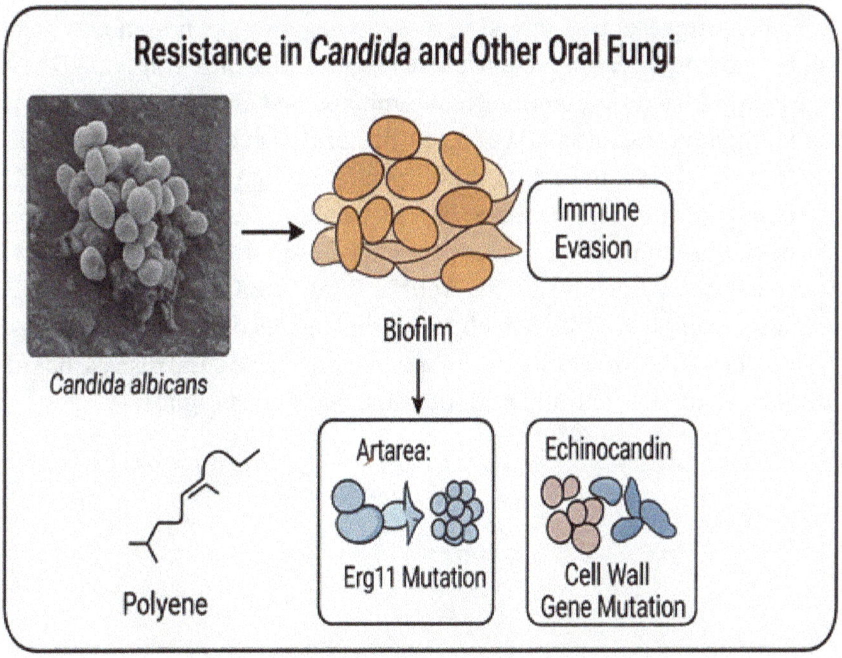

4.2 Resistance Mechanisms in Oral Bacteria

The bacteria that cause periodontitis are gram-negative. Porphyromonas gingivalis is this. The characteristics of this bacterium, which is the subject of periodontitis study, keeps scientists alert. An article in 2015's "Current Status of Periodontitis" by Claycamp states that "infections caused by P. gingivalis are known to shrug off several drugs, making this already complex disease even trickier." There is one advantage this bacterium has over others. It can go beyond the host's defenses. Because of this, researchers refer to P. gingivalis as a genuine pathogen. Ironically, the efflux pump of this drug-resistant bacterium plays a major role in P. gingivalis pathogenesis. Compared to bacteria whose main mechanism of drug resistance is the efflux pump, this process is distinctly different. P. gingivalis's effects are not limited to periodontitis. They're systemic.PG_0285, PG_0538, PG_0539, and PG_1797 are among the genes in the bacterial genome that have been identified as prospective candidates for therapeutic intervention. According to a study by Ash Bolt et al. (2013), targeting the genes PG_0539 and PG_1797 is linked to improved efflux pumps and pathogens. This suggests that targeting these genes may open up a new treatment control option for three very prevalent and resistant strains of P. gingivalis. Prevotella species, Aggregatibacter actinomycetemcomitans, and Fusobacterium nucleatum are the other main periodontopathogens, or bacteria, that cause periodontitis in the human oral cavity. It is known that these species contain bacterial strains that are resistant to amoxicillin, clindamycin, and metronidazole. Geographical access to drugs has been a problem, even if rates of resistance are still around 10% worldwide (European Medicines Agency, 2015). Antibiotic-resistant bacteria are predicted to become more common in 2025, which highlights the need of maintaining susceptibility to antibacterial medications. Although human periodontal disease has already been linked to virulence, chronic periodontitis, and poor prognosis,.

Figure 2. Resistance Mechanisms in Oral Bacteria

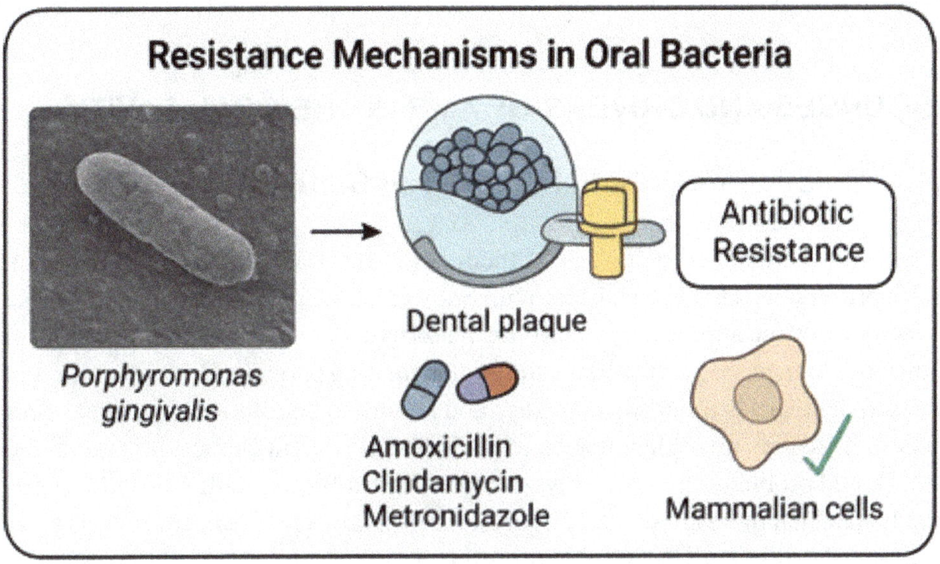

4.3. Novel Antimicrobial Strategies and Compounds

Mechanical debridement is still the tried-and-true treatment for periodontitis, though it may occasionally be combined with antibiotics or other antimicrobials if needed. However, the hunt for alternatives is still fueled by the shortcomings of existing treatments, the ongoing problem of antibiotic resistance, or both (Chang et al., 2015). Because of this, AM404, an antibacterial acetaminophen derivative, is relevant. Because it can inhibit the growth of Porphyromonas gingivalis and prevent biofilm formation, particularly on titanium, it has great potential for treating peri-implantitis. It works by diffusion across the bacterial carbon chain.

At concentrations up to four times the minimum inhibitory concentration (MIC), AM404 was demonstrated to have cytotoxic effects on mammalian cells, indicating potential therapeutic benefits (Lee et al., 2020). According to a twenty-year regional study conducted in the United States, the prevalence of bacterial resistance to amoxicillin and clindamycin in 1999 and 2000 was fifteen to twenty-eight times lower than the number of cases with chronic gingivitis.

These kinds of results must be carefully examined, accounting for reduced sample sizes within certain populations and any differences in analysis techniques. However, the isolates did not change their sensitivity or resistance to amoxicillin, metronidazole, and doxycycline, either separately or in combination. When it comes to the possibility of drug-resistant strains, care is essential because several therapies have a known set of resistance genes.

5 SOURCES AND DRIVERS OF AMR IN THE ORAL CAVITY

5.1 Antibiotic Prescribing Practices in Dentistry

Even for patients who don't need them, antibiotics are employed in the dental health profession. This is consistent with Sao et al. (2022), who argue that a variety of factors impact antibiotic prescribing patterns and that dentists need the right knowledge to manage medications safely when treating patients. One of the emerging issues in dentistry is mouthwash misuse and its link to antibiotic resistance. In conclusion, if there is no logical reason to prescribe or use antibiotics, it is not a good idea. Dental problems are not always treated with antibiotics. Gillieatt and Coleman (2024) state that there are several circumstances in the dental context, such as avoiding complications from bacterial endocarditis or other infections following surgery.

5.2 Co-Selection of Antibiotic Resistance by Non-Antibiotic Agents

Instead, recent studies have looked at the function of non-antibiotic antimicrobials, such as biocides, disinfectants, antiseptics, and preservation chemicals, and the consequences of their impact on biological habitats contaminated with metals and the development of drug-resistant organisms. The use of copper and zinc compounds in mouthwashes, cleansers, and other dental accessories has gained popularity recently because of their established antibacterial qualities. Specifically, bacterial cells can be killed by copper ions via membrane-based, ROS-mediated, or enzymatic processes.

By blocking glycolytic enzymes, zinc ions' antibacterial and anti-inflammatory qualities can help avoid gum disease, according to Ng et al. (2024). By acting on Streptococcus mutans, the primary cariogenic bacterium, zinc supplements such as zinc acetate, zinc oxide, and zinc chloride may prevent tooth cavities. According to Gerits et al. (2017), the antibacterial qualities of the copper ion can enhance the functionality of dental materials that contain copper.

However, sensitivity and resistance become issues when these applications are expanded. A phenomenon known as co-resistance occurs when antibiotic-resistant bacteria coexist with metal resistance genes (MRGs) or antibiotic resistance genes (ARGs) in the form of a plasmid. When Zn and Cu are utilized in dental materials, resistance risks must be evaluated because plasmids containing numerous ARGs have been found in oral microbiomes and environmental isolates exhibit resistance to silver.

6. DEVELOPMENT AND IDENTIFICATION NEW ANTIBIOTICS AND REPURPOSING OF EXISTING ANTIBIOTIC

We must keep an eye on the current use of antibiotics in order to prevent resistance given the impending reality of MDR and XDR illnesses. In order to do this, basic scientific research into new target materials must be accelerated, or existing ones must be modified. Research may concentrate on developing entirely new antimicrobial drugs with improved physiochemical characteristics or novel chemical structures, refining existing antibiotics, or exploring novel possibilities such phage proteins. The lengthy licensing process for antibiotics is the main obstacle, lengthening the time lag and reducing the pharmaceutical return on investment. The possibility that nanotechnology or nano-functionalization could boost the antibacterial effectiveness of existing antibiotics is a topic of continuous discussion.

Vass et al., however, divided nanoparticles into two functional groups in their 2022 study on the use of nanotechnology to fight multidrug resistance: chemically generated nanoparticles and biologically derived nanoparticles with antibacterial qualities. It is anticipated that several forms of resistance will decline because the antimicrobial activity mechanism is mostly focused on interaction with the bacteria. The method by which antibiotic-producing actinomycetes evolve resistance to NPs was covered by James et al. (2017). According to a 2023 study, filamentous bacteria can form a symbiotic relationship with the hosts they rely on for sustenance and defense. It is thought that the host's environmental stimuli influence the gene regions that produce NPs to create novel drugs. Murray et al. (2024) highlighted the use of prokaryotes for a number of applications, including post-translational models of peptides, polyketides, and ribosome-associated models. As we continue to search for new antibacterial medicines, these technologies play a crucial role in the identification of new and enigmatic biosynthetic gene clusters. The approach used in this instance may not move quickly, but it is powerful since it combines ecological and genetic data. Not only can we find and reexamine new antibiotics and gene clusters for new compounds as genome sequencing resolution advances, but we may also set the stage for determining which specific medical conditions will benefit most from the use of those medicines. The incorporation of genetic data regarding mechanisms of action will undoubtedly be important.

Specifically focusing on human defensins like LL-37 and analogs, Grass et al. (2011) explore the function of defensins as a developing field of novel antibacterial therapy. Cost, toxicity, and stability are the three issues that Uwitonze et al. (2020)

address when utilizing host-based techniques to prevent infections. This page explains what they are and how they function.However, we still face modern issues brought on by traditional antibacterial substances and the growing threat of drug-resistant strains as a result of scientific inquiry's never-ending quest for knowledge. We need more funding in our research initiatives to advance both fronts.

7. ACTIONS TO FIGHT ANTIBIOTIC RESISTANCE

Antibacterial resistance arises when harmful bacteria learn to avoid the drugs that will kill them. To prevent infections and halt their spread, certain criteria must be adhered to. Careful and strict regulation of antibiotic use and ongoing monitoring can lead to better antibiotic administration and efforts to reduce resistance.

8. FACTORS CONTRIBUTING TO ANTIBIOTIC RESISTANCE AND ITS TRANSFER

Antibiotic resistance is already recognized as a persistent innate characteristic of bacterial cells, and human behavior is contributing to it. The main causes are the speed at which new chemical antibiotics are created, overprescription, inappropriate use, and occasionally the use of medicines to promote the development of cattle bred on farms.

According to Van der Meij et al. (2017), these are significant considerations. Having three children may possibly be a contributing factor, according to recent studies, however this is unclear. The widespread use of antibiotic as boosters of growth in agriculture, prescription overuse, and abuse are human factors that encourage the development of resistance to antibiotics. Bacteria create defense mechanisms in their natural environment (Tracanna et al., 2017).

Emerging theories and theories of education According to some study, the difficulties associated with antibiotic distribution and schedule adherence may be lessened with better communication with healthcare practitioners. Students seeking health-related careers may benefit from taking undergraduate courses that provide knowledge to tackle antimicrobial resistance (AMR) (Pachón-Ibáñez et al., 2017). Figures 2A and 2B in Razzaque's study illustrate the crucial elements and strategies used by medical professionals to get past the microbiological and health issues related to the usage of antibiotics. These strategies can be incorporated into the curriculum for undergraduates pursuing health professions and assist alleviate the health risks associated with elevated incidence levels of AMR (Ventola, 2015). ATRIC (Atrium) Razzaque outlines the fundamental mechanics that underpin an effective AMR strategy in order to make all of these ideas more understandable. Resistance occurs when the disease or target bacterial species has evolved a defense against the antibiotic's effects. Changes to the bacterial cell wall and/or enzymes that break down the antibiotic may cause this. Others include modifying and blocking the antibiotic's bacterial receptor, preventing bacterial uptake, and causing an increase in efflux. It should be noted that the abuse of broad-spectrum antibiotics contributes to the emergence of antimicrobial resistance, or AMR. Due to their weakened immune systems, patients are more vulnerable to infections after surgery (knees, dialysis, and cancer).

Antimicrobial resistance (AMR) is a condition that primarily affects individuals who are dealing with many health issues at the same time. Patients who use antibiotics as a "last resort" end up needing longer inpatient stays, being admitted more frequently, and having their treatment expenses further increase (Reygaert, 2018). As more and more evidence suggests that drug use is the root cause of the rise in antibiotic resistance, it is critical to integrate normal treatment facility management into the patient's care, returning to this point on a regular basis. Campaigns for health awareness should disseminate accurate information regarding illness prevention, transmission, and immunization. Comprehensive wound and infection prevention plans are necessary for patients getting multiple diagnosis care in order to lower the number of inpatient hospitalizations and avoid infections. Together, a defined course of therapy for the use of antibiotics and an accurate diagnosis that isn't deceptive are required. One of the main causes of the rising issue of antibiotic resistance is the overuse of antibiotics, which is brought on by individuals living in poor nations' reliance on their own medicines for viral diseases.

The pharmaceutical industry must eliminate any financial incentive for healthcare providers to overprescribe antibiotics in order for them to be prescribed appropriately. It is obvious that "superbugs" may spread from animals to people with ease. Finding the source of infections would be essential in the future to prevent such incidents. Based on their composition, viruses can readily spread from one species to another, as demonstrated by the COVID-19 pandemic.

9. APPLICATIONS OF TECHNOLOGY AGAINST ANTIBIOTIC RESISTANCE

The results suggest that the genes causing antibiotic resistance are diverse and that mapping microbial diversity requires cutting-edge methods (CDC, 2013). Thanks to techniques like next-generation sequencing, advanced bioinformatics, and big dynamic databases, this research has expedited and is now required.

According to Dadgostar (2019), the data also indicate that the mechanisms of resistance are not static, but rather vary and necessitate the use of cutting-edge instruments to distinguish between bacterial strains.

Genetic research advances go hand in hand with figuring out what causes AMR, and new technology improve surveillance and risk reduction initiatives. Chaw et al. (2018) claim that innovative techniques that combine deep genetic understanding with AMR enable fully informed, preventive measures. According to a number of scientists, metagenomics now holds the most promise for resistance detection. Over the past ten years, several studies have proposed and thoroughly validated three technical pillars: shotgun metagenomics, also called functional metagenomics, also called and targeted gene sequencing.

Transgenic libraries have developed resistances to 14 out of 18 antibiotics from eight different drug families, specifically targeting the juvenile resistome in the gut microbiome.

Genes linked to efflux pumps, resistant folate pathway reductases, chloramphenicol acetyltransferases, and beta-lactamases have been identified as resistance-related factors. Additionally, there is some data that suggests the transfer of certain resistance genes (Perry et al., 2014). The most advanced method for analyzing resistance these days is metagenomics. Shotgun sequencing, targeted gene sequencing, and functional metagenomics are the three methods that have so far seen extensive and ongoing use. The resistome of the young intestine was discovered by isolating antibodies for 14 of 18 antibiotics in eight classes using the metagenomic recombinant library technique. Important discoveries included acetyltransferases, dihydrofolate reductases, beta-lactamases, and multidrug efflux transporters.

10. PROBIOTICS

Probiotics are live bacteria. They could enhance health and sanitation. The FAO and WHO describe probiotics as live bacteria "which, when supplied in adequate quantity, may benefit the host."

" Probiotics are said to be the most interesting bacteria to learn about since they could help us achieve our goals for cleanliness and wellness. Their history started in 1908 when Nobel winner and Russian scientist Elie Metchnikoff postulated that meals high in lactic acid bacteria would have health benefits and be utilized medicinally. Since then, additional data has supported Metchnikoff's original theory on the therapeutic benefits of probiotics, according to a Healthline Daily article.

Since these early findings, several studies have validated the positive effects of probiotics, which has helped to explain their increasing appeal in recent decades.

Millions of individuals worldwide are thought to use probiotics on a daily basis for health-related purposes, either through food sources or pills. The FAO/WHO document from 2002 outlines standards for judging the legitimacy of probiotics, such as their capacity to attach to tissue, withstand competition from harmful microbes, and ensure host safety. Competitive exclusion is used in some methods of tissue repair to prevent the growth of bacteria in the gastrointestinal system (Fang & Polk, 2011).

The therapeutic use of probiotics is supported by more recent evidence from the human and animal literature, which covers a wide range of different illnesses and has been published in numerous research reviews. The ability of probiotics to stick to the surface, interact with host cells safely, and prevent infections through competitive antagonistic interactions are the most crucial aspects of their therapeutic application. In certain probiotics, the gut microbial flora is balanced in part by the mechanism of competitive exclusion. According to Ouwehand et al. (2002), probiotics have been effectively used to treat inflammation, diarrhea, and infections in both human and animal models.

11. FUTURE PERSPECTIVES

AMR research is, in fact, entering a new age. The next ten years will focus on pinpointing the exact causes and development of antibiotic resistance, building on a decade of significant advancements. The one-health discussions, which have already highlighted the limitations and challenges in our understanding of how resistance genes transfer from animals to humans, will define researchers' next concerns. This research aims to shed light on how resistance genes spread and how we can stop the emergence of antibiotic resistance. According to current research, an economically viable biological system could improve hospital hygiene and minimize patient infection rates while also reducing contamination by microbes and the emergence of antibiotic resistance.

Probiotic programs catered to the specific microbiomes of hospital patients may also help to explain the low occurrence of infections and related conditions associated with healthcare. Regardless of the cleaning strategy used, ultra-sensitive molecular methods for detecting and quantifying bacterial communities may become essential for tracking the spread of diseases across hospitals and their human hosts. With the development of new, culture-independent methods of microbe monitoring, we may soon be able to identify the key members of a population of microorganisms responsible for specific outcomes, monitor potentially harmful changes in a population, and take corrective action before damage is done. This could have a big impact on emerging medical cleaning methods to reduce infection rates.

12.CONCLUSION

The human microbiome is a living, breathing reservoir of resistance genes found in our bodies. From a One Health perspective, it is impossible to overstate how crucial the surroundings is to the emergence, persistence, and spread of antibiotic resistance. The significance of the microbiome that exists in our systems, especially in the dental and colon microbiomes, is demonstrated by our bodies' responses to environmental stressors, the usage of antibiotics, and the intricate network of helpful and harmful bacteria.

According to the One Health viewpoint, horizontal gene transfer causes resistance genes to spread from one location to another.

The last ten years have seen advances in the fields of metagenomics, functional genomics, and bioinformatics that have improved our understanding of how the microbiome contributes to the development of infections. Probiotics, person-specific strategies, enhanced antimicrobial stewardship, and other antimicrobial strategies are some of the recommendations put forth for preventing resistance while preserving the microbiome. The mechanism of antimicrobial resistance is still rife with uncertainties, hazards, and monitoring difficulties. Global cooperation is needed to address the problem of antibiotic resistance caused by the human microbiome. Understanding how the human microbiome contributes to antimicrobial resistance is essential to the ongoing battle against antibacterial resistance.

13. REFERENCES

Ahlstrom, C. A., Bonnedahl, J., Woksepp, H., Hernandez, J., Olsen, B., & Ramey, A. M. (2018). Acquisition and dissemination of cephalosporin-resistant E. coli in migratory birds sampled at an Alaska landfill as inferred through genomic analysis. *Scientific Reports*, *8*(1), 7361. DOI: 10.1038/s41598-018-25474-w PMID: 29743625

Ashbolt, N. J., Amézquita, A., Backhaus, T., Borriello, P., Brandt, K. K., Collignon, P., Coors, A., Finley, R., Gaze, W. H., Heberer, T., Lawrence, J. R., Larsson, D. G. J., McEwen, S. A., Ryan, J. J., Schönfeld, J., Silley, P., Snape, J. R., Van den Eede, C., & Topp, E. (2013). Human health risk assessment (HHRA) for environmental development and transfer of antibiotic resistance. *Environmental Health Perspectives*, *121*(9), 993–1001. DOI: 10.1289/ehp.1206316 PMID: 23838256

Berendonk, T. U., Manaia, C. M., Merlin, C., Fatta-Kassinos, D., Cytryn, E., Walsh, F., Bürgmann, H., Sørum, H., Norström, M., Pons, M.-N., Kreuzinger, N., Huovinen, P., Stefani, S., Schwartz, T., Kisand, V., Baquero, F., & Martinez, J. L. (2015). Tackling antibiotic resistance: The environmental framework. *Nature Reviews. Microbiology*, *13*(5), 310–317. DOI: 10.1038/nrmicro3439 PMID: 25817583

Chang, S.-K., Lo, D.-Y., Wei, H.-W., & Kuo, H.-C. (2015). Antimicrobial resistance of Escherichia coli isolates from canine urinary tract infections. *The Journal of Veterinary Medical Science*, *77*(1), 59–65. DOI: 10.1292/jvms.14-0009 PMID: 25720807

Chaw, P. S., Hopner, J., & Mikolajczyk, R. (2018). The knowledge, attitude and practice of health practitioners towards antibiotic prescribing and resistance in developing countries—A systematic review. *Journal of Clinical Pharmacy and Therapeutics*, *43*(5), 606–613. DOI: 10.1111/jcpt.12730 PMID: 29959783

Claycamp, H. G. (2015). Risk assessment of antimicrobial resistance. In Chen, C.-Y., Yan, X., & Jackson, C. R. (Eds.), *Antimicrobial Resistance and Food Safety* (pp. 283–302). Academic Press., DOI: 10.1016/B978-0-12-801214-7.00014-3

Dadgostar, P. (2019). Antimicrobial resistance: Implications and costs. *Infection and Drug Resistance*, *12*, 3903–3910. DOI: 10.2147/IDR.S234610 PMID: 31908502

Dolejska, M., & Literak, I. (2019). Wildlife is overlooked in the epidemiology of medically important antibiotic-resistant bacteria. *Antimicrobial Agents and Chemotherapy*, *63*(8), e01167–e19. DOI: 10.1128/AAC.01167-19 PMID: 31209001

European Medicines Agency. (2015). *Reflection paper on the risk of antimicrobial resistance transfer from companion animals* (EMA/CVMP/CHMP/682198/2014). https://www.ema.europa.eu/en/documents/scientific-guideline/reflection-paper-risk-antimicrobial-resistance-transfer-companion-animals_en.pdf

Food and Agriculture Organization of the United Nations & World Health Organization. (2002). *Guidelines for the evaluation of probiotics in food*. FAO/WHO. ftp://ftp.fao.org/es/esn/food/wgreport2.pdf

Gerits, E., Spincemaille, P., De Cremer, K., De Brucker, K., Beullens, S., Thevissen, K., Cammue, B. P. A., Vandamme, K., Fauvart, M., Verstraeten, N., & Michiels, J. (2017). Repurposing AM404 for the treatment of oral infections by *Porphyromonas gingivalis*. *Clinical and Experimental Dental Research*, *3*(2), 69–76. DOI: 10.1002/cre2.61 PMID: 29744181

Gillieatt, B. F., & Coleman, N. V. (2024). Unravelling the mechanisms of antibiotic and heavy metal resistance co-selection in environmental bacteria. *FEMS Microbiology Reviews*, *48*(2), fuae017. Advance online publication. DOI: 10.1093/femsre/fuae017 PMID: 38897736

Grass, G., Rensing, C., & Solioz, M. (2011). Metallic copper as an antimicrobial surface. *Applied and Environmental Microbiology*, *77*(5), 1541–1547. DOI: 10.1128/AEM.02766-10 PMID: 21193661

Guiyoule, A., Gerbaud, G., Buchrieser, C., Galimand, M., Rahalison, L., Chanteau, S. P., & Carniel, E. (2001). Transferable plasmid-mediated resistance to streptomycin in a clinical isolate of Yersinia pestis. *Emerging Infectious Diseases*, *7*(1), 43–48. DOI: 10.3201/eid0701.010106 PMID: 11266293

Guo, J., Li, J., Chen, H., Bond, P. L., & Yuan, Z. (2017). Metagenomic analysis reveals wastewater treatment plants as hotspots of antibiotic resistance genes and mobile genetic elements. *Water Research*, *123*, 468–478. DOI: 10.1016/j.watres.2017.07.002 PMID: 28689130

Guzman, J., & Vilcinskas, A. (2020). Bacteria associated with cockroaches: Health risk or biotechnological opportunity? *Applied Microbiology and Biotechnology*, *104*(24), 10369–10387. DOI: 10.1007/s00253-020-10973-6 PMID: 33128616

Hokken, M. W. J., Zwaan, B. J., Melchers, W. J. G., & Verweij, P. E. (2019). Facilitators of adaptation and antifungal resistance mechanisms in clinically relevant fungi. *Fungal Genetics and Biology*, *132*, 103254. DOI: 10.1016/j.fgb.2019.103254 PMID: 31326470

James, C., James, S. J., Onarinde, B. A., Dixon, R. A., & Williams, N. (2017). A critical review of AMR risks arising as a consequence of using biocides and certain metals in food animal production. *Antibiotics (Basel, Switzerland)*, *12*(10), 1569. DOI: 10.3390/antibiotics12101569 PMID: 37998771

Kmet, V., Cuvalová, A., & Stanko, M. (2018). Small mammals as sentinels of antimicrobial-resistant staphylococci. *Folia Microbiologica, 63*(5), 665–668. DOI: 10.1007/s12223-018-0602-7 PMID: 29524153

Mathur, S., & Singh, R. (2005). Antibiotic resistance in food lactic acid bacteria—A review. *International Journal of Food Microbiology, 105*(3), 281–295. DOI: 10.1016/j.ijfoodmicro.2005.03.025 PMID: 16289406

Moossavi, S. (2014). The necessity for an Iranian gut microbiome initiative. *Middle East Journal of Digestive Diseases, 6*(2), 109–110. PMID: 24872871

Morio, F., Jensen, R. H., Le Pape, P., & Arendrup, M. C. (2017). Molecular basis of antifungal drug resistance in yeasts. *International Journal of Antimicrobial Agents, 50*(5), 599–606. DOI: 10.1016/j.ijantimicag.2017.05.012 PMID: 28669835

Morton, E. R., Lynch, J., Froment, A., Lafosse, S., Heyer, E., Przeworski, M., Segurel, L., & Quintana-Murci, L. (2015). Variation in rural African gut microbiota is strongly correlated with colonization by entamoeba and subsistence. *PLOS Genetics, 11*(11), e1005658. DOI: 10.1371/journal.pgen.1005658 PMID: 26619199

Mulani, M. S., Kamble, E. E., Kumkar, S. N., Tawre, M. S., & Pardesi, K. R. (2019). Emerging strategies to combat ESKAPE pathogens in the era of antimicrobial resistance: A review. *Frontiers in Microbiology, 10*, 539. DOI: 10.3389/fmicb.2019.00539 PMID: 30988669

. Murray, L. M., Hayes, A., Snape, J., Kasprzyk-Hordern, B., Gaze, W. H., & Murray, A. K. (2024). Co-selection for antibiotic resistance by environmental contaminants. *npj Antimicrobials and Resistance, 2*(1), 9. https://doi.org/DOI: 10.1038/s44259-024-00030-x

Nasirian, H. (2017). Infestation of cockroaches (Insecta: Blattaria) in the human dwelling environments: A systematic review and meta-analysis. *Acta Tropica, 167*, 86–98. DOI: 10.1016/j.actatropica.2016.12.019 PMID: 28012906

Ng, E., Tay, J. R. H., Boey, S. K., Laine, M. L., Ivanovski, S., & Seneviratne, C. J. (2024). Antibiotic resistance in the microbiota of periodontitis patients: An update of current findings. *Critical Reviews in Microbiology, 50*(2), 329–340. DOI: 10.1080/1040841X.2023.2201411 PMID: 37140235

Ouwehand, A. C., Salminen, S., & Isolauri, E. (2002). Probiotics: An overview of beneficial effects. *Antonie van Leeuwenhoek, 82*(1), 279–289. DOI: 10.1023/A:1020620607611 PMID: 12369194

Oyeyemi, O. T., Agbaje, M. O., & Okelue, U. B. (2016). Food-borne human parasitic pathogens associated with household cockroaches and houseflies in Nigeria. *Parasite Epidemiology and Control*, *1*(1), 10–13. DOI: 10.1016/j.parepi.2015.12.001

Pachón-Ibáñez, M. E., Smani, Y., Pachón, J., & Sánchez-Céspedes, J. (2017). Perspectives for clinical use of engineered human host defense antimicrobial peptides. *FEMS Microbiology Reviews*, *41*(3), 323–342. DOI: 10.1093/femsre/fux012 PMID: 28521337

Pai, H.-H. (2013). Multidrug resistant bacteria isolated from cockroaches in long-term care facilities and nursing homes. *Acta Tropica*, *125*(1), 18–22. DOI: 10.1016/j.actatropica.2012.08.016 PMID: 22960645

Pai, H.-H., Chen, W.-C., & Peng, C.-F. (2005). Isolation of bacteria with antibiotic resistance from household cockroaches (Periplaneta americana and Blattella germanica). *Acta Tropica*, *93*(3), 259–265. DOI: 10.1016/j.actatropica.2004.11.005 PMID: 15716054

Perry, J. A., & Wright, G. D. (2013). The antibiotic resistance "mobilome": Searching for the link between environment and clinic. *Frontiers in Microbiology*, *4*, 138. DOI: 10.3389/fmicb.2013.00138 PMID: 23755047

Razzaque, M. S. (2021). Implementation of antimicrobial stewardship to reduce antimicrobial drug resistance. *Expert Review of Anti-Infective Therapy*, *19*(5), 559–562. DOI: 10.1080/14787210.2021.1858802 PMID: 33084432

Reygaert, W. C. (2018). An overview of the antimicrobial resistance mechanisms of bacteria. *AIMS Microbiology*, *4*(3), 482–501. DOI: 10.3934/microbiol.2018.3.482 PMID: 31294229

Saidi, B., Mafirakureva, P., & Mbanga, J. (2013). Antimicrobial resistance of Escherichia coli isolated from chickens with colibacillosis in and around Harare, Zimbabwe. *Avian Diseases*, *57*(1), 152–154. DOI: 10.1637/10268-060412-ResNote.1 PMID: 23678746

Sao, P., Vats, S., & Singh, S. (2022). *Porphyromonas gingivalis* resistance and virulence: An integrated functional network analysis. *Gene*, *839*, 146734. DOI: 10.1016/j.gene.2022.146734 PMID: 35835406

Tracanna, V., de Jong, A., Medema, M. H., & Kuipers, O. P. (2017). Mining prokaryotes for antimicrobial compounds: From diversity to function. *FEMS Microbiology Reviews*, *41*(3), 417–429. DOI: 10.1093/femsre/fux014 PMID: 28402441

Uwitonze, A. M., Ojeh, N., Murererehe, J., Atfi, A., & Razzaque, M. S. (2020). Zinc adequacy is essential for the maintenance of optimal oral health. *Nutrients*, *12*(4), 949. DOI: 10.3390/nu12040949 PMID: 32235426

van der Meij, A., Worsley, S. F., Hutchings, M. I., & van Wezel, G. P. (2017). Chemical ecology of antibiotic production by Actinomycetes. *FEMS Microbiology Reviews*, *41*(3), 392–416. DOI: 10.1093/femsre/fux005 PMID: 28521336

Ventola, C. L. (2015). The antibiotic resistance crisis: Part 1: Causes and threats. *P&T : a Peer-Reviewed Journal for Formulary Management*, *40*(4), 277–283. PMID: 25859123

Warnes, S. L., Highmore, C. J., & Keevil, C. W. (2012). Horizontal transfer of antibiotic resistance genes on abiotic touch surfaces: Implications for public health. *mBio*, *3*(6), e00489–e12. DOI: 10.1128/mBio.00489-12 PMID: 23188508

Yu, V. L. (2011). Guidelines for hospital-acquired pneumonia and health-care-associated pneumonia: A vulnerability, a pitfall, and a fatal flaw. *The Lancet. Infectious Diseases*, *11*(3), 248–252. DOI: 10.1016/S1473-3099(10)70306-5 PMID: 21371658

Zurek, L., & Ghosh, A. (2014). Insects represent a link between food animal farms and the urban environment for antibiotic resistance traits. *Applied and Environmental Microbiology*, *80*(12), 3562–3567. DOI: 10.1128/AEM.00600-14 PMID: 24705326

Chapter 2
Antimicrobial Resistance: Global Threats, Challenges, and Strategic Approaches for Prevention

M. Thirupathi
Department of Microbiology, Sacred Heart College, Tirupattur, India

S. Monisha
https://orcid.org/0009-0003-0742-8843
Department of Microbiology, Sacred Heart College, Tirupattur, India

M. Sandeep Kumar
Department of Microbiology, Sacred Heart College, Tirupattur, India

P. Saranraj
https://orcid.org/0000-0002-5052-6532
Department of Microbiology, Sacred Heart College, Tirupattur, India

M. Manigandan
https://orcid.org/0000-0002-8115-2713
Department of Microbiology, Sacred Heart College, Tirupattur, India

ABSTRACT

Antimicrobial resistance (AMR) represents a major threat to global public health, driven by the overuse and misuse of antibiotics across human and animal health sectors. Its emergence followed the discovery of penicillin, and the rise of multidrug-resistant organisms now significantly complicates treatment, leading to therapeutic failure, increased morbidity and mortality, and substantial economic burdens. This chapter provides a comprehensive overview of contemporary strategies to mitigate

DOI: 10.4018/979-8-3373-3825-5.ch002

AMR. Key approaches include the promotion of antimicrobial stewardship programs, which are essential for optimizing antibiotic use and preserving their efficacy. Complementary tools such as vaccination, antimicrobial peptides, bacteriophage therapy, monoclonal antibodies, and the development of new antibiotics also form a critical part of the response. The chapter concludes that combating AMR requires a multifaceted and system-wide approach, integrating these diverse strategies to address this complex challenge.

1. INTRODUCTION

The ability of microorganisms to resist antimicrobial agents is referred to as antimicrobial resistance (AMR), which makes conventional treatment ineffective. One of the major constituents of this crisis is multidrug-resistant bacterial isolates that are resistant to a wide range of therapeutics due to a variety of defences (Biswas et al., 2012). AMR is a serious world health risk, directly resulting in a fatality figure of about 1.27 million as well as 4.95 million in 2019 alone. The main cause of AMR is the selection pressure in Favor of evolution is an excessive use of antibiotics and misuse. This includes prescribing practices like non-adherence to treatment regimens, self-medication of the patients and inappropriate prescribing. This was noted during the COVID -19 pandemic, in which widespread use of antibiotics in treating viral infections was probably a contributor to the acceleration of resistance. This abuse is not new and warnings have been given as early as 1945 on the irresponsible use of penicillin which creates resistant strains.

A case in point is specific national issues of concern, including those witnessed in Saudi Arabia, which can be used to describe the intricate inter-play of factors. Although in 2018 the regulations became stricter on the prescription of the antimicrobials, the accessibility of over-the-counter drugs and large population migrations, such as the Hajj pilgrimage, promote cross-border distribution of resistant organisms, including the species of *Acinetobacter baumannii* and *Escherichia coli*. The implications are serious, and it is possible to roll back a century of medical advances. These antibiotics have highly decreased mortality since the advent of the antibiotic revolution changed medicine to be more diagnostic rather than therapeutic. Nevertheless, this basis is currently threatened by the gradual increase of pan-resistant bacteria (Clancy & Nguyen, 2020).

There should be a multifaceted approach in addressing AMR. Some of the essential interventions are the enhancement of antimicrobial stewardship programmes to enable effective use, the introduction of strict infection prevention and control protocols to curb the transmission of resistant strains and improvement of global surveillance. Finally, the AMR crisis can only be reduced with regard to preventing the selective pressure generated by the antimicrobial misuse, which requires policy, regulation, and international collaboration.

2. ANTIMICROBIAL RESISTANCE

Antimicrobial resistance (AMR) is a complex and urgent health, economic, and technological challenge of worldwide health, economies, and medical systems. Recent studies highlight its extreme and increasing weight over the range of geographic and socioeconomic environments. In the low- and middle-income countries (LMICs), the crisis is more exaggerated. Systematic reviews in Somalia indicate very high levels of resistance, with methicillin-resistant *Staphylococcus aureus* 97.4 per cent and widespread multidrug resistance in Gram-negative bacteria, with 100 per cent resistance to rescue antibiotics, including carbapenems (Hassan et al., 2025; Saranraj and Manigandan, 2025). Similarly, a national study in Iran between 2000 and 2021 concluded that mortality caused by carbapenem-resistant *Klebsiella pneumoniae* had more than doubled, resulting in an economic burden of 291.1 to 873.31mm USD (PPP) in 2021 alone (Shahsavand et al., 2025; Kolanjinathan et al., 2024).

The AMR burden does not solely lie in the field of human health but also in veterinary medicine and environmental reservoirs giving rise to conditional sources of resistance. A study on Australian cattle showed that there was minimal AMR in the Enterococcus spp. implying that livestock do not undoubtedly contribute to the clinically important strains of interventions in the animal production setting (Abraham et al., 2026), whereas a study in Indonesia clarified the complexity of interventions in the production of livestock. The longitudinal study of broiler farms showed that even with the decline in the total use of antimicrobials, the resistance of commensal *E. coli* did not decrease, which highlights the persistence of AMR in the environment (Sani et al., 2025). This is an essential environmental aspect, since scoping reviews in Canada have shown that there is a lot of missing data on AMR spread by water, soil, and bioaerosol, especially in wastewater treatment plants and livestock facilities (Perez Maldonado et al., 2025).

To deal with this international burden, bottom-up approaches are required to produce localized data to make sound policy. In Brazil, the health care stakeholders have underscored the significance of the subnational burden estimates to reflect both clinical, economic, and social effects of both the public and the private health care sectors to inform specific interventions (Keenan et al., 2025). At the same time, the initial efforts in LMICs are education and stewardship; research in Somalia and Bangladesh shows that although educational programmes may increase knowledge, the very poor practices and the misconceived values have deep roots in the population and require long-term, context-specific measures (Hassan et al., 2025; Sakib et al., 2025).

3. MECHANISMS OF ANTIMICROBIAL RESISTANCE

When we explore the details of the microbial defence mechanisms, we find a beautiful, but powerful symphony of biochemical defence mechanisms used by bacteria to resist antimicrobial agents. The tactics can be classified into four broad categories namely limiting drug uptake, modifying drug targets, inactivating drugs and actively refluxing drugs. All these strategies can be either inherent, a natural quality of the organism, or can be gained by genetic mutation or horizontal gene transfer (HGT), in the latter case, resistance can spread rapidly in bacteria populations (Rice, 2010; Hussein et al., 2023).

3.1. Limiting Drug Uptake

This natural or learnt process decreases the intracellular concentration of an antimicrobial. The first approach should be the down-regulation or mutation of outer membrane porin channels within Gram-negative bacteria, which should physically limit antibiotic access. Subsequent decreased permeability is among the major factors that lead to resistance in the pathogen *Acinetobacter baumannii* and *Pseudomonas aeruginosa* (Hoffmann et al., 2025).

Table 1. Molecular Mechanisms of Antimicrobial Resistance (AMR) in Bacteria

Mechanism of AMR	Methodology	Major sources of example	references
Enzymatic Inactivation or Modification	Bacteria produce enzymes that chemically modify or degrade the antibiotic, rendering it inactive before it can reach its target.	β-lactamases (e.g., ESBLs, carbapenemases) that hydrolyze penicillins, cephalosporins, and carbapenems.	(Tamma & Cosgrove, 2011)
Target Site Modification	The bacterial target of the antibiotic (e.g., ribosome, cell wall synthesis enzyme) is altered through mutation or enzymatic modification, reducing the drug's ability to bind effectively.	Methicillin-resistant *Staphylococcus aureus* (MRSA) with altered penicillin-binding proteins (PBP2a). MDR-TB with mutations in RNA polymerase.	(Littmann & Viens, 2015)
Reduced Drug Permeability/ Accumulation	Changes in the bacterial outer membrane or cell wall reduce the uptake and internal accumulation of the antibiotic.	Porin loss in *Pseudomonas aeruginosa* and *Enterobacteriaceae*, preventing carbapenem entry.	(Tamma & Cosgrove, 2011)
Active Efflux Pumps	Bacterial membrane proteins actively pump antibiotics out of the cell, preventing intracellular concentrations from reaching effective levels.	Multidrug efflux pumps (e.g., AcrAB-TolC in *E. coli*) that export a wide range of drug classes.	(Littmann & Viens, 2015)
Biofilm Formation	Bacteria form structured, surface-attached communities encased in a protective extracellular matrix. This creates a physical and physiological barrier that limits antibiotic penetration and induces a tolerant, slow-growing state.	Biofilms formed by *Pseudomonas aeruginosa* and *Staphylococcus epidermidis* in chronic infections (e.g., cystic fibrosis, device-related).	(Hussein et al., 2023)

continued on following page

Table 1. Continued

Mechanism of AMR	Methodology	Major sources of example	references
Horizontal Gene Transfer (HGT)	The acquisition of resistance genes from other bacteria via mobile genetic elements such as plasmids, transposons, and integrons. This is the primary driver for the rapid dissemination of multidrug resistance.	Plasmid-borne genes encoding ESBLs (*bla* genes) and carbapenemases (e.g., *bla*_{KPC}, *bla*_{NDM}).	(Rice, 2010; Hussein et al., 2023)
Bypass of Metabolic Pathway	Bacteria develop alternative metabolic pathways that circumvent the step inhibited by the antibiotic, allowing survival despite the drug's presence.	Acquisition of a resistant dihydrofolate reductase enzyme to bypass trimethoprim inhibition.	(Littmann & Viens, 2015)

3.2 Drug Target Modification

Bacteria also have the ability to change the particular cellular structures (targets) to which antibiotics bind, hence reduce the effects of the drugs. Such change can be through mutations of the chromosomes, as in the case of *Mycobacterium tuberculosis*, which causes multi-drug resistance to TB (MDR-TB), or through gene acquisition by means of alternative and low-affinity targets. The most commonly recognized is a methicillin-resistant *Staphylococcus aureus* (MRSA); it gains access to the mecA or mecC genes, thus producing an altered penicillin-binding protein (PBP2a) and is unreachable by the β-lactam antibiotics (Zhang et al., 2025).

3.3. Drug Inactivation

A number of these bacteria become resistant to the action of producing enzymes that directly alter or break down antimicrobial molecules. This is one of the leading mechanisms of acquired resistance to β -lactam antibiotics. The pathogens have enzymes like extended -lactamases (ESBLs) and carbapenemases that breakdown these drugs. Resistance to high level is disseminated rapidly through the horizontal transfer of plasmid encoded genes which encode these enzymes like bla genes in ESBL producing *E. coli* or carbapenemase genes in CRE (Tamma & Cosgrove, 2011).

3.4 Active Drug Efflux

To prevent the drug to reach a lethal concentration, microorganisms use membrane-associated efflux pumps to actively remove antibiotics out of the cell. Some pumps are very specific, whereas others have broad spectrum, which is able to export more than one, structurally unrelated, drug class, thus granting multidrug resistance (MDR). They can be constitutively expressed or up-regulated upon exposure to drugs and are still of importance in pathogens like *Neisseria gonorrhoeae* and *Candida* species.

Outside of these main mechanisms, bacteria tend to engage in synergistic modes. Protective biofilms formation creates a physical and metabolic obstacle which increases antimicrobial tolerance. Besides, the interaction of the mechanisms, namely decreased uptake, alteration of the target, and efflux, may lead to pan-drug resistance, which is a daunting challenge to modern therapy (Littmann and Viens, 2015). The adaptive ability of the microbes to resist antimicrobial pressure is highlighted by the clinical appearance of MDR pathogens.

Figure 1. Mechanism of Antimicrobial Resistance in Bacteria

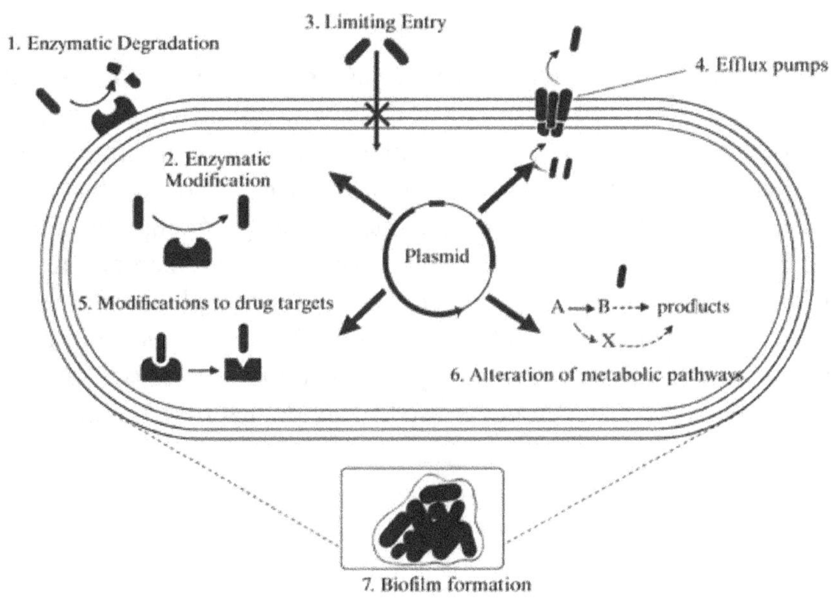

4. NOVEL APPROACHES FOR COMBATING AMR

The unabated emergence of antimicrobial resistance (AMR) requires the creation of innovative therapeutic measures. The bacteriophage (phage) therapy, antimicrobial peptides (AMPs), monoclonal antibodies (mAbs), and nanoparticle-based delivery system are promising alternatives to the traditional antibiotics (Hatfull et al., 2022).

Phage therapy has great specificity and activity against biofilms, but its use in clinical practice is limited by a limited range of strain-specific activity and rapid elimination by the immune system (Guo et al., 2024). AMPs offer an exquisite pathogen selectivity and a low likelihood of resistance but there are problems of protease vulnerability, possible toxicity, and expensive production costs that must be addressed (Leptihn & Loh, 2022). mAbs are costly, incapable of attacking intracellular proteins, and induce immune responses. Engineered nanoparticles allow targeted multi-drug delivery and the improvement of drug stability but the issues of cytotoxicity, biocompatibility, and scalability of manufacturing remain (Kususzewicz et al., 2021; Doran, 2024).

4.1 Phage therapy

Together, these novel solutions can be seen as significant facets of the strategic arsenal that is necessary to tackle the AMR crisis with each having its mechanism of bypassing the already known resistance pathways. Phage therapy, the application of bacteriophages to treat bacterial diseases is a 100-year-old concept that had been almost entirely replaced by antibiotics with the discovery of penicillin (Strathdee et al., 2023; Saranraj et al., 2023). However, the recent antimicrobial resistance epidemic has led to its re-emergence in a big way as a potential therapeutic option. Phages are viruses, which are highly specific to infect and replicate in bacterial hosts, ultimately lysing them during the lytic replication process (Dissanayake et al., 2019). It is based on this natural bactericidal action that they are used.

Figure 2. Phage therapy for antimicrobial resistance

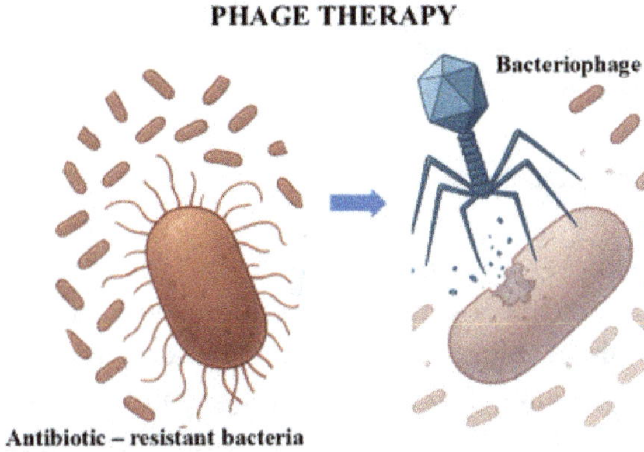

The major clinical benefit of phage therapy is its specificity to the target pathogens and, therefore, reduces the disturbance of the commensal microbiota. Lytic phages developed to treat particular bacterial infections are used in patients in a clinical environment (Umansky & Fortier, 2023). This limited host range is a major challenge that leads to the need to ensure that the causative pathogen is identified using adequate diagnosis before treatment. Therapeutic cocktails of several phages are one of the major strategies to overcome this and preempt phage resistance (Youssef et al., 2024). In burns, multidrug-resistant (MDR) pathogens, products such as Pyophage and PhagoBurn have been used successfully in the treatment of the invasive species of burns, including, but not limited to, *Pseudomonas aeruginosa*, MDR *Staphylococcus aureus*, and *Escherichia coli*. Phage therapy is a powerful and specific weapon in the strategic tool of AMR despite the regulatory and production challenges.

4.2 Antimicrobial peptides

Antimicrobial peptides (AMPs) are short molecules, naturally occurring molecules, which are part of innate immunity in a wide range of taxa (Ganesan et al., 2023). Their main action is to interfere with the microbial cytoplasmic membranes through the formation of pores which make the cells lysed. Alternatively, other AMPs prevent critical cell functions like nucleic acid and protein synthesis (de-Souza et al., 2023). One huge therapeutic benefit is that they are both broad-spectrum active and have a low tendency to induce resistance, which is a result of high fitness cost of such adaptations to the pathogen. Cyclic peptides approved by the FDA, including polymyxins, have clinical use, and new entrants, including Pexiganan (diabetic foot ulcers) and Murepavadin (targeting *Pseudomonas aeruginosa) are in research (Gomes et al., 2020; Jain et al., 2023). Although they are promising, such issues as protease vulnerability, possible poisoning, and costly production require additional optimisation of pharmaceuticals.

4.3 Monoclonal antibodies

Monoclonal antibodies (mAbs) provide a very specific therapeutic means since they target highly conserved pathogen epitopes or virulence factors, including toxins, and hence produce minimal collateral damage to the microbiota and can reduce such selective pressure (Mazur et al., 2023). Regulatory approvals have been granted to oncology dominant mAbs like bezlotoxumab (targeting *Clostridium difficile toxin B) and raxibacumab (targeting *Bacillus anthracis) (Lee et al., 2017; Esposito et al., 2023). Their specificity constrains off-target reaction but limitations each mAb to a constrained pathogen range as well. The obstacles to large-scale use are high costs of manufacture, intravenous route of administration, and immunogenicity. The further evolution of the topic is aimed at cost-cutting measures and creating synergistic solutions to improve efficacy and avoid resistance.

4.4 Nanoparticles

Nanoparticles (1-100nm) are a flexible tool to deal with AMR via improved drug delivery and inherent antimicrobial action. They may be designed so as to enhance drug solubility, stability, and local delivery at points of infections to enhance efficacy and minimize side effects (Chakraborty et al., 2023). One of the mechanisms is the production of reactive oxygen species (ROS) which destroy bacterial membranes and destroy biofilms. AgNPs in particular have a very strong and general activity with pathogens, such as multidrug-resistant strains of both Pseudomonas aeruginosa and *Escherichia coli* (Sahli et al., 2022). Their size and concentration affect their efficacy, and the larger the surface area, the higher the action of antibacterial (Elumalai et al., 2024). The positive aspects are low propensity to cause resistance and eco-friendly possibility of pivoting to green synthesis. But, there are also issues which pertain to possible cytotoxicity, biocompatibility, and scalable manufacturability to address clinical translation.

5. IMPLEMENTING EFFECTIVE ANTIBIOTICS

Prescription practices with regard to antimicrobial agents should be guided by the following principles: (1) make an accurate diagnosis; (2) use appropriate antibiotics and dosage schedule; (3) when empirical therapy is required (Fridkin, 2001), revise the plan based on patient progression or laboratory results; (4) avoid unapproved use of antimicrobials in the case of a viral infection; (5) when empirical therapy is necessary, educate patients how to administer the drug correctly and the need to adhere to the entire treatment The medical history and dental history are also necessary to provide accurate diagnosis and preclude or prevent complications, including allergies or drug interactions. The identified risks of antimicrobial toxicity and hypersensitivity, the emergence, selection, and spread of resistant organisms should be weighed against possible prophylactic advantages. This is a moral responsibility of us as health professionals, and in my case as a dentist, to prescribe antimicrobials responsibly and in an adequate manner. Most treatment programs that are designed to treat a variety of infectious diseases will succeed when the guidelines that are outlined in this cornerstone are observed.

6. ROUTES OF ANTIMICROBIAL RESISTANCE

There is a complex interaction between biological, behavioural, economic and systemic determinants that lead to the proliferation and escalation of resistant infections.

6.1 Overuse in Healthcare

The major cause of AMR is excessive use of antibiotics in human medicine. It has been shown that 3050 percent of the prescriptions given to treat respiratory infections bronchitis or common cold are unnecessary because of the etiological importance of these diseases which are predominantly viral. According to the report provided by the Centres of Disease Control and Prevention (CDC), 90 percent of these prescriptions are made by general practitioners in the United States (Llor and Bjerrum, 2014). This practice is often based on time limitations, pressure exerted by the patients, or vague diagnoses. Excessive prescribing of the fluoroquinolones and other broad-spectrum agents increases the development of resistance to more than two medications, including MRSA and *C. difficile*. Self-medication, easy access to prescription medications, and inadequate healthcare facilities have worsened the problem of in Southeast Asia, where up to 80 percent of antibiotic use does not come with a prescription (Spellberg et al., 2008; Saranraj et al., 2025).

6.2 Agricultural Antibiotic Use

Antimicrobial resistance is a phenomenon that has been greatly driven by the use of antibiotics in agriculture especially as a growth promoter among livestock. According to Van -Boeckel et al. (2017), in the United States, agriculture is the largest consumer of antibiotics, with a large part of it being dedicated to non-therapeutic purposes. The antibiotics added to animal feed are tetracyclines and macrolides, which are released into meat, milk, and eggs and as a result, they create a favourable environment in the human microbiome to develop resistance (Marshall and Levy, 2011). Surveys carried around Chinese poultry farms have proved that livestock waste pollution to the environment employs the resistance gene mutations, including tet genes, to the soil, water, and crops. In this way, the resistant bacteria, including *Salmonella* and *E. coli*, can spread along the food chain, and the outbreaks related to the contaminated pork and poultry. Although the European Union banned the use of growth promoters in the year 2006, most LMICs continue using them because of laxity in regulations and the monetary benefits.

6.3 Poor Infection Control

Lack of proper Infection Prevention and Control (IPC) measures contributes to the spread of resistant bacteria. Hospitals are centres of resistant infections due to widespread usage of antibiotics, invasive practices and patients who are immuno-compromised (Allegranzi et al., 2011). Poor hand hygiene and poor sterilisation methods facilitate proliferation of organisms like *Acinetobacter baumannii*, carbapenem resistant Enterobacteriaceae (CRE), and MRSA. According to World Health Organization estimates, the prevalence of healthcare-associated infections (HAIs) is 710 percent in most parts of the world, and more than 20 percent in the LMICs since most countries do not fund IPC programmes.

Communities are more susceptible to diseases like tuberculosis that is Multidrug Resistant (MDR-TB) when there is inadequate sanitation, a shortage of fresh water, and overcrowding.

6.4 Lack of New Antibiotics

AMR is aggravated by economic barriers that are the high cost of drug development and the comparatively low profitability of antibiotics. Antibiotics are usually used in short-courses, unlike chronic-disease drugs which generate long-term revenue, so the financial motivation of producers is less. In developing and middle-income nations, this use of cheaper, older antimicrobials to reduce costs of resistance, and low-capacity diagnostic systems to support correct prescribing (Plackett, 2020).

There are also obstacles to innovation in the form of regulatory hiccups, especially lengthy approval processes. Therefore, the global AMR coordination to implement the Global Plan of Action on AMR (2015) is being done in a piecemeal, or disjointed manner, which is indicative of the absence of a global coordination, within resource-limited environments, particularly.

6.5 Economic and Systemic Challenges

The AMR is exacerbated by economic issues, the most significant being the poor profitability of antibiotics as opposed to the high cost of their development. The shortness of antibiotic courses limits the amount of revenue compared to the chronic-disease therapeutics. In the lower- and middle-income countries, the trend of using cheaper, older antimicrobials reinforces the resistance, and the lack of diagnostic services hampers wise use of prescribing (O'Neill, 2016). Along with regulatory hurdles (long approval processes) are another deterrent to innovation. In addition, the Global Action Strategy on AMR (2015) provided by the WHO is being followed in a disjointed fashion, which is indicative of its general lack of coordination at an international level (especially in under-resource-rich areas).

7. THE IMPACT OF AMR ON HUMAN AND ANIMAL POPULATIONS

The problem of antimicrobial resistance (AMR) is a great crisis in the interrelationship of the One Health framework, as it affects human, animal, and environmental health. Its main cause is the widespread misuse of antimicrobials in clinical medicine, veterinary practice, and agriculture which increases the rate of the development of multi-drug-resistant pathogens. This degradation of first-line therapies compels the adoption of inferior, more toxic and expensive options, which predispose patients to more risks and impose more health care costs (Arnold et al., 2024). Most importantly, AMR endangers the health of the most basic medical practices including surgery, chemotherapy, and neonatal care.

The magnitude is noteworthy as AMR caused 1.27 million and caused or contributed to 4.95 million deaths worldwide in 2019 (Murray et al., 2022). The financial cost is very high, as it is based on the long hospitalisation, the complicated infection control, and the lost productivity. In farming, the use of antimicrobials results in reservoir of resistance, and food-borne pathogens including Campylobacter and Salmonella are directly threatening the human health (Tesema and Birhanu, 2024). Such issues as animal welfare, food security, and economic stability also face risk because of resistant infections in livestock (Kiggundu et al., 2024). Mitigation efforts ought to be based on One Health surveillance, stewardship, as well as intervention measures across all sectors.

7.1 Prevalence of AMR

Antimicrobial resistance is a widespread, increasing issue on the planet, which has existed since the dawn of antibiotic usage but has increased over the past decades. The first mechanisms of resistance emerged nearly as soon as penicillin was distributed in large quantities, which dictated the beginning of a further development of an evolutionary arms race. Resistance organisms have gained prominence in the mid-20th century including the methicillin-resistant Staphylococcus aureus (MRSA), and it is an indication of an impending health hazard to the populace. The use of agriculture and livestock antibiotics has also increased the spread of the resistance genes among the ecological niches (Kiggundu et al., 2019). This shows a shocking worldwide load due to surveillance. In the US, 2019 report by the Centres for Disease Control and Prevention reported an annual prevalence of over 2.8million antibiotic-resistant infections, which led to the deaths of over 35,000 persons. In the European Union the prevalence of resistant infections is seen to be more than 700,000 cases per annum, resulting into nearly 33,000 deaths and incurring a healthcare expenditure of more than EUR 1.5billion.

International monitoring efforts, including the World Health Organization Global Antimicrobial Resistance Surveillance System (GLASS) are essential in giving meaningful insights to the current situation. Evidence of 22 countries reveals shocking resistance levels which comprise inconsistent and aggressive rates of resistance in common bacterial pathogens. In the case of *Escherichia coli*, ciprofloxacin, a first-line treatment used in the treatment of urinary tract, has a resistance of between 8.4 92.9 per cent among countries. In the case of Klebsiella pneumoniae, the rate of resistance to ciprofloxacin ranges between 4.1 -79.4 (WHO GLASS report).

7.2 AI in Combating AMR

Machine Learning (ML) and Artificial Intelligence (AI) are more and more considered as transformative technologies in the global attempt to face antimicrobial resistance with new methods that will supplement traditional stewardship and enhance drug discovery. In clinical practice, AI can make clinical medicine more precise, by quickly processing highly complex data, such as patient history, local microbiological trends, and real-time clinical presentation, predicting high-probability infections and yielding the most empirical choice of antibiotic. These AI-based clinical decision support systems can potentially reduce the excessive prescription of broad-spectrum agents, which is one of the main causes of resistance, by prescribing specific therapy at an earlier stage of the treatment process (Akova, 2016).

In addition to stewardship, there is a significant future potential in artificial intelligence in helping to revive the stagnant antibiotic development pipeline. With the help of deep-learning algorithms to screen large genomic, metagenomic, and chemical libraries, AI can discover new antimicrobial compounds and new bacterial targets with remarkable efficiency, circumventing the more conventional, slow methods of discovery (Theuretzbacher, 2009). Epidemiological models driven by AI can also monitor and predict the appearance and spread of resistant strains, on local and global levels, guiding adaptable interventions that can be applied to the population, and formulary control. However, there is still a lot to overcome. The AI model performance depends on the quality, quantity, and variety of the training data, and biases can be caused by datasets that are disproportionately biased towards the population of high-income nations, thus limiting extrapolation to other world conditions (Subramaniam and Girish, 2020). Furthermore, the black box character of certain intricate algorithms is an obstacle to clinical implementation, since medics intend to have recommendations that are interpretable and explainable, in order to develop trust. These obstacles notwithstanding, AI, once carefully validated and carefully incorporated into healthcare systems, can become the important technological development in the multifaceted approach to maintain the antimicrobial efficacy and address the crisis of Antimicrobial Resistance (AMR).

7.3 AMR Burden and Associated Issues

Antimicrobial resistance has far-reaching effects that go beyond direct death to include devastating economic, healthcare, and societal effects that jeopardize the existence of modern medicine. Recent projections are simply astounding: bacterial AMR was directly connected to 1.27 million deaths and was linked to 4.95 million deaths worldwide in 2019 (Murray et al., 2022). It is projected to be following a dismal course, and one concurrently review estimates that by 2050 AMR will be as many as 10 million deaths a year without intervention, the highest impact occurring in the low- and middle-income nations whose healthcare resources are the most limited. The economic burden is also significant due to the fact that it is associated with sustainable hospitalisation, the necessity to spend more and intensive care, and disability. In the European Union alone, AMR causes cost and productivity losses in healthcare estimated at more than over EUR 1.5 billion/annum.

The problems connected to it are complex. To begin with, the decline of effective antibiotics compromises the basis of modern medical practice. Normal operations, chemotherapy of some types of cancer, organ transplant, and work with preterm babies are also becoming increasingly risky exponentially without effective infection prevention and control, which can undo decades of medical progress (Kofteridis et al., 2020). Second, pan-resistant infections may cause the re-emergence of bacterial diseases that have traditionally been considered treatable, and thus has a greater impact on the global disease burden of diseases like tuberculosis, pneumonia, and gastrointestinal infections. There are thirdly, the environmental aspect of AMR provides a reservoir effect because the resistant genes and bacteria spread to waters, soil, and even animals, and the cycle continues. Lastly, the absence of a strong pipeline of new antimicrobials in addition to the speed at which bacteria evolve puts the entire situation in a perilous imbalance. This situation, sometimes called a post-antibiotic era, foreshadows the situation in which common infections and minor injuries would be deadly again, and the overall increase in life expectancy and quality of life attained over the last 100 years would be put at risk (Ahmed, 2024). The burden is complex and therefore demands unprecedented coordination on an international level, continued investment in alternative forms of medicine and increased stewardship both in the human and animal health domains.

8. STRATEGIC INTEGRATION OF IMMUNIZATION, RAPID TESTING, AND STEWARDSERSHIP MODELS

The problem of antimicrobial resistance (AMR) has been deemed a significant problem that needs a concerted effort in its resolution by global policy frameworks. The 2015 World Health Organization (WHO) Global Action Plan has a cornerstone that promotes a multisectoral approach of One Health in all three domains (human, animal and environmental health) and as a strategy, its objectives will focus on awareness, surveillance, infection prevention, optimal use of antimicrobial products and sustainable investment (WHO, 2015). More recent high-level efforts such as reports on AMR by the United Nations Interagency Coordination Group (IACG) and the 2024 political declaration by the UN General Assembly have reinforced this blueprint, calling on the need to implement national action plans more quickly and to decouple the cost of research-and-development of antibiotics and their sales to achieve effective equitable access.

Although this policy consensus is rather strong, there remains a gap in implementation that is especially acute in the countries of low-and-middle-income (LMICs). The effects of the global frameworks are severely restricted by structural and informational obstacles. Surveillance systems are also inadequate, and data reporting is inconsistent, and the burden of AMR in a region is high when compared to the local capacity to conduct research (Mukherjee & Sahay, 2023; Borromeo et al., 2025). Some of the essential instruments of stewardship are not readily available, such as diagnostics, such as point-of-care tests, are commonly not cost-effective and sustainable in the context of the real LMIC environment (Modgil et al., 2025). In the same vein, the concept of strategic dependencies, e.g., the almost complete dependence of Africa on imported vaccines, does not comply with the principle of equitable access and compromises the prevention objectives (Akegbe et al., 2023).

Therefore, the next step in the correct AMR mitigation is to go beyond the universal policy support and allow contextually-oriented, equity-based measures. This requires simultaneous investment in the development of underlying health systems, such as laboratory systems, human capacity building, and data integration, and the emergence of local diagnostics and vaccine innovations ecosystems. The most important issue of sustainable prevention is bridging the gap between global governance and local capacity.

9. APPLICATIONS OF AMR

In the control of the initial phases of AMR, there are no simple solutions. The gravity of the problem lies in the fact that it is difficult to diminish the enormous consumption of drugs because they are used in medicine and food animal production economy (Rahman et al., 2022). Farming systems commonly deliver antimicrobials to animals to prevent infection and stimulate growth and clinicians commonly use empirical antibiotic prescriptions to protect against bacterial infection despite the absence of rapid and point-of-care diagnostics. Although the dangers of antibiotic resistance associated with excessive use are known, the effectiveness of antimicrobial stewardship programmes in healthcare and change in animal husbandry regulations are not properly adopted (Manigandan, 2014; Du Plessis, 2017). The failure of the antibiotic drug-development pipeline to keep up with the current evolution of Multidrug-Resistant (MDR) microorganisms increases these problems. Pharmaceutical firms are also abandoning costly research on antibiotics in large numbers due to low financial incentives. In addition to it, with the extended phase-trial times, it seems questionable that in the nearest future, any solution will be discovered, despite the policy extensions that finance the creation of antibiotics being a step in the right direction (Ferri et al., 2017).

10. CHALLENGES AND LIMITATIONS OF COMBATTING ANTIBIOTIC RESISTANCE STRATEGIES

Antimicrobial resistance remains a potent issue affecting health worldwide and negatively impacting treatment outcomes and propagating resistant infections. Even though there is no one-fit-all intervention that can completely address this issue, there are a number of measures that can help lessen the effect and spread of resistance. It has been proven by epidemiological studies that the use of antibiotics is directly related to the development of resistance to the bacteria and the overuse of antibiotics is viewed as one of the main causes of resistance. The resistance genes may occur by natural mutations or be transferred between the bacterial species horizontally through the transfer of genes; this is enhanced by poor prescription methods and insufficient dosages. The factors increase the rate of resistance determinants diffusion and increase the pathogenicity of the disease (Park et al., 2022). To solve these problems, it is necessary to improve antibiotic stewardship, reinforce infection prevention measures, and come up with alternative therapeutic measures, which include phage therapy and immunotherapies. Education and campaigns to create awareness of the community about the responsible use of antibiotics are also crucial. There are alternative antimicrobial measures that are being explored due to the decreasing efficacy of traditional antibiotics. Disrupting bacterial communication networks with quorum -quenching models, microbial-based therapies, stem-cell applications, immunotherapeutic modalities, photodynamic anti-microbial techniques, CRISPR -Cas systems and interaction with resistance mechanisms, bacteriophage therapy, and bioactive compounds of animal venoms are emerging approaches that are discussed in this section.

10.1 Immunotherapeutic Approaches

The use of methods that bypass the immune system can also give even the antibiotic-vulnerable bacteria a chance to escape treatment. The goal of immunotherapeutic approaches is to address this challenge by using and boosting the immunity against bacterial infection (McCulloch et al., 2022).

The orchestration of innate immunity that includes Natural Killer (NK) cells, Innate Lymphoid Cells (ILCs), and adaptive lymphocytes in the form of T and B cells is one of the pillars of pathogen eradication. These cellular protectors carry out cytotoxic attacks on infected cells in conjunction with the release of a set of inflammatory mediators which either initiate or maintain myeloid antibacterial activities. The PD-1 /PD-L1 axis as well as other modulatory checkpoints regulate this balance so as to avoid collateral tissue destruction. An example is to prevent immunopathology in case of an infection by the immunopathogen, PD -1 is up-regulated on T cells, which inhibits overactive effecter action.

Tim3-Gal9 pathway has become a key controller in antimicrobial immunity. Tim3 is a T-cell immunoglobulin and mucin domain protein that has a negative regulatory effect by suppressing TH1-type responses (Wang et al., 2022). Although this attenuation helps to reduce inflammatory damage, excessive Tim3 activation induces T0 cells exhaustion. Gal9 (a galactoside) in the form of its Tim3-ligand interacting with Tim3 receptors on TH1 cells induces macrophages to increase their bactericidal capabilities; caspase-1 is activated by this interaction that ultimately triggers the release of IL-1B which is one of the foundations of innate defenses. Empirical evidence indicates that combined Tim3-Gal9 interaction promotes host antimicrobial action through the regulation of immunity and prompting macrophages.

One example of a futuristic therapeutic approach is the use of engineered nanovesicles, which entrap bacterial toxins and, under ultrasound stimulation, produce ROS. This approach combines anti-virulence immunotherapy and antibacterial sonodynamic therapy, which is an evolved point of convergence between nanotechnology and immunology.

Macrophages which are part of innate defence also exhibit great plasticity, becoming differentiated functional phenotypes based on stimuli by the microbes. The pro-inflammatory pathways and the clearance of the pathogen are coordinated by the classically activated M1 phenotype, which is generated as a result of cytokine induction (Mitton & Ackroyd, 2008). On the other hand, the alternatively activated M2 type is involved in the repair of tissues, resolution of inflammation as well as anti-inflammatory mechanisms. The immunotherapeutic application of macrophage polarization Therapeutic control of macrophage polarization is therefore on the rise: initial pathogen eradication is achieved by M1 induction, and tissue healing is supported by restoration of M2 polarization.

10.2 Antibacterial Photodynamic Therapy

Photo-dynamic therapy is a method of antibacterial treatment that involves light administration and employs a photoswitchable reagent to react with oxygen to generate a potent radical, which destroys bacterial cells. Photo-dynamic therapy is also a type of antibacterial therapy that uses light to treat bacteria and uses a photo switchable to reaction to oxygen to form a powerful radical to destroy bacteria (Davies and Powers 342).

The accidental discovery of Photodynamic Therapy (PDT) at the beginning of the twentieth century highlighted the immense promise of light-activated compounds to cause cellular death. Modern PDT combines molecular biology, photochemistry and customized treatment regimens (Mitton & Ackroyd, 2008). Its effectiveness depends on three mutually dependent factors, i.e. a biocompatible Photosensitizer (PS), light of a specific wavelength and physiological oxygen supply. The activation of light causes the PS to transition to an excited triplet state, which drives a multi-step photochemical radical cascade that ultimately results into the production of highly reactive ROS such as hydroxyl radicals and singlet oxygen, which cause oxidative stress to vital biomolecules, cellular structures, and drug-resistant pathogens.

The generation of ROS is also enhanced when iodide anions are present whereby the formation of triiodide and hydrogen peroxide cascades zinc-free iodide radicals, which enhances cellular injury pathways. However, the effectiveness of PDT is closely related to the oxygen level in tissues, which dictates the treatment outcomes and also the feasibility of the procedure, including the prolonged exposure duration and poor photoadherence.

The innovation to overcome these hurdles has included conjugation of PDT and traditional antibiotics thus creating synergies. As an example, Gentamicin (GEN) conjugated with Toluidine Blue-mediated PDT have shown high potency to inhibit both susceptible and multidrug resistant in vitro and in vivo against Staphylococcus aureus over 15 hours. This dual modality takes advantage of the oxidative attack of PDT to weaken the membranes of bacteria and inhibition of ribosome by gentamicin to speed up the removal of pathogens. The subsequent multiplicity of attacks oxides on membrane lipids and proteins as well as the disruption of ribosomal functioning significantly reduces bacterial virulence and promotes the healing of the tissues (Liu et al., 2022).

In addition to direct antimicrobial action, oxidative processes of PDT regulate host reactions, including by reducing bacterial growth and colonization, modulating inflammatory mediators, and up-regulating the growth factor expression. With the continued evolution of research, the future of infectious disease control is bright with the development of photosensitizer chemistry and precision therapy measures, especially in the context of rising antibiotic resistance.

11. CONCLUSION

Antimicrobial resistance (AMR) constitutes one of the foremost global health crises of the 21st century, threatening to reverse decades of medical progress. The convergence of relentless microbial evolution and pervasive antimicrobial misuse across human and animal health sectors has propelled us towards a perilous post-antibiotic era, where common infections and routine medical procedures could become life-threatening. Effectively countering this multifaceted threat demands an integrated, multi-pronged strategy anchored in a One Health framework. This requires robust antimicrobial stewardship to optimize use, accelerated innovation in novel therapeutics and rapid diagnostics, and stringent infection prevention and control measures globally. Simultaneously, addressing the economic and policy barriers that stifle antibiotic development is critical. There is an urgent need for coordinated international action, sustained investment, and political commitment to implement these strategies. Only through such concerted and collaborative efforts can we safeguard the efficacy of existing antimicrobials, restore the pipeline for new ones, and ensure these life-saving drugs remain effective for future generations.

REFERENCES

Abraham, R., Sahibzada, S., Lee, T., Jordan, D., McMillan, K., Mellor, G., Duffy, L., Lugsomya, K., O'Dea, M., Abraham, S., & Barlow, R. (2026). Antimicrobial resistance, genomic, and public health insights into *Enterococcus* spp. from Australian cattle. *Veterinary Microbiology, 312*, 110788. PMID: 41308245

Ahmed, S. K. (2024). Artificial intelligence in nursing: Current trends, possibilities and pitfalls. *Journal of Medicine, Surgery, and Public Health, 3*, 100072.

Akegbe, H., Onyeaka, H., Mazi, I. M., Olowolafe, O. A., Omotosho, A. D., Oladunjoye, I. O., Tajudeen, Y. A., & Ofeh, A. S. (2023). The need for Africa to develop capacity for vaccinology as a means of curbing antimicrobial resistance. *Vaccine: X, 14*, 100320. PMID: 37293248

Akova, M. (2016). Epidemiology of antimicrobial resistance in bloodstream infections. *Virulence, 7*(3), 252–266. PMID: 26984779

Allegranzi, B., Bagheri Nejad, S., Combescure, C., Graafmans, W., Attar, H., Donaldson, L., & Pittet, D. (2011). Burden of endemic health-care-associated infection in developing countries: Systematic review and meta-analysis. *Lancet, 377*(9761), 228–241. PMID: 21146207

Arnold, K. E., Laing, G., McMahon, B. J., Fanning, S., Stekel, D. J., Pahl, O., Coyne, L., Latham, S. M., & McIntyre, K. M. (2024). The need for One Health systems-thinking approaches to understand multiscale dissemination of antimicrobial resistance. *The Lancet. Planetary Health, 8*(2), e124–e133. PMID: 38331529

Biswas, S., Brunel, J.-M., Dubus, J.-C., Reynaud-Gaubert, M., & Rolain, J.-M. (2012). Colistin: An update on the antibiotic of the 21st century. *Expert Review of Anti-Infective Therapy, 10*(8), 917–934. PMID: 23030331

Borromeo, A. S., Manaloto, A. M., & Antonio, R. P. (2025). Southeast–Asian landscape of antimicrobial resistance research (2014–2024): A bibliometric analysis. *Journal of Global Antimicrobial Resistance, 45*, 125–133. PMID: 40983143

Chakraborty, A., Diwan, A., & Tatake, J. (2023). Prospect of nanomaterials as antimicrobial and antiviral regimen. *AIMS Microbiology, 9*(3), 444–466. PMID: 37649798

Clancy, C., & Nguyen, M. (2020). Coronavirus disease 2019, superinfections, and antimicrobial development: What can we expect? *Clinical Infectious Diseases, 71*(10), 2736–2743. PMID: 32361747

De Souza, G. H., Rossato, L., de Oliveira, A. R., & Simionatto, S. (2023). Antimicrobial peptides against polymyxin-resistant Klebsiella pneumoniae: A patent review. *World Journal of Microbiology & Biotechnology, 39*(3), 1–10. PMID: 36720739

Dissanayake, U., Ukhanova, M., Moye, Z. D., Sulakvelidze, A., & Mai, V. (2019). Bacteriophages reduce pathogenic Escherichia coli counts in mice without distorting gut microbiota. *Frontiers in Microbiology, 10*, 1984. PMID: 31551950

Doran, P. M. (2024). Foreign protein degradation and instability in plants and plant tissue cultures. *Trends in Biotechnology, 24*(9), 426–432. PMID: 16843560

Du Plessis, G. M. (2017). *Microbial geopolitics: Living with danger and the future of security* [Doctoral dissertation, University of Pretoria].

Elumalai, K., Srinivasan, S., & Shanmugam, A. (2024). Review of the efficacy of nanoparticle-based drug delivery systems for cancer treatment. *Biomedical Technology, 5*, 109–122.

Esposito, S., Amirthalingam, G., Bassetti, M., Blasi, F., De Rosa, F. G., Halasa, N. B., Huttner, A., Martin-Loeches, I., Pollard, A. J., Rello, J., Schultsz, C., Tumbarello, M., & Kantele, A. (2023). Monoclonal antibodies for prophylaxis and therapy of respiratory syncytial virus, SARS-CoV-2, human immunodeficiency virus, rabies and bacterial infections. *Frontiers in Immunology, 14*, 1172054. PMID: 37256125

Ferri, M., Ranucci, E., Romagnoli, P., & Giaccone, V. (2017). Antimicrobial resistance: A global emerging threat to public health systems. *Critical Reviews in Food Science and Nutrition, 57*(13), 2857–2876. PMID: 26464037

Fridkin, S. K. (2001). Vancomycin-intermediate and -resistant Staphylococcus aureus: What the infectious disease specialist needs to know. *Clinical Infectious Diseases, 32*(1), 108–115. PMID: 11118389

Ganesan, N., Mishra, B., Felix, L., & Mylonakis, E. (2023). Antimicrobial peptides and small molecules targeting the cell membrane of Staphylococcus aureus. *Microbiology and Molecular Biology Reviews : MMBR, 87*(2), e0003722. PMID: 37129495

Gomes, D., Santos, R., Soares, R. S., Reis, S., Carvalho, S., Rego, P., Peleteiro, M. C., Tavares, L., & Oliveira, M. (2020). Pexiganan in combination with nisin to control polymicrobial diabetic foot infections. *Antibiotics (Basel, Switzerland), 9*(3), 128. PMID: 32244862

Guo, Z., Yuan, M., & Chai, J. (2024). Advantages and limitations of lytic phages compared with chemical antibiotics to combat bacterial infections. *Heliyon, 10*(7), e34849. PMID: 39148970

Hassan, S. A., Isak, M. J., Osman, A. M., Hassan, Y. M., Ahmed, A. M., Mire, S. A., Jimale, K. A., Omar, A. I., & Ahmed, N. R. (2025). Effectiveness of an e-Bug–based antimicrobial resistance education intervention: A prospective quasi-experimental study among Grade 12 students in Mogadishu, Somalia. *IJID Regions*, *17*, 100771. PMID: 41143070

Hatfull, G. F., Dedrick, R. M., & Schooley, R. T. (2022). Phage therapy for antibiotic-resistant bacterial infections. *Annual Review of Medicine*, *73*, 197–211. PMID: 34428079

Hoffmann, A., Grubwieser, P., Bumann, D., Haschka, D., & Weiss, G. (2025). Tackling microbial iron homeostasis: Novel antimicrobial strategies. *Trends in Pharmacological Sciences*, *46*(10), 1004–1017. PMID: 40914687

Hussein, S., Qurbani, K., & Ahmed, S. K. (2023). Potential increase in Crimean–Congo hemorrhagic fever incidence in Iraq post Eid-al-Adha, 2023. *New Microbes and New Infections*, *54*, 101175. PMID: 37727502

Jain, M., Stitt, G., Son, L., & Enioutina, E. Y. (2023). Probiotics and their bioproducts: A promising approach for targeting methicillin-resistant Staphylococcus aureus and vancomycin-resistant Enterococcus. *Microorganisms*, *11*(10), 2393. PMID: 37894051

Keenan, K., Kiffer, C. R. V., Carmo, É. V. S., Corrêa, J. S., Abreu, A. L. d., Massuda, A., Gales, A. C., & Colombo, A. L. (2025). Antimicrobial resistance burden estimates from the bottom-up: Research priorities for estimating the impact of antimicrobial resistance in Brazil. *IJID Regions*, *14*, 100558. PMID: 39911748

Kiggundu, R., Waswa, J. P., Konduri, N., Kasujja, H., Murungi, M., Vudriko, P., Akello, H., Lugada, E., Muiva, C., Were, E., Tjipura, D., Kajumbula, H., Kikule, K., Nfor, E., & Joshi, M. P. (2019). [Title of 2019 article needed for citation].

Kiggundu, R., Waswa, J. P., Konduri, N., Kasujja, H., Murungi, M., Vudriko, P., Akello, H., Lugada, E., Muiva, C., Were, E., Tjipura, D., Kajumbula, H., Kikule, K., Nfor, E., & Joshi, M. P. (2024). A One Health approach to fight antimicrobial resistance in Uganda: Implementation experience, results, and lessons learned. *Biosafety and Health*. PMID: 40078942

Kofteridis, D. P., Andrianaki, A. M., Maraki, S., Mathioudaki, A., Plataki, M., Alexopoulou, C., Ioannou, P., Samonis, G., & Valachis, A. (2020). Treatment pattern, prognostic factors, and outcome in patients with infection due to pan-drug-resistant gram-negative bacteria. *European Journal of Clinical Microbiology & Infectious Diseases*, *39*(5), 965–970. PMID: 31933017

Kolanjinathan, K., Rajasekar, M., Harinathan, B., Saranraj, P., & Manigandan, M. (2024). Assessment of the antimicrobial and mosquito larvicidal efficacy of medicinal herb *Elytraria acaulis*. *International Journal of Entomological Research*, *9*(11), 225–228.

Lee, Y., Lim, W. I., Bloom, C. I., Moore, S., Chung, E., & Marzella, N. (2017). Bezlotoxumab (Zinplava) for Clostridium difficile infection: The first monoclonal antibody approved to prevent the recurrence of a bacterial infection. *P&T : a Peer-Reviewed Journal for Formulary Management*, *42*(12), 735–738. PMID: 29234211

Leptihn, S., & Loh, B. (2022). Complexity, challenges and costs of implementing phage therapy. *Future Microbiology*, *17*(8), 643–646. PMID: 35400196

Littmann, J., & Viens, A. M. (2015). The ethical significance of antimicrobial resistance. *Public Health Ethics*, *8*(3), 209–224. PMID: 26566395

Liu, X., Liu, S., Mai, B., Su, X., Guo, X., Chang, Y., Dong, W., Wang, W., & Feng, X. (2022). Synergistic gentamicin-photodynamic therapy against resistant bacteria in burn wound infections. *Photodiagnosis and Photodynamic Therapy*, *39*, 103034. PMID: 35882288

Llor, C., & Bjerrum, L. (2014). Antimicrobial resistance: Risk associated with antibiotic overuse and initiatives to reduce the problem. *Therapeutic Advances in Drug Safety*, *5*(6), 229–241. PMID: 25436105

Manigandan, M. (2014). Mass cultivation and determination of biochemical composition of Spirulina platensis in three different medium. *International Journal of Pharmacy and Biological Sciences*, *5*(3), 847–854.

Marshall, B. M., & Levy, S. B. (2011). Food animals and antimicrobials: Impacts on human health. *Clinical Microbiology Reviews*, *24*(4), 718–733. PMID: 21976606

Mazur, N. I., Terstappen, J., Baral, R., Bardají, A., Beutels, P., Buchholz, U. J., Cohen, C., Crowe, J. E., Cutland, C. L., Eckert, L., Feikin, D., Fitzpatrick, T., Graham, B. S., Heikkinen, T., Higgins, D., Hirve, S., Klugman, K. P., Kragten-Tabatabaie, L., Lemey, P., & Bont, L. J. (2023). Respiratory syncytial virus prevention within reach: The vaccine and monoclonal antibody landscape. *The Lancet. Infectious Diseases*, *23*(1), e2–e21. PMID: 35952703

McCulloch, T. R., Wells, T. J., & Souza-Fonseca-Guimaraes, F. (2022). Towards efficient immunotherapy for bacterial infection. *Trends in Microbiology*, *30*(2), 158–169. PMID: 34253452

Mitton, D., & Ackroyd, R. (2008). A brief overview of photodynamic therapy in Europe. *Photodiagnosis and Photodynamic Therapy*, *5*(2), 103–111. PMID: 19356640

Modgil, V., Sahay, S., Taneja, N., Mukherjee, A., Joshi, N., Mitra, A., Soman, B., Singh, R., Sinha, O., & Surial, R. (2025). Enhancing access to antimicrobial resistance diagnostics for the marginalised: Challenges and opportunities of point-of-care technologies. *Journal of Global Antimicrobial Resistance*, *44*, 281–286. PMID: 40645328

Mukherjee, A. S., & Sahay, S. (2023). Systems thinking based approaches to engage with health inequities shaping Antimicrobial Resistance in low and lower-middle-income countries. *Journal of Infection and Public Health*, *16*, 129–133. PMID: 37977980

Murray, C. J. L., Ikuta, K. S., Sharara, F., Swetschinski, L. R., Aguilar, G. R., Gray, A., Han, C., Bisignano, C., Rao, P., Wool, E., Johnson, S. C., Browne, A. J., Chipeta, M. G., Fell, F., Hackett, S., Haines-Woodhouse, G., Hamadani, B. H. K., Kumaran, E. A. P., McManigal, B., & Naghavi, M. (2022). Global burden of bacterial antimicrobial resistance in 2019: A systematic analysis. *Lancet*, *399*(10325), 629–655. PMID: 35065702

O'Neill, J. (2016). *Tackling drug-resistant infections globally: Final report and recommendations*. Review on Antimicrobial Resistance.

Park, A. R., Kim, S. B., Jung, S. W., Chun, J. W., Kim, J. H., Kim, J., Lazarte, Y. R., Jang, J. M. S., Jang, H. B., Thompson, K. D., Jung, T. S., & Cha, I. S. (2022). Membrane vesicles from antibiotic-resistant Staphylococcus aureus transfer antibiotic resistance to antibiotic-susceptible Escherichia coli. *Journal of Applied Microbiology*, *132*(4), 2746–2759. PMID: 35019198

Pérez Maldonado, M., Ofori-Darko, D., Nichols, V., French, J., Spence, K., Reid-Smith, R. J., & Parmley, E. J. (2025). Investigating the occurrence of antimicrobial resistance in the environment in Canada: A scoping review. *Canadian Journal of Microbiology*, *71*, 1–13. PMID: 40279669

Plackett, B. (2020). Why big pharma has abandoned antibiotics. *Nature*, *586*, S50–S52.

Rahman, M. M., Alam Tumpa, M. A., Zehravi, M., Sarker, M. T., Yamin, M., Islam, M. R., Harun-Or-Rashid, M., Ahmed, M., Ramproshad, S., Mondal, B., Dey, A., Damiri, F., Berrada, M., Rahman, M. H., & Cavalu, S. (2022). An overview of antimicrobial stewardship optimization: The use of antibiotics in humans and animals to prevent resistance. *Antibiotics (Basel, Switzerland)*, *11*(5), 667. PMID: 35625311

Rice, L. B. (2010). Progress and challenges in implementing the research on ESKAPE pathogens. *Infection Control and Hospital Epidemiology*, *31*(S1), S7–S10. PMID: 20929376

Sahli, C., Moya, S. E., Lomas, J. S., Gravier-Pelletier, C., Briandet, R., & Hémadi, M. (2022). Recent advances in nanotechnology for eradicating bacterial biofilm. *Theranostics*, *12*(5), 2383–2405. PMID: 35265216

Sakib, M. A. N., Mitro, P., Oishee, F. Y., Talukdar, P. R., Mazumder, Z., Islam, R., Khaiat, S. B., Hossain, M. Z., & Hossain, M. M. (2025). Assessing knowledge, attitudes, and preventive practices of smallholder livestock farmers toward antimicrobial use, resistance, and sources in Bangladesh. *IJID One Health*, *2025*, 100101.

Sani, R. A., Rachmawati, A., Sunandar, S., Pertela, G., Jahja, E. J., Suandy, I., van den Broek, J., de Wit, S. J., Wagenaar, J. A., Speksnijder, D. C., & Velkers, F. C. (2025). Longitudinal evaluation of interventions on antimicrobial use and antimicrobial resistance on broiler farms in West Java, Indonesia. *Poultry Science*, *104*(12), 106010. PMID: 41274108

Saranraj, P., & Manigandan, M. (2025). Antibacterial Efficacy of Moringa oleifera Leaf Extract against Salmonella typhimurium in a Rat Model: An Experimental Study on Infection Treatment. *Al-Anbar Journal of Veterinary Sciences*, *18*(1), 19–23.

Saranraj, P., Sayyed, R. Z., Kokila, M., Salomi, V., Sivasakthivelan, P., Manigandan, M., & Mawar, R. (2023). Evolving concepts of biocontrol of phytopathogens by endophytic Pseudomonas fluorescence. In *Plant growth promoting microorganisms of arid region* (pp. 365–388). Springer Nature Singapore.

Saranraj, P., Singh, S., Manigandan, M., Nisha, R., Lokeshwari, B., & Gayathri, K. (2025). Pharmacological Effects of Medicinal Herbs: Recent Development and Progress. In Pharmacology of Plants and Plant Derived Biologically Active Molecules (pp. 30-45). CRC Press.

Shahsavand, A., Golestani, A., Akbarpour, S., Salehi, M., Seifi, A., Mohammadi, K., & Shafaati, M. (2025). Burden of antimicrobial resistance and estimated economic impact of Klebsiella pneumoniae in Iran—A 2000 to 2021 analysis. *New Microbes and New Infections*, *68*, 101675. PMID: 41377034

Spellberg, B., Guidos, R., Gilbert, D., Bradley, J., Boucher, H. W., Scheld, W. M., Bartlett, J. G., & Edwards, J. (2008). The epidemic of antibiotic-resistant infections: A call to action for the medical community from the Infectious Diseases Society of America. *Clinical Infectious Diseases*, *46*(2), 155–164. PMID: 18171244

Strathdee, S. A., Hatfull, G. F., Mutalik, V. K., & Schooley, R. T. (2023). Phage therapy: From biological mechanisms to future directions. *Cell*, *186*(1), 17–31. PMID: 36608652

Subramaniam, G., & Girish, M. (2020). Antibiotic resistance: A cause for re-emergence of infections. *Indian Journal of Pediatrics*, *87*(11), 937–944. PMID: 32026301

Tamma, P. D., & Cosgrove, S. E. (2011). Antimicrobial stewardship. *Infectious Disease Clinics of North America*, *25*(1), 245–260. PMID: 21316003

Tesema, M. Y., & Birhanu, A. G. (2024). One Health initiative to mitigate the challenge of antimicrobial resistance in the perspectives of developing countries. *Bulletin of the National Research Center*, *48*(1), 14.

Theuretzbacher, U. (2009). Accelerating resistance, inadequate antibacterial drug pipelines and international responses. *International Journal of Antimicrobial Agents*, *33*(3), 195–199. PMID: 22341298

Umansky, A. A., & Fortier, L. C. (2023). The long and sinuous road to phage-based therapy of Clostridioides difficile infections. *Frontiers in Medicine*, *10*, 1259427. PMID: 37680620

United Nations Interagency Coordination Group on Antimicrobial Resistance. (2019). *No time to wait: Securing the future from drug-resistant infections.*

Van Boeckel, T. P., Glennon, E. E., Chen, D., Gilbert, M., Robinson, T. P., Grenfell, B. T., Levin, S. A., Bonhoeffer, S., & Laxminarayan, R. (2017). Reducing antimicrobial use in food animals. *Science*, *357*(6358), 1350–1352. PMID: 28963240

Wang, H., Wang, D., Huangfu, H., Lv, H., Qin, Q., Ren, S., Zhang, Y., Wang, L., & Zhou, Y. (2022). Branched AuAg nanoparticles coated by metal–phenolic networks for treating bacteria-induced periodontitis via photothermal antibacterial and immunotherapy. *Materials & Design*, *224*, 111401.

World Health Organization. (2015). Global action plan on antimicrobial resistance.

World Health Organization. (2015). *Global action plan on antimicrobial resistance.*

Youssef, R. A., Sakr, M. M., Shebl, R. I., Saad, B. T., & Aboshanab, K. M. (2024). Genomic characterization, in vitro, and preclinical evaluation of two microencapsulated lytic phages VB_ST_E15 and VB_ST_SPNIS2 against clinical multidrug-resistant Salmonella serovars. *Annals of Clinical Microbiology and Antimicrobials*, *23*(1), 1–17. PMID: 38360595

Zhang, J., Chu, A., Yang, P., Ouyang, X., Li, B., Mao, W., Wu, X., Zhong, C., Gou, S., Zhang, Y., Liu, H., & Ni, J. (2025). De novo design of mirror-image dimeric antimicrobial peptides with low drug resistance and in vivo efficacy. *Journal of Medicinal Chemistry*, *68*(19), 20304–20323. PMID: 41023587

Chapter 3
Mechanistic Insights Into Antimicrobial Resistance: A Medical Microbiology Perspective

Amina Hayat
https://orcid.org/0009-0000-6459-5945
International Islamic University, Islamabad, Pakistan

Areeba Khubaib
https://orcid.org/0009-0005-8880-3119
King Abdulaziz University, Jeddah, Saudi Arabia

Huzaif Khan
COMSATS University, Islamabad, Pakistan

Nayab Qayyum
https://orcid.org/0009-0009-9624-8994
University of Poonch, Rawalakot, Pakistan

Farman Alam
Bahauddin Zakariya University, Multan, Pakistan

Javaria Khatoon
https://orcid.org/0009-0006-9869-8487
University of Poonch, Rawalakot, Pakistan

ABSTRACT

Antimicrobial resistance (AMR) is considered to be one of the most significant ongoing crises in global healthcare, as it jeopardizes the effectiveness of contemporary medicine and control of infectious diseases. This chapter is a detailed review of the molecular and mechanistic pathogenesis of AMR in the context of medical microbiology. It explains the mechanisms of adaptations and survival of bacterial populations in antimicrobial pressure. Major molecular mechanisms, including enzymatic inactivation of antibiotics, alteration of target sites, overexpression of efflux pumps, and decreased membrane permeability, are thoroughly explained. The chapter goes on to discuss the resistance occurring within biofilms, and horizontal gene transfer, which provides conjugation, transformation, and transduction, is in-

DOI: 10.4018/979-8-3373-3825-5.ch003

vestigated as a path of utmost importance. New alternative approaches are required to cope with this current issue. Knowledge of these molecular bases is important in creating successful antimicrobial stewardship initiatives.

1. INTRODUCTION AND CORE CONCEPTS OF ANTIMICROBIAL RESISTANCE

Antimicrobial resistance denotes the capability of microorganisms to withstand antibiotics and other antimicrobial interventions. The escalation of AMR has severely undermined the utility of many persistent antimicrobial therapies for treating infections, posing a significant obstacle to clinical care and public health. Bacterial pathogens (those causing human disease) that are impervious to available antibiotics may account for 1.27 million of the estimated 7.7 million deaths due to bacterial infections (Rush et al. 2019). Costly payment for antimicrobial resistance continues to increase. AMR is frequently presented as a single, abstract problem and, as a result, remains unseen by many stakeholders. It has evolved into a pervasive threat to the health, well-being, and prospects of most humans and other species on Earth. Today, individuals face substantial odds of encountering an antimicrobial-resistant infection at some point in life, while their ability to access effective treatment is diminishing. The health burden of resistant bacterial infections competes with or exceeds that of HIV and malaria and is a global phenomenon. AMR jeopardizes the control of infectious diseases across age groups and restricts drug development (Murray, et al. 2022). Addressing AMR requires multi-sectoral, cross-disciplinary cooperation, improved diagnostics, assessment of impacts, and effective scientific communication. Frontline defenders include clinicians, pharmacists, clinical microbiologists, and infection prevention specialists. Advances in diagnostic technology enable advanced pathogen identification and appropriate management of bloodstream infections (Peri, et al. 2024).

The threat of antimicrobial resistance is now widely regarded as the most serious hazard to human health globally. Political attention has been urged by declarations from the World Health Organization (WHO) and the U.S. Centers for Disease Control and Prevention (CDC), warning of a crisis and the prospect of reverting to a pre-antibiotic era. Patterns of antimicrobial resistance can be exploited to identify microorganisms by various phenotypic profiles (Carlet, et al. 2014). An organism resistant to at least three antibiotics representing different classes (e.g., aminoglycosides, carbapenems, cephalosporins, and/or fluoroquinolones) is classified as multidrug-resistant (MDR). Strains that remain susceptible to only one or two agents from different classes are termed extensively drug-resistant (XDR). Strains resistant to all available antimicrobial agents are considered pandrug-resistant (PDR) (Magiorakos, et al. 2012).

1.1 Multidrug Resistance and Its Implications

The rise of MDR bacteria poses complicated problems to clinical care and health in the population. The effect of the conventional antibiotics may be affected by resistance mechanisms such as efflux pumps, enzymatic degradation, and target modification, resulting in the need to use alternative or combination therapies. It is imperative to understand these mechanisms in order to be able to prescribe proper treatment. There are a number of new strategies that are being considered to resist MDR. The efflux pump inhibitors increase the sensitivity of the already existing antibiotics, biofilm disruptors are used to target innately resistant bacterial communities, and enzyme inhibitors (β-lactamase inhibitors) are used to reestablish the activity of weakened drugs (Kincses, Nové et al. 2025). Combined, these measures provide some hopeful alternatives of decreasing use of last-resort antibiotics. In addition to clinical environments, human, animal, and environmental reservoirs are the determinants of the spread of resistance. The spread of the resistant bacteria and genes is caused by zoonotic transmission, use of antibiotics in agriculture and contamination of the environment. The adoption of One Health perspective highlights such links and the significance of interventions based on the coordination of interventions in human, veterinary, and environmental areas. There are new technologies that offer more solutions (Al-Khalaifah, et al. 2025). Models of artificial intelligence and machine learning can be used to forecast the resistance pattern and optimize the choice of antibiotics, and CRISPR-based antimicrobials allow targeting resistance genes specifically. These inventions present a progressive outlook of interventions to fight MDR. Zoonotic and environmental pathways are also very important in the spread of resistance. The transmission of the resistance bacteria can be performed by contaminated water, soil, food products, as well as direct contact with animals. Knowing these levels of transmission, as well as horizontal transfer of genes between environmental and clinical strains, is critical towards the overall monitoring and control of MDR pathogen (Pandey, et al. 2024).

2. ANTIBIOTIC CLASSIFICATION:

Antibiotics can be classified by their mechanism of action; some inhibit bacterial cell wall synthesis, others disrupt protein synthesis, nucleic acid synthesis, or disturb metabolism. Alternatively, antibiotics may be grouped by the spectrum of activity: for instance, broad-spectrum agents are active against both Gram-positive and Gram-negative organisms (Dyary, et al. 2023). Major classes of antibiotics, along with their examples, primary targets, and mode of action, are summarized in Table 1. Figure 1 gives us a visual representation of the key antibiotic classes, identifying each group by name and showing the representative examples. The figure is a sort of roadmap of all the key classes presented in the text.

Table 1. Overview of Antibacterial Agents and Their Targets

Antibiotic Class	Examples	Primary Targets	Mechanism of Action	Common Resistance Mechanisms
β-lactams	Penicillin, Cephalosporin, Imipenem	Penicillin-Binding Proteins (PBPs)	Inhibits cell wall synthesis by blocking peptidoglycan cross-linking	β-lactamase production, PBP modification, reduced permeability
Aminoglycosides	Gentamicin, Amikacin, Tobramycin	30S Ribosomal Subunit	Causes mRNA misreading and protein synthesis disruption	Enzymatic modification, efflux pumps, ribosomal mutation
Fluoroquinolones	Ciprofloxacin, Levofloxacin	DNA Gyrase and Topoisomerase IV	Inhibits DNA replication and supercoiling	Target mutations, efflux pumps, plasmid-mediated resistance
Macrolides	Erythromycin, Azithromycin	50S Ribosomal Subunit	Blocks translocation in protein elongation	Methylation of rRNA, efflux, and target site mutation
Tetracyclines	Doxycycline, Tetracycline	30S Ribosomal Subunit	Prevents tRNA binding, halting protein synthesis	Efflux, ribosomal protection proteins
Glycopeptides	Vancomycin, Teicoplanin	Peptidoglycan Precursors (D-Ala-D-Ala)	Inhibits cell wall synthesis in Gram-positive bacteria	D-Ala-D-Lac alteration, decreased binding affinity
Sulfonamides	Sulfamethoxazole	Dihydropteroate Synthase	Inhibits folic acid synthesis	Enzyme mutation, metabolic bypass
Trimethoprim	Trimethoprim	Dihydrofolate Reductase	Blocks tetrahydrofolate synthesis, hindering DNA synthesis	Target site mutation, overproduction of target enzyme

Figure 1. Various classes of antibiotics based on their action mechanism

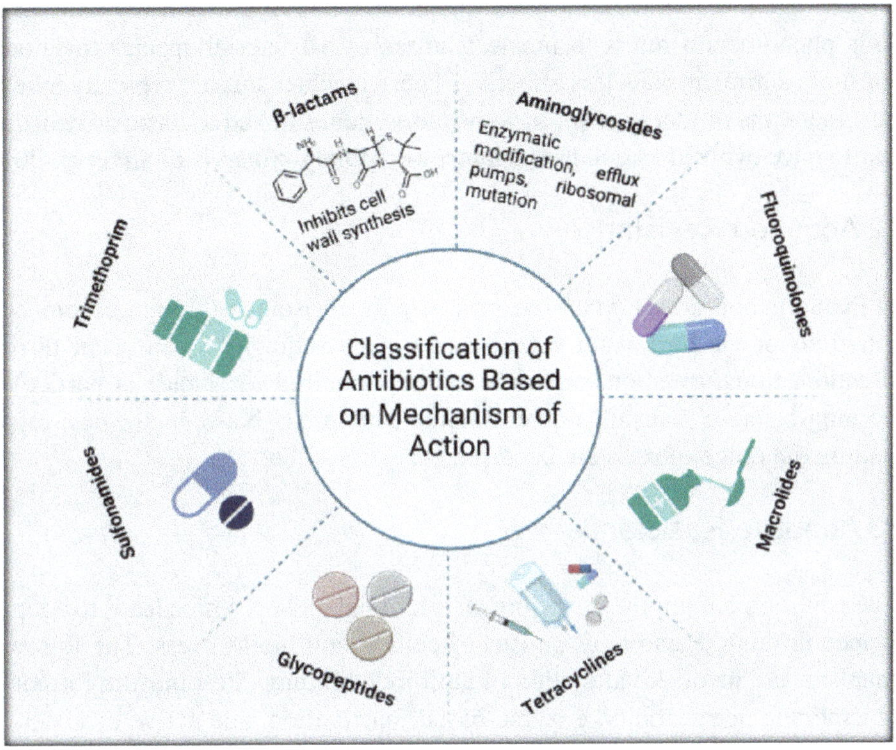

3. BACTERIAL ADAPTATION TO ANTIMICROBIAL PRESSURE

Multidrug-resistant pathogens are increasing to alarming proportions, and the traditional antibiotics are ineffective. Therefore, to eliminate this issue, it is of urgent necessity to develop alternative treatment methods. In that aspect, it is highly necessary to explain the mechanisms of resistance.

3.1 Types of Resistance Mechanisms

Bacterial resistance mechanisms can be classified into intrinsic, acquired, and adaptive resistance, distinct strategies bacteria employ to tolerate antibiotic exposure.

3.1.1 Intrinsic Resistance

This phenomenon refers to innate features of a bacterial species that render one or more antimicrobials less effective. These mechanisms are typically inherent to most members of that species. In some cases, genes linked to intrinsic resistance appear to have evolved as defenses against microbial toxins. (Liu, Shi et al. 2019)

3.1.2 Acquired Resistance

A Phenomenon arises when bacteria acquire resistance through chromosomal mutations or via horizontal gene transfer. This acquisition can occur through conjugation, transformation, or transduction. Acquired resistance is particularly concerning because resistance determinants can spread between species, rapidly expanding the range of resistant bacteria.

3.1.3 Adaptive Resistance

The environment imposes pressure on microbial niches, which leads to adaptive resistance through dynamic responses of cells to antibiotic stress. The following mechanisms are involved: alteration of antibiotic binding sites, biofilm formation, low membrane permeability, enzyme-based inactivation, and active efflux of antimicrobial agents, which may interact synergistically to enhance drug resistance, making treatment more difficult (Tavares-Carreon, De Anda-Mora et al. 2023).

4. RESISTANCE MOLECULAR MECHANISMS

First, antibiotic resistance was reported in 1930, and it was inevitable, although fatal pathogens were present. The strains of microbes end up developing resistance genes by other bacteria via transgenes, phages, plasmids, or chromosomal mutations. The bacteria have, over the years, evolved several ways of neutralizing the effects of the different classes of antibiotics, such as interfering with the synthesis of proteins, disintegration of components of the bacterial cell wall, disruption of the metabolic processes, or the release of nucleic acids (Darby, et al. 2023).

4.1. Antibiotic Enzyme Inactivation

The ability of bacteria to break down antibiotics using enzymes is one of the main mechanisms of resistance to β-lactam, aminoglycosides, and chloramphenicol.

These enzymes are often expressed in transposable factors and plasmids, which promotes the propagation of resistance (Elshobary, et al. 2025).

4.1.2 β-Lactam Hydrolyzing Enzymes

Part of the β-lactam group, carbapenems is structurally related to penicillin but with a broad spectrum against Gram-negative and Gram-positive bacteria. The principal properties of carbapenems are stability against most β-lactamases and cell wall penetration into bacterial cells (Codjoe and Donkor 2017). The β-lactam antibiotics may be categorized into penicillin, cephalosporins, monobactams, and carbapenems, and each of them includes a β-lactam ring, a different additional ring, and side chains. β-lactamases cause enzyme-mediated resistance (Kim, Kim et al. 2023). β-lactamase, which has been further divided into serine β-lactamases (SBLs) and metallo-β-lactamases (MBLs) depending on the type of catalytic component, is one such common resistance mechanism against the β-lactams, particularly in problematic Gram-negative bacteria, according to (Naas, et al. 2017). Hydrolyzing nucleophilic residue of serine that the SBLs use is quite interesting from a therapeutic viewpoint. The MBLs, which use zinc ions to activate water molecules to catalyze the hydrolysis of β-lactam antibiotics, have gained a lot of attention recently, partly due to their potent carbapenem action and extremely broad substrate specificity (Tehrani and Martin 2018)s; (Mora-Ochomogo and Lohans 2021).

4.1.3 ESBLs

The proliferation of extended-spectrum β-lactamases (ESBLs) complicates AMR, heightening morbidity, raising the hospital stays, and increasing treatment costs (Maslikowska, Walker et al. 2016). Many *enterobacteriaceae* produce β-lactam-hydrolyzing enzymes encoded on plasmids or chromosomes and are identified by the WHO as especially problematic pathogens. ESBL-producing *Enterobacteriaceae* (ESBL-E) do not hydrolyze cephamycins or carbapenems but are resistant to penicillins, aztreonam, and primary third-generation cephalosporins (Castanheira, et al. 2021). Due to the common carriers of Enterobacteriaceae to the gastrointestinal tract of humans and animals, ESBL genes are freely distributed among clinical, community, agricultural, and environmental ecosystems. Recent studies represent the ESBL spreading among food animals, wastewater, and fresh produce, which adds to the growth of mobile ESBL reservoirs (Bevan et al. 2020; Hafez et al. 2023; Chen et al. 2024). These plasmid-associated genes, especially those in the blaCTX-M, blaTEM and blaSHV categories, are often accompanied by mobile genetic elements like insertion sequences (e.g. ISEcp1), which increase cross-species and cross-environmental transmission. One Health perspective is thus essential to ESBL spread control because environmental and foodborne methods are now equal in control, or even more than the hospital-based control (Lak Hondori, Mohammadi-Sichani et al. 2025).

4.1.4 Comparison of ESBLs and Carbapenemases

Carbapenemases are more advanced stages of evolution in β-lactam resistance, and their hydrolytic patterns are more extensive and have more dire consequences, although ESBLs are highly problematic. Their comparison with ESBLs is presented below in Table 2.

Table 2. Comparison of key characteristics, hydrolytic activity, inhibitor susceptibility, and clinical impact of ESBLs and carbapenemases.

Feature	ESBLs	Carbapenemases
Hydrolytic spectrum	Hydrolyze extended-spectrum cephalosporins; cannot hydrolyze carbapenems	Hydrolyze all β-lactams, including carbapenems
Major families	CTX-M, SHV, TEM	KPC, NDM, OXA-48-like, VIM, IMP
Location	Mostly plasmid-borne	Plasmid and chromosome
Inhibitor susceptibility	Often inhibited by clavulanic acid, sulbactam, tazobactam; newer inhibitors (e.g., avibactam) are highly effective	Extremely limited inhibitor options; only a few inhibitors (e.g., avibactam for KPC and some OXA-48 variants) show activity
Clinical impact	Limits cephalosporin use; carbapenems remain effective	Associated with extreme drug resistance, high mortality, and treatment failures
WHO priority	Critical	Highest critical

ESBLs are the main ones that affect the effectiveness of extended-spectrum cephalosporins. Carbapenems, in their turn, destroy the final defense of β-lactam, and, in most cases, only toxic or less efficient agents (e.g., colistin, tigecycline) are left. According to the recent surveillance studies, such a convergence is an alarming occurrence. *K. pneumoniae* ST258 and *E. coli* ST131 clones, in particular, tend to co-harbour carbapenemase genes along with ESBL-producing strains (Olaitan, Orababa et al. 2025).

4.1.5 ESBLs in the Context of Other Resistance Mechanisms

Although combinations of β-lactam/β-lactamase inhibitors prove effective with certain ESBLs, such inhibitors are not effective due to co-resistance mechanisms. ESBL-producing Gram-negative bacteria are mostly involved in increased efflux pumps (AcrAB-TolC) expression, loss or mutation of porins (e.g., OmpK35,

OmpK36), and co-administration of aminoglycoside-modifying enzymes, Fosfomycin resistance genes, and fluoroquinolone mutations (Katsarou, et al. 2025).

4.1.6 Modifying Enzyme-Aminoglycoside

Aminoglycosides are actinomycete-derived natural or semisynthetic antibiotics. The aminoglycosides were the first class of antibiotics to find clinical use, and a number of them were incorporated into humans. In the initial phases of antimicrobial chemotherapy, the aminoglycosides were usually taken as the first-line therapy. They, however slowly abolished in the 1980s when they were replaced by cephalosporins, carbapenems, and fluoroquinolones. Aminoglycosides are synergistic with a variety of other antibacterial classes. The recent renewal of interest in broad-spectrum and rapidly bactericidal antibiotics is itself the result of a complex of causes. These are the increased prevalence of MDR bacteria and the possibility of increasing the effectiveness and safety of this group of antibiotics by an enhanced dosing schedule (Krause, et al. 2016). Aminoglycosides are the most important antimicrobial agents used in dual therapy against various diseases in humans and animals. These drugs are made from the genus *Streptomyces* and *Micromonospora*. These are bactericidal agents that disrupt bacterial translation and are active against other Gram-positive and Gram-negative bacteria (Breijyeh, et al. 2020). Other mutations in genetic materials that encode ribosomal RNA and ribosomal proteins also lead to aminoglycoside resistance, but the mechanism is not as prevalent in *E. coli* because it has many copies of the rRNA gene (Foudraine, et al. 2021). Aminoglycosides are: tobramycin, amikacin, gentamicin, netilmicin, and so on. They may be resisted at the high level by the methylation of certain residues at 16S rRNA (AL-Tameemi, Almanaseer et al. 2023).

For many years, aminoglycosides have been an important part of the treatment of severe illnesses. Unfortunately, their utility has been limited by the appearance and development of resistance. In other cases, the insusceptibility was so extreme that it was almost insignificant. The most prevalent mechanism of aminoglycoside resistance in the clinical setting is enzymatic modification. Aminoglycoside-altering enzymes, such as nucleotidyl transferases, phosphotransferases, and acetyltransferases, catalyze the alteration of many OH or NH2 residues found in the nucleus or sugar components of the 2-deoxystreptamine (Ramirez and Tolmasky 2010). Antibiotics known as aminoglycosides are not typically utilized as a first-line treatment for *H. pylori* infections. Instead, separate antibiotics like metronidazole, amoxicillin, or clarithromycin are often recommended in combination with a proton pump inhibitor. In a less resource-intensive approach, scientists are exploring repurposing medications to inhibit aminoglycoside-modifying enzymes (AMEs). However, resistance to these inhibitors is expected to occur, which raises the issue of antibiotic resistance.

Strategies to develop inhibitors against enzymes and make modified antibiotics resistant are crucial. When used with antibiotics, natural plant extracts may help address the issue of bacterial resistance (AL-Tameemi, et al. 2023).

The efflux pumps have been reported as one of the main factors contributing to the clinical treatment dilemma since they actively export antibiotics beyond bacterial cells so that effective intracellular concentrations become diminished and bacteria can survive the therapeutic intervention. Here, even though the mere overexpression of efflux pumps does not necessarily increase minimum inhibitory concentrations (MICs) above clinical breakpoints, bacteria with increased efflux activity may be able to survive at the site of infection with subinhibitory drug concentrations, giving rise to a pool of bacteria with high-level resistance and resulting in the failure in treatment of patients undergoing standard therapy. This has been observed in chronic lung infections, including in patients with cystic fibrosis undergoing many different classes of antibiotics, and where efflux-mediated persistence allows adaptation and subsequent clinical resistance, leading to the long-term persistence of the infection and subsequent changes in the therapeutic choice. Efflux pumps also contribute to multidrug-resistant hospital pathogens like *Acinetobacter baumannii*, where elevated efflux activity is linked to resistance to various antibiotic classes and is also linked with increased rates of mortality in susceptible patients and in severe nosocomial infections, often exceeding 50-60% in diseased patients. There is a high rate of resistance to fluoroquinolones and other important antibiotics in clinical isolates of *Enterococcus faecium* with efflux pump determinants, and the efflux pump inhibitor has been demonstrated to decrease MICs, which is even more compelling evidence of its role in therapeutic failure. In combination, these results demonstrate how efflux pumps not only decrease the efficacy of antibiotics, but also enhance chronic infections, prolonged hospitalization, higher healthcare expenditures, and worse patient outcomes in clinical practice. (Chandal, Sharma et al. 2025)

4.2 Antibiotic Target Modification

One of the first strategies used by bacteria to avoid b-lactam antibiotics was to change the structure of penicillin-binding proteins (PBPs). Drug affinity at the target site may be decreased by modifications in PBPs. Similar to this, members of the erythromycin ribosome methylase (erm) gene family methylate 16S rRNA, changing binding sites to prevent the binding of lincosamide and macrolide. The primary targets of b-lactam antibiotics, peptidoglycan production and remodeling, are regulated by a collection of PBPs encoded by each bacterial family. Despite the protracted recognition of PBPs, little is known about how they regulate activity, where they are found, and how they interact with other proteins during cell growth and division. One of the four to sixteen PBP homologues that some bacteria have is frequently necessary for their survival (Carlson, et al. 2025).

Regardless of cell wall density, PBP changes are caused by intricate cell wall remodeling and related modifications in wall-associated polypeptides. PBPs promote cell turgor and provide structural integrity by catalyzing the formation of peptidoglycan. Multidrug-resistant (MDR) types of pathogenic bacteria have been linked to mutations in PBPs, which present a significant challenge to infection control. Treatment of bacterial infections is made more difficult by the emergence of MDR strains and the prevalence of PBP-mediated resistance (Dabhi, Patel et al. 2024).

4.2.1 Mutation in DNA Gyrase/Topoisomerase (Fluoroquinolones)

Fluoroquinolones target DNA gyrase and topoisomerase IV, two essential enzymes. However, after roughly twenty-five years of clinical use, target-mediated resistance has eroded the clinical utility of this vital antibiotic class for certain infections.

Target alteration, such as alterations in penicillin-binding proteins (PBPs) and DNA gyrase / topoisomerase IV mutations, has a direct negative impact on the efficacy of antibiotics and is a cause of disease failures under clinical practice. The changes in PBP, which are observed in MRSA and penicillin-resistant *Streptococcus pneumoniae*, reduce β-lactam binding, and this can lead to chronic infections and 20-35 percent mortality in bloodstream infections. In the same manner, the resistance of fluoroquinolone caused by mutations in DNA gyrase and topoisomerases reduces therapy of *E. coli* and *Klebsiella* infections, relying on a last-resort therapy and combination therapy. These changes increase hospitalization, increase healthcare expenses, and the probability of serious complications, which is why it is necessary to urgently conduct diagnostics and specific therapeutic methods (Isuranga and Danthanarayana 2025).

4.3 Efflux Pumps

Efflux pumps are membrane transporters necessary for bacterial metabolism, pathogenicity, and multidrug resistance. These pumps prevent the obstruction of exogenous chemicals (detergents, disinfectants, and antibiotics) within the cells by actively reducing the concentration of these chemicals at their respective biological sites. Consequently, efflux transporters become a new object of investigation of inhibitors to combat MDR-based infectious diseases (De Gaetano, et al. 2023). Activity of the efflux pump is illustrated in Figure 2, which gives a simplified schematic of the working of the efflux pumps, where the antibiotics entering the bacterial cell are taken out and returned into the bacterial cell instantly using these membrane proteins. The graph is a graphical support of the explanation, with focus on the directional movement of drugs and the contribution of efflux systems to reduce the concentration of antibiotics in the cell.

Figure 2. Efflux pump activity to flush out antibiotics outside the cell.

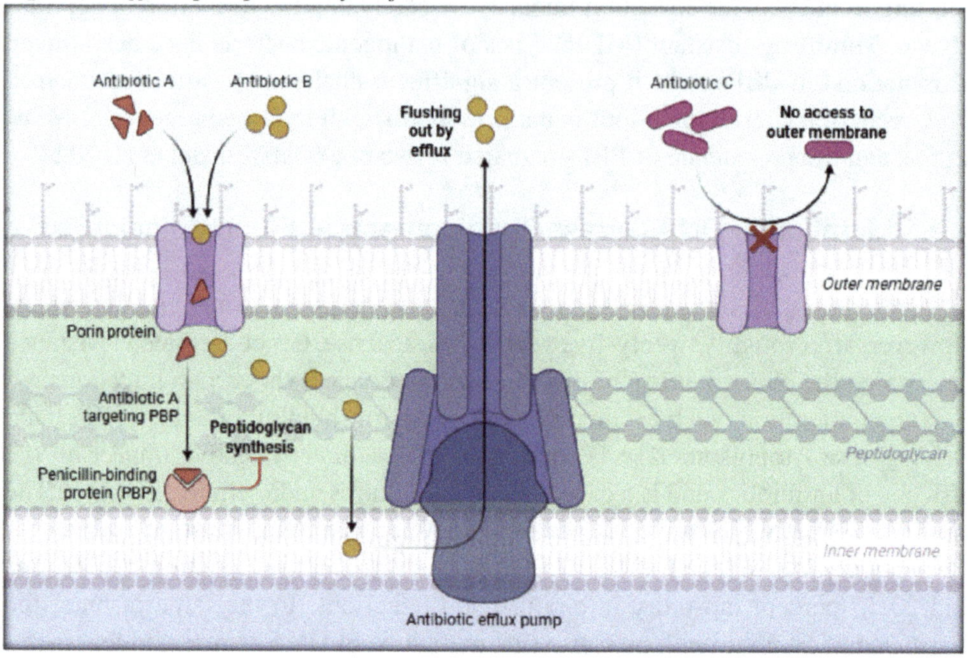

4.3.1 Key Efflux Families

As membrane transport systems are highly active in establishing the extracellular levels of antimicrobial chemicals, reducing their intracellular concentration to levels below the effective therapeutic dose, it has also been shown that they contribute significantly to antibiotic resistance in bacteria.

These systems are resistant to antibiotics because they are made up of different super families with different structural and functional traits. Lineages to five major super families, the multidrug and toxic compound extrusion (MATE) superfamily, the small multidrug resistance (SMR) superfamily, the ATP-binding cassettes (ABC) superfamily, the resistance nodulation and cell division (RND) superfamily, and the major facilitator superfamily (MFS), describe the substrate specificity, structural traits, energy sources, and efflux transporters. (De Gaetano, Lentini et al. 2023)

4.3.2 ATP-Driven Efflux Pumps (ABC)

The ABC family of proteins is widely distributed in bacteria and aids in both nutrient absorption and xenobiotic efflux. These transporters have two transmembrane domains (TMDs) that form a substrate transport channel and two nucleotide-binding domains (NBDs) that enable efflux by ATP hydrolysis. The role of periplasmic binding proteins in gram-negative bacteria in providing substrate identification and initiating the transportation process is well known. ABC transporters are involved in both virulence and antibiotic resistance (Scoffone, Trespidi et al. 2025). Antibiotics are pumped out by export systems. *Escherichia coli's* tripartite efflux mechanism contributes to *Enterobacteriaceae* macrolide resistance and virulence factor secretion. When eliminated, aminoglycosides and cationic antimicrobial peptides (CAPs) are more efficient against *Serratia marcescens* than other antibiotics. The ABC transporters are regulated by two-component regulatory systems as well as substrate-sensitive transcriptional regulators (Zakaria, fakharul zaman raja Yahya et al. 2023). Recently, ABC transporter inhibitors have been developed as antibiotic adjuvants, but this is hard to achieve as bacterial efflux systems are redundant and hard to control (Belay, Getachew et al. 2024).

4.3.3 Major Facilitator Superfamily (MFS)

The MFS is the largest and best-characterized family of transmembrane secondary transporters in prokaryotes and eukaryotes. MFS proteins mediate substrate movement via secondary active transport mechanisms, i.e., symport, antiport, and uniport. Their substrate range is broad, including ions, sugars, amino acids, metabolites, and antimicrobials (Henderson, Fendler et al. 2019). MFS transporter gene SCO4121 in *Streptomyces coelicolor* is implicated in multidrug resistance; its overexpression confers resistance to many antibiotics, including ciprofloxacin and chloramphenicol, while its deletion increases susceptibility. MFS-family efflux pumps (e.g., SA09310 and SCO4121) lower intracellular antibiotic concentrations and promote bacterial survival in the presence of antimicrobials. The evolutionary adaptability and broad substrate profile of MFS transporters make them attractive targets for efflux pump inhibitors (EPIs) aimed at enhancing existing antibiotics and overcoming MDR (Elshobary, et al. 2025).

4.3.4 Small Multidrug Resistance (SMR Family)

SMR proteins were found to take part in the production and release of different lipophilic substances such as antiseptics, detergents, antibiotics, and other medicines. The SMR family is very heterogeneous in terms of structure and function by being highly protein-coded in plasmids and bacterial chromosomes. This heterogeneity makes SMR proteins resistant to most antibiotic agents, including b-lactams like cephalosporins. The proximity of SMR genes to the antimicrobial resistance (AMR) genes in bacterial genomes has been reported as the cause of such resistance, and thus, the genetic amplification of multidrug resistance in bacterial cells. The most recent use of the SMR capability is the A1S0710 gene that encodes an SMR transporter protein in *Acinetobacter baumannii* (Vrancianu, Gheorghe et al. 2020). The deletion of this gene has been experimentally done and it has been observed that deletion of this gene has two effects on the deleting cells; firstly removal of this gene leads to reduced motility of the deleting cells and secondly removal of this gene leads to increased virulence of the deleting cells. The role of the SMR proteins in the determination of bacterial survival and pathogenicity is facilitated by the combined action of the SMR proteins (Pérez-Varela, Corral et al. 2019).

4.3.5 Multidrug and Toxic Compound Extrusion (MATE) Family

The MATE family was identified in 2008 in relation to microorganisms that were resistant to many drugs. One of the first to be described was the *Neisseria gonorrhoeae* NorM, a multidrug efflux pump that has the capacity to produce fluoroquinolone and other harmful chemicals extracellularly. The secondary active transporters known as MATE transporters are essential for the efflux of cationic substrates and for lowering the sensitivity of bacteria to the majority of antimicrobial medications. These are, but are not limited to, tetraphenylphosphonium, norfloxacin, berberine, and ethidium bromide, which would accumulate in bacterial cells unless they were expelled by these pumps. Implementing ethambutol does not require a particularly complex approach (Miyauchi, et al. 2017).

4.3.6 Independent Family - Proteobacterial Antimicrobial Compound Efflux (PACE) Family

Another group of recently discovered bacterial membrane transport proteins, which deal with antimicrobial resistance, is termed efflux of proteobacterial antimicrobial chemicals. As of 2013, numerous *Proteobacteria* have been found to have PACE family transporters, particularly in the clinically significant pathogenic species (Kim, et al. 2021).

The prototype AceI (Acinetobacter chlorhexidine efflux protein I) of this family was the first to be identified in *Acinetobacter baumannii*. It has been demonstrated that AceI is resistant to chlorhexidine, which is an essential antiseptic in a healthcare setting (Migliaccio, et al. 2022). Despite the lack of research on the mechanism of PACE transporters, the currently existing evidence indicates that the transporter is a proton-dependent efflux pump. So as to reduce the levels of medication in the bacterial cell and eliminate resistance, they are thus likely to actively expel anti-microbial chemicals out of the cell by using the force of the proton motive force (Javed 2020).

With the continued familiarity with the PACE family, it is becoming very clear that these transporters are a major source of bacterial antimicrobial resistance. Further studies relating to the same are essential in the development of measures that can be used to overcome the increasing jeopardy of antibiotic-related infections.

4.3.7 Resistance Nodulation Cell Division Superfamily (RND)

The RND superfamily encompasses bacteria, archaea, and some eukaryotes, and bacterial RND pumps are major contributors to antibiotic resistance. RND systems actively express a wide array of antibiotics and other toxic compounds from Gram-negative bacteria, supporting tolerance to pH changes, metal ions, bile acids, fatty acids, and host antimicrobial peptides (Nikaido 2018). These systems are central to bacterial survival under hostile conditions. Periplasmic adaptor proteins (PAPs) facilitate assembly of outer membrane protein (OMP)-bound pumps. RND multidrug efflux pumps have been extensively studied in human-associated bacteria, though less so in other taxa (Yamasaki, Zwama et al. 2023). Major Bacterial Efflux Pump Families along with their functions are summarized in following table:

Table 3. Comparative Summary of Major Bacterial Efflux Pump Families and Their Functional Attributes in Multidrug Resistance

Efflux Pump Family	Energy Source	Key Structural Features	Representative Examples	Primary Substrates / Role in Resistance
ATP-Binding Cassette (ABC)	ATP hydrolysis	Two transmembrane domains (TMDs) + two nucleotide-binding domains (NBDs); often involve periplasmic binding proteins in Gram-negative bacteria	MacB, LmrA, *E. coli* MacAB-TolC	Efflux of macrolides, aminoglycosides, cationic antimicrobial peptides; involved in virulence and nutrient transport
Major Facilitator Superfamily (MFS)	Proton motive force (secondary active transport)	Typically 12–14 transmembrane helices; uniport/symport/antiport mechanisms	EmrB, TetA, SCO4121	Broad substrate range including antibiotics (chloramphenicol, ciprofloxacin), sugars, ions; major contributor to MDR in many species
Small Multidrug Resistance (SMR)	Proton motive force	Small proteins (≈110 aa) forming homo/heterodimers; encoded on plasmids and chromosomes	EmrE, A1S_0710	Efflux of antiseptics, detergents, b-lactams, and lipophilic compounds; associated with AMR gene clusters and MDR amplification
Multidrug and Toxic Compound Extrusion (MATE)	Na^+ gradient or proton motive force	12-transmembrane domain secondary transporters	NorM, MepA	Efflux of fluoroquinolones, berberine, ethidium bromide, cationic drugs; overexpression linked to tigecycline resistance
Proteobacterial Antimicrobial Compound Efflux (PACE)	Proton motive force	Recently discovered family; structurally less characterized	AceI (A. baumannii)	Efflux of chlorhexidine and other biocides; linked with MDR in Proteobacteria, major concern for hospital infection control
Resistance Nodulation Division (RND)	Proton motive force	Tripartite system: inner membrane pump + periplasmic adaptor protein (PAP) + outer membrane channel (e.g., TolC)	AcrAB-TolC, MexAB-OprM	Broad-spectrum efflux of b-lactams, fluoroquinolones, dyes, bile salts, metals; dominant efflux system in Gram-negative bacteria

The efflux pumps decrease the amount of intracellular antibiotics, which results in chronic infections and multidrug resistance in the pathogenic bacteria, including *Acinetobacter baumannii*, *E. coli*, and *Staphylococcus aureus*. The efflux pump contributes to the failures in treatment, extended hospitalization, and mortality (30-

60% in severe nosocomial infections), which should lead to the use of efflux pump inhibitors and strict antibiotic stewardship.

4.4 Reduced Permeability

The capacity of bacteria to decrease membrane permeability is one of the main processes of antibiotic resistance as it decreases the concentration of antibiotics inside the cell. Gram-negative bacteria, especially, have the outer membrane, which is a selective barrier that does not allow harmful compounds to enter it. Hydrophilic antibiotics, including β-lactams, fluoroquinolones, and aminoglycosides, enter the cell by the main route of penetration via porin proteins: a channel-like structure on the outer membrane. Resistance can be caused by the mutation or downregulation of porins, which greatly decreases uptake of antibiotics. Indicatively, Pseudomonas aeruginosa does not permeate easily to carbapenem because of mutations in the OprD porin that serve to absorb imipenem and meropenem. On the same note, cephalosporin-resistant Escherichia coli strains have been observed to suppress OmpF and OmpC porins, resulting in reduced drug uptake. These alterations are usually accompanied by other resistance mechanisms, e.g. efflux pumps overexpression or β-lactamases production, leading to multidrug resistance.

Also, the lipid composition of bacterial membranes may change, which may also change permeability and influence the diffusion of antibiotics. There is evidence that changes in the structure of lipopolysaccharide (LPS) have the potential to further increase resistance through the reduction of membrane fluidity and the strength of repulsion between charges associated with cationic antibiotics in *Acinetobacter baumannii* (Elshobary, et al. 2025).

Clinical isolates have been observed to have a few mutations in the porin genes, which disrupt protein production. The mutated gene sequence containing these mutations contains stop codons, deletions, or insertions in the sequence, resulting in early protein translation. Notably, it has also been stated that a mutation in position 25 of the OmpK36 gene, cytosine-thymine, causes a change in the mRNA structure that creates an interaction between the produced uracil and the first adenine of the Shine-Dalgarno sequence. This mutated RNA stem conceals the ribosome binding site and, consequently, it inhibits effective translation that resulting in insufficient OmpK36 expression (Wong, David et al. 2022). Potential antimicrobial resistance mechanisms are summarized in Figure 3.

Figure 3. Major Mechanisms of Action that cause antimicrobial resistance

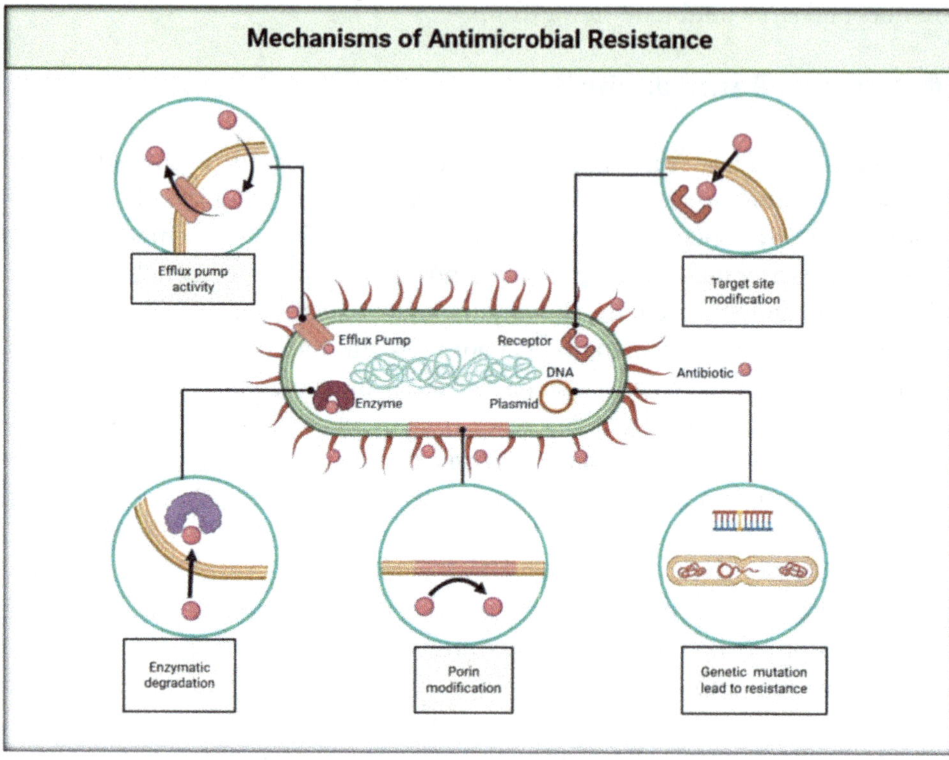

4.5 Biofilm-Mediated Resistance: Architecture and Resistance of Biofilms

Self-synthesized extracellular polymeric substance (EPS) matrix envelops organized microbial communities are termed as biofilms, which are crucial in microbial illnesses and healthcare-associated infections (HAIs) (Fleming and Rumbaugh 2018). Bacteria in biofilms create EPS, a multicomponent matrix, to provide structural support and protection. Bacterial adhesion, nutrition sequestration, and resistance to external stimuli, such as antibiotics and immune reactions, are all improved by EPS, a polysaccharide, protein, extracellular DNA (eDNA), and lipid-based structure. Because it contributes to antibiotic resistance, it is a pathogen of great interest to methods that try to break up biofilms to treat related illnesses. Recent studies also observes that during infection the EPS composition is dynamically altered which increases biofilms even more resistant to last-line antibiotics like carbapenems and colistin. One of the causes of antimicrobial resistance is biofilm, which has a special structure and adaptive processes that offer resistance against antimicrobial agents. Crucial elements, including bacterial cell density, quorum-sensing communication, and genetic adaptations like efflux pump activation, mutations, and so on increase their resistance to therapy, making treatment more difficult (Rao, et al. 2021). Recent evidence reveals that quorum-sensing blockers and efflux pump inhibitors are currently being explored as adjuncts therapy because they have the potential to make biofilm resilience less strong. Complex structure, hierarchical growth, and connections to various human diseases are characteristics of biofilms. It is necessary to regulate their growth in terms of physiological processes and alterations in cell composition. Heterogeneous biofilms can enhance resilience and adaptability by promoting genetic variety. Microorganisms like *Candida albicans* and *Listeria monocytogenes* use many signaling pathways and transcription factors to form biofilms (Kember, et al. 2022). Also, multi-omics research demonstrates that the heterogeneity of biofilms is a significant cause of ineffective antibiotic treatment of chronic infections (Pandrangi, et al. 2025).

Additionally, they play a crucial role in the pathophysiology of chronic rhinosinusitis, periodontal disorders, and infections linked to urinary catheters (Pentland, et al. 2020; Nowak, et al. 2021). *P. aeruginosa* is commonly seen in the biofilms of chronic wounds, including venous leg ulcers and diabetic foot (Standyło, et al. 2022). By producing persistent inflammation and erecting a physical barrier to immune cells and medications, these biofilms have a detrimental effect on wound healing. Device-associated infections arise as a result of *S. aureus* biofilms on implantation devices, including implants, prosthetic joints, and catheters. It is often necessary to extricate the devices from such biofilms because of their high level of antibiotic resistance. Implant and catheter biofilms are also responsible of recurrent infections despite proper antibiotic treatment and approaches aimed at eliminating biofilms must be used urgently in hospitals (Mishra, et al. 2024). Compared to their planktonic counterparts, organisms found in biofilms exhibit noticeably higher levels of antibiotic resistance. Compromised medication penetration, restricted nutrition availability, and adaptive stress response can all be used to explain this enhanced resistance. Furthermore, bacteria take advantage of biofilm formation in several ways, such as defense against the host's immune system, antibiotic resistance, and recurrent infection (Chakraborty, et al. 2021). A 2024 update of WHO GLASS also reports that biomimicking pathogens have 10-1,000 times increased MIC values compared to planktonic cells which makes infection control in the world a big challenge (Sati, Carrara et al. 2025).

4.5.1 The Molecular Changes that Underlie Biofilm Resistance to Antimicrobial Agents

There is a strong connection between biofilm and the rise in microbial cell resistance to antibiotics. Certain genes influence the development of antibiotic resistance, which is a sign of the phenomenon's genetic foundation, and regulate the formation of biofilms. Furthermore, bacterial cells that separate from biofilms still exhibit the phenotype of antibiotic resistance, suggesting that antibiotic resistance endures even after the cells change to a planktonic state (Das and Samal 2018). Recently, genes that are involved in the regulation of efflux pumps (e.g., acrAB-tolC) and stress-response regulators had been reported to be upregulated despite dispersal, which provides continued resistance (HUDA, et al. 2025).

The capacity of bacteria in biofilms to withstand antimicrobial treatments is superior to that of bacteria that are free to survive. Their increased resistance makes it difficult to treat them at all and significantly lowers their susceptibility to antibiotics (Hayet, et al. 2023). This inertial tolerance has now been associated with the existence of metabolically dormant so-called persister cells, surviving large doses of antibiotics and eventually reestablishing the infection site.

Even at low concentrations, biofilms have been shown to exhibit a remarkable ability to react rapidly to antibiotics. This demonstrates the strong selection pressure imposed by antimicrobial medications, which accelerates the development of resistance mechanisms. This flexibility might be challenging in therapeutic interventions. Additionally, resistance is strengthened because the biofilm matrix, which is rich in proteins and eDNA, sticks to antibiotics and reduces their efficacy. This mixture decreases the effects of specifically designed antibiotics that do have anti-biofilm properties while protecting bacterial cells. New discoveries also suggest that eDNA in the matrix is a chelating agent to positively charged antibiotics, that further reduces penetration and leads to failure of treatment (Sivalingam, et al. 2025).

The formation of biofilm plays a major role in the clinical failure of treatment of clinical infections due to the creation of a protective scaffold that restricts penetration of antibiotics and the protection of metabolically dormant persister cells. Recurrent and chronic infections are linked to this mechanism, especially in device-associated infection like catheters, implants and prosthetic joints, and in the chronic wound. Biofilm-related pathogens may have 10-1000 times increased MICs as compared to planktonic cells and result in an increased duration of stay, repeated courses of antibiotics, and increased morbidity, underscoring the significance of anti-biofilm agents in healthcare facilities (Vatansever, et al. 2025). The detailed summary of potential resistance mechanisms is presented in Table 4.

Table 4. "Comparative Analysis of Antimicrobial Resistance Mechanisms in Major Pathogens"

Pathogen (syndromes)	Drugs/classes most impacted	Dominant resistance mechanisms	Key marker genes	Notes
Escherichia coli (UTI, sepsis)	b-lactams, FQs, AGs	ESBLs; carbapenemases; porin ↓ + efflux; FQ target mutations; PMQR	**bla**CTX-M, **bla**TEM/ **SHV**; **bla**NDM/**KPC**/ **OXA-48-like**; **gyrA**/ **parC** QRDR; **qnr**, **aac(6′)-Ib-cr**	ESBL → 3GC failure; combo mechanisms raise MICs sharply
Klebsiella pneumoniae (HAP/VAP, BSI)	Carbapenems, 3GC, FQs	Carbapenemases (Class A KPC, B NDM/VIM/IMP, D OXA-48-like); ESBLs + porin loss; efflux	**bla**KPC, **bla**NDM, **bla**OXA-48-like; **ompK35/36** loss; **acrAB-tolC**	High clonal spread; OXA-48-like common in South Asia/ MENA
Pseudomonas aeruginosa (HAP/VAP, CF)	Carbapenems, FQs, AGs	OprD porin loss; inducible **AmpC**; multiple RND efflux pumps; target mutations; AG-modifying enzymes	**oprD** inactivation; **ampC** derepression; **MexAB-OprM/MexXY-OprM**; **gyrA/parC**; **aac/ aph/ant**	Intrinsically low permeability; multi-mechanistic
Acinetobacter baumannii (ICU infections)	Carbapenems, AGs, FQs	OXA-type carbapenemases; porin/penicillin-binding changes; efflux; AG-modifying enzymes	**bla**OXA-23/**-24/-58**, **IS**Aba1-**bla**OXA-51; **AdeABC/AdeIJK**; **aac/ aph/ant**	CRAB often pan-resistant; ISAba1 promoter boosts OXA
Staphylococcus aureus (SSTI, BSI)	b-lactams (esp. anti-staph), others	**mecA/mecC** → PBP2a (low b-lactam affinity); b-lactamase (**blaZ**); target changes (e.g., **gyrA**, **grlA** for FQs)	**SCCmec (mecA)** encoding **PBP2a**; **blaZ**	Newer cephalosporins active vs some MRSA, but PBP2a allostery matters
Enterococcus faecium/faecalis (VRE)	Glycopeptides, b-lactams	Altered cell-wall termini → van gene clusters; HLAR via enzymes	**vanA/vanB** (D-Ala-D-Lac), **vanC** (D-Ala-D-Ser); **aac(6′)-aph(2″)**	**vanA** → high-level VAN+TEI resistance; infection-control critical
Streptococcus pneumoniae (CAP, meningitis)	Penicillins, cephalosporins, macrolides	Mosaic PBPs (↓ b-lactam affinity); **erm/mef** (MLS_B, efflux)	Altered **pbp2x/pbp2b/ pbp1a**; **erm(B)**, **mef(A/E)**	Stepwise PBP changes raise MICs; macrolide resistance common
Mycobacterium tuberculosis (TB)	RIF, INH, EMB, FQs, AMKs	Target-gene mutations (drug activation/target)	**rpoB** (RIF), **katG/inhA** (INH), **embB** (EMB), **gyrA/B** (FQs), **rrs/eis** (AGs)	WGS increasingly used for rapid resistance prediction

Abbreviations: 3GC = third-gen cephalosporins; FQs = fluoroquinolones; AGs = aminoglycosides; CF = cystic fibrosis; HAP/VAP = hospital/ventilator-acquired pneumonia; BSI = bloodstream infection.

4.6 Global Trends in Antimicrobial Resistance Across Key Pathogens and Mechanisms

Recent surveillance data demonstrate that AMR patterns have changed significantly over the past several years. According to the WHO Global Antimicrobial Resistance and Use Surveillance System (GLASS), resistance to key antibiotic–pathogen combinations has increased in many contexts between 2018 and 2023, with carbapenem-resistant *Enterobacteriaceae* showing notable annual increases. Over 40% of monitored pathogen-antibiotic combinations exhibited rising resistance trends during this period. These trends are reflected across multiple pathogens, including *E. coli*, *K. pneumoniae*, *Acinetobacter* spp., and *Neisseria gonorrhoeae*, underscoring the dynamic evolution of resistance mechanisms and their growing clinical impact worldwide. The following table summarizes recent global trends in antimicrobial resistance among key pathogens, highlighting the evolving prevalence of major resistance mechanisms and their clinical implications.

Table 5. "Trends in Antimicrobial Resistance"

Pathogen / Mechanism	Trend Observed (2020–2025)	Source / Notes
Carbapenem-resistant *Acinetobacter* **spp.**	Resistance ~54.3% globally and **increasing annually** (~5.3% per year)	WHO GLASS 2025 surveillance data showing rising resistance in the bloodstream and other infections. (Tosas Auguet, et al. 2025)
Third-generation cephalosporin-resistant *E. coli*	~44.8% global resistance; trend relatively **stable, but high prevalence**	(Pfeifer, et al. 2025)
Carbapenem-resistant *E. coli*	Low baseline (~2.4%) but **increasing rapidly** (~12.5% annually)	(Sheng, et al. 2025)
Carbapenem-resistant *K. pneumoniae*	~16.7% globally; **increasing annually** (~15.3% per year)	(Maldonado, et al. 2025)
MRSA (*S. aureus* **resistant to methicillin)**	~27.1% global resistance; **stable or slightly decreasing in some regions**	(Elmongui, et al. 2025)
Fluoroquinolone-resistant *N. gonorrhoeae*	Very high (~75%); remains persistently elevated	(Nekahiwot 2024)
ESBL-producing *E. coli*	Pooled global prevalence ~25.4% in humans; remains **high and persistent**	(Sema, et al. 2025)
ESBL-producing *E. coli* **(clinical trend)**	Reported increases in resistance rates (e.g., from ~42% in 2019 to ~68% in 2022 in some studies)	(Goleanu, et al. 2025)
MDR Gram-negative bloodstream and urinary tract pathogens	Enterobacteriaceae resistance to third-gen cephalosporins increased (e.g., from ~59% to ~71% over 2020–2024 in Malawi)	(Bwanali, et al. 2025)

5. HORIZONTAL GENE TRANSFER AND GENETIC BASIS

Genetic mutation is one of them, and it leads to resistance and results in primary resistance in the absence of any drug exposure; the other is the mutations in the ribosomal RNA 23S sequences that cause macrolide resistance or the modified DNA gyrase genes gyrA and gyrB that cause fluoroquinolone resistance. The substitution, inversion, deletion, or addition can be used to bring about these changes. Another means through which resistance-carrying genes are transferred to different bacteria and their descendants is through plasmid transfer (Rajakumari, et al. 2024). These changes may also modify the structure of the target site, and this would make the antibiotic less potent and specific. Rifampicin is an antibiotic that attaches to the RNA polymerase gene, and a mutation in the gene leads to the inhibition of *Mycobacterium tuberculosis* (Muteeb, et al. 2023). Other important effects of these mutations include the overexpression of efflux pumps, special protein transporters that are able to actively take out the antibiotics from the cells. This mechanism leads to antimicrobial resistance that makes the antibiotics ineffective since they cannot reach their intracellular targets. The MexAB-OprM efflux pump of the *P. aeruginosa* strains can release fluoroquinolones and aminoglycosides. Also, *Acinetobacter baumannii* has a high number of efflux pumps, thereby making it resistant to a number of b-lactam antibiotics, aminoglycosides, fluoroquinolones, trimethoprim, tetracyclines, and chloramphenicol (Mancuso, et al. 2021).

Another way through which bacteria acquire antibiotic resistance is through lateral or horizontal gene transfer. The case of blaNDM-1 gene diffusion within the family of *Enterobacteriaceae* is an exact instance that can be applied in this scenario. The gene secretes the enzyme carbapenemase that further weakens the otherwise effective antibiotic carbapenem. The three most common methods of transmitting genes horizontally include conjugation, transduction, and transformation. The easiest way to facilitate conjugation is via exposure to heavy metals or antibiotics, which may stimulate the transfer of genetic material between bacteria (Urban-Chmiel, Marek et al. 2022).

During conjugation, DNA is passed on between cells via adhesion with the pili or a cell surface. The whole process is facilitated by conjugative machinery, which is encoded by chromosome conjugative components or plasmid genes. In the *Enterobacteriaceae* and *Pseudomonas* families, the mechanism of the spread of extended-spectrum b-lactam resistance genes is through conjugation on plasmids (Martin, Phan et al. 2017). Transduction is done by the use of bacteriophages. They can enhance their survival and pass positive genes to a different host. The extraction of bacteriophages that cause hospital-acquired diseases has been found to effectively transfer antibiotic-resistant genes (ARGs) to susceptible strains of MRSA infections. Also, plasmids contribute to transduction and conjugation. (Bello-López, Cabrero-

Martínez et al. 2019) Plasmids are circular DNA molecules that are circular and can be transferred by bacteriophage when transferring through transduction or by Cells-to cells when transferred through bacterial conjugation. Under the latter-mentioned technique, through metamorphosis, the bacteria absorb extracellular pieces of DNA, leading to their functional expression. *Helicobacter pylori* have been discovered to be able to transform, acquire genes via natural competence, and later become a virulent pathogen (Johnston, Martin et al. 2014).

6. CLINICAL, ENVIRONMENTAL DRIVERS OF RESISTANCE

6.1 Selection Pressure and Hospital-Acquired Infection

A significant healthcare issue, formerly referred to as nosocomial infection, has been evolving into a primary healthcare burden in most healthcare systems worldwide. The length of hospital stays as well as the usage of antibiotics to treat the patients have increased due to HAIs. Subsequently, HAIs may prove to be very costly to health systems and may also have a huge effect on the choice of resistant bacteria. Recent literature has identified a prevalence rate of at least one type of HAI as one-in-seven patients in (more) high-income countries and 10-in-100 patients in (low- and middle-income countries), and ten percent of infected patients die of the infection (Antonelli, Ales et al. 2024).

MDR (multidrug-resistant) microorganisms can be minimized by means of adequate infection prevention and control (IPC) policies and measures impacting the effect of HAIs on individuals, communities, and society across the world. HAIs may, however, easily move rapidly within and outside of medical facilities when there is no IPC infrastructure, and due to the abuse of antibiotics in the industrial and clinical environment, which contaminates the environment. Offering an emission of antibiotics and pesticides, considerable ecological imbalance in the reaction to human actions, such as the dramatic land transformations, pollution, and loss of biodiversity, provides advantages to the spread of HAI (Watts, Amann et al. 2021; Goniewicz, Burkle et al. 2025).

The rise in heavy metal or biocide levels in soil and water, which contribute to antimicrobial resistance (AMR) through co-/cross-resistance mechanisms, has been linked to the climate crisis, according to recent data. Currently, the focus is on investigating new technologies that may be used to detect and resolve the current issues that may prevent vaccinations and therapies against resistant strains from being produced (Zhao, et al. 2024).

Environmental pollution, which creates selective pressures that favor resistant bacteria and enable the horizontal spread of resistance genes to all ecosystems, is a universal contributor to evolutionary change and the proliferation of antimicrobial resistance (AMR). Air pollution, agricultural runoff, untreated sewage, and pharmaceutical and industrial waste are the primary environmental factors that affect AMR selection, persistence, and transmission in each area in a different way (Sastalla, et al. 2025).

6.2 The Major Pollutants and Their Locations in the World

6.2.1 Pharmaceutical Waste

Accordingly, a global assessment revealed that antibiotics can be discovered in rivers in more than 100 nations, and that pharmaceutical industry effluents in India and Europe contain up to 31 mg/L of ciprofloxacin and 1.2 mg/L of the antibiotic in the Danube River, respectively. Sulfonamide concentrations in the surface waters of Chinese manufacturing plants can reach 2.5 mg/L. These sub-inhibitory quantities (10100 ng/L or more) are unique to environmental bacteria's blaCTX-M, qnrS, and mcr-1 resistance genes (Kelbrick, et al. 2023).

6.2.2 Industrial Waste and Microplastics

Microplastics and their releases into the environment from industrial processes, such as the manufacturing of textiles, are worldwide problems. High levels of the genes sul1, ermB, and marA are found in estuaries with industrial legacy pollution in China and the United Kingdom. ARGs prefer the development of biofilm in resistant bacteria and are present in microplastics in rivers throughout Europe, Asia, and Africa (Li, et al. 2018).

6.2.3 Wastewater (Partially Treated and Untreated)

Untreated and insufficiently treated urban wastewater, particularly in low- and middle-income nations, is the primary source of ARB and ARGs on Earth. AMR genes are abundant in urban sewage in 60 nations, with Asia, Africa, and South America having the largest geographical prevalence of AMR genes. ARG concentrations reach 108 copies/mL, and both treated and untreated wastewater discharge significant numbers of integrons (intI1), van A-positive *Enterococcus*, and carbapenem-resistant *Enterobacteriaceae* (CRE) into the water. Both coastal and inland water may be impacted by the released water (Larsson and Flach 2022).

6.2.4 Synergies Between Pollutants

Although antibiotics, metals, and microplastics have been shown to have distinct impacts on AMR, new studies have demonstrated that the combined effects of these substances may have a greater cumulative effect than the cumulative individual effects. Numerous selection, retention, and horizontal transfer of resistance genes may result from these interactions, posing a new risk to human and environmental health (Sassi, et al. 2025).

Co-contamination with metals and medicines, for instance, can dramatically raise the expression of resistance genes. A recent investigation showed that when zinc (10 mg/L) and oxytetracycline (0.1 mg/L) were combined, *Bacillus* species in soil expressed the tetA gene over 100 times more than when the two pollutants were exposed separately. According to this finding, metals and antibiotics are probably going to accelerate the evolution and spread of resistance in contaminated soils (Knapp, et al. 2011).

Gene transfer is facilitated and carried by microplastics. Recent findings indicate that microplastics in the form of 1 μm polystyrene particles may have an active role in promoting horizontal resistance gene transfer, in contrast to their performance as passive carriers in the preceding sections. In the marine population, the presence of these particles specifically doubled the rate of blaTEM gene transfer between *Vibrio* species. This is the ability of microplastics to selectively produce microenvironmental conditions that facilitate bacterial gene transfer (Arias-Andres, et al. 2018).

In the context of environmental determinants of AMR, these data generally indicate the necessity to comprehend pollutant mixtures and interactions rather than assessing individual pollutants. Future mitigation plans must take these synergies into account to better control the spread of resistance (Han, et al. 2022).

6.3 AMR LINKS-Quantitative Evidence of Pollution

The occurrence and dissemination of AMR genes in the environment, including soil, water, and air, is increasingly posing a threat to human health. The worst of these is waterborne resistance. Ciprofloxacin has been demonstrated to have low levels of antibiotic concentration, which has a selection pressure on aquatic microbial communities. The survival of bacterial taxa with plasmid-encoded quinolone resistance and the maintenance of plasmid-mediated quinolone resistance (PMQR) genes, such as qnrS, were promoted in manure-amended soil at lower concentrations of ciprofloxacin (0.04-0.4 mg/kg) and prevented at a higher concentration of ciprofloxacin (0.4mg/kg) (Huang, et al. 2016).

Similarly, it has been observed that manure increases the amount of sul1, a gene that resists sulfonamide, in agricultural soils. Within a year of applying manure, the amount of sul1 in the soil can increase to 103 copies per gram, demonstrating the rapid and lasting effects of agricultural operations on the soil resistome. Furthermore, AMR spreads widely through agricultural settings or airborne transmission (Heuer, Schmitt et al. 2011). It has been discovered that there is a lot of ARBS in the air near animal farms. The study that discovered airborne MRSA CC398 in pig farms serves as another illustration of the possibility of resistant germs spreading through the air (Masclaux, et al. 2013).

5. CONCLUSION

Antimicrobial resistance (AMR) is a multifaceted health threat to the world, the emergence of which is the result of a complex interaction of molecular, cellular, and environmental components. This chapter has outlined the major ways that bacteria can circumvent antibiotics, such as through enzyme inactivation, target site alterations, overexpression of efflux pumps, decreased membrane permeability, as well as biofilm-based defense. Multidrug-resistant pathogens in environmental and clinical settings are enhanced via genetic transfer. In addition, environmental pollutants such as antibiotics, heavy metals, and microplastics are also selection forces that increase the persistence and spread of resistance genes, and it is important to highlight that the evolution of microbes is linked to human activity.

These mechanistic insights are of great significance for antimicrobial stewardship practices, the production of effective diagnostic tools, and alternative therapeutic options. One Health orientation, which combines clinical, environmental, and molecular research, is needed to halt the development of resistant strains and protect the effectiveness of the existing and future antimicrobial treatment of AMR.

REFERENCES

Al-Khalaifah, H.. (2025). A One-Health Perspective of Antimicrobial Resistance (AMR): Human, Animals and Environmental Health. *Life (Chicago, Ill.)*, *15*(10), 1598.

AL-Tameemi, Z. A., et al. (2023). Systematic study of aminoglycoside group antibiotics drug resistance. *WORLD (Oakland, Calif.)*, *2*(6).

Antonelli, A.. (2024). Healthcare-associated infections and antimicrobial use in acute care hospitals: A point prevalence survey in Lombardy, Italy, in 2022. *BMC Infectious Diseases*, *24*(1), 632.

Arias-Andres, M.. (2018). Microplastic pollution increases gene exchange in aquatic ecosystems. *Environmental Pollution*, *237*, 253–261.

Belay, W. Y.. (2024). Mechanism of antibacterial resistance, strategies and next-generation antimicrobials to contain antimicrobial resistance: A review. *Frontiers in Pharmacology*, *15*, 1444781.

Bello-López, J. M.. (2019). Horizontal gene transfer and its association with antibiotic resistance in the genus Aeromonas spp. *Microorganisms*, *7*(9), 363.

Breijyeh, Z.. (2020). Resistance of gram-negative bacteria to current antibacterial agents and approaches to resolve it. *Molecules (Basel, Switzerland)*, *25*(6), 1340.

Bwanali, A. N.. (2025). Trends and patterns of antimicrobial resistance among common pathogens isolated from adult bloodstream and urinary tract infections in public health facilities in Malawi, 2020–2024. *BMC Infectious Diseases*, *25*(1), 946.

Carlet, J.. (2014). Antibiotic resistance: A geopolitical issue. *Clinical Microbiology and Infection*, *20*(10), 949–953.

Carlson, E. E.. (2025). Decoding the Penicillin-Binding Proteins with Activity-Based Probes. *Accounts of Chemical Research*, *58*(11), 1754–1763.

Castanheira, M.. (2021). Extended-spectrum β-lactamases: An update on their characteristics, epidemiology and detection. *JAC-Antimicrobial Resistance*, *3*(3), dlab092.

Chakraborty, P.. (2021). Biofilm formation in the lung contributes to virulence and drug tolerance of Mycobacterium tuberculosis. *Nature Communications*, *12*(1), 1606.

Chandal, N.. (2025). In Vitro and In Vivo Investigations into the Potential of Quinazoline and Quinoline Derivatives as NorA Efflux Pump Inhibitors Against Resistant Staphylococcus aureus Strains. *Antibiotics (Basel, Switzerland)*, *14*(4), 339.

Codjoe, F. S., & Donkor, E. S. (2017). Carbapenem resistance: A review. *Medical Science*, *6*(1), 1.

Dabhi, M.. (2024). Penicillin-binding proteins: The master builders and breakers of bacterial cell walls and its interaction with β-lactam antibiotics. *Journal of Proteins and Proteomics*, *15*(2), 215–232.

Darby, E. M.. (2023). Molecular mechanisms of antibiotic resistance revisited. *Nature Reviews. Microbiology*, *21*(5), 280–295.

Das, P. K., & Samal, S. (2018). Microbial biofilms: Pathogenicity and treatment strategies. *PharmaTutor*, *6*(1), 16–22.

De Gaetano, G. V.. (2023). Antimicrobial resistance: Two-component regulatory systems and multidrug efflux pumps. *Antibiotics (Basel, Switzerland)*, *12*(6), 965.

Dyary, H.. (2023). History, current situation, and future perspectives on antibiotics and antibiotic Resistance. *International Journal of Agriculture and Biosciences*, *2*, 109–118.

Elmongui, E.. (2025). Evaluating anti-MRSA antibiotic stewardship with a focus on trends in consumption and resistance in a tertiary hospital in Alexandria, Egypt from 2019 to 2023. *Archives of Public Health = Archives Belges de Santé Publique*, *83*(1), 133.

Elshobary, M. E.. (2025). Combating antibiotic resistance: Mechanisms, multidrug-resistant pathogens, and novel therapeutic approaches: An updated review. *Pharmaceuticals*, *18*(3), 402.

Fleming, D., & Rumbaugh, K. (2018). The consequences of biofilm dispersal on the host. *Scientific Reports*, *8*(1), 10738.

Foudraine, D. E.. (2021). Exploring antimicrobial resistance to beta-lactams, aminoglycosides and fluoroquinolones in E. coli and K. pneumoniae using proteogenomics. *Scientific Reports*, *11*(1), 12472.

Goleanu, C. D.. (2025). Trends in antibiotic resistance of Escherichia coli strains isolated from clinical samples (2019–2023): A hospital-based retrospective analysis. *Pathogens (Basel, Switzerland)*, *14*(9), 927.

Goniewicz, K.. (2025). Transforming global public health: Climate collaboration, political challenges, and systemic change. *Journal of Infection and Public Health*, *18*(1), 102615.

Han, B.. (2022). The source, fate and prospect of antibiotic resistance genes in soil: A review. *Frontiers in Microbiology*, *13*, 976657.

Hayet, S.. (2023). Titanium complexes affect Bacillus subtilis biofilm formation. *RSC Medicinal Chemistry*, *14*(5), 983–991.

Henderson, R. K.. (2019). Coupling efficiency of secondary active transporters. *Current Opinion in Biotechnology*, *58*, 62–71.

Huang, T.. (2016). Low-concentration ciprofloxacin selects plasmid-mediated quinolone resistance encoding genes and affects bacterial taxa in soil containing manure. *Frontiers in Microbiology*, *7*, 1730.

HUDA, M., et al. (2025). "Prevalence of ACRA, ACRB, and TOLC efflux pump genes among multiple-drug resistant escherichia coli strains in isolates obtained from patients with diabetes mellitus." Laboratory diagnostics. Eastern Europe Учредители: УП" Профессиональные издания", ООО «Вилин–Профессиональные издания» 14(1): 63-74.

Isuranga, M., & Danthanarayana, D. N. (2025). Antimicrobial Potential of Phytochemicals from Coccinia grandis Leaves: A Molecular Docking Study Against Penicillin-Binding Protein 5 of Escherichia coli and DNA Topoisomerase IV Subunit B (ParE 24kDa) of Staphylococcus aureus and Escherichia coli. *Biology, Medicine, & Natural Product Chemistry*, *14*(1), 541–552.

Javed, W. (2020). *Study of the conformational states of a bacterial multidrug ABC transporter BmrA*. Université Grenoble Alpes. [2020-....]

Johnston, C.. (2014). Bacterial transformation: Distribution, shared mechanisms and divergent control. *Nature Reviews. Microbiology*, *12*(3), 181–196.

Katsarou, A.. (2025). β-lactam/β-lactamase inhibitor combination antibiotics Under development. *Pathogens (Basel, Switzerland)*, *14*(2), 168.

Kelbrick, M.. (2023). Cultivating antimicrobial resistance: How intensive agriculture ploughs the way for antibiotic resistance. *Microbiology*, *169*(8), 001384.

Kim, D.. (2023). Structural insights for β-lactam antibiotics. *Biomolecules & Therapeutics*, *31*(2), 141.

Kim, J.. (2021). Structural insights into transporter-mediated drug resistance in infectious diseases. *Journal of Molecular Biology*, *433*(16), 167005.

Kincses, A.. (2025). Repurposed Drugs and Efflux Pump Inhibitors Against Gram-Negative Urinary Tract Pathogenic Bacteria. *Antibiotics (Basel, Switzerland)*, *14*(10), 988.

Knapp, C. W.. (2011). Antibiotic resistance gene abundances correlate with metal and geochemical conditions in archived Scottish soils. *PLoS One*, *6*(11), e27300.

Krause, K. M.. (2016). Aminoglycosides: An overview. *Cold Spring Harbor Perspectives in Medicine*, *6*(6), a027029.

Lak Hondori, M.. (2025). Frequency of Beta-lactamase Genes (blaSHV, blaTEM, blaCTX-M-15, blaKPC, blaOXA-48) in Multidrug-resistant Klebsiella pneumoniae. *International Journal of Molecular and Clinical Microbiology*, *15*(1), 2180–2189.

Larsson, D. J., & Flach, C.-F. (2022). Antibiotic resistance in the environment. *Nature Reviews. Microbiology*, *20*(5), 257–269.

Li, J.. (2018). Global survey of antibiotic resistance genes in air. *Environmental Science & Technology*, *52*(19), 10975–10984.

Liu, J.. (2019). Mutations in efflux pump Rv1258c (Tap) cause resistance to pyrazinamide, isoniazid, and streptomycin in M. tuberculosis. *Frontiers in Microbiology*, *10*, 216.

Magiorakos, A.-P.. (2012). Multidrug-resistant, extensively drug-resistant and pandrug-resistant bacteria: An international expert proposal for interim standard definitions for acquired resistance. *Clinical Microbiology and Infection*, *18*(3), 268–281.

Maldonado, K. V. M.. (2025). Widespread Distribution of Carbapenem-Resistant Klebsiella spp. in Clinical and Environmental Settings. *Antibiotics (Basel, Switzerland)*, *14*(11), 1140.

Mancuso, G.. (2021). Bacterial antibiotic resistance: The most critical pathogens. *Pathogens (Basel, Switzerland)*, *10*(10), 1310.

Martin, J.. (2017). Covert dissemination of carbapenemase-producing Klebsiella pneumoniae (KPC) in a successfully controlled outbreak: Long-and short-read whole-genome sequencing demonstrate multiple genetic modes of transmission. *The Journal of Antimicrobial Chemotherapy*, *72*(11), 3025–3034.

Masclaux, F. G.. (2013). Concentration of airborne Staphylococcus aureus (MRSA and MSSA), total bacteria, and endotoxins in pig farms. *The Annals of Occupational Hygiene*, *57*(5), 550–557.

Maslikowska, J.. (2016). Impact of infection with extended-spectrum β-lactamase-producing Escherichia coli or Klebsiella species on outcome and hospitalization costs. *The Journal of Hospital Infection*, *92*(1), 33–41.

Migliaccio, A.. (2022). Inhibition of AdeB, AceI, and AmvA efflux pumps restores chlorhexidine and benzalkonium susceptibility in Acinetobacter baumannii ATCC 19606. *Frontiers in Microbiology*, *12*, 790263.

Mishra, A.. (2024). Medical device-associated infections caused by biofilm-forming microbial pathogens and controlling strategies. *Antibiotics (Basel, Switzerland), 13*(7), 623.

Miyauchi, H.. (2017). Structural basis for xenobiotic extrusion by eukaryotic MATE transporter. *Nature Communications*, *8*(1), 1633.

Mora-Ochomogo, M., & Lohans, C. T. (2021). β-Lactam antibiotic targets and resistance mechanisms: From covalent inhibitors to substrates. *RSC Medicinal Chemistry*, *12*(10), 1623–1639.

Murray, C. J.. (2022). Global burden of bacterial antimicrobial resistance in 2019: A systematic analysis. *Lancet*, *399*(10325), 629–655.

Muteeb, G.. (2023). Origin of antibiotics and antibiotic resistance, and their impacts on drug development: A narrative review. *Pharmaceuticals*, *16*(11), 1615.

Naas, T.. (2017). Beta-lactamase database (BLDB)–structure and function. *Journal of Enzyme Inhibition and Medicinal Chemistry*, *32*(1), 917–919.

Nekahiwot, S. (2024). "Multi-drug resistant gonorrhea: an emerging global threat." Multi-Drug Resistant Gonorrhea: An Emerging Global Threat.

Nikaido, H. (2018). RND transporters in the living world. *Research in Microbiology*, *169*(7-8), 363–371.

Nowak, J.. (2021). Inactivation of the gene encoding the cationic antimicrobial peptide resistance factor MprF increases biofilm formation but reduces invasiveness of Listeria monocytogenes. *Journal of Applied Microbiology*, *130*(2), 464–477.

Olaitan, M. O.. (2025). Prevalence of ESBL-producing Escherichia coli in sub-Saharan Africa: A meta-analysis using a One Health approach. *One Health*, *20*, 101090.

Pandey, S.. (2024). Antibiotic resistance in livestock, environment and humans: One Health perspective. *Journal of Animal Science and Technology*, *66*(2), 266.

Pandrangi, S. L., ... (2025). Omics Approaches in Diagnosis of Polymicrobial Biofilms and Identification of Novel Therapeutic Drugs. Omics Approaches in Biofilm Research: Perspectives and Applications, Springer: 369-389.

Pentland, D. R., ... (2020). "CO2 enhances the ability of Candida albicans to form biofilms, overcome nutritional immunity and resist antifungal treatment." bioRxiv: 2020.2003. 2031.018200.

Pérez-Varela, M.. (2019). Roles of efflux pumps from different superfamilies in the surface-associated motility and virulence of Acinetobacter baumannii ATCC 17978. *Antimicrobial Agents and Chemotherapy*, *63*(3), 02190–02118. DOI: 10.1128/aac

Peri, A. M.. (2024). Rapid diagnostic tests and antimicrobial stewardship programs for the management of bloodstream infection: What is their relative contribution to improving clinical outcomes? A systematic review and network meta-analysis. *Clinical Infectious Diseases*, *79*(2), 502–515.

Pfeifer, N. M.. (2025). Escherichia coli resistant to the highest priority critically important fluoroquinolone or 3rd and 4th generation cephalosporin antibiotics persist in pigsties. *Applied and Environmental Microbiology*, •••, 01386–01324.

Rajakumari, K.. (2024). Comprehensive review of DNA gyrase as enzymatic target for drug discovery and development. *European Journal of Medicinal Chemistry Reports*, *12*, 100233.

Ramirez, M. S., & Tolmasky, M. E. (2010). Aminoglycoside modifying enzymes. *Drug Resistance Updates*, *13*(6), 151–171.

Rao, H.. (2021). Approaches for mitigating microbial biofilm-related drug resistance: A focus on micro-and nanotechnologies. *Molecules (Basel, Switzerland)*, *26*(7), 1870.

Rush, L.. (2019). Communicating antimicrobial resistance and stewardship in the national press: Lessons from sepsis awareness campaigns. *The Journal of Infection*, *78*(2), 88–94.

Sassi, A.. (2025). The Role of the Environment (Water, Air, Soil) in the Emergence and Dissemination of Antimicrobial Resistance: A One Health Perspective. *Antibiotics (Basel, Switzerland)*, *14*(8), 764.

Sastalla, I.. (2025). *NIAID workshop report: systematic approaches for ESKAPE bacteria antigen discovery*. MDPI.

Sati, H., et al. (2025). "The WHO Bacterial Priority Pathogens List 2024: a prioritisation study to guide research, development, and public health strategies against antimicrobial resistance." The Lancet infectious diseases.

Scoffone, V. C.. (2025). The evolution of antimicrobial resistance in Acinetobacter baumannii and new strategies to fight it. *Antibiotics (Basel, Switzerland)*, *14*(1), 85.

Sema, T.. (2025). Global Prevalence and Risk Factors of Multidrug Resistance Escherichia Coli in Human and Animal Samples (2015-2023): A Systematic Review and Meta-Analysis. *J Gastro Endosc*, *3*(2), 1–10.

Sheng, J.. (2025). Global geographic and genomic epidemiology analysis of carbapenem-resistant Escherichia coli carrying bla NDM-9. *MSphere*, •••, 00704–00725.

Sivalingam, P.. (2025). Microplastics, Nanoplastics and Nanoparticles: Emerging Dynamic Carriers of Extracellular DNA Antibiotic Resistance Genes in the Environment. *BioNanoScience*, *15*(1), 198.

Standyło, A.. (2022). The correlation between second-hand tobacco smoke exposure and biofilm formation in chronic rhinosinusitis. *Journal of Education, Health and Sport*, *12*(6), 268–275.

Tavares-Carreon, F.. (2023). Serratia marcescens antibiotic resistance mechanisms of an opportunistic pathogen: A literature review. *PeerJ*, *11*, e14399.

Tehrani, K. H., & Martin, N. I. (2018). β-lactam/β-lactamase inhibitor combinations: An update. *MedChemComm*, *9*(9), 1439–1456.

Tosas Auguet, O., et al. (2025). "Global antibiotic resistance surveillance report 2025."

Urban-Chmiel, R.. (2022). Antibiotic resistance in bacteria—A review. *Antibiotics (Basel, Switzerland)*, *11*(8), 1079.

Vatansever, C.. (2025). Evaluating the Antibiofilm Effects of Antibiotics on Staphylococcus Species from Pediatric Hematology–Oncology Patients. *Microbial Drug Resistance (Larchmont, N.Y.)*, *31*(6), 178–188.

Vrancianu, C. O.. (2020). Antibiotic resistance profiles, molecular mechanisms and innovative treatment strategies of Acinetobacter baumannii. *Microorganisms*, *8*(6), 935.

Watts, N.. (2021). The 2020 report of The Lancet Countdown on health and climate change: Responding to converging crises. *Lancet*, *397*(10269), 129–170.

Wong, J. L.. (2022). Recurrent emergence of Klebsiella pneumoniae carbapenem resistance mediated by an inhibitory ompK36 mRNA secondary structure. *Proceedings of the National Academy of Sciences of the United States of America*, *119*(38), e2203593119.

Yamasaki, S.. (2023). Drug resistance and physiological roles of RND multidrug efflux pumps in Salmonella enterica, Escherichia coli and Pseudomonas aeruginosa. *Microbiology*, *169*(6), 001322.

Zakaria, N. F. S.. (2023). Multiple bacterial strategies to survive antibiotic pressure. *RE:view*.

Zhao, W.. (2024). Increased risk of antibiotic resistance in surface water due to global warming. *Environmental Research*, *263*, 120149.

Chapter 4
Mechanisms of Antimicrobial Resistance: Genetic and Phenotypic Insights

Zahid Ahmad Thoker
https://orcid.org/0009-0002-6897-5835
Lovely Professional University, India

Lovleen Marwaha
https://orcid.org/0000-0002-5175-2590
Lovely Professional University, India

ABSTRACT

AMR is a problem of significant global health concern, which threatens to reduce decades of medical advancement by weakening the efficacy of antibiotics, as well as other antimicrobials. The genetic mechanisms of AMR are spontaneous mutations and horizontal gene transfer of plasmids and transposons and phenotypic adaptation, such as biofilm formation, efflux pumps, and persister cell states which increase bacterial survival. Improper use of antibiotics in healthcare and agriculture such as environmental contamination aids the transmission of resistant strains within the ecosystems. Global surveillance should be conducted with advanced diagnostic tools, such as PCR, CRISPR-based, and whole genome sequencing. The fight against AMR needs combined measures, antibiotic stewardship, new therapeutics, alternative solutions, like bacteriophages and the One Health approach, which involves the connection of human, animal, and environmental health to maintain antimicrobial activity across the globe.

DOI: 10.4018/979-8-3373-3825-5.ch004

INTRODUCTION

Antimicrobial resistance (AMR) is one of the most significant global public health threats of the twenty-first century. It has given rise to a threat to the effectiveness of antibiotics and other antimicrobial agents, to which the transformation of modern medicine owes. According to the World Health Organization, antimicrobial resistance is one of the top 10 global health threats, accounting for approximately 1.27 million fatalities each year and indirectly contributing to around 5 million deaths worldwide (Murray et al., 2022; WHO, 2024). The crisis threatens treatment of common infectious diseases, major surgery, and immunosuppressive medical treatment, including chemotherapy and organ transplant (O'Neill, 2020). When it goes uncontrolled, AMR-related mortality encompasses the entire globe and is expected to surpass cancer-related mortalities by 2050; the financial cost is estimated to be more than USD 100 trillion (World Bank, 2023).

The major mechanism of AMR development is the evolutionary flexibility of microorganisms that may resist antimicrobial exposure due to genetic mutations or acquisition of resistance genes via horizontal gene transfer. This plasticity supports the concept of a microorganism-environment interaction. Under antibiotic pressure, resistant variants have the advantage of selective survival, which is facilitated by horizontal gene transfer through transposons, plasmids, integrons, and bacteriophages (Partridge et al., 2018). Such mobile genetic elements are implicated in increasing the horizontal spread of resistance genes between bacterial populations, thereby crossing the species and even genus barriers. The prevalence of so-called superbugs (methicillin-resistant Staphylococcus aureus, carbapenem-resistant Enterobacteriaceae, and vancomycin-resistant Enterococcus) further elucidates how much genetic alteration can contribute to clinical resistance (Holmes et al., 2019).

In addition to genetic changes, microorganisms are phenotypically plastic, that is, they can develop transient resistance without undergoing permanent changes to their genome. These adaptations involve biofilm formation, overexpression of efflux pumps, lowered membrane permeability, and the acquisition of persister cell states-a dormant state that gives tolerance against antibiotics (Balaban et al., 2019). Microsystem Biofilms, especially, offer a protective microenvironment to restrict drug entry and increase cell-cell communication by quorum sensing, and survive together (Flemming & Wuertz, 2019).

Genetic-phenotypic continuum of AMR represents a complicated combination between genetic inheritance and physiological adaptations (reversible). Although the genetic factors that dictate the occurrence of resistance determinants, the phenotypic responses influence the manifestation, regulation, and maintenance of the resistance traits. As an example, the expression of efflux systems like AcrAB-TolC in Escherichia coli and MexAB-OprM in Pseudomonas aeruginosa may be programmed and regulated by the environment (Du et al., 2018). Equally, the biofilm phenotype may provoke horizontal gene exchange, and the mechanism of resistance more strongly supports the genetic background (Hall & Mah, 2017). Thus, the study of AMR requires an integrative model that can consider both genomic factors and cellular responses to antimicrobial pressure.

Table 1. Major Mechanisms of Antimicrobial Resistance and Their Biological Basis

Mechanism Type	Specific Mechanism	Biological Process	Representative Pathogens
Genetic	Spontaneous mutations	Alteration of antibiotic target sites	Mycobacterium tuberculosis
Genetic	HGT	Exchange of resistance genes through plasmids, transposons, and phages	Escherichia coli, Klebsiella pneumoniae
Genetic	Integron-mediated resistance	Capture and expression of resistance gene cassettes	Pseudomonas aeruginosa
Phenotypic	Efflux pump overexpression	Active extrusion of antibiotics	Staphylococcus aureus
Phenotypic	Biofilm formation	Surface-associated multicellular communities	Pseudomonas species
Phenotypic	Persister cell formation	Dormant, non-dividing survival phenotype	Salmonella enterica
Phenotypic	Reduced permeability	Loss or modification of porins alters membrane permeability	Acinetobacter baumannii

The resistance genes are propagated by environmental and anthropogenic factors. Massive abuse and overdose of antibiotics in healthcare, veterinary, and agricultural industries have contributed to the extensive pollution of water, soil, and food systems with resistant bacteria and antimicrobial residues (Kraemer et al., 2019). Multi-resistant infectious agents can breed in environmental reservoirs, e.g., wastewater treatment plants and aquaculture systems, and promote the spread of genes between ecological niches (Hendriksen et al., 2019). The philosophy is the One Health, which has been endorsed by WHO, FAO, and OIE, and that emphasizes the interaction between human, animal as well and environmental health and promotes combined surveillance and stewardship policies to mitigate the spread of AMR (WHO, 2023).

The modern trends in the field of molecular diagnostics and bioinformatics have transformed the AMR detection and surveillance. Some of the methods that can be applied to determine the resistance determinants precisely and trace the global trends of spread include PCR (polymerase chain reaction), WGS (whole genome sequencing), and metagenomic analysis (Tagini and Greub, 2020). CRISPR-based technologies can be applied in the diagnosis the treatment and offer a genome-wide solution to the target resistance genes (Bikard & Barrangou, 2020). Such technological advances can be applied to understand the resistome, the entirety of known and potential resistance genes, and can be used to design interventions.

Irrespective of these developments, the rising prevalence of multidrug-resistant (MDR), extensively drug-resistant (XDR), and pan-drug-resistant (PDR) pathogens is becoming a challenge that is increasingly becoming a burden on health care systems all over the world. The economic costs of AMR are not limited to the medical treatment, and they also include its impact on productivity, hospitalization, and mortality (OECD, 2022). Consequently, the prevention of AMR must be interdisciplinary, which means that microbiology, genomics, pharmacology, and the sphere of the policy of population health policy must be merged.

The rationale of this chapter is to achieve a deep understanding of the mechanisms of antimicrobial resistance at the genetic and phenotypic levels. By describing how the phenotypes of resistance in bacteria are acquired, expressed, and maintained, this chapter aims to balance the knowledge in the spheres of molecular research with the clinical and environmental points of view. It also puts forth the new approaches, such as CRISPR-based antimicrobials, bacteriophage therapy, antimicrobial peptides, and genomic surveillance, which may possibly reverse or contain the AMR crisis. It is important to understand how genetic inheritance and phenotypic adaptation interplay dynamically and to come up with novel interventions that can manage the efficacy of the current antimicrobials and lead to the discovery of new therapeutic agents. Figure 1 also depicts a schematic illustration of multidisciplinary interventions of CRISPR-based technologies, molecular diagnostics, One Health approaches, and interdisciplinary frameworks.

Figure 1. Integral strategies for combatting antimicrobial resistance

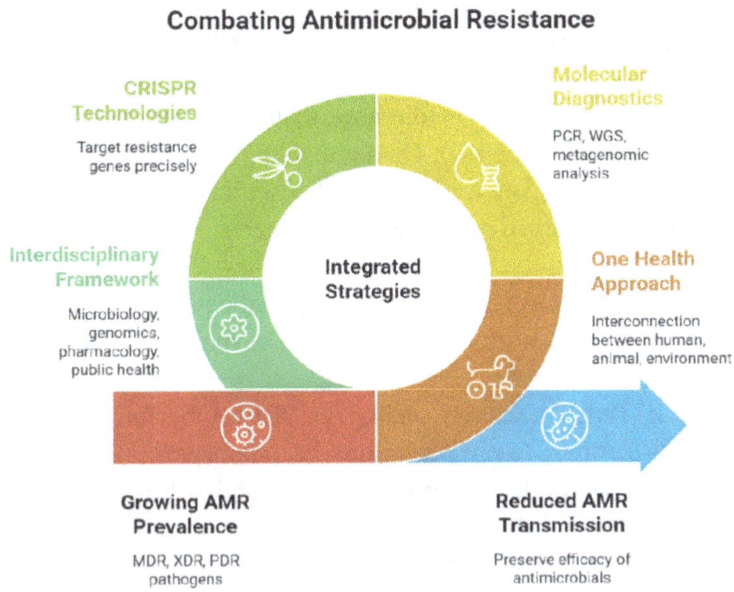

2. BASIC CONCEPTS IN ANTIMICROBIAL RESISTANCE

AMR is the ability of a microorganism to withstand the effects of an antimicrobial agent to which it was previously sensitive. This resistance can occur because of the intrinsic aspects or focus acquired changes of genetic material that alter the drug's efficiency to some extent, even to a complete degree (WHO 2020). Antimicrobial is used to refers to agents that are effective against a variety of pathogens, such as antibiotics (against bacteria), antivirals, antifungals, and antiparasitic. When microorganisms evolve defences against these agents that make standard treatments become ineffective by making infections recurrent and possibly spreading, while standard care is rendered useless. Terminologies in this field include:

- **Intrinsic resistance:** It is a resistance in the normal and natural structure or functional traits of a species (e.g., Gram-negative bacteria's outer membrane inhibits antibiotics from penetrating the bacterial cell).
- **Acquired resistance:** Acquired resistance due to mutations or the gain of foreign genetic material.

- **Multidrug-resistant (MDR):** Resistance to at least one agent from at least three different antimicrobial categories.
- **Extensively drug-resistant:** Antimicrobial resistance across all but one or two categories.
- **Pan-drug-resistant:** There is tolerance to all antimicrobial substances available (Magiorakos et al., 2012). Distinguishing these terms is critical for clinical decision-making, surveillance, and research, as they guide diagnostic classification and inform public health strategies.

Antimicrobial agents are classified according to the type of microorganisms that they attack as well as the nature of their action. The main classes include:

- **Antibiotics:** Target bacterial pathogens; Target bacterial pathogens; subgroups – β-lactams (e.g., penicillins, cephalosporins), aminoglycosides, tetracyclines, macrolides, fluoroquinolones, and sulfonamides. Each of the classes has an impact on a different aspect of bacterial physiology, for example, synthesis of a cell wall, protein synthesis, or DNA replication.
- **Antivirals:** Inhibit viral replication or entry; Prevent transmission to the baby or other infants; examples in breastfeeding include antiretroviral drugs in ART (e.g., Nevirapine, Ritonavir), maternal vaccines, etc.
- **Antifungals:** Target fungal membranes or cell wall components; Target fungal membranes or parts of the cell wall; examples include azoles, echinocandins, and polyenes.
- **Antiparasitics:** Act against protozoa and helminths; Antiparasitic drugs work against protozoa and helminths; for example, metronidazole, chloroquine, and ivermectin. Each class has a specific mechanism of action, and resistance often emerges through mechanisms that either neutralize this action or prevent the drug from reaching its target. For instance, β-lactam resistance may involve the production of β-lactamases that hydrolyze the antibiotic's active site (Bush & Bradford, 2016). Knowing these classifications is essential in proper prescription, antimicrobial stewardship, and in creating new therapeutic agents. Microorganisms have a wide range of antimicrobial evasion strategies, which can be roughly divided into genetic and phenotypic approaches. These can be shown graphically in Figure 2.

Figure 2. Antimicrobial evasion strategies of microorganisms

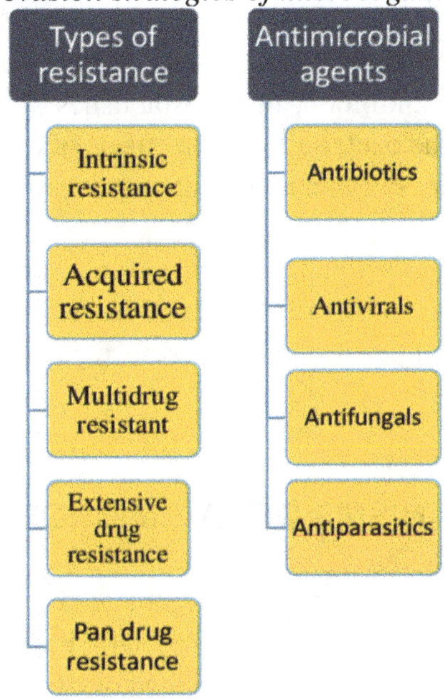

Genetic resistance is permanent and heritable, whereas the phenotypic resistance could be reversible and is modulated by the environment. Some of the key mechanisms of resistance include:

- **Enzymatic inactivation:** Enzymes that degrade or alter the antibiotic are produced by microbes. Some commonly cited examples include β-lactamases that cleave β-lactam antibiotics, as well as aminoglycoside-modifying enzymes.
- **Alteration of target sites:** Mutations or enzymatic modifications in the binding site of the antibiotic provide reduced drug efficacy. For example, a mutation in DNA gyrase leads to fluoroquinolone resistance.
- **Reduced permeability:** Gram-negative organisms commonly exhibit changes, such as membrane porins that prevent antibiotics from entering the bacterial cell.
- **Efflux pumps:** These transport proteins actively throw antibiotics out of the cell before they can hit their target. Multidrug efflux pumps such as AcrAB-TolC in E. coli are particularly difficult to deal with.
- **Bypass mechanisms:** The organism bypasses the inhibited pathway through another path or acquires an enzyme that can be resistant. For instance,

methicillin-resistant Staphylococcus aureus (MRSA) expresses a different penicillin-binding protein (PBP2a) that is synthesized because of mecA.

- **Biofilm formation:** This is not a straightforward form of genetic resistance encountered by the antibiotic, but it establishes a protective microenvironment that prevents the bacteria from the effects of the antibiotic and the host's defense and promotes chronic and recurring infection.

The interaction of these mechanisms provides microorganisms with the ability to adapt quickly to selective pressure (impact of drugs, biocides, and other factors), particularly in areas with high antibiotic exposure, e.g., hospitals, farms, and wastewater plants (Munita & Arias, 2016).

3. GENETIC MECHANISMS OF ANTIMICROBIAL RESISTANCE

AMR is caused by genetic changes within the microbial populations at its bedrock. This modification allows microbes, especially bacteria, to exist and develop as the antibiotics would have otherwise inhibited or destroyed them. There are two major processes of genetic mechanisms of AMR: 1) Mutation-generated resistance and 2) horizontal gene transfer (HGT).

3.1 Mutation-Driven Resistance

Microorganisms, specifically bacteria, have an amazing ability to adapt even in a very hostile environment in which antibiotics are present. One of the simplest and effective ways in which they do it is by using the spontaneous violation of their genetic code. These are random changes that occur naturally in the bacterial DNA, more particularly during replication. Even though most mutations do not affect survival, very few yield a survival advantage under conditions of antibiotics (Munita & Arias, 2016). This is a kind of resistance that is not the same as that which is obtained by horizontal gene transfer. Within bacterial chromosome evolution, there is the development of mutation-driven resistance without the contribution of external genetic content. These mutations may affect the genes that code for the target of the drugs, control elements, or members of the efflux systems (Blair et al., 2015). For example, many antibiotics target essential enzymes or structures in bacteria. When such a mutation changes these targets, the drug may fail to bind effectively. One of the well-documented examples is rifampin resistance in Mycobacterium tuberculosis, often due to mutations of the rpoB gene changing the RNA polymerase enzyme (Sandgren et al., 2009). In the same way, fluoroquinolone resistance in Escherichia coli and Salmonella enterica is often explained by mutations that target the gyrA and parC genes, responsible for DNA gyrase and topoisomerase IV subtypes (Hooper 2001). Other mutations influence the permeability of the membrane by transforming genes that encode for porin proteins, such as ompF, that inhibit the entrance of drugs into the cell. Moreover, certain mutations cause overproduction of efflux pump systems, for example, the AcrAB-TolC system in Enterobacteriaceae, which actively pumps antibiotics away from the bacterial cell (Li et al., 2015).

Mutations also alter intrinsic enzymes that break or neutralize antibiotics in some cases. Although a mutation may only provide a low level of resistance, bacteria can pile up several mutations over time. These resistant strains can proliferate in the presence of the selective pressure of antibiotic use (especially inadequate dosages and long exposure), when common strains are also killed (Blair et al., 2015). Even though the initial reductions in fitness initiated by mutations can be reversed rapidly by means of compensatory mutations that make resistant strains persistently resistant and permit their dissemination (Sandgren et al., 2009). Clinically, this kind of resistance is particularly problematic in the case of chronic infections, such as tuberculosis, nosocomial infections, and tuberculosis in patients with cystic fibrosis. Such infections typically require prolonged antibiotic use, and, during that process, resistant mutants can evolve and become dominant, causing a failure in treatment and narrow therapeutic tools (Munita & Arias, 2016). The emphasis on understanding mutation-driven resistance is on the need for careful utilization of antibiotics, firm diagnostics, along with the development of new drugs that target less mutable aspects of bacterial functions.

3.2 Horizontal Gene Transfer

Horizontal gene transfer is a decisive reproductive strategy employed by bacteria to gain different new features, including antimicrobial resistance. As opposed to vertical transmission via replication, HGT enables the direct transfer of genes between organisms within a single organism, across species or genera, which makes it a fast spreading of resistance, environmental, and clinical (von Wintersdorff et al., 2016; Thomas & Nielsen, 2005). The three main strategies of HGT are transformation, transduction, and conjugation.

3.2.1 Transformation: Uptake of Free DNA

Transformation encompasses the bacterial cell capturing naked DNA fragments from the surrounding through the process of competent bacterial uptake. This DNA is normally extracted from bacteria that have been lysed. However, there are certain bacteria, including Streptococcus pneumonia, Neisseria gonorrhoeae, and Bacillus subtilis, that are naturally competent and can bring in foreign DNA into their genome

(Johnston et al. 2014). This process allows for the insertion of resistance genes such as changed penicillin-binding proteins (PBPs), which help in β-lactam resistance. This tool of gene acquisition increases flexibility, particularly in a biofilm or an environment that is favorable to antibiotics.

3.2.2 Transduction: Viral-Mediated Gene Transfer

The member cell of a bacterial population during transduction is infected by bacteriophages that are actually viruses which infect bacteria, and the genetic materials of the member cell and that of the donor cell are exchanged. There are times when these viruses carry fragments of bacterial DNA, including resistance genes, during the assembly. The next bacterium gets infected by the viral infection, wherein the DNA is injected into it and promotes genetic recombination (Penadés et al., 2015). This can be generalized that involve all genes or particularized that involve genes near a phage site for integration. Transduction is one of the key limits of gene spread among resistance genes, particularly in polymicrobial communities and environmental reservoirs.

3.2.3 Conjugation: Plasmid-Mediated Transfer

Sometimes, the most clinically significant form of HGT is conjugation. It includes contact between cells directly via a pilus and through which plasmids or circular DNA molecules are transferred. These plasmids (which are frequently gene-unique for multiple resistance genes or R-plasmids) can be transferred among the various bacterial species with utmost velocity, increasing the circulation of resistance (Carattoli 2013; Thomas & Nielsen, 2005). For example, the resistance to carbapenem or extended-spectrum β-lactams in Escherichia coli or Klebsiella pneumoniae is often related to conjugative plasmids containing genes like bla_NDM and bla_CTX-M, which, along with transformation and transduction, are one of the potent mechanisms through which resistance genotypes spread among bacterial species. These mechanisms emphasize the constant fact of the evolution of microbes, and they point to the critical need for stewardship and surveillance as sources of control of antimicrobial resistance Gillings, 2014; von Wintersdorff et al., 2016). These three mechanisms of horizontal gene transfer and the main points of difference can be shown in Figure 3 as well.

Figure 3. Three mechanisms of horizontal gene transfer and the main points of difference

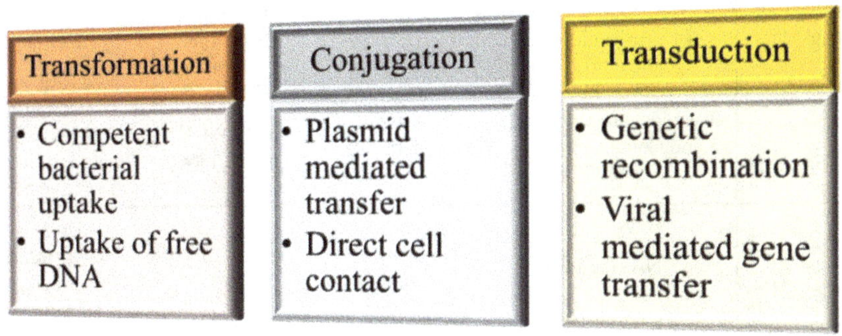

3.3 Role of Mobile Genetic Elements

Plasmids, Integrons, transposons, and insertion sequences (IS elements) are mobile genetic elements (MGEs) that are essential both in the architecture of resistance genes as well as their mobility. The role of these mobile genetic elements is given below:

- **Plasmids:** These are DNA segments that exist outside the chromosome, and they replicate independently; also, they carry a variety range of resistance determinants. They tend to be vectors of gene transfer and exist on both gram-positive and gram-negative bacteria.
- **Transposons:** They are also referred to as jumping genes and can move from chromosomal to plasmid DNA and vice versa. They often have resistance genes and can help them integrate into a variety of genomic environments. For example, the Tn1546 transposon contains the vanA gene cluster for vancomycin resistance in Enterococcus faecium (Arthur et al., 1996).
- **Integrons:** These are resistance platforms that can multiplex gene cassettes, including resistance genes. Class 1 Integrons, usually found in Gram-negative pathogens, are commonly associated with other MGEs, increasing multi-resistance potential (Gillings, 2014).

The co-selection as such is not only feasible due to the acquisition of resistance but also because of the paired use of one antimicrobial that selects for resistance against multiple and unrelated drugs due to physical linkage on the same genetic element. Table 3 below also depicts the mechanisms of Horizontal Gene Transfer (Conjugation, Transformation, and Transduction), Mobile Genetic Elements, and Their Role in AMR.

Table 2. Mechanisms of Horizontal Gene Transfer (Conjugation, Transformation, and Transduction), Mobile Genetic Elements, and Their Role in AMR

Mechanism	Genetic Vehicle	Representative Species	Example Resistance Genes	Remarks
Conjugation	Plasmids, Integrative and Conjugative Elements (ICEs)	Escherichia coli, Klebsiella pneumoniae	blaNDM-1, mcr-1, tetA	Direct cell-to-cell DNA transfer; dominant in Gram-negative bacteria
Transformation	Free DNA fragments	Streptococcus pneumoniae, Neisseria gonorrhoeae	Altered pbp, erm	Uptake of environmental DNA; facilitated by competence systems
Transduction	Bacteriophages	Staphylococcus aureus, Salmonella spp.	mecA, ermC	Phage-mediated gene packaging and transfer
Mobile Genetic Elements (MGEs)	Transposons, Integrons	Enterococcus, Pseudomonas, Escherichia coli	vanA, aadA, sul1	Enable integration and recombination of ARGs across species

3.4 Genetic Clustering and Co-selection

Co-selection is an important and often underrated phenomenon of genetic resistance. Resistance genes are rarely isolated; they tend to be clustered or found in operons, particularly on plasmids or integrons. This high genomic relatedness enables the multiple resistance traits to be sustained concurrently by the selective pressures of a single antimicrobial, or even a heavy metal or biocide. For instance, studies have reported the co-selection of a β-lactam or aminoglycoside resistance through associated plasmid genes following copper use in agriculture (Baker-Austin et al., 2006). This is of particular concern in wastewater treatment plants, animal husbandry, and aquaculture, where a selective agent in place of the antibiotics can be used to promote the emergence of resistance. Overall, the genotypes of antimicrobial resistance are suggestive of an interacting web of mutation, gene acquisition, and regulatory changes, which is dynamic. The systems make AMR not only a clinical hazard but also a great ecological and evolutionary one.

4. PHENOTYPIC MECHANISMS OF ANTIMICROBIAL RESISTANCE

Although genetic processes predispose antimicrobial resistance (AMR), phenotypic resistance is a non-permanent and temporary group of traits that shield microorganisms from facing antimicrobial pressure. These mechanisms are so significant, since they are, quite often, early and/or parallel to genetic adaptations and a keystone for persistence and recurrence of the infections in suboptimal treatment or conditions of environmental pressure. Phenotypic resistance could be reversible and does not require mutations or gene acquisition. Rather, it entails modifications in cellular physiology, metabolic condition, or microenvironment that diminish the efficacy of antimicrobials. This section explains the main phenotypic adaptations that microbes employ to escape antivirus activity.

4.1 Biofilm Formation

Biofilms are structured communities that are integrated in a secreted extracellular matrix. This matrix adheres to both biotic and abiotic surfaces, such as catheters, prosthetic joints, and tissue, and significantly halts antibiotic penetration almost completely. Within biofilms, there is a possibility that antibiotics may be chemically inactivated or trapped. Cells enter a non-growing state with decreased metabolic activity that makes them less prone to antibiotics that target ongoing processes, like quinolones and aminoglycosides. Persister cells, or a subpopulation of metabolically inactive cells, survive doses of high antibiotics and repopulate after the cessation of treatment (Hall & Mah, 2017). The most common biofilm-associated pathogens are Pseudomonas aeruginosa, Staphylococcus epidermidis, and Candida albicans, which are often implicated in non-healing infections of cystic fibrosis, endocarditis, and device-associated infections.

4.2 Efflux Pumps and Membrane Permeability

Microorganisms can develop resistance by increasing drug efflux or decreasing drug influx, which means that there are lower intracellular drug concentrations than therapeutic levels. Efflux pumps are proteins situated in the transmembrane that actively pump antibiotics out of the cell. It drives out β-lactams, fluoroquinolones, and tetracyclines, for example, in E. coli, the AcrAB-TolC efflux system. Downregulation of porins or changes in membrane lipids reduce permeability so that the drug cannot get in. A loss of OprD porin in Pseudomonas aeruginosa offers imipenem resistance (Poole, 2007). Not all of these mechanisms are genetically programmed; Environmental stimuli such as low pH, nutrient deprivation, or antibiotic exposure may induce these genes. Some of these bacteria can escape the antibiotics by entering into a dormant, non-replicating state called persistence. Persister cells are not like resistant strains in that they do not propagate in the presence of antibiotics, but are not killed by them. After they remove the antibiotic, these cells can "wake up" and lead to an outbreak of the infection. Persistence in infections such as tuberculosis and urinary tract infections is often encountered and is often found in Nutrient limitation, Oxidative stress, and Antibiotic pressure. For instance, the bacterium Mycobacterium tuberculosis can become latently infected in host macrophages and evade treatment, causing a long-term illness (Zhang et al., 2012).

4.3 Adaptive Resistance

An example of adaptive resistance is when there is a temporary increase in resistance due to factors such as exposure to sub-MIC concentrations of an antibiotic, the presence of host immune cells, or osmotic stress. This phenotype is usually controlled by: 1) Regulatory pathways (e.g., two-component systems), 2) Global stress responses, and 3) Inducible efflux systems. However, one has to note that adaptive resistance only occurs when the stimulus is present and gets washed out as soon as it is withdrawn from the system. This mechanism is particularly important in polymyxin and aminoglycoside antibiotics case, where transient resistance can make the treatment course unpredictable (Fernández et al., 2010).

5. EFFECT OF ANTIBIOTIC RESISTANCE MECHANISMS

AMR has emerged gradually by means of a serious threat to human health due to the genetic as well as phenotypic changes. Apart from the abovementioned laboratory processes, these mechanisms reflect themselves in practical clinical outcomes, from treatment failure up to increased mortality. This passage explains the implications of AMR mechanisms on the diagnosis, therapy, and public health strategies.

5.1 Impact on Treatment Outcomes

The resistance of antimicrobials to treatments considerably reduces the efficiency of the normal treatment, compelling health care professionals to resort to the second or third-line antibiotics, which are rather more lethal, less effective, and significantly more costly. Not only is this change harmful to patient outcomes, but it has to imposes a heavy burden on healthcare systems. As an example, the cure of infections caused by carbapenem-resistant Enterobacteriaceae (CRE) has a limited number of options, and it has a mortality rate exceeding 50% in a certain health care setting (van Duin & Doi, 2017). In the same way, multidrug-resistant tuberculosis, i.e, MDR-TB treatment, necessitates the use of medications such as linezolid or bedaquiline, which presuppose long-term usage and are associated with toxicity and suboptimal outcomes. Among them are, but are not limited to, ESBL production, resistance to methicillin (observed in MRSA), and microbial biofilm formation, which are strongly related to extending the hospital stay, slowing the healing process, and surgical re-infection (Magill et al., 2014). The implications depict the urgent need to have robust AMR mitigation strategies, surveillance, and new therapeutic agents.

5.2 Challenges in Diagnosis and Treatment Choices

The importance of antimicrobial resistance (AMR) is generating significant issues in clinical diagnostics, which prevents the correct diagnosis and successful treatment of infectious diseases. Though the conventional culture-based methods are still common in most of the laboratories, they are likely to overlook those that may grow slowly or not grow at all, like the persister that, in a non-metabolic state, may be reactivated following the treatment (Lewis, 2010). Although being more sensitive, molecular diagnostics are not devoid of their limitations, and could only identify resistance genes (e.g., bla KPC or mecA), whereas these genes do not always result in expressed phenotypic resistance in the context of such mechanisms as increased efflux pump activity or permeability change (Ellington et al., 2017). Other than this, bacterial biofilms are another diagnostic barrier. Such hierarchical communities of bacteria, when grown on indwelling medical devices, can severely affect inaccurate culture outcomes, often resulting in false negatives (Donlan and Costerton, 2002). This backfires particularly in low-resource healthcare facilities where there is limited access to such diagnostics. The number of empirical treatments is high in such environments, and the therapy is more likely to fail, or there is a risk of more resistant strains emerging (Okeke et al., 2005). Thus, designing and introducing rapid, low-cost, and effective diagnostic tools is also important in terms of worldwide AMR control.

5.3 Multidrug-Resistant Organisms (MDROs)

MDROs are standards for pathogens resistant to up to three classes of antimicrobial agents. They represent the blend of several resistance modalities (plasmid-mediated genes + efflux + biofilm) and are commonly referred to as superbugs. Examples include

- MRSA (Methicillin-Resistant Staphylococcus aureus): through the mecA gene that creates an altered penicillin-binding protein (PBP2a) gene
- VRE (Vancomycin-Resistant Enterococci): harboring vanA or vanB operons
- MDR/XDR-TB: sensitive to isoniazid, rifampin, and often to second-line drugs

- NDM-1 and KPC producers: enzymes that cleave carbapenems and numerous β-lactams

MDROs are infamous for nosocomial outbreaks, especially within ICUs, transplant units, and among immunocompromised patients (Tacconelli et al., 2018).

5.4 Implications for Public Health Policies and Antibiotic Stewardship

The transmission of AMR is no longer restricted to the hospital or clinical setting, but has spread to the general environment, forming ecological reservoirs of resistive genes. This may be carried out in various modes, including by way of wastewater outflow, agricultural overload, and global transportation, thereby enabling the movement of the resistance determinants between humans, animals, and the ecosystems. Worryingly enough, surveillance data indicate that resistance mechanisms are evolving even quickly than the formation of new antibiotics (World Health Organization [WHO], 2020), and as a danger not just to the health of the entire population but also to the treatment strategies worldwide. Policy frameworks must, in response to this new crisis, make use of an integrative, multisectoral approach. Laying down the Antimicrobial Stewardship Programs (ASPs) has been among the major interventions as they are strategized to maximize the utilization of antibiotics in clinical facilities, aiming to minimize unwarranted exposure, as well as delay resistance development. Infection Prevention and Control activities meant to curb the transmission of resistant pathogens, particularly in high-risk settings like hospitals and long-term care, are also important. There should also be powerful surveillance and reporting mechanisms, like those of the WHO, the Global Antimicrobial Resistance Surveillance System (GLASS), and others, to follow the trends and inform the evidence-based policy. The core of all these strategies is the One Health approach, whereby we realize the natural interdependency of human health and animal/ environmental health. By addressing the AMR at this stage of system interconnectedness, the One Health approach represents the long-term and final path (WHO, 2020).

6. DETECTION AND DIAGNOSTIC APPROACHES IN ANTIMICROBIAL RESISTANCE

Timely and useful diagnosis of antibiotic resistance (AMR) is a significant part of patient care, and it is only a reasonable reaction to the antibiotic resistance that will result in success in controlling infections and managing the use of antimicrobials. As genetic mutations become more and more a part of the resistance mechanisms, and more diverse and complex, so too must our resistance to TB strategies in making diagnoses. The section gives a summary of the conventional and the modern techniques of identifying AMR in clinical and research studies. The timely diagnosis and its use are of paramount importance to the effective cure of infectious diseases and to preventing the emergence of antimicrobial resistance (AMR). Convention culture-based diagnostics remain the gold standard in clinical microbiology. These methods are used to verify the identity of pathogens and test antimicrobial susceptibility using phenotypic assays. Standard methods include the disk diffusion method (Kirby-Bauer test), broth dilution, and E-tests, with which the Minimum Inhibitory Concentration (MIC) can be established directly, so one can see what a certain antimicrobial can do. Modern systems, such as VITEK 2, MicroScan, use colorimetric and turbidimetric techniques that automate and hasten this process. However, these tests are usually time-consuming (usually 24-72 hours) and may not reliably detect resistant organisms in cases of slow-growing bacteria, mixed infections, or an infection caused by biofilm-associated pathogens (Jorgensen & Ferraro, 2009).

Molecular diagnostics have appeared as reliable instruments of quick and sensitive resistance gene detection in order to overcome the limitations of phenotypic testing. Polymerase Chain Reaction (PCR), including its derivatives, namely the multiplex and the real-time PCR, is regularly employed to detect specific genetic markers such as mecA (methicillin resistance), bla ND M (carbapenem resistance), and vanA/B (vancomycin resistance). These methods are more sensitive and faster than culture-based methods, with results coming within hours. Nevertheless, the molecular tests usually fail to answer the question of whether a gene is actively expressed or if it translates into phenotypic resistance. Also, they might follow the correct treatment procedures but miss novel or rare resistance mechanisms that are not included in the test panel (Liesenfeld et al., 2014).

Whole Genome Sequencing (WGS) provides a comprehensive answer in the form of mapping of the whole resistome, i.e., the entire resistome contained within a microbial genome. It enables one to detect chromosomal mutations that are related to Resistance, including gyrA, rpoB, and katG, that trigger Resistance to fluoroquinolones and rifampin. WGS also helps in surveillance, monitoring of outbreaks, and tracing the spread of resistant genes from species to ecosystems. Despite its enormous potential, application of WGS in routine clinical workflows remains restrained by its high costs, high need for specialized equipment and bioinformatics knowledge, and dependence on curated databases such as CARD (Comprehensive Antibiotic Resistance) and ResFinder (Ellington et al., 2017).

New innovative phenotypic screening tools are now being formulated to bridge the gap between conventional and molecular diagnostics. There are quick responses, such as lateral flow immunoassays, which can be used to detect resistance proteins, such as the carbapenemases, from clinical samples. Bacterial identification and some resistance can be detected using MALDI-TOF MS (Matrix-Assisted Laser Desorption/Ionization Time-of-Flight Mass Spectrometry), depending on different protein imprints. Moreover, new technologies such as microfluidic chips and biosensors can infer real-time growth inhibition and resistance-associated metabolic changes. These tools are especially useful in point-of-care settings, with potential to widen diagnostic capacity within resource-limited regions (Chin et al, 2017). Together, these diagnostic tools form a critical foundation for effective antimicrobial stewardship, personalized therapy, and global AMR surveillance.

7. STRATEGIES FOR COMBATING ANTIMICROBIAL RESISTANCE

AMR is a contemporary medical existential challenge that needs to be approached using multiple-pronged strategies that involve the use of molecular innovations, policy reactions, and global cooperation. AMR implies that resistance determinants, both genetic and phenotypic, should be addressed to counter it, and the reasonable use of antimicrobials ought to be approved. Scientific and translational methodologies that can be employed to minimize the resistance and restore the efficacy of existing therapies will be described in the following strategies.

7.1 Genomic Surveillance and Predictive Epidemiology

Genomic surveillance represents an inevitable part of modern AMR control because it may provide real-time data on the dynamics of pathogen evolution, gene transfer, and outbreak mechanisms. Genomic data is utilized in the form of the WHO Global Antimicrobial Resistance and Use Surveillance System (GLASS) and the Antibiotic Resistance Laboratory Network, which is provided by the Centers for Disease Control (Munk et al., 2022; WHO, 2023). The mapping out of resistance determinants, such as blaNDM-1, mecA, and mcr-1, in bacterial populations can also be performed through the use of whole genome sequencing (WGS) in a more detailed way (Didelot et al., 2019). Genomic surveillance systems are gradually becoming pervaded with artificial intelligence (AI) and machine learning (ML) to enhance predictive capabilities and forecasting of outbreaks (Schwartz, Ritchie, and Smith, 2023).

7.2 CRISPR-Based Antimicrobials

The CRISPR-Cas system has been recognized as a bacterial adaptive immune system, which has revolutionized genome editing and introduced new perspectives on AMR control. CRISPR-based antimicrobials can selectively cleave antibiotic resistance genes (ARGs) and also select resistant strains, but not beneficial microbiota (Citorik, Mimee, and Lu, 2019). The CRISPR-Cas constructs of interest have been engineered to such a degree that they can be employed to silence plasmids harboring blaCTX-M or mecA, therefore, restoring 8-lactam antibiotic sensitivity in pathogens (Bikard et al., 2020). Delivery is still a major issue, and developments in bacteriophage-based CRISPR-delivery systems present a feasible solution to targeted in vivo systems (Dong et al., 2021). The flexibility of CRISPR antimicrobials has potential in precision medicine, especially in addressing multidrug-resistant (MDR) infections that are not readily managed using traditional treatment regimens.

7.3 Bacteriophage Therapy

As a natural and very specific alternative to antibiotics, bacteriophages, which are viruses that infect bacteria, are an option. Phage therapy has resurfaced as one of the prospective approaches to the treatment of MDR pathogens like Pseudomonas aeruginosa, Acinetobacter baumannii, and Staphylococcus aureus (Abedon et al., 2021). Contrary to antibiotics, phages are able to coevolve with bacteria and reduce the chances of resistance development in the long term (Lin et al., 2022). What is more, phage-enzymes such as endolysins and depolymerases can destroy bacterial biofilm and cell walls, improving the action of antibiotics (Gordillo Altamirano & Barr, 2019). There are improvements in clinical applications, with the use of custom phage cocktails and compassionate-use therapy demonstrating promising results in chronic infections. Standardization of regulation and the ability to scale manufacturing are also key to mainstream clinical integration (Pirnay et al., 2022).

7.4 Antimicrobial Peptides (AMPs) and Novel Therapeutics

The constituents of the innate immunity are antimicrobial peptides (AMPs), which have a wide-spectrum effect on bacteria, fungi, and viruses. They are useful candidates due to their mechanisms, including membrane disruption, the suppression of nucleic acid synthesis, and immunomodulation, which make them valuable against MDR organisms (Mahlapuu et al., 2020). Developing synthetic and engineered AMPs, namely, peptide mimetics and lipopeptides, to address the limitations of toxicity and instability is underway (Li et al., 2021). The systems of AMP delivery based on nanotechnology also provide an increased level of stability and bioavailability

(Tiwari et al., 2023). Also, antimicrobial adjuvants, quorum-sensing preventors, and antivirulence compounds are under consideration to recover antibiotic sensitivity without subjecting to heavy selection pressure (Allen, Traxler, and Barker, 2021).

7.5 Antibiotic stewardship and policy interventions

The innovative advancement of science should be supplemented with effective antibiotic stewardship programmes (ASPs) to provide responsible use of the available antimicrobials. ASPs are aimed at reducing the development of resistance and preventing adverse effects by optimising the choice of drugs, dose, and duration (Baur et al., 2019). One Health integrated systems (between human, animal, and environmental health) play a key role in the reduction of antibiotic abuse in livestock and aquaculture (Chokshi, Sifri, Cennimo, and Horng, 2019). It still requires education, regulatory control, and international collaboration in the form of organizations like WHO, FAO, and OIE to achieve long-term success (WHO, 2023). The application of real-time diagnostics, surveillance-based prescriptions, and national awareness campaigns can all help to reduce the tide of resistance until new treatment options are created. An overview of key translational strategies, their mechanisms, clinical uses, and recent limitations, with an emphasis on integrated scientific, clinical, and policy innovations in the fight against AMR, is also presented in Table 3.

Table 3. Comparative overview of key strategies for combating antimicrobial resistance

Strategy	Mechanism	Applications	Limitations
Genomic Surveillance	Tracking resistance genes and outbreaks via WGS, bioinformatics, and AI	Early detection, outbreak prevention, and resistance mapping	Resource-intensive, requires data infrastructure
CRISPR-Based Antimicrobials	Precision genome editing to disrupt ARGs	Rdesensitization of pathogens, control of MDR infections	Delivery challenges, regulatory issues
Bacteriophage Therapy	Use of phages to target and lyse resistant bacteria	Treatment of MDR/ XDR infections, biofilm disruption	Host specificity, regulatory/scale-up barriers
Antimicrobial Peptides	Broad-spectrum membrane disruption and immunomodulation	Alternative therapeutics for MDR organisms	Stability, toxicity, and delivery
Antibiotic Stewardship	Responsible use of antimicrobials, stewardship programs	Optimized therapy, slowed resistance emergence	Compliance, education, global coordination

8. EMERGING RESISTANCE THREATS AND FUTURE DIRECTIONS

Antimicrobial resistance (AMR) remains increasing rapidly, whereas there is an acute lag in developing new antibiotics. This increasing difference is a serious threat to the world's public health, food safety, and sustainable development. The increase in the number of multidrug-resistant organisms (MDROs), which are being linked with failed treatment, prolonged duration of stay in the hospital, and growing rates of mortality, is a special concern. The interplay between AMR clinical, agricultural, and environmental drivers has expedited the spread of resistance mechanisms across borders. Those are the most frightening aspects of AMR, which are the horizontal exchange of resistance genes promoted by mobile genetic elements (MGEs) such as plasmids, transposons, and integrons. These provide the potential for the quick spread and dissemination of resistance qualities among heterogeneous bacterial populations. An excellent example of this concept includes the mcr-1 gene, which imparts colistin resistance (a last resort) on a plasmid. First identified in nature in animals, mcr-1 is now emerging globally in human clinical isolates and in food products, which is of immediate concern for public health with potential for zoonotic transmission and agricultural use of antibiotics (Liu et al., 2016). Moreover, resultant emerging resistance genes such as tet (X4) and cfr confer resistance to tetracyclines and oxazolidinones (eg, linezolid) in respectively. These genes have been found in clinical and agricultural settings, suggesting the synthesis of resistance within these sectors. The fact that these genes co-locate with great frequency on combinatorial plasmids makes them particularly worrisome as they give co-resistance to several classes of antibiotics and speed up their global dispersal (Wang et al., 2020). The persistence and convergence of such interpretations of mobile resistance determinants suggest a need for synergy in surveillance, containment measures, and investigation of next-generation therapeutics.

In the ever-growing threats of pathogens, it is now becoming more and more rampant for the pathogens to become multidrug resistant (MDR), extensively drug resistant (XDR), and even pan-drug resistant (PDR). Hence, there is a particular urgency to address this scourge in the world of health systems. Such diachronic classification illustrates the overall decay of efficacy across classes of antimicrobial agents. For example, anticipated to be a common etiology of hospital-acquired infections, Acinetobacter baumannii is seen in XDR forms that are resistant to nearly all β-lactams, fluoroquinolones, and aminoglycosides, with polymyxins as the only available treatment. Perhaps more alarming, strains of Klebsiella pneumoniae for which PDR has been reported have been encountered in India and various regions of Europe. These are all multi-drug resistant strains, and therefore, there are no treatment options. This results in a higher mortality rate by far (Nordmann, Naas,

& Poirel, 2012). Failure to contain such resistant organisms is not merely in part due to selective drug pressure alone; it also depends on the evolutionary plasticity of bacteria. In most cases, the resistance mechanisms are likely to involve a biological fitness cost, for example, a reduced growth rate or the virulence. However, most of the resistant pathogens attain compensatory mutations that will ease these disadvantages, thus restoring the fitness and sustaining the long-term presence of such pathogens in clinical settings. Consequently, these fearsome strains not only survive in environments rich in antibiotics but also essentially dominate the susceptible counterparts in such settings, thereby causing endemic or epidemic situations worldwide within healthcare institutions.

Actions to combat antimicrobial resistance (AMR) must be holistic and integrated, that is, where one health surveillance model links human, animal, and environmental health sectors. GLASS, which is one of the pillars of this methodology, is a Global Anti-microbial Resistance Surveillance System created by WHO to monitor global trends of resistance and trends in antimicrobial use in countries and sectors. Over 120 countries have formulated and are starting to execute National Action Plans towards this effort of harmonization of AMR strategies into a coordinated model. Moreover, environmental surveillance has also gone up, displaying detection of resistance genes in wastewaters, livestock farms, and aquaculture environments and explaining the role of non-clinical ecosystems in the transmission of AMR. These findings demonstrate the necessity of cross-cutting interventions outside of the traditional healthcare settings. Since resistance mechanisms are transboundary, and a global governance model with data sharing in real-time, collaborative research, and fair funding strategies to appreciate the low and middle-income layers of the world disproportionately vulnerable to AMR is necessary to make the containment and mitigation efforts successful (Robinson et al, 2016).

Due to the rapid increase in the threat of antimicrobial resistance (AMR), the current research efforts are becoming more focused on the development of new therapeutics and next-generation tests. Phage therapy is the most promising of the innovations to exploit the specificity of bacteriophages to kill the specific type of pathogenic bacteria, and this is a precision-related alternative compared to using the whole spectrum of antibiotics. Both natural and synthetic antimicrobial peptides (AMPs) are also getting attention due to their rapidity and multidrug-resistant range of bactericidal activity. The other frontier is the use of CRISPR-Cas systems, which can enable to performance of directed editing of genes to eliminate resistance-conferring genes of the microbial genomes, which, with permissive therapeutic and preventive uses, are a legitimate alternative to antibiotics. Artificial intelligence (AI) is being used in drug discovery to predict antimicrobial activity, to rank new potential drug candidates, and to predict pharmacology profiles faster and with higher precision than ever before. Meanwhile, new technologies in the field of point-of-care diagnostics, during rapid innovations, including portable microfluidics and mobile-based technologies, are changing the AMR detection in low-resource environments, which enables rapid, cheap, and decentralized testing. Such technological innovations must be followed by an investment in the long-term in the area of antibiotic stewardship, such as awareness among populations, education of healthcare providers, and the restrictive regulatory environment to deter the excessive use of antimicrobials in human, veterinary, and agricultural practice (de la Fuente-Núñez et al, 2017; Torres-Barcelo, 2018).

9. CONCLUSION

Multifactorial genetic and phenotypic processes have resulted in AMR becoming one of the most urgent issues of public health over the last one hundred years. The distribution and amplification of resistance genes, most often encoded in the mobile genetic elements, are further complicated by adaptive bacterial behaviours, such as biofilm formation and the development of persister cells, which have made most first-line antibiotics still more ineffective. Clinical implications of these resistance mechanisms in this chapter are far-reaching, with the failure to treat them, increased hospital stay, high mortality, and significant economic burden to the entire world being a result of these mechanisms. Researchers, clinicians, and even policy-makers need the basic conceptual knowledge of AMR (in terms of its nomenclature and classification based on the mechanisms of resistance). The same can be said about the development of diagnostic methods (including traditional culture-based tests to molecular and whole-genome) that can be called upon to detect resistant pathogens in time and to inform proper treatment. The mcr-1 and pan-drug-resistant pathogens are new threats that are changing the global health community towards integrated approaches of One Health. These are interrelations between people, animals, and the environment in resistance ecology. These are phage therapy, CRISPR-based architecture, or even AI-based drug discovery, which can potentially reverse the resistance tide. Ultimately, the way to go is not just that of scientific and technological breakthrough, but also of international collaboration, individual engagement, and stringent antibiotic stewardship throughout the board. Chapter priority is, then, to provide an in-depth background on the mechanisms of AMR and urge further research, awareness, and policy restructuring, which can put a stop to this increasingly serious crisis.

REFERENCES

Abedon, S. T., García, P., Mullany, P., & Aminov, R. (2021). Editorial: Phage therapy: Past, present, and future. *Frontiers in Microbiology*, *12*, 658218. DOI: 10.3389/fmicb.2021.658218

Allen, H. K., Traxler, M. F., & Barker, M. (2021). Mechanisms and ecological impacts of antibiotic resistance evolution. *Nature Reviews. Microbiology*, *19*(7), 416–429. DOI: 10.1038/s41579-021-00530-6

Arthur, M., Molinas, C., & Courvalin, P. (1996). The vanS and vanR genes of *Tn1546* are required for glycopeptide resistance in *Enterococcus faecium* BM4147. *Journal of Bacteriology*, *175*(1), 117–127. DOI: 10.1128/jb.175.1.117-127.1993

Baker-Austin, C., Wright, M. S., Stepanauskas, R., & McArthur, J. V. (2006). Co-selection of antibiotic and metal resistance. *Trends in Microbiology*, *14*(4), 176–182. DOI: 10.1016/j.tim.2006.02.006

Balaban, N. Q., Helaine, S., Lewis, K., Ackermann, M., Aldridge, B., Andersson, D. I., & Levin, B. R. (2019). Definitions and guidelines for research on antibiotic persistence. *Nature Reviews. Microbiology*, *17*(7), 441–448. DOI: 10.1038/s41579-019-0196-3

Baur, D., Gladstone, B. P., Burkert, F., Carrara, E., Foschi, F., Döbele, S., & Tacconelli, E. (2019). Effect of antibiotic stewardship on the incidence of infection and colonisation with antibiotic-resistant bacteria and Clostridium difficile infection: A systematic review and meta-analysis. *The Lancet. Infectious Diseases*, *19*(9), 998–1008. DOI: 10.1016/S1473-3099(19)30038-3

Bikard, D., & Barrangou, R. (2020). Using CRISPR–Cas systems as antimicrobials. *Nature Biotechnology*, *38*(2), 143–155.

Bikard, D., Euler, C. W., Jiang, W., Nussenzweig, P. M., Goldberg, G. W., Duportet, X., & Fischetti, V. A. (2020). Exploiting CRISPR-Cas nucleases to combat antimicrobial resistance. *Nature Reviews. Microbiology*, *18*(10), 611–622. DOI: 10.1038/s41579-020-0386-z

Blair, J. M., Webber, M. A., Baylay, A. J., Ogbolu, D. O., & Piddock, L. J. (2015). Molecular mechanisms of antibiotic resistance. *Nature Reviews. Microbiology*, *13*(1), 42–51. DOI: 10.1038/nrmicro3380

Bush, K., & Bradford, P. A. (2016). β-Lactams and β-lactamase inhibitors: An overview. *Cold Spring Harbor Perspectives in Medicine*, *6*(8), a025247. DOI: 10.1101/cshperspect.a025247

Carattoli, A. (2013). Plasmids and the spread of resistance. *International Journal of Medical Microbiology*, *303*(6-7), 298–304. DOI: 10.1016/j.ijmm.2013.02.001

Chin, C. D., Linder, V., & Sia, S. K. (2017). Commercialization of microfluidic point-of-care diagnostic devices. *Lab on a Chip*, *12*(12), 2118–2134. DOI: 10.1039/C2LC21204H

Chokshi, A., Sifri, Z., Cennimo, D., & Horng, H. (2019). Global contributors to antibiotic resistance. *Journal of Global Infectious Diseases*, *11*(1), 36–42. DOI: 10.4103/jgid.jgid_110_18

Citorik, R. J., Mimee, M., & Lu, T. K. (2019). CRISPR-based antimicrobials. *Nature Reviews. Microbiology*, *17*(3), 153–164. DOI: 10.1038/s41579-018-0135-3

Didelot, X., Bowden, R., Wilson, D. J., Peto, T. E., & Crook, D. W. (2019). Transforming clinical microbiology with bacterial genome sequencing. *Nature Reviews. Genetics*, *20*(10), 601–612. DOI: 10.1038/s41576-019-0153-6

Dong, H., Xiang, Y., & Fang, W. (2021). Phage-delivered CRISPR-Cas systems for precision antimicrobial applications. *Trends in Biotechnology*, *39*(10), 1049–1062. DOI: 10.1016/j.tibtech.2021.03.008

Du, D., Wang-Kan, X., Neuberger, A., van Veen, H. W., Pos, K. M., Piddock, L. J., & Luisi, B. F. (2018). Multidrug efflux pumps: Structure, function and regulation. *Nature Reviews. Microbiology*, *16*(9), 523–539.

Ellington, M. J., Ekelund, O., & Aarestrup, F. M.. (2017). The role of whole genome sequencing in antimicrobial susceptibility testing of bacteria: Report from EUCAST Subcommittee. *Clinical Microbiology and Infection*, *23*(1), 2–22. DOI: 10.1016/j.cmi.2016.11.012

Fernåndez, L., Gooderham, W. J., & Hancock, R. E. W. (2010). Adaptive resistance to the "last hope" antibiotics colistin and polymyxin B in Pseudomonas aeruginosa is mediated by activation of the arn operon. *Antimicrobial Agents and Chemotherapy*, *54*(8), 3372–3377. DOI: 10.1128/AAC.00216-10

Flemming, H. C., & Wuertz, S. (2019). Bacteria and archaea on Earth and their abundance in biofilms. *Nature Reviews. Microbiology*, *17*(4), 247–260.

Gillings, M. R. (2014). Integrons: Past, present, and future. *Microbiology and Molecular Biology Reviews : MMBR*, *78*(2), 257–277. DOI: 10.1128/MMBR.00056-13

Gordillo Altamirano, F. L., & Barr, J. J. (2019). Phage therapy in the postantibiotic era. *Clinical Microbiology Reviews*, *32*(2), e00066–e18. DOI: 10.1128/CMR.00066-18

Hall, C. W., & Mah, T.-F. (2017). Molecular mechanisms of biofilm-based antibiotic resistance and tolerance in pathogenic bacteria. *FEMS Microbiology Reviews*, *41*(3), 276–301. DOI: 10.1093/femsre/fux010

Hendriksen, R. S., Munk, P., Njage, P., van Bunnik, B., McNally, L., Lukjancenko, O., & Aarestrup, F. M. (2019). Global monitoring of antimicrobial resistance based on metagenomics analyses of urban sewage. *Nature Communications*, *10*(1), 1124.

Holmes, A. H., Moore, L. S., Sundsfjord, A., Steinbakk, M., Regmi, S., Karkey, A., & Piddock, L. J. (2019). Understanding the mechanisms and drivers of antimicrobial resistance. *Lancet*, *387*(10014), 176–187.

Jorgensen, J. H., & Ferraro, M. J. (2009). Antimicrobial susceptibility testing: A review of general principles and contemporary practices. *Clinical Infectious Diseases*, *49*(11), 1749–1755. DOI: 10.1086/647952

Kraemer, S. A., Ramachandran, A., & Perron, G. G. (2019). Antibiotic pollution in the environment: From microbial ecology to public policy. *Microorganisms*, *7*(6), 180.

Li, J., Koh, J. J., Liu, S., Lakshminarayanan, R., Verma, C. S., & Beuerman, R. W. (2021). Membrane-active antimicrobial peptides: Translating mechanistic insights to design. *Frontiers in Neuroscience*, *15*, 633625. DOI: 10.3389/fnins.2021.633625

Liesenfeld, O., Lehman, L., Hunfeld, K. P., & Kost, G. (2014). Molecular diagnosis of sepsis: New aspects and recent developments. *European Journal of Microbiology & Immunology*, *4*(1), 1–25. DOI: 10.1556/EuJMI.4.2014.1.1

Lin, D. M., Koskella, B., & Lin, H. C. (2022). Phage therapy: An alternative to antibiotics in the age of multidrug resistance. *World Journal of Gastrointestinal Pharmacology and Therapeutics*, *13*(3), 77–91. DOI: 10.4292/wjgpt.v13.i3.77

Liu, Y.-Y., Wang, Y., & Walsh, T. R.. (2016). Emergence of plasmid-mediated colistin resistance mechanism MCR-1 in animals and human beings in China: A microbiological and molecular biological study. *The Lancet. Infectious Diseases*, *16*(2), 161–168. DOI: 10.1016/S1473-3099(15)00424-7

Magill, S. S., Edwards, J. R., & Bamberg, W.. (2014). Multistate point-prevalence survey of health care-associated infections. *The New England Journal of Medicine*, *370*(13), 1198–1208. DOI: 10.1056/NEJMoa1306801

Magiorakos, A. P., Srinivasan, A., Carey, R. B., Carmeli, Y., Falagas, M. E., Giske, C. G., & Monnet, D. L. (2012). Multidrug-resistant, extensively drug-resistant, and pandrug-resistant bacteria: An international expert proposal for interim standard definitions for acquired resistance. *Clinical Microbiology and Infection*, *18*(3), 268–281. DOI: 10.1111/j.1469-0691.2011.03570.x

Mahlapuu, M., Björn, C., & Ekblom, J. (2020). Antimicrobial peptides as therapeutic agents: Opportunities and challenges. *Critical Reviews in Biotechnology*, *40*(7), 978–992. DOI: 10.1080/07388551.2020.1796576

. Munita, J. M., & Arias, C. A. (2016). Mechanisms of antibiotic resistance. *Microbiology Spectrum*, 4(2), . https://doi.org/DOI: 10.1128/microbiolspec.VMBF-0016-2015

Munk, P., Brinch, C., Synnott, A., & Hendriksen, R. S. (2022). Global genomic surveillance of antimicrobial resistance: A One Health approach. *Nature Microbiology*, *7*(9), 1291–1304. DOI: 10.1038/s41564-022-01149-4

Murray, C. J., Ikuta, K. S., Sharara, F., Swetschinski, L., Robles Aguilar, G., & Gray, A.Global Burden of Disease 2021 AMR Collaborators. (2022). Global burden of bacterial antimicrobial resistance in 2019: A systematic analysis. *Lancet*, *399*(10325), 629–655.

Nordmann, P., Naas, T., & Poirel, L. (2012). Global spread of carbapenemase-producing Enterobacteriaceae. *Emerging Infectious Diseases*, *17*(10), 1791–1798. DOI: 10.3201/eid1710.110655

O'Neill, J. (2020). *Tackling drug-resistant infections globally: Final report and recommendations*. UK Government.

OECD. (2022). *Stemming the Superbug Tide: Just a Few Dollars More*. OECD Publishing., DOI: 10.1787/9789264307599-

Pal, C., Bengtsson-Palme, J., Kristiansson, E., & Larsson, D. G. J. (2015). Co-occurrence of resistance genes to antibiotics, biocides, and metals reveals novel insights into their co-selection potential. *BMC Genomics*, *16*(1), 964. DOI: 10.1186/s12864-015-2153-5

Partridge, S. R., Kwong, S. M., Firth, N., & Jensen, S. O. (2018). Mobile genetic elements associated with antimicrobial resistance. *Clinical Microbiology Reviews*, *31*(4), e00088–e17.

Pirnay, J. P., Verbeken, G., Rose, T., Jennes, S., Zizi, M., Huys, I., & Merabishvili, M. (2022). Introducing phage therapy to Western medicine. *Emerging Infectious Diseases*, *28*(1), 16–23. DOI: 10.3201/eid2801.210157

Poole, K. (2007). Efflux pumps as antimicrobial resistance mechanisms. *Annals of Medicine*, *39*(3), 162–176. DOI: 10.1080/07853890701195262

Robinson, T. P., Bu, D. P., & Carrique-Mas, J.. (2016). Antibiotic resistance is the quintessential One Health issue. *Transactions of the Royal Society of Tropical Medicine and Hygiene*, *110*(7), 377–380. DOI: 10.1093/trstmh/trw048

Sandgren, A., Strong, M., Muthukrishnan, P., Weiner, B. K., Church, G. M., & Murray, M. B. (2009). Tuberculosis drug resistance mutation database. *PLoS Medicine, 6*(2), e1000002. DOI: 10.1371/journal.pmed.1000002

Schwartz, D. C., Ritchie, A., & Smith, M. A. (2023). AI-driven diagnostic models for predicting antimicrobial resistance. *Nature Biotechnology, 41*(2), 254–266. DOI: 10.1038/s41587-023-01750-5

Tacconelli, E., Carrara, E., & Savoldi, A.. (2018). Discovery, research, and development of new antibiotics: The WHO priority list of antibiotic-resistant bacteria and tuberculosis. *The Lancet. Infectious Diseases, 18*(3), 318–327. DOI: 10.1016/S1473-3099(17)30753-3

Tagini, F., & Greub, G. (2020). Bacterial genome sequencing in clinical microbiology: A pathogen-oriented review. *European Journal of Clinical Microbiology & Infectious Diseases, 39*(5), 785–802.

Tiwari, G., Tiwari, R., & Srivastava, P. (2023). Nanocarrier-assisted delivery of antimicrobial peptides: A frontier in combating multidrug resistance. *Drug Delivery and Translational Research, 13*(2), 234–248. DOI: 10.1007/s13346-023-01198-z

van Duin, D., & Doi, Y. (2017). The global epidemiology of carbapenemase-producing Enterobacteriaceae. *Virulence, 8*(4), 460–469. DOI: 10.1080/21505594.2016.1222343

World Bank. (2023). *Pulling together to beat superbugs: Knowledge and implementation gaps in addressing antimicrobial resistance.* Washington, DC.

World Health Organization. (2020). *Global antimicrobial resistance and use surveillance system (GLASS) report 2020.* https://www.who.int/glass

World Health Organization. (2023). *One Health Joint Plan of Action 2022–2026.* WHO Press.

World Health Organization. (2024). *Global Antimicrobial Resistance and Use Surveillance System (GLASS) Report 2024.* WHO.

World Health Organization (WHO). (2020). *Antimicrobial resistance: A global threat.* https://www.who.int/antimicrobial-resistance/en/

Zhang, Y., Yew, W. W., & Barer, M. R. (2012). Targeting persisters for tuberculosis control. *Antimicrobial Agents and Chemotherapy, 56*(5), 2223–2230. DOI: 10.1128/AAC.06288-11

Chapter 5
Biofilm Formation and Its Contribution to Antibiotic Resistance

M. Anushiya
Department of Microbiology, Sacred Heart College, Tirupattur, India

P. Saranraj
https://orcid.org/0000-0002-5052-6532
Department of Microbiology, Sacred Heart College, Tirupattur, India

J. Nancy
Department of Microbiology, Sacred Heart College, Tirupattur, India

G. Vithiya
https://orcid.org/0009-0001-0729-4318
Department of Microbiology, Sacred Heart College, Tirupattur, India

P. Prakathi
https://orcid.org/0009-0000-4457-9008
Department of Microbiology, Sacred Heart College, Tirupattur, India

M. Manigandan
https://orcid.org/0000-0002-8115-2713
Department of Microbiology, Sacred Heart College, Tirupattur, India

ABSTRACT

Biofilm production is one of the biological modes of bacterial survival, prolonged existence, and resistance to various forms of antimicrobial agents. A biofilm refers to a self-made polymer matrix that encloses a microbial body of organized bacteria, referred to as Exopolysaccharides (EPS), which adheres to both biological or non-biological surfaces. This unique structural organization makes it difficult for antibiotics to work effectively by inhibiting the functioning of this shielded environment. The physical barrier provided by the EPS matrix further enhances the sequestration or deactivation of antimicrobial drugs and limits the penetration

DOI: 10.4018/979-8-3373-3825-5.ch005

of medicines. Due to this fact, biofilm-associated bacteria can express antibiotic resistance several hundred times higher than that of their free-living counterparts, hence biofilms are a major cause of recurring and chronic infections.

Combatting Antimicrobial Resistance Through Medical Microbiology

1. INTRODUCTION

Antibiotic resistance a severe global public health concern because the main vectors for its causation are the unnecessary discriminatory use of antibiotics in medicine, veterinary care, aquaculture, and agriculture (Zhao et al., 2021). Antimicrobial Resistant bacteria have spread due to this trend it becomes tougher to fight against infectious diseases. Despite efforts to develop novel pharmaceutical interventions, pathogens such as *Pseudomonas aeruginosa* and multidrug-resistant Enterobacteriaceae have become increasingly resistant to available antibiotics for treating infections caused by these microbes (El-Sapagh et al., 2023). The World Health Organization (WHO) includes antibiotic resistance in its top ten threats to global health. This issue underlines the urgent need for new therapeutic modalities, conscientious use of antibiotics, and continuous research for halting the dissemination of Antimicrobial Resistance (AMR). Multidrug-resistant bacteria are an emerging concern, while *in vitro* susceptibility testing was the backbone in defining resistance. The natural process of antibiotic resistance is very complex due to environmental factors, microbial community density, and extensive use of antimicrobials in medicine, agriculture, or food production (Osei Sekyere et al., 2023). Through various Horizontal Gene Transfer (HGT) methods, including transformation, conjugation, and transduction, the genes of Antibiotic Resistance are distributed among resistant microorganisms. In addition, Outer Membrane Vesicles (OMVs) are used as carriers to facilitate genetic exchange and promote the spread of resistance genes within bacterial populations. In 1928, the discovery of penicillin in a new era of drug development, yielding the current estimated annual production of approximately 100,000 tonnes of the antibiotic (Gunther et al., 2022). However, this is the numerous bacterial species developing resistance to multiple medications, leading to multidrug resistance. The fact that it is increasing from the discovery of penicillin to the current widely developed resistance that creative approaches against antimicrobial resistance need to be developed to protect public health characteristics of bacteria and the continuous use of antibiotics make the issue of resistance so complex and require novel strategies for maintaining effective therapies against infectious diseases. Multiple Drug Resistance (MDR) bacteria are commonly referred to as those resistant to at least three classes of different antibiotics (Zhou et al., 2022).

New antibiotic research faces significant scientific, financial, and regulatory hurdles, making the battle against antimicrobial resistance quite challenging. The low financial returns or high costs of development, pharmaceutical corporations have been increasingly withdrawing from antibiotic research. Estimates suggest that it takes 10 to 15 years and approximately USD 1 billion to bring a new antibiotic to market (Alam et al., 2021). The complex regulatory environment, strict safety rules, and commercial incentives significantly discourage pharmaceutical innovation. Newly developed antibiotics quickly become ineffective because of the rapid establishment of bacterial resistance mechanisms; this further decreases the economic viability of antibiotic research (Hosny et al., 2025). Scientifically, the discovery of new antimicrobial chemicals is rather challenging because of the complexity of bacterial adaptability and the increasing sophistication of resistance mechanisms. More sophisticated methodologies like computer drug design, metagenomic exploration, or interdisciplinary approaches that combine microbiology, genetics, and sophisticated computer techniques are required because traditional screening methods have produced declining returns (Sakagianni et al., 2024).

Inactivation or enzymatic modification of the antibiotic, decreased affinity for binding to bacterial molecular targets, horizontal gene transfer between species through plasmids carrying Multidrug Resistance (MDR) related genes, alterations in bacterial cell surface permeability, overexpression of efflux pumps that can recognize and expel a variety of antibiotics with different mechanisms of action, and genetic variations as polymorphisms or insertions at DNA sequences encoding transcriptional regulators are some of the mechanisms of bacterial antibiotic resistance (Kakoullis et al., 2021). Efflux pumps are essential membrane transporters that are involved in metabolism, multidrug resistance, and bacterial pathogenicity. These pumps stop exogenous chemicals like antibiotics, disinfectants, or detergents from reaching their primary biological targets by actively lowering their intracellular concentrations. Consequently, efflux transporters have emerged as interesting targets for the creation of novel inhibitors to fight infectious disorders linked to Multidrug Resistance (MDR) (De Gaetano et al., 2023).

2. FORMATION OF BIOFILMS

Adsorption, Adhesion, Microcolony development, Maturation, and Dispersion are the steps involved in the three-dimensional architecture in Biofilm (Figure - 1). The solid liquid interface of a biofilm surface with an aqueous medium provides an ideal environment for microbe adhesion and growth. The cells of the biofilm colony are closely related to each other, which promotes establishing a gradient in Quorum Sensing (QS), gene exchange, and nutrition availability. Biofilms originate from a turbulent flow condition with a Reynolds number (Re). In fluid mechanics, the Reynolds number is a non-dimensional number that helps in predicting fluid flow patterns in a wide range of situations by measuring the ratio of inertial to viscous forces. A low number of Re< suggests laminar flow, while a high value Re> indicates turbulent flow. Turbulent flow enhances biofilm formation (Wassmann et al., 2017). Reports suggest that bacteria can easily colonize smooth and rough surfaces, the physical nature of a biofilm surface has a negligible impact on bacterial adhesion. Limited research tools in the 1970s restricted the studies conducted to understand the mechanism of biofilm growth. Development of sophisticated instrumentation and technologies unfolded that biofilms are adaptive structures used by microorganisms as a defensive shield that build an advantageous environment which lets them retain nutrients and ensure survival in an unfavourable environment. Moreover, though the biofilms produced by different microbes are highly similar, they may also have little characteristics that are specific to a species. Research conducted in the first decades of the 21st century has explained how physiological processes and natural forces regulate biofilm production (Sonderholm et al., 2017).

Figure 1. Biofilm formation

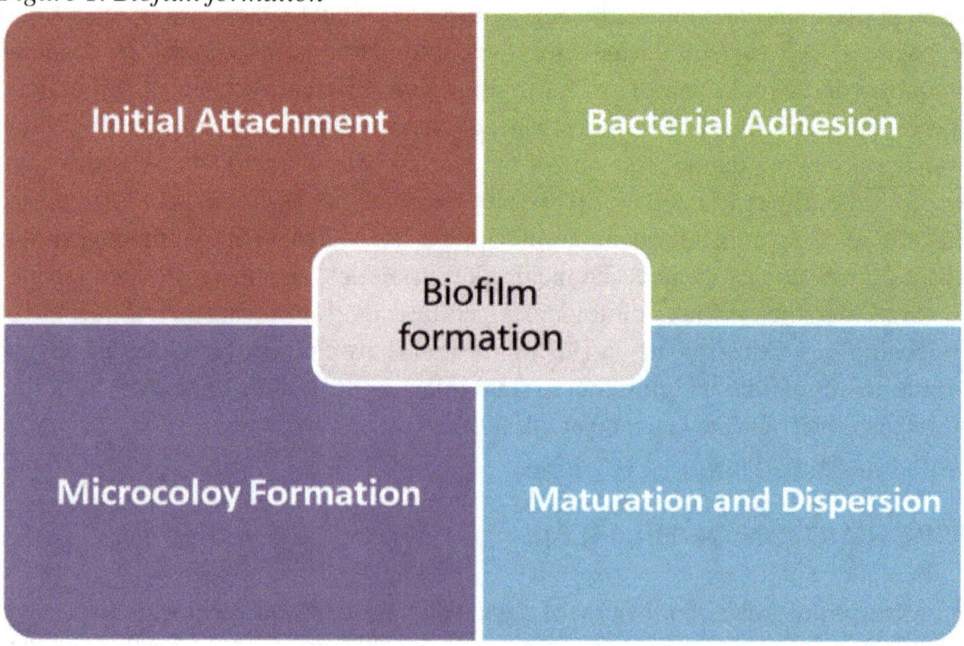

2.1. Initial Attachment

The planktons, the initial stages of attachment begin. These planktons attach to any surface they meet via physical forces or bacterial appendages such as flagellum or pili (Gupta et al., 2016). At this point, it is only a temporal bond that is easily reversed, with chances of it happening through fortuitous encounter. Several variables, including material properties of the substrate, bacterial cell surface properties, temperature, or pressure, determine the degree of adherence by bacteria to any surface they meet. Hydrophobic, steric, electrostatic, van der Waals, and protein adhesions are some of the forces responsible for bacterial adherence. These bacteria are able to resist forces of attraction and remain attached to any surface they meet through the combined effects of the mentioned forces, which result in the formation of an irreversible bacterial monolayer (Veerachamy et al., 2014).

2.2. Bacterial Adhesion and Aggregation

The second phase of adhesion referred to as the anchor or latching phase that involves a molecularly coordinated binding of some of these adhesins to the outermost layer. At this stage, the adhesion process consolidates the loosely attached organisms through the production of Extracellular Polysaccharides (EPS), which reacts with surface materials and receptor-specific ligands that exist in the form of pili, fimbriae, fibrillae, or a combination of both. At this stage, without any form of intervention through physical or chemical means, it is able to make the organisms more tightly adhere to the surface to which they are attached (Paharik & Horswill 2016). At the end of this phase, the organism would be found in a stable, irreversible manner to the surface, much like a cocoon would adhere to a leaf. Some of these organisms would be using a number of various adhesins that would stick them to surfaces dependent on the situation at this phase of adhesion, planktonic forms of microorganisms would adhere to other surface-bound forms of microorganisms as well as each other, resulting in the formation of aggregates on the surface. According to (Lebeaux et al., 2013), it is interesting to point out that the presence of some form of a certain bacterium on an outer layer would influence the adherence of some other forms of bacteria. Several forms of adhesins for these bacteria are produced differently, with some of these adhesins being transcriptionally regulated. This allows organisms to transform from their aquatic, sessile state to becoming planktonic dependent on their environmental stimuli.

2.3. Microcoloy Formation

Bacterial adhesion is followed by cell division and proliferation to create micro-colonies. Certain chemical signals within the EPS and micro communities initiate this process (Anderson et al., 2015). Bacterial colonies usually contain a range of micro-communities in a biofilm. These micro-communities work together in a variety of ways. The interchange of substrates, the movement of important metabolic products, and the removal of metabolic waste all depend on this collaboration. Anaerobic digestion and the breakdown of complex organic matter into CH_4 and CO_2 need the presence of at least three distinct types of bacteria. After complex organic components are broken down, fermenting bacteria start to produce alcohol and acid. These substrates are subsequently eaten by acetogenic bacteria, while methanogens produce methane from acetate, carbon monoxide and hydrogen to provide energy. A complete environment for the development of syntrophic association is provided by biofilm.

2.4. Biofilm Maturation and Dispersion

The linked cells mature and continue to develop during the fourth stage of biofilm formation, known as maturation. The connected bacterial cells secrete molecules that facilitate maturation and lead to the expression of genes specific to biofilms. To increase the virulence of bacteria, factors assist change the regulation of genes. The first step in the process is the cells production of EPS, which protects the biofilm from antimicrobial agents and stabilizes its structure (Joo & Otto 2012). For instance, during maturation, *Pseudomonas aeruginosa* produces distinct saccharides that provide biofilm durability. A paper claims that environmental DNA, or e-DNA, is in charge of biofilm strength and intracellular signaling. The epidermidis polysaccharide intercellular adhesion (PIA) antigen protects the growing bacteria against polymorphonuclear leukocytes in addition to promoting initial attachment (Vuong et al., 2004). When cells accumulate and aggregate on the surface, numerous layers of cell clusters are formed. The EPS, which is where Quorum Sensing (QS) & intercellular signaling take place, also encases these clusters as they finally grow into microcolonies. In general, maturation happens in two phases Cell-to-cell contact and the production on neural signal molecules, such as N-acylated homoserine lactone (AHL), are part of stage I, while the expansion of the microcolony size and thickness to approximately 100 μm, which is the definition of an established microcolony, is part of stage II). The bacteria in the biofilm work together to form connections, and the degree of connectedness between them is determined by their distance from one another. In the maturation phase, bacteria can identify the size and proximity of neighbouring groups, which helps them form clusters that can more successfully make bonds with neighbouring cells (Gu et al., 2013). Instead of regulating gene and protein expression through individual bacterial cells, the entire bacterial colony in the biofilm does so. The production of EPS, cellular aggregation, chemical bonding, QS, and the formation of micro and macro-colonies comprise the second stage. One crucial stage in the creation of biofilms is dispersion, the process by which bacteria move from one area of an infected person's body to another to spread infection. Two distinct layers are usually present in a biofilm. There are two layers, the base layer, where the bacteria are present in greater quantities, and the top layer, which serves as a dispersal zone where the bacteria spread and remain in the environment. This stage causes severe illnesses such embolic issues and chronic infections, which need for immediate medical attention. This method is therefore commonly referred to as metastatic seeding (Chao et al., 2014) become limited as a biofilm ages, and hazardous metabolic byproducts accumulate. Thus, in order to proliferate, acquire nutrients, and eliminate stressful circumstances and waste products, the microbial cells disperse to different regions of the diseased host or the medical implant (Oppenheimer-Shaanan et al., 2013). To start the dispersion process, single cells or groups of cells that have been separated from the biofilm are assembled and that for the case of aerobic bacteria, it is triggered by either an oxygen level or a nutritional deficit. Tiny molecules like the fatty acid DSF (cis-11-methyl-2-dodecenoic acid) become activated in auto phosphorylation in reaction to the deficit. Cyclic diguanylate Guanosine Monophosphate (c-di-GMP) is broken down by the cyclic diguanylate phosphodiesterase, which is activated by this auto phosphorylation. When Cyclic diguanylate Guanosine Monophosphate (c-di-GMP) breaks down, shear pressures or planktonic cell discharge tear apart biofilm clusters, which subsequently dissolve portions of EPS (Grande et al., 2014). There are more processes engaged in the death of EPS than gene regulatory networks. An example of such a process is the enzymes produced by the bacterial cells to help in the degradation of saccharides. This process release the top layer of bacteria as it helps break down the polysaccharide matrix that traps the biofilm.

3. QUORUM SENSING (QS) IN BIOFILM DEVELOPMENT

In order to manage their cell density, biofilms employ the use of QS, which is a cell communication system. Using the approach of signals called autoinducers, biofilms manage this complex process to ensure that the density of biofilm tissues does not exceed the threshold. It is bacterial cells that produce autoinducers, with their production rising with the increase in cell density. It is argued that by (Erkihun et al., 2024), the threshold or critical amount of autoinducers reached by a given concentration of microbial cells determines the coordination of the cells. Binding with autoinducers either triggers or inhibits various genes of targets at that given time. At that time, by inducing maximum biofilm development and maximum coordination of virulence factors, this regulation of the QS system allows bacteria to collectively act for the development of the whole microbial community (Mahto et al., 2022). This collective functioning causes the biofilm to work just like an organism that is multicellular, making it feasible for the bacteria to live under various conditions. Apart from managing the number of bacteria, the role of the QS system helps various beneficial mutations for microbes spread through the biofilm colony of microbes, assists development of antibiotic resistances, and manages the availability of nutrients for bacteria. In addition to that, the system is of great importance for the development of biofilms as it influences genes of motilities, production of EPS, and cell surfaces of biofilms (Daquila et al., 2024). This system by producing various metabolites and virulence factors helps bacteria work collectively for defending themselves from other microbes as well as immune systems of hosts. These biofilms that consist of more microbes work for advancing cross-species interactions as well as communications between species since various bacterial species employ various signals of QS.

4. BIOFILM ANTIBIOTIC TOLERANCE (BAT)

Compared to their counterparts forming planktonic environments, bacteria in biofilms are actually more resistant to antibiotic intervention (Shree et al., 2023). While the mechanisms underlying antibiotic resistance in planktonic bacteria are generally well understood, it is unclear how this resistance develops in biofilms. Biofilms contribution to antimicrobial tolerance appears to function in a different way. Interestingly, even though the same cells showed antibiotic resistance earlier in the biofilm mode, antimicrobial sensitivity is rapidly restored shortly as the biofilm-residing cells separate from the main population (Dutt et al., 2022). Thus, alternative routes to antimicrobial resistance from bacteria are anticipated to be included in Biofilm Antibiotic Tolerance (BAT) (Verderosa et al., 2019). These characteristics imply that additional or altered resistance tactics may be a part of biofilm-associated tolerance. The main way that antibiotics work is by blocking the production of proteins, nucleic acids, & cell walls, which increases the permeability of the membranes of cells and produces antimetabolites. bacteria have developed a variety of resistance mechanisms to offset these effects. These tactics include altering the target to stop antibiotic binding, degrading or modifying drugs to render them inactive, employing efflux pumps to actively remove antibiotics from the cell, and avoiding the target through other metabolic pathways. The development of efficient antibiotic therapies and tactics to address the escalating problem of antibiotic resistance depends on elucidating these intricate linkages. The ability of the bacterial pathogens integrated into biofilms to resist antimicrobial treatment by utilizing their pre-existing gene complement is known as BAT. The two forms of BAT observed are induced BAT (from the antimicrobial treatment response) and innate BAT (from biofilm formation). Since antibiotics mostly affect cells that are actively dividing, persistent cells that show high levels of antibiotic resistance while at rest, restricted antibiotic penetration due to the prevalence of EPS (Davenport et al., 2014), and decreased growth rate due to oxygen and nutrient deprivation in internal areas of biofilms all are currently identified as major innate factors that directly influence BAT. Additionally, biofilms show significant horizontal gene transfer, allowing antibiotic resistance traits to spread rapidly across the population. Subsequently, biofilms' three-dimensional structure produces chemical gradients and microenvironments that have the ability to block or neutralize antimicrobial agents. Extracellular DNA (eDNA), which can bind or sequester antimicrobial chemicals, is another component of the biofilm matrix that contributes to resistance (Wood et al., 2013). Increased production of efflux pumps and additional defense mechanisms can be triggered by stress responses inside biofilms. Furthermore, the presence of metabolically dormant "persisted cells" after antimicrobial treatment acts as an arsenal for biofilm regrowth.

5. BIOFILMS IN MEDICAL DEVICE-ASSOCIATED INFECTIONS

5.1. Device-Related Infections

Medical Device-related infections were among the first clinical infections linked to biofilm formation. There is currently no substitute for these devices, patients cannot live without pacemakers, electrical dialysers, joint prosthesis, intravenous catheters, and urine catheters. Additionally, there is an increased risk of infection linked to biofilms using these devices. Most often, *Pseudomonas* and *Staphylococcus* species enter the host via opportunistically infecting a medical equipment. These days, these infections are known as chronic polymer-associated infections (Gotz 2002).

5.1.1 Urinary Tract Infection (UTI)

UTIs, which are the most commonly diagnosed urological infections, are the most common bacterial illnesses. It is believed that women are more susceptible to UTIs than men. Catheter placement during hospital stays is a common cause of UTIs. Additionally, they may arise from bacteria moving from the urethra to a bladder. Some people are predisposed to getting UTIs due to their genetic makeup.

This infection is more often caused by Gram-negative bacterial strains (Walsh & Collyns 2017). UPEC (Uropathogenic *Escherichia coli*) strains are present in the intestinal region but have the potential to move to the urinary system and become pathogenic, they have been reported to be most frequently responsible for straight-forward cases. Bacterial cell surface virulence factors include type 1 fimbriae, flagellum, capsular lipopolysaccharide, or proteins linked to the outside side of the cell membrane. Siderophores and hemolysin are virulence agents that are secreted (Shah et al., 2019).

5.1.2 Catheter-Related Bloodstream Infection

Catheter-related bloodstream infections (CRBSIs) are a major concern in healthcare settings because they increase rates of morbidity, death, and medical costs. They are thought to be the most prevalent nosocomial infections, and longer hospital stays raise the risk of infection (Bouza et al., 2014). Every year, about 400,000 instances of CRBSIs are reported. One of the main causes of CRBSIs is the formation of biofilm on the outside of intravascular catheters, such as Artery Catheters (Acs) and Central Venous Catheters (CVCs). Within the biofilm matrix, microbes are able to reside better. This makes microbes more resistant to antimicrobial agents. As a physical barrier, microbes protect themselves from antimicrobial agents. Moreover, they protect the bacteria from the host immune systems. Eradication of CRBSIs is often achieved by removing the infected catheters since biofilms formed are very tough (Zhang et al., 2016). Several factors contribute to biofilm formation in catheters. Some of the factors that influence biofilm formation include catheter material, procedure of inserting the catheters, the length of time spent with the catheters, or any previous medical ailment of the patient. *Staphylococcus epidermis, Staphylococcus aureus, Enterococcus species, Candida species* (Esposito et al., 2013) namely *Candida albicans, Candida parapsilosis* are some of the microbial species that show association with CRBSIs. Biofilms pose detrimental effects on catheters. These biofilms generate chronic bloodstream infections, septicems, systemic infections such as endocarditis, among various other severe infections. These biofilms also provide a reservoir for microbes to migrate to other body areas, adding to the complexities of present infections among patients. It is important to provide strict asepsis while inserting catheters or to invariably make the hands clean while dealing with the catheters. This should ensure less formation of biofilms in the catheters. Even using antimicrobial impregnated catheters is not enough. There are studies that show application of anti-infective materials to significantly reduce microbial contaminations of the catheters. These findings reveal that application of anti-infective materials significantly prevents microbial contaminations of the catheters. Key elements of biofilm-based therapeutic techniques are shorter residence times of the microbial species, altering microbial species properties for effective destruction, disrupting microbial species cell walls. These elements would contribute to development of effective therapeutic approaches for CRBSIs (Bruenke et al., 2016).

5.1.3 Ventilator-Associated Pneumonia (VAP)

VAP is a dangerous infection that can affect patients on mechanical ventilation. The formation of biofilms on the surfaces of ventilators and endotracheal tubes is a major part of developing and maintaining VAP, according to (Khazaal et al., 2020). VAP manifestations appear after 48 hours of mechanical breathing. A biofilm matrix allows bacteria to stick to a surface and build complex structures, enabling their growth in a favorable environment. Microorganisms most commonly related to biofilm-related VAP include *Staphylococcus aureus, Klebsiella pneumoniae, Pseudomonas aeruginosa,* and *Acinetobacter baumanii.* According to Farzi et al. (2023), these biofilms can lead to a number of bad results longer lengths of hospital stay, higher mortality rates, and persistent infection are all possible. These biofilms on the surface of the ventilator and endotracheal tube represent a source for continuous bacterial colonization and promote aspiration of bacteria into the lower respiratory tract. Consequently, lung function is compromised, thus triggering an inflammatory response. The presence of biofilm further complicates the management of VAP due to its ability to evade treatment from antimicrobials. Biofilm-related VAP necessitates the realization of preventive measures and strategies against it. Preventive strategies include closely monitoring infection control policies, regular checking of endotracheal tubes, and the formation of biofilms, along with good oral hygiene. Moreover, for potential treatment of the conditions, research related to surface modification employing different antimicrobial coatings on ETT and biofilm disruption technologies are under consideration (Zangirolami et al., 2020).

5.1.4. Other Device-Related Infections

Biofilm-related diseases can also be observed in contact lenses as well as Intra-Uterine Devices (IUDs). *Lactobacilli plantarum, Staphylococcus epidermis, Candida albicans, Staphylococcus aureus,* and a few species of *Corynebacterium, Enterococci,* etc. can potentially contaminate the tail of IUDs. Even the surface of the contact lenses gets colonized by bacteria Variety of lenses, electrolyte levels, or lens polymer materials, and the type of bacterial strain influence the microbes' ability of attraction. *Staphylococcus epidermis, Escherichia coli,* a few species of *Proteus* sp., *Serratia* sp., *Candida* sp., *Pseudomonas aeruginosa,* and *Staphylococcus aureus* get adhered to the surface of the contact lens, creating biofilm-related illnesses. Biofilm-related diseases can also be observed in contact lenses as well as Intra-Uterine Devices (IUDs) (Hong et al., 2024).

5.1.5. Cystic Fibrosis

Cystic fibrosis is an autosomal recessive genetic condition that affects how well the lungs normally function. Patients with this illness typically have abnormal discharges in the respiratory epithelium due to a malfunction in the Cystic Fibrosis Transmembrane Conductance Regulator protein (CFTR). This causes the epithelium to produce viscous mucus, which makes breathing difficult (Yu et al., 2024). The key factor in patient's bacterial infections is the existence of such a mucus layer. *Staphylococcus aureus, Haemophilus influenzae*, and *Pseudomonas aeruginosa* have been linked to lung infections in persons with cystic fibrosis. The lung area that has been affected with *Haemophilus influenzae* is also more susceptible to subsequent *Pseudomonas aeruginosa* infections. In the lower respiratory tract of young patients, the CFTR gene mutation also harbours lung colonies of *Staphylococcus aureus* or *Haemophilus influenzae*, which are replaced in adulthood by colonies of *Pseudomonas aeruginosa* biofilms have a detrimental effect on the lungs in individuals with cystic fibrosis, and their presence is determined by looking for the bacteria's secreted Homoserine lactone (HSL) in the patients' sputum (Azzaya et al., 2020).

5.1.6. Osteomyelitis

Both bacteria and fungi can cause osteomyelitis, a disease of the bone. Trauma, a prior infection, or a direct route (bloodstream) can all facilitate bacterial entrance into the bone. When drawn in through the bloodstream, leucocytes reach the area after the bone's metaphysic becomes contaminated. By releasing enzymes that lyse the bone, these leucocytes attempt to absorb the infection Thus, pus develops and permeates through the blood vessels of the bone, thereby impeding normal blood flow through the bone and causing the death of the bone, or devitalization. Interestingly enough, *Staphylococcus aureus* often emerges as the offending organism in such cases. Due to the presence of fibrin receptors, *Staphylococcus aureus* can adhere to the fibrin present in the bone matrix and subsequently start to form biofilms (Ziran, 2007).

5.1.7. Periodontitis

A gum illness called periodontitis damages both the soft tissues and the bones supporting the teeth. Tooth loss can also result from periodontitis. It is typically caused by inadequate dental and oral hygiene. *Fusobacterium nucleatum* and *Pseudomonas aerobicus*, which may grow on a range of surfaces, including the mucosal surfaces of the oral cavity, are the microorganisms responsible for periodontitis. Colonization facilitates the release of toxins, invasion of mucosal cells, and modification of the calcium flux. Within two to three weeks of bacterial infection, plaque, which consists of a biofilm community, appears. Saliva, which has bactericidal qualities, is unable to reach or permeate the whole biofilm as plaque levels rise, causing dental cavities to form in teeth (Overman, 2007).

5.1.8. Biofilm and Drug Resistance

The microorganisms that make up the biofilm and its structural features are what cause antibiotic resistance. Biofilms may play a major role in the exceedingly complex phenomenon of drug resistance linked to biofilms. Treatment options for biofilms and related infections include antibiotics, disinfectants, and germicidal chemicals. Comparing bacteria in biofilms to their planktonic stage, the former exhibit 10 – 1000 times greater drug resistance, particularly to antibiotics. It has been observed, for instance, that all *Staphylococcus epidermidis* biofilm isolates were sensitive to vancomycin when analyzed planktonically (Wang et al., 2006). Nevertheless, almost 75% of the bacteria were resistant to the same medicines when they were isolated from a biofilm. *Klebsiella pneumoniae* was observed in a similar manner. This strain is highly resistant to several antibiotics when tested from a biofilm, but it is vulnerable when isolated from an aqueous solution.

The development of antimicrobial resistance can be attributed to a variety of factors, including varying growth rates of biofilm microbiological organisms, delayed or insufficient diffusion of antimicrobial drugs through the biofilms, and other functional changes. It is known that bacteria in the planktonic condition can evolve resistance to medications by using mutations, efflux pumps, or enzymes (Sharma et al., 2019). These investigations do not, however, rule out the possibility that antibiotic resistance is influenced by typical biofilm resistance mechanisms. The traditional form of antibiotic resistance was previously noted in *Pseudomonas aeruginosa* that was isolated from a biofilm that was repeatedly exposed to ceftazidime. Drug effectiveness is reduced or eliminated entirely by a variety of unique components within a biofilm, which further fuels resistance. A subgroup of microorganisms in a biofilm that display a form of differentiation akin to spore formation, the biofilm's altered chemical microenvironment and reduced drug penetration are all strategies associated with drug resistance in bacterial biofilm colonies. This condition, which is also known as recalcitrance, happens when bacteria in the biofilm are able to withstand large antibiotic dosages because of a number of independent processes. The development of antibiotic resistance in biofilms is also facilitated by the maintenance of a large number of bacterial cells that survive antibiotic treatment due to tolerance of the slow-growing population and the presence of persisters, a rapid mutation rate, the presence of antimicrobial-selective pressure, and localized competition between mutants in the compartmentalized structure of the biofilms. These investigations do not, however, rule out the possibility that antibiotic resistance is influenced by typical biofilm resistance mechanisms. The traditional form of antibiotic resistance was previously noted in *Pseudomonas aeruginosa* that was isolated to a biofilm that was repeatedly exposed to ceftazidime. The activity of medications that spread via biofilms can be inhibited by EPS through the diffusion-reaction inhibition phenomena. This may in the antibiotics in being destroyed by enzymatic degradation or chelated and forming complexes (Singh et al., 2007).

6. BIOFILM ENHANCES ANTIBIOTIC RESISTANCE

In many parts of the world, antibiotic resistance has surfaced. From 2013 to 2023, the most recent meta-analysis showed an increasing tendency. Southeast Asia, Europe, and Africa had the highest rate of metronidazole resistance, next to clarithromycin. In the majority of places, amoxicillin resistance is not common (Dan et al., 2023). But it started to increase, especially in Mongolia and the DR Congo. One possible explanation for this result is the existence of a biofilm. According to (Pinheiro et al., 2014) a previous study, germs that can form biofilms have a higher level of resistance Increasing the minimum inhibitory doses of antibiotics as of a permanent alteration in cells, such as mutations or the acquisition of resistant functions by horizontal gene transfer, is known as antibiotic resistance (Welch et al., 2005).

6.1. The Barrier of Extracellular Polysaccharide

Increased antibiotic resistance has been linked to exopolysaccharides found in biofilms. They accomplish this by creating a barrier that stops the host's immune cells from phagocytosing antibiotics. Exopolysaccharides contribute to antibiotic resistance by both restricting the entry of drugs and offering structural support during the formation of biofilms. Antibiotics may be introduced gradually to promote adaptive phenotypic responses and possibly increase tolerance (Walsh, 2000).

6.2. The Roles of eDNA and Horizontal Gene Transfer

By changing the surrounding environment, eDNA may also have an impact on antibiotic resistance. An anionic macromolecule called eDNA has the ability to chelate cations like magnesium ions, lowering the atmospheric actual level of Mg_2^+. Antimicrobials and eDNA can also physically interact, with the latter attempting to remove the agent form the sequence targets. Additionally, it promotes the horizontal transmission of resistance genes among the biofilm's competent cells (Kumar et al., 2013). Nonetheless, for a deeper comprehension, the direct processes of eDNA on antibiotic resistance in *Helicobacter pylori* Another important factor in biofilm associated antibiotic resistance is horizontal gene transfer, which points to an evolutionary tactic for environmental adaptation. vertical gene transfer of poles or plasmids by cell division can be energy costly, horizontal gene transfer is more advantageous (Lata et al., 2015). *Haemophilus pylori* possesses conjugation tools such pilis and the Type IV secretion system. Genes that confer antibiotic resistance and other advantageous characteristics can be exchanged between bacterial cells through this procedure, which entails the transfer of genetic material. Bacteria can share antibiotic-resistant genes because biofilms include vesicles that shield nucleic acids from deterioration. A point mutant in locus 2142 or 2143 of 23S rRNA was linked to enhanced biofilm development when exposed to clarithromycin, according to (Magnet et al., 2001) a prior study.

6.3. Relationship Between CRISPR CAS and Antibiotic Resistance

An adaptive immunity mechanism called CRISPR-Cas (clustered routinely interspaced short periodic repeats and its associated Cas proteins) helps defend bacteria against foreign genetic material like plasmids and bacteriophages. Horizontal gene transfer, a frequent way that antibiotic resistance spreads, is naturally inhibited by it. This implies that CRISPR-Cas may be involved in preventing bacterial populations from acquiring and spreading antibiotic resistance genes (Nikaido et al., 2003). Moreover, in more complex bacterial communities, CRISPR-Cas systems can effectively and selectively identify antibiotic resistance genes (ARGs) and destroy pathogenic bacteria without disturbing other bacteria, unlike conventional antibiotics that often lack selectivity and destroy beneficial bacteria. This is to ensure that the CRISPR-Cas systems can effectively target the ARGs, which would ensure that CRISPR-Cas targets the genes using RNA molecules complementary to some DNA sequences.

Due to their selectivity, CRISPR-Cas systems provide a novel means for combating antibiotic-resistance (Sharma et al., 2019). Furthermore, CRISPR-Cas systems can improve the treatment of bacterial infections by making antibiotics effective again through the selection of ARGs for destruction. Due to the ability of CRISPR-Cas systems to target multiple ARGs concurrently, they would provide effective means for combating bacteria that resist multiple medications simultaneously. Research using CRISPR-Cas systems for therapeutic purposes is still in progress. These systems provide novel means for improving health statuses globally and revolutionizing approaches for the treatment of antibiotic-resistant illnesses (Liu et al., 2022). Horizontal gene transfer (HGT) for antibiotic resistance genes is among the factors that contribute to the increase in multidrug-resistant bacteria. CRISPR loci along with CRISPR-associated (Cas) genes, which are found in about 30 – 40% of bacteria in repeated sequences, constitute CRISPR-Cas systems that provide adaptive immunity. These immunity systems utilize the spacers as a form of 'memory' of previous encounters with the attacker. These systems utilize the matching Cas enzymes for cutting down and destroying any sequences that earlier attacked the bacteria (Mah et al., 2001). This is aimed at ensuring that the cell does not let more expensive Mobile Genetic Elements (MGEs) into their tissues to attack their defend by Bacteriophages. *Acinetobacter baumannii* stops the propagation of antibiotic resistance genes by using the I-Fb CRISPR-Cas system. This highly conserved CRISPR-Cas system successfully stops the horizontal transmission of gene elements. The outer membrane permeability of AB43 strains decreased when any part of the CRISPR-Cas system was removed, which is consistent with earlier research on membrane permeability (Cochran et al., 2000). The CRISPR Cas system is associated with a large decrease in virulence variables and a decrease in genes that confer resistance to antibiotics. On the other hand, multidrug resistance was discovered to be associated with the lack of the CRISPR locus. Moreover, the presence of the CRISPR-Cas system is inversely correlated with the incidence of bacterial resistance (Davies, 2003).

The quorum-sensing regulatory las R mRNA has also demonstrated potential in lowering *Pseudomonas aeruginosa* bacterial pathogenicity, especially when the I-F CRISPR-Cas system is used. It's interesting to note that a section of the QS synthase gene aba I, specifically nucleotides 29 to 39 in aba I and its repetitions, largely matches spacer 101 of the CRISPR system. This points to a possible mechanism for the regulation of quorum sensing and pathogenicity in *Pseudomonas aeruginosa* by CRISPR. *Pseudomonas aeruginosa* bacterial pathogenicity has been demonstrated to decrease when the quorum sensing regulator las R mRNA is targeted, especially when the I-F CRISPR-Cas system is employed. It's interesting to note that a section of the QS synthase gene aba I, specifically nucleotides 29 to 39 in aba I and its repetitions, largely matches spacer of the CRISPR system. The strain becomes extremely resistant to most of the drugs examined when any component of the CRISPR-Cas system is removed. The lower quantity of AHLs, the I-Fb CRISPR-Cas system could additionally target and destroy aba I (QS synthase) mRNA, lowering biological characteristics and genes linked to drug resistance (Li et al., 2014). Cas3 cleavage activity was also discovered to be essential for regulating the breakdown of aba I mRNA. Strains susceptible to gentamicin, teicoplanin, erythromycin, and tetracycline were shown to have a much higher number of CRISPR loci. A negative correlation between CRISPR-Cas loci and antibiotic resistance was found, however, as fewer CRISPR loci were found in strains that tested positive for vancomycin (van A), tetra cycline (tet M), macrolides (erm B), aminoglycosides (aac 6'-aph 2”), streptogramins (aad E), and streptothricin (ant 6). Type IIC CRISPR-Cas systems and the absence of antibiotic resistance genes were present in most methicillin-susceptible *Staphylococcus coagulans* isolates. This implies that the acquisition of Antibiotic-resistant genes (ARG) with mobile genomic elements may be impeded by the Type II CRISPR–Cas system in *Staphylococcus coagulans* strains (Fux et al., 2005).

Table 1: Demonstrated various functions of CRISPR-Cas systems in controlling antibiotic resistance and bacterial defense. By keeping intervening sequences and cleaving invasive genetic elements like plasmids and bacteriophages, CRISPR-Cas limits the entry of foreign DNA and offers adaptive protection. CRISPR-Cas systems lessen the acquisition and dissemination of antibiotic resistance genes within bacterial populations by preventing horizontal gene transfer. Their sequence-specific targeting allows for the simultaneous targeting of several resistance determinants, the selective removal of ARGs, and the restoration of antibiotic susceptibility. Furthermore, CRISPR-Cas systems reduce pathogenicity, biofilm formation, and species-specific resistance features by interfering with regulatory genes like as las R and aba I, which affect virulence and quorum sensing.

Table 1. Role of CRISPR–Cas Systems in Controlling Antibiotic Resistance and Virulence

Aspect	Mechanism	Primary Targets	Biological Impact	References
Adaptive immunity	CRISPR loci store spacers as immune memory; Cas enzymes cleave matching invasive DNA	Plasmids, bacteriophages, MGEs	Protection from foreign genetic invasion	(Khangai et al., 2023)
Inhibition of HGT	Sequence-specific targeting of mobile genetic elements	ARG-carrying plasmids	Limits spread of antibiotic resistance	(Fauzia et al., 2020)
Selective ARG targeting	crRNA guides Cas proteins to complementary ARG sequences	Antibiotic resistance genes	Eliminates resistance without harming commensals	(Tseng et al., 2009)
Restoration of antibiotic efficacy	Simultaneous targeting of multiple ARGs	Multidrug resistance determinants	Resensitizes bacteria to antibiotics	(Reighard., 2015)

continued on following page

Table 1. Continued

Aspect	Mechanism	Primary Targets	Biological Impact	References
Virulence regulation	Cas-mediated interference with virulence gene expression	Virulence-associated genes	Reduced pathogenicity	(Hall & Mah., 2017)
Quorum sensing interference	Cas3-dependent cleavage of *lasR* and *abaI* mRNA	QS regulatory genes	Decreased AHL production and biofilm virulence	(Lewis, 2008)
species-specific resistance control	Conserved Type I-F/I-Fb CRISPR-Cas activity	Horizontally transferred genes	Reduced membrane permeability and resistance	(Grande et al., 2012)

7. FUTURE PERSPECTIVES

Future research on illnesses connected to biofilms could go in a number of different areas. The following areas are where improvements can be made: Various Advanced Biofilm Imaging and Detection Methods. In order to diagnose infections linked to biofilms and track the effectiveness of treatment, it will be essential to develop better methods for early detection and precise imaging of biofilms (Khan et al., 2010). To visualize biofilm structures other dynamics in real time, this may include using sophisticated imaging modalities such molecular imaging, high-resolution microscopy, and non-invasive imaging techniques. The development of tailored and customized therapies that take into account the unique properties of biofilms, the makeup of microorganisms, and host variables is crucial for the advancement of biofilm treatment. To isolate the markers for biofilm infections, it would mean using the latest genomes, proteomics, and metabolomics. Combination Therapies: Using a combination of therapies, such as biofilm-dissolving drugs and regular antimicrobials, Future studies on diseases caused by biofilm could progress in a number of ways. These are areas that would see development Various advanced techniques for biofilm imaging and detection. In order to provide a proper diagnosis of infections caused by biofilms and monitor the efficiency of treatment, it is important that more effective techniques of biofilm detection be devised. This would include using advanced techniques of biofilm imaging, such as high-resolution microscopes, molecular imaging, and non-invasive imaging techniques (Xu et al., 2000).

It is important that personalized or customized therapy that takes into account the properties of biofilms, the composition of microbes, and host factors become important for biofilm therapy development. To isolate the markers for biofilm infections, it would mean using the latest genomes, proteomics, and metabolomics techniques. Combination Treatments Greater biofilm destruction could potentially become possible through using multiple treatment options, such as antimicrobials and biofilm-dissolving compounds. It is likely that efforts aimed at disrupting the biofilm matrix and fighting antibiotic resistance would be incorporated into complementary approaches focusing on different phases of biofilm development (orazi & otoole 2019). Nanotechnology and Biomaterials, New solutions for biofilm management would emerge from current research work being done here. It is possible to produce nanoparticles, nanocoating, and material modifications that selectively attack biofilms, destroy it, and release antimicrobial medications in a controlled manner. A significant amount of attention would be given to biofilm engineering as well as research into strategies for either inhibiting or promoting biofilm development. This would mean developing antimicrobial nanocoatings, biofilm-resistant materials, and innovative techniques for preventing biofilm adhesion and subsequent development. Clinical Trials, Validation Studies Well-structured clinical studies and validations are required for effective testing of innovative therapeutic approaches targeting biofilms for testing (Billings et al., 2015). These studies would provide critical evidence for the establishment of standardized procedures for biofilm management as well as the integration of alternative medicines into practice. Finally, areas that could experience improvement with respect to biofilm engineering, combination therapy, personalized therapy, biofilm detection, and clinical validation research include biofilm engineering, combination therapy, personalized therapy, biofilm detection, and clinical validation research significant progress with regard to the management of biofilm-related diseases (Oubekka et al., 2012).

8. CONCLUSION

Biofilm formation represents a highly sophisticated survival strategy that significantly contributes to the persistence and escalation of antibiotic resistance in microbial populations. Through the production of extracellular polymeric substances, quorum sensing–mediated coordination, and the establishment of complex three-dimensional structures, biofilms create protective microenvironments that limit antibiotic penetration, promote metabolic dormancy, and facilitate horizontal gene transfer. These features collectively enable biofilm-associated microorganisms to exhibit markedly higher tolerance and resistance to antimicrobial agents compared with their planktonic counterparts. The clinical implications of biofilms are profound, particularly in chronic and device-associated infections such as catheter-related bloodstream infections, ventilator-associated pneumonia, urinary tract infections, cystic fibrosis, and osteomyelitis, where conventional antibiotic therapies often fail to achieve complete eradication. Understanding the molecular mechanisms underlying biofilm development and biofilm antibiotic tolerance is essential for designing effective intervention strategies. Emerging approaches, including quorum quenching, biofilm-disrupting agents, nanotechnology-based delivery systems, and CRISPR-Cas–mediated targeting of resistance genes, offer promising alternatives to traditional antibiotics. However, translating these strategies into clinical practice requires extensive validation and interdisciplinary collaboration. Overall, combating biofilm-driven antibiotic resistance demands an integrated approach combining prudent antimicrobial use, improved diagnostic tools, innovative therapeutic strategies, and sustained research efforts to mitigate its growing threat to global public health.

9. REFERENCES

Alam, M. M., Islam, N., Hossain Hawlader, M. D., Ahmed, S., Wahab, A., Islam, M., Uddin, K. R., & Hossain, A. (2021). Prevalence of multidrug resistance bacterial isolates from infected wound patients in Dhaka, Bangladesh: A cross-sectional study. *International Journal of Surgery Open*, *28*, 56–62. DOI: 10.1016/j.ijso.2020.12.002

Anderson, J. K., Huang, J. Y., Wreden, C., Sweeney, E. G., Goers, J., Remington, S. J., & Guillemin, K. (2015). Chemorepulsion from the quorum signal autoinducer-2 promotes *Helicobacter pylori* biofilm dispersal. *Molecular Biology*, *6*(4), e00379–e15. DOI: 10.1128/mBio.00379-15 PMID: 26152582

Azzaya, D., Gantuya, B., Oyuntsetseg, K., Davaadorj, D., Matsumoto, T., Akada, J., & Yamaoka, Y. (2020). High antibiotic resistance of *Helicobacter pylori* and its associated novel gene mutations among the Mongolian population. *Microorganisms*, *8*(7), 1062. DOI: 10.3390/microorganisms8071062 PMID: 32708761

Billings, N., Birjiniuk, A., Samad, T. S., Doyle, P. S., & Ribbeck, K. (2015). Material properties of biofilms A review of methods for understanding permeability and mechanics. *Reports on Progress in Physics*, *78*(3), 036601. DOI: 10.1088/0034-4885/78/3/036601 PMID: 25719969

Bouza, E., Guinea, J., & Guembe, M. (2014). The role of antifungals against *Candida* biofilm in catheter-related candidemia. *Antibiotics (Basel, Switzerland)*, *4*(1), 1–17. DOI: 10.3390/antibiotics4010001 PMID: 27025612

Bruenke, J., Roschke, I., Agarwal, S., Riemann, T., & Greiner, A. (2016). Quantitative comparison of the antimicrobial efficiency of leaching versus nonleaching polymer materials. *Macromolecular Bioscience*, *16*(5), 647–654. DOI: 10.1002/mabi.201500370 PMID: 26806336

Chao, Y., Marks, L. R., Pettigrew, M. M., & Hakansson, A. P. (2014). *Streptococcus pneumoniae* biofilm formation and dispersion during colonization and disease. *Frontiers in Cellular and Infection Microbiology*, *4*, 194. DOI: 10.3389/fcimb.2014.00194 PMID: 25629011

Cochran, W. L., McFeters, G. A., & Stewart, P. S. (2000). Reduced susceptibility of thin *Pseudomonas aeruginosa* biofilms to hydrogen peroxide and monochloramine. *Journal of Applied Microbiology*, *88*(1), 22–30. DOI: 10.1046/j.1365-2672.2000.00871.x PMID: 10735239

D'Aquila, P., De Rose, E., Sena, G., Scorza, A., Cretella, B., Passarino, G., & Bellizzi, D. (2024). Quorum quenching approaches against bacterial-biofilm-induced antibiotic resistance. *Antibiotics (Basel, Switzerland), 13*(7), 619. DOI: 10.3390/antibiotics13070619 PMID: 39061301

Dan, B., Dai, H., Zhou, D., Tong, H., & Zhu, M. (2023). Relationship between drug resistance characteristics and biofilm formation in *Klebsiella pneumoniae* strains. *Infection and Drug Resistance, 16*, 985–998. DOI: 10.2147/IDR.S395098 PMID: 36824066

Davenport, E. K., Call, D. R., & Beyenal, H. (2014). Differential protection from tobramycin by extracellular polymeric substances from *Acinetobacter baumannii* and *Staphylococcus aureus* biofilms. *Antimicrobial Agents and Chemotherapy, 58*(8), 4755–4761. DOI: 10.1128/AAC.03071-14 PMID: 24913166

Davies, D. (2003). Understanding biofilm resistance to antibacterial agents. *Nature Reviews. Drug Discovery, 2*(2), 114–122. DOI: 10.1038/nrd1008 PMID: 12563302

De Gaetano, G. V., Lentini, G., Famà, A., Coppolino, F., & Beninati, C. (2023). Antimicrobial resistance: Two-component regulatory systems and multidrug efflux pumps. *Antibiotics (Basel, Switzerland), 12*(5), 965. DOI: 10.3390/antibiotics12050965 PMID: 37370284

Dutt, Y., Dhiman, R., Singh, T., Vibhuti, A., Gupta, A., Pandey, R. P., Raj, V. S., Chang, C.-M., & Priyadarshini, A. (2022). The association between biofilm formation and antimicrobial resistance with possible ingenious bio-remedial approaches. *Antibiotics (Basel, Switzerland), 11*(7), 930. DOI: 10.3390/antibiotics11070930 PMID: 35884186

El-Sapagh, S., El-Shenody, R., Pereira, L., & Elshobary, M. (2023). Unveiling the potential of algal extracts as promising antibacterial and antibiofilm agents against multidrug-resistant *Pseudomonas aeruginosa*: In vitro and in silico studies including molecular docking. *Plants, 12*(19), 3324. DOI: 10.3390/plants12193324 PMID: 37765485

Erkihun, M., Asmare, Z., Endalamew, K., Getie, B., Kiros, T., & Berhan, A. (2024). Medical scope of biofilm and quorum sensing during biofilm formation: Systematic review. *Bacteria, 3*(2), 118–135. DOI: 10.3390/bacteria3020009

Esposito, S., Purrello, S. M., Bonnet, E., Novelli, A., Tripodi, F., Pascale, R., Unal, S., & Milkovich, G. (2013). Central venous catheter-related biofilm infections: An up-to-date focus on meticillin-resistant *Staphylococcus aureus*. *Journal of Global Antimicrobial Resistance, 1*(2), 71–78. DOI: 10.1016/j.jgar.2013.04.003 PMID: 27873581

Farzi, N., Oloomi, M., Bahramali, G., Siadat, S. D., & Bouzari, S. (2023). Antibacterial properties and efficacy of LL-37 fragment GF-17D3 and scolopendin A2 peptides against resistant clinical strains of *Staphylococcus aureus, Pseudomonas aeruginosa*, and *Acinetobacter baumannii* in vitro and in vivo model studies. *Probiotics and Antimicrobial Proteins, 15*(5), 1–19. DOI: 10.1007/s12602-023-10053-x PMID: 37148452

Fauzia, K. A., Miftahussurur, M., Syam, A. F., Waskito, L. A., Doohan, D., Rezkitha, Y. A. A., Matsumoto, T., Tuan, V. P., Akada, J., Yonezawa, H., & Yamaoka, Y. (2020). Biofilm formation and antibiotic resistance phenotype of *Helicobacter pylori* clinical isolates. *Toxins, 12*(8), 473. DOI: 10.3390/toxins12080473 PMID: 32722296

Fux, C. A., Costerton, J. W., Stewart, P. S., & Stoodley, P. (2005). Survival strategies of infectious biofilms. *Trends in Microbiology, 13*(1), 34–40. DOI: 10.1016/j.tim.2004.11.010 PMID: 15639630

Götz, F. (2002). *Staphylococcus* and biofilms. *Molecular Microbiology, 43*(6), 1367–1378. DOI: 10.1046/j.1365-2958.2002.02827.x PMID: 11952892

Grande, R., Campli, E. D., Bartolomeo, S. D., Verginelli, F., Giulio, M. D., Baffoni, M., Bessa, L. J., & Cellini, L. (2012). *Helicobacter pylori* biofilm: A protective environment for bacterial recombination. *Journal of Applied Microbiology, 113*(3), 669–676. DOI: 10.1111/j.1365-2672.2012.05366.x PMID: 22639839

Grande, R., Nistico, L., Sambanthamoorthy, K., Longwell, M., Iannitelli, A., Cellini, L., Di Stefano, A., Hall Stoodley, L., & Stoodley, P. (2014). Temporal expression of *agrB, cidA*, and *alsS* in the early development of *Staphylococcus aureus* UAMS-1 biofilm formation and the structural role of extracellular DNA and carbohydrates. *Pathogens and Disease, 70*(3), 414–422. DOI: 10.1111/j.1365-2672.2012.05350.x PMID: 24535842

Gu, H., Hou, S., Yongyat, C., De Tore, S., & Ren, D. (2013). Patterned biofilm formation reveals a mechanism for structural heterogeneity in bacterial biofilms. *Langmuir, 29*(35), 11145–11153. DOI: 10.1021/la402608z PMID: 23919925

Gunther, T., Kramer-Schadt, S., Fuhrmann, M., & Belik, V. (2022). Environmental factors associated with the prevalence of ESBL/AmpC-producing *Escherichia coli* in wild boar (*Susscrofa*). *Frontiers in Veterinary Science, 9*, 980554. DOI: 10.3389/fvets.2022.980554 PMID: 36311652

Gupta, P., Sarkar, S., Das, B., Bhattacharjee, S., & Tribedi, P. (2016). Biofilm, pathogenesis and prevention A journey to break the wall: A review. *Archives of Microbiology, 198*(1), 1–15. DOI: 10.1007/s00203-015-1148-6 PMID: 26377585

Hall, C. W., & Mah, T.-F. (2017). Molecular mechanisms of biofilm-based antibiotic resistance and tolerance in pathogenic bacteria. *FEMS Microbiology Reviews*, *41*(3), 276–301. DOI: 10.1093/femsre/fux010 PMID: 28369412

Hong, T. C., El-Omar, E. M., Kuo, Y. T., Wu, J. Y., Chen, M. J., Chen, C. C., Fang, Y. J., Leow, A. H. R., Lu, H., Lin, J. T., & Wu, M. S. (2024). Primary antibiotic resistance of *Helicobacter pylori* in the Asia-Pacific region between 1990 and 2022: An updated systematic review and meta-analysis. *The Lancet. Gastroenterology & Hepatology*, *9*(1), 56–67. DOI: 10.1016/S2468-1253(23)00306-9 PMID: 37972625

Hosny, S., Elshobary, M. E., & El-Sheekh, M. M. (2025). Unleashing the power of microalgae: A pioneering path to sustainability and achieving the sustainable development goals. *Environmental Science and Pollution Research International*, *32*, 1–31. DOI: 10.1007/s11356-025-36181-1 PMID: 39920498

Joo, H.-S., & Otto, M. (2012). Molecular basis of in vivo biofilm formation by bacterial pathogens. *Chemistry & Biology*, *19*(12), 1503–1513. DOI: 10.1016/j.chembiol.2012.10.022 PMID: 23261595

Kakoullis, L., Papachristodoulou, E., Chra, P., & Panos, G. (2021). Mechanisms of antibiotic resistance in important Gram-positive and Gram-negative pathogens and novel antibiotic solutions. *Antibiotics (Basel, Switzerland)*, *10*(4), 415. DOI: 10.3390/antibiotics10040415 PMID: 33920199

Khan, W., Bernier, S. P., Kuchma, S. L., Hammond, J. H., Hasan, F., & O'Toole, G. A. (2010). Aminoglycoside resistance of *Pseudomonas aeruginosa* biofilms modulated by extracellular polysaccharide. *International Microbiology*, *13*(4), 207–212. DOI: 10.2436/20.1501.01.123 PMID: 21404215

Khangai, A., Saruuljavkhlan, B., Azzaya, D., Gantuya, B., Oyuntsetseg, K., Akada, J., Matsumoto, T., & Yamaoka, Y. (2023). Exploring alternative treatment choices for multidrug-resistant clinical strains of *Helicobacter pylori* in Mongolia. *Microorganisms*, *11*(12), 2852. DOI: 10.3390/microorganisms11122852 PMID: 38137996

Khazaal, S. S., Al-Saryi, N., & Ibrahim, S. A. (2020). Immunomodulation by *Acinetobacter baumannii* of endotracheal tube biofilm in ventilator-associated pneumonia. *Meta Gene*, *24*, 100672. DOI: 10.1016/j.mgene.2020.100672

Kumar, B., Sharma, D., Sharma, P., Katoch, V. M., Venkatesan, K., & Bisht, D. (2013). Proteomic analysis of *Mycobacterium tuberculosis* isolates resistant to kanamycin and amikacin. *Journal of Proteomics*, *94*, 68–77. DOI: 10.1016/j.jprot.2013.08.025 PMID: 24036035

Lata, M., Sharma, D., Deo, N., Tiwari, P. K., Bisht, D., & Venkatesan, K. (2015). Proteomic analysis of ofloxacin-mono resistant *Mycobacterium tuberculosis* isolates. *Journal of Proteomics, 127*(Pt A), 114–121. https://doi.org/DOI: 10.1016/j.jprot.2015.07.031

Lebeaux, D., Chauhan, A., Rendueles, O., & Beloin, C. (2013). From in vitro to in vivo models of bacterial biofilm-related infections. *Pathogens (Basel, Switzerland), 2*(2), 288–356. DOI: 10.3390/pathogens2020288 PMID: 25437038

Lewis, K. (2008). Multidrug tolerance of biofilms and persister cells. *Current Topics in Microbiology and Immunology, 322*, 107–131. DOI: 10.1007/978-3-540-75418-3_6 PMID: 18453274

Li, L., Mendis, N., Trigui, H., Oliver, J. D., & Faucher, S. P. (2014). The importance of the viable but non-culturable state in human bacterial pathogens. *Frontiers in Microbiology, 5*, 258. DOI: 10.3389/fmicb.2014.00258 PMID: 24917854

Liu, Q., Yin, L., Zhang, X., Zhu, G., Liu, H., Bai, F., Cheng, Z., Wu, W., & Jin, Y. (2022). Reversion of ceftazidime resistance in *Pseudomonas aeruginosa* under clinical setting. *Microorganisms, 10*(12), 2395. DOI: 10.3390/microorganisms10122395 PMID: 36557649

Magnet, S., Courvalin, P., & Lambert, T. (2001). Resistance-nodulation-cell division-type efflux pump involved in aminoglycoside resistance in *Acinetobacter baumannii* strain BM4454. *Antimicrobial Agents and Chemotherapy, 45*(12), 3375–3380. DOI: 10.1128/AAC.45.12.3375-3380.2001 PMID: 11709311

Mah, T.-F., & O'Toole, G. A. (2001). Mechanisms of biofilm resistance to antimicrobial agents. *Trends in Microbiology, 9*(1), 34–39. DOI: 10.1016/S0966-842X(00)01913-2 PMID: 11166241

Mahto, K. U., Kumari, S., & Das, S. (2022). Unraveling the complex regulatory networks in biofilm formation in bacteria and relevance of biofilms in environmental remediation. *Critical Reviews in Biochemistry and Molecular Biology, 57*(3), 305–332. DOI: 10.1080/10409238.2021.2015747 PMID: 34937434

Nikaido, H. (2003). Molecular basis of bacterial outer membrane permeability revisited. *Microbiology and Molecular Biology Reviews : MMBR, 67*(4), 593–656. DOI: 10.1128/MMBR.67.4.593-656.2003 PMID: 14665678

Oppenheimer-Shaanan, Y., Steinberg, N., & Kolodkin-Gal, I. (2013). Small molecules are natural triggers for the disassembly of biofilms. *Trends in Microbiology, 21*(11), 594–601. DOI: 10.1016/j.tim.2013.08.005 PMID: 24080023

Oubekka, S. D., Briandet, R., Fontaine-Aupart, M.-P., & Steenkeste, K. (2012). Correlative time-resolved fluorescence microscopy to assess antibiotic diffusion-reaction in biofilms. *Antimicrobial Agents and Chemotherapy, 56*(6), 3349–3358. DOI: 10.1128/AAC.00216-12 PMID: 22450986

Overman, P. R. (2007). Biofilm: A new view of plaque. *The Journal of Contemporary Dental Practice, 1*(3), 18–29. DOI: 10.5005/jcdp-1-3-18 PMID: 12167880

Paharik, A. E., & Horswill, A. R. (2016). The staphylococcal biofilm: Adhesins, regulation, and host response. *Microbiology Spectrum, 4*(2). Advance online publication. DOI: 10.1128/microbiolspec.VMBF-0022-2015 PMID: 27227309

Pinheiro, L., Brito, C. I., Pereira, V. C., Oliveira, A., Camargo, C. H., & Cunha, M. L. R. S. (2014). Reduced susceptibility to vancomycin and biofilm formation in methicillin-resistant *Staphylococcus epidermidis* isolated from blood cultures. *Memorias do Instituto Oswaldo Cruz, 109*(7), 871–878. DOI: 10.1590/0074-0276140128 PMID: 25410990

Reighard, K. P. (2015). Antibacterial action of nitric oxide-releasing chitosan oligosaccharides against *Pseudomonas aeruginosa* under aerobic and anaerobic conditions. *Antimicrobial Agents and Chemotherapy, 59*(10), 6506–6513. DOI: 10.1128/AAC.01208-15 PMID: 26239983

Sakagianni, A., Koufopoulou, C., Koufopoulos, P., Kalantzi, S., Theodorakis, N., Nikolaou, M., Paxinou, E., Kalles, D., Verykios, V. S., & Myrianthefs, P. (2024). Data-driven approaches in antimicrobial resistance: Machine learning solutions. *Antibiotics (Basel, Switzerland), 13*(12), 1052. DOI: 10.3390/antibiotics13121052 PMID: 39596745

Shah, C., Baral, R., Bartaula, B., & Shrestha, L. B. (2019). Virulence factors of uropathogenic *Escherichia coli* (UPEC) and correlation with antimicrobial resistance. *BMC Microbiology, 19*(1), 204. DOI: 10.1186/s12866-019-1587-3 PMID: 31477018

Sharma, D., Misba, L., & Khan, A. U. (2019). Antibiotics versus biofilm: An emerging battleground in microbial communities. *Antimicrobial Resistance and Infection Control, 8*, 76. DOI: 10.1186/s13756-019-0533-3 PMID: 31131107

Shree, P., Singh, C. K., Sodhi, K. K., Surya, J. N., & Singh, D. K. (2023). Biofilms: Understanding the structure and contribution towards bacterial resistance in antibiotics. *Medicine in Microecology, 16*, 100084. DOI: 10.1016/j.medmic.2023.100084

Singh, P. K., Schaefer, A. L., Parsek, M. R., Moninger, T. O., Welsh, M. J., & Greenberg, E. P. (2007). Quorum-sensing signals indicate that cystic fibrosis lungs are infected with bacterial biofilms. *Nature*, *407*(6805), 762–764. DOI: 10.1038/35037627 PMID: 11048725

Sonderholm, M., Bjarnsholt, T., Alhede, M., Kolpen, M., Jensen, P. Ø., Kuhl, M., & Kragh, K. N. (2017). The consequences of being in an infectious biofilm: Micro-environmental conditions governing antibiotic tolerance. *International Journal of Molecular Sciences*, *18*(12), 2688. DOI: 10.3390/ijms18122688 PMID: 29231866

Tseng, Y. S., Wu, D. C., Chang, C. Y., Kuo, C. H., Yang, Y. C., Jan, C. M., Su, Y. C., Kuo, F. C., & Chang, L. L. (2009). Amoxicillin resistance with beta-lactamase production in *Helicobacter pylori*. *European Journal of Clinical Investigation*, *39*(9), 807–812. DOI: 10.1111/j.1365-2362.2009.02166.x PMID: 19614952

Veerachamy, S., Yarlagadda, T., Manivasagam, G., & Yarlagadda, P. K. (2014). Bacterial adherence and biofilm formation on medical implants: A review. *Proceedings of the Institution of Mechanical Engineers. Part H, Journal of Engineering in Medicine*, *228*(10), 1083–1099. DOI: 10.1177/0954411914556137 PMID: 25406229

Verderosa, A. D., Totsika, M., & Fairfull-Smith, K. E. (2019). Bacterial biofilm eradication agents: A current review. *Frontiers in Chemistry*, *7*, 824. DOI: 10.3389/fchem.2019.00824 PMID: 31850313

Vuong, C., Voyich, J. M., Fischer, E. R., Braughton, K. R., Whitney, A. R., DeLeo, F. R., & Otto, M. (2004). Polysaccharide intercellular adhesin (PIA) protects *Staphylococcus epidermidis* against major components of the human innate immune system. *Cellular Microbiology*, *6*(3), 269–275. DOI: 10.1046/j.1462-5822.2004.00367.x PMID: 14764110

Walsh, C. (2000). Molecular mechanisms that confer antibacterial drug resistance. *Nature*, *406*(6797), 775–781. DOI: 10.1038/35021219 PMID: 10963607

Walsh, C., & Collyns, T. (2017). The pathophysiology of urinary tract infections. *Surgery (Oxford)*, *35*(6), 293–298. DOI: 10.1016/j.mpsur.2017.03.007

Wang, G., Yang, H., Olczak, A. A., Maier, S. E., & Maier, R. J. (2006). Dual roles of *Helicobacter pylori* NapA in inducing and combating oxidative stress. *Infection and Immunity*, *74*(12), 6839–6846. DOI: 10.1128/IAI.00991-06 PMID: 17030577

Wassmann, T., Kreis, S., Behr, M., & Buergers, R. (2017). The influence of surface texture and wettability on initial bacterial adhesion on titanium and zirconium oxide dental implants. *International Journal of Implant Dentistry*, *3*(1), 32. DOI: 10.1186/s40729-017-0093-3 PMID: 28714053

Welch, K. T., Virga, K. G., Whittemore, N. A., Ozen, C., Wright, E., Brown, C. L., Lee, R. E., & Serpersu, E. H. (2005). Discovery of non-carbohydrate inhibitors of aminoglycoside-modifying enzymes. *Bioorganic & Medicinal Chemistry*, *13*(22), 6252–6263. DOI: 10.1016/j.bmc.2005.06.059 PMID: 16140014

Wood, T. K., Knabel, S. J., & Kwan, B. W. (2013). Bacterial persister cell formation and dormancy. *Applied and Environmental Microbiology*, *79*(23), 7116–7121. DOI: 10.1128/AEM.02636-13 PMID: 24038684

Yu, Y., Xue, J., Lin, F., Liu, D., Zhang, W., Ru, S., & Jiang, F. (2024). Global primary antibiotic resistance rate of *Helicobacter pylori* in recent 10 years: A systematic review and meta-analysis. *Helicobacter*, *29*(1), e13103. DOI: 10.1111/hel.13103 PMID: 38898622

Zangirolami, A. C., Dias, L. D., Blanco, K. C., Vinagreiro, C. S., Inada, N. M., Arnaut, L. G., Pereira, M. M., & Bagnato, V. S. (2020). Avoiding ventilator-associated pneumonia: Curcumin-functionalized endotracheal tube and photodynamic action. *Proceedings of the National Academy of Sciences of the United States of America*, *117*(37), 22967–22973. DOI: 10.1073/pnas.2006759117 PMID: 32868444

Zhang, L., Gowardman, J., Morrison, M., Runnegar, N., & Rickard, C. M. (2016). Microbial biofilms associated with intravascular catheter-related bloodstream infections in adult intensive care patients. *European Journal of Clinical Microbiology & Infectious Diseases*, *35*(2), 201–205. DOI: 10.1007/s10096-015-2532-5 PMID: 26610337

Zhao, X., Chen, Z., Yang, T., Jiang, M., Wang, J., Cheng, Z., Yang, M., Zhu, J., Zhang, T., Li, H., Li, A., Chen, H., & Wang, H. (2021). Glutamine promotes antibiotic uptake to kill multidrug-resistant uropathogenic bacteria. *Science Translational Medicine*, *13*(625), eabj0716. Advance online publication. DOI: 10.1126/scitranslmed.abj0716 PMID: 34936385

Zhou, Y., Zhong, Z., Hu, S., Wang, J., Deng, Y., Li, X., Chen, X., Li, X., Tang, Y., Li, X., Zheng, Z., & Li, B. (2022). A survey of *Helicobacter pylori* antibiotic-resistant genotypes and strain lineages by whole-genome sequencing in China. *Antimicrobial Agents and Chemotherapy*, *66*(4), e02188–e21. DOI: 10.1128/aac.02188-21 PMID: 35652644

Ziran, B. H. (2007). Osteomyelitis. *The Journal of Trauma and Acute Care Surgery*, *62*(6), S59. DOI: 10.1097/TA.0b013e318065abb6 PMID: 17556977

Chapter 6
Multidrug-Resistant Pseudomonas aeruginosa in Nosocomial Infections

Kehinde Adewole Oyeniran
https://orcid.org/0000-0003-1754-6184
International Centre for Genetic Engineering and Biotechnology, Cape Town, South Africa

Ayoigbala Monioluwa Lawal
https://orcid.org/0009-0003-5243-5401
Federal University, Oye Ekiti, Nigeria

Olubukola Helen Oyeniran
https://orcid.org/0000-0001-5262-7487
Federal University, Oye Ekiti, Nigeria

Busayo Mutiat Olowe
https://orcid.org/0000-0003-0953-4140
Bamidele Olumilua University of Education, Science, and Technology, Ikere-Ekiti, Nigeria

Lara Donaldson
International Centre for Genetic Engineering and Biotechnology, Cape Town, South Africa

ABSTRACT

Pseudomonas aeruginosa is a rod-shaped, Gram-negative bacterium in the family Pseudomonadaceae that is native to soil and water environments. It is also found in other unlikely places, including surgical equipment and on the hands of hospital

DOI: 10.4018/979-8-3373-3825-5.ch006

personnel. This chapter discusses how multidrug-resistant (MDR) P. aeruginosa plays a significant role in hospital-associated opportunistic infections. MDR P. aeruginosa strains are primarily responsible for the high global prevalence of opportunistic pneumonia, bloodborne, and surgical wound infections, particularly in immunocompromised patients. Key mechanisms of resistance in MDR P. aeruginosa can be intrinsic, acquired, and genetic. Addressing antimicrobial drug resistance requires stewardship, hygiene practices, and combining antimicrobials due to limited therapeutic options. Future attempts may involve leveraging multidisciplinary techniques in molecular biology, bioinformatics, and machine learning to improve understanding and management of drug resistance. Novel therapies, vaccine development, and global surveillance are also useful.

1.0 INTRODUCTION

Pseudomonas aeruginosa is a Gram-negative rod-shaped bacterium that is naturally found in soil and water environments (Pei et al., 2025). Soil, as the universal reservoir of microorganisms, plays a key role in maintaining the biogeochemical cycle and in the distribution and redistribution of different microorganisms via a support system that continuously moves them between long-term storage and the transient, temporary airborne-like state (Kästner et al., 2021).

Despite being predominantly found in soil and water environments, *P. aeruginosa* can also thrive in other environments and unlikely places, such as on medical devices and on the hands of healthcare workers, as a result of which it is commonly associated with nosocomial, or hospital-associated infections. Nosocomial diseases are mild to life-threatening iatrogenic conditions – predisposed hospital-acquired infections that have emerged as a critical global concern in healthcare settings (Elfadadny et al., 2024). The prevalence of *P. aeruginosa*-associated infections in intensive care units (ICU) is particularly concerning, ranking as the third most frequently isolated bacterium from infections acquired within these critical care environments (Ahmed, 2022).

The ability of *P. aeruginosa* to colonise both biotic and abiotic surfaces within hospital environments contributes greatly to its persistent spread and uncanny capability to infect nearly all body systems, further exacerbating its clinical significance (Letizia et al., 2025). Infections caused by *P. aeruginosa* often result in pneumonia, septicaemia, urinary tract infections, and difficult-to-treat surgical site infections (Reynolds & Kollef, 2021). The internal resistance mechanism driving resistance to multiple antibiotics in this bacterium via the acquisition of resistance genes not only promotes the emergence of multidrug-resistant strains but also significantly complicates treatment and handling strategies (Sindeldecker & Stoodley, 2021).

Furthermore, genome-encoded virulence factors and resistance determinants are valid virulence drivers conferring key adaptive traits to different conditions and host immunity (Jurado-Martín et al., 2021; Sathe et al., 2023). Based on the few applicable therapeutic options for infections caused by multi-strains of multidrug-resistant *P. aeruginosa,* it has been identified by the World Health Organisation (WHO) as a critical pathogen requiring urgent development of new antibiotics because of its very many innate, acquired, and adaptive resistance mechanisms (Chen et al. 2023).

P. aeruginosa is highly prevalent and can be found in most unexpected places, including healthcare facilities, mostly as a result of its ability to produce biofilms that support its persistence in the environment (Fernández-Billón et al., 2023). Unlike the fastidious *Lactobacillus* sp., for instance, *P. aeruginosa* can utilise a variety of carbon sources like simple carbohydrates, organic acids, and even complex polymers (Matuszewska et al., 2021). Lastly, its ability to mount resistance to multiple antibiotics and the evolutionary advantages this confers also position it as a progressing virulence evolution in multiple hosts. Therefore, understanding the mechanisms, epidemiology, and management strategies of multidrug-resistant *P. aeruginosa* in nosocomial infections relative to current practices and techniques may provide better ways for control.

Here, we examine the incidence of multidrug-resistant *P. aeruginosa* in nosocomial infections, resistance mechanisms, and their management in the context of modern practices, result-orientated future treatment and control perspectives.

2.0 EPIDEMIOLOGY AND PREVALENCE

2.1 Opportunistic Pathogen and a Major Nosocomial Threat

The frequent rate of *P. aeruginosa*-associated nosocomial infections stems from its many adaptive mechanisms conferring genetics that make both antimicrobial resistance and ubiquitous status in the healthcare settings possible. The continuous sustenance of *P. aeruginosa* in moist healthcare settings and its very common recovery from surfaces and medical equipment may further showcase its versatile metabolism, water activity requirement, and drug resistance profile (Morin et al., 2021).

Factors contributory to the transmission of *P. aeruginosa* in healthcare settings are contaminated equipment, workers' hygiene, and environmental sources like water and fomites (e.g., respiratory equipment). For a fact, *P. aeruginosa* exhibits a preponderance for colonising medical devices such as catheters and ventilators, with biofilm production playing a key role in antibiotic resistance and weakened host defences, producing persistent infections in immunocompromised, cystic fibrosis and organ transplant patients (Maurice et al., 2018; Sole et al., 2025) *P. aeruginosa* can cause a broad range of infections in patients with serious underlying medical conditions and is a leading cause of healthcare-associated secondary infections worldwide (Sathe et al., 2023). Patients in intensive care and burn units, and those undergoing mechanical ventilation, are twice as vulnerable to *P. aeruginosa* infections (Reynolds & Kollef, 2021).

As an opportunistic pathogen of particular concern to WHO, *P. aeruginosa* can cause and exacerbate most iatrogenic, nosocomial infections in immunocompromised patients recovering from procedures such as organ transplants, a condition that may be further complicated by graft-versus-host reactions and multi-drug resistance (Flores-Vega et al., 2025; Sanya et al., 2023). The bacterium often exploits vulnerabilities in host defences to establish infections in various sites, leading to significant morbidity and mortality (Elfadadny et al., 2024; Liao, 2023). In addition to its role in hospital-acquired infections (Figure 1), *P. aeruginosa* can also be found in community settings, particularly in individuals with chronic respiratory conditions or those who have frequent exposure to water sources. However, acute respiratory infections with *P. aeruginosa* may be transiently cleared by the host immune response or antibiotic treatment, but failure to control the infection may result in bacteraemia or respiratory failure from a full-blown infection or excessive immune-mediated damage (Nickerson et al., 2024).

Figure 1. An overview of Pseudomonas aeruginosa dissemination as an opportunistic pathogen in nosocomial infection. Soil and water serve as its natural reservoirs, facilitating its spread through interactions with living organisms. The ubiquitous nature of P. aeruginosa is strongly supported by its non-fastidious nutritional status. However, the long-term implications for the dissemination of multidrug-resistant strains to natural habitats remain unclear

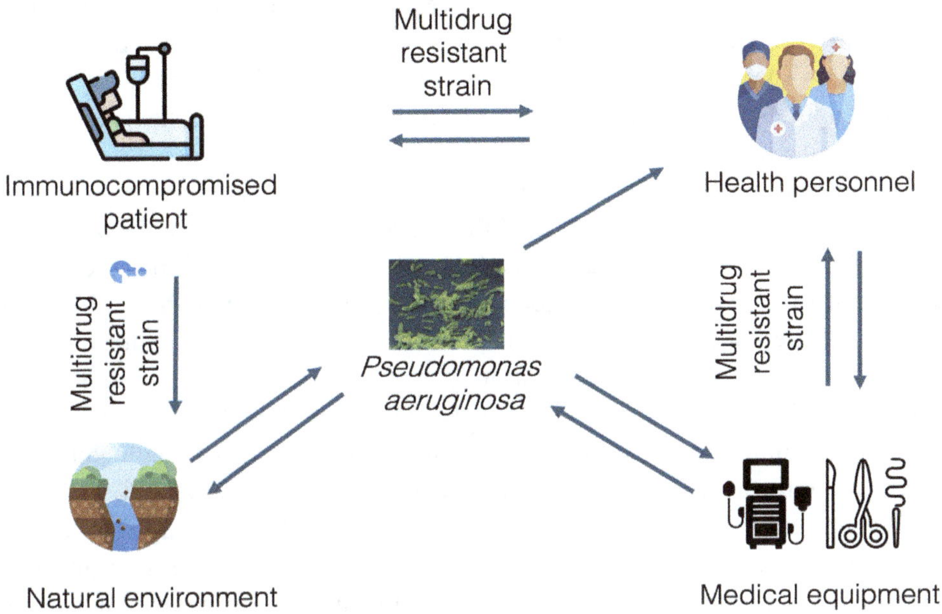

2.2 Hospital Prevalence

In global terms, resistance to high-end broad-spectrum antibiotics is rapidly increasing. Antibiotics such as carbapenems and polymyxin B that are central to treating ICU-associated strains. In a developed country like the United States, approximately 7% of hospital-associated infections are caused by *P. aeruginosa* (Reynolds & Kollef, 2021). Brazil and Poland have experienced approximately 48.7% and 66.7% of nosocomial infection-associated *P. aeruginosa* isolates with multidrug resistance to a diverse range of both broad- and narrow-spectrum antibiotics, respectively, with notable elevated incidence in critically ill and immunocompromised patients or those with problematic anatomical barriers (Ribeiro et al., 2019;Shortridge et al., 2018).

The overall global economic burden of antimicrobial resistance sits at a median estimate of US$693 billion in hospital costs and almost US$194 billion in productivity losses (Naylor et al., 2025). Relative to sensitive strains, the increase in hospital stays for resistant strains could be between 1.37- and 1.77-fold (Morales et al., 2012). The specific attributable cost of infection with a resistant strain, in addition to a length of stay of 7.4 days and a 49.2% higher odds of readmission is likely between -US$2,371.4 and +US$29,289.1 per patient episode (Sendra et al., 2024).

About ten years ago in Europe, multidrug resistance was 13% of *P. aeruginosa* isolates; this observation has since been on the increase (Polemis et al., 2024). A bothersome discovery revealed increasing prevalence of multidrug-resistant strains in hospitals worldwide, with some regions reporting rates as high as 30-40% (Karruli et al., 2023). These high prevalence rates are pointers to the concerns of limited treatment options available for managing infections caused by resistant strains and the likely spike in morbidity, mortality, and healthcare costs.

A recent study from a tertiary care hospital in Saudi Arabia, from data spanning between 2013 and 2022, reported that 37.5% of *P. aeruginosa* isolates were multidrug-resistant, 5.3% were extensively drug-resistant, and 3.5% met the criteria for difficult-to-treat resistance (Shabi et al., 2025). In like manner, the China Antimicrobial Surveillance Network (CHINET) 2024 surveillance report for hospitals across China shows that *P. aeruginosa* imipenem and meropenem resistance rates in 2024 were 21.3% and 17.3%, respectively (Guo et al., 2025).

In sub-Saharan Africa, multidrug-resistant *P. aeruginosa* is a leading cause of nosocomial infections. *P. aeruginosa* incidence rates are between 20% and 70%, with higher rates in ICUs and surgical wards (Kothari et al., 2022). In Nigeria, 43% of *P. aeruginosa* isolates from clinical samples were resistant to all tested antibiotic categories, with research facilities in tertiary healthcare settings finding higher rates of MDR isolates in clinical samples (Awanye et al., 2022; Olalekan et al., 2023). In Zambia, Kenya, and Ethiopia, resistance to carbapenems by MDR *P. aeruginosa* is on the rise, making it a major contributor to hospital-acquired infections in these countries (Asamenew et al., 2023; Kaluba et al., 2021; Ramatla et al., 2025)

3.0 RESISTANCE MECHANISMS

As part of their evolution, pathogens continuously devise means to restore the natural balance amidst the chaos caused mostly by anthropogenically induced changes. One such means is the evolution of resistance genes that have become a major threat to modern healthcare. *P. aeruginosa* shows remarkable adaptability through various resistance mechanisms that foster better ability to tolerate and resist antimicrobial agents (Elfadadny et al., 2024). These resistance mechanisms can be innate or intrinsic, acquired, and adaptive in nature, each contributing to its ability to evade antibiotic action (Figure 2).

Figure 2. The underlying molecular-driven processes responsible for antibiotic resistance in Pseudomonas aeruginosa work complementarily towards achieving a common target. These processes are at the interplay of various core interconnected processes that include inactivation of antibiotics via enzymatic breakdown, pump systems that prevent antibiotics from reaching recommended intracellular concentrations, genetic mutations and gene transfer, alteration of cell membrane permeability and quorum sensing-guided biofilm formation.

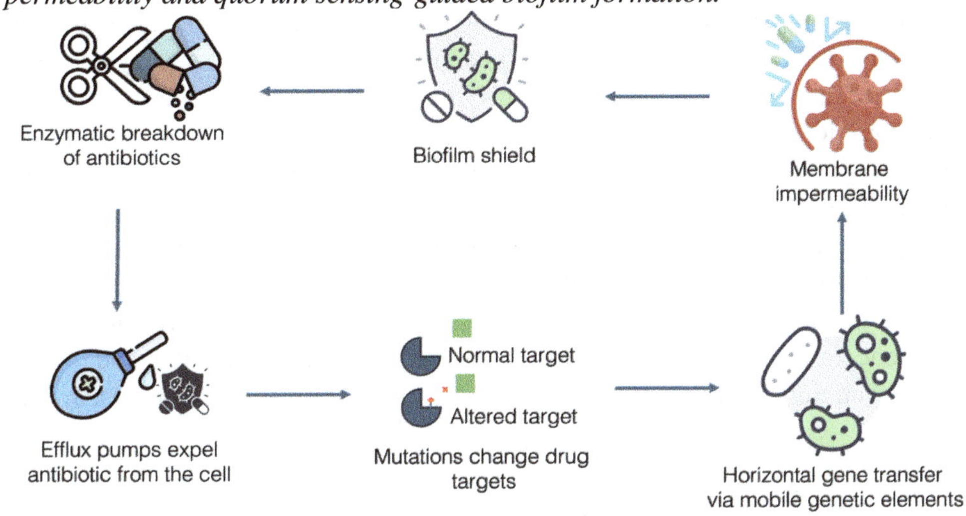

3.1 Intrinsic Resistance

These are mostly internally regulated measures that have evolved as both defensive and adaptive strategies to either evade or prevent antibiotic cell entry and subsequent accumulation. In addition to active efflux pump systems, these measures may also involve a partial alteration or complete loss of outer membrane permeability. Outer membrane modifications specifically involve lowering or lessening the expression of porins or completely disrupting the lipopolysaccharide to prevent antibiotic entry into the cell. While efflux pumps simultaneously pump antibiotics out of the cell, preventing the right intracellular concentration (Yin et al., 2024). Furthermore, several other chromosomally encoded efflux pumps, such as MexAB-OprM, MexCD-OprJ, and MexEF-OprN, which actively expel a wide range of antibiotics from the cell, are also common (Pang et al., 2019). Because these processes provide a fundamental level of resistance to multiple antibiotics, they make *P. aeruginosa* difficult to control.

3.2 Acquired Resistance

This occurs when previously drug-sensitive bacteria develop resistance over time due to long-term exposure to such a drug. *P. aeruginosa* can mount resistance to most broad-spectrum antibiotics through many subsystems of horizontal gene transfer. Horizontal gene transfer, which includes molecular processes like transduction, transformation, and conjugation, allows *P. aeruginosa* or any other bacteria to acquire resistance genes from different bacteria of varying backgrounds (Pepi et al., 2021). These horizontally transferred genes may encode enzymes such as beta-lactamases, aminoglycoside-modifying enzymes, and carbapenemases that render antibiotics useless (Pei et al., 2025). For example, beta-lactamases attack the beta-lactam ring of penicillin and cephalosporins via hydrolysis, rendering them ineffective. Aminoglycoside-modifying enzymes add new chemical groups to aminoglycosides, which causes a critical structural change that can be disruptive to their ability to bind to ribosomes and prevent protein synthesis. Antibiotic-degrading enzymes like metallo-beta-lactamases and serine carbapenemases are particularly more concerning due to their broad substrate range activities on carbapenems, our last-line antibiotic defence for many Gram-negative bacterial infections (Dettori et al., 2023).

3.3 Genetic Mutation-Mediated Resistance

Genetic mutations as a key driver of evolution in pathogens may from time to time cause the emergence of resistant strains. Mutations in chromosomal genes can confer traits that may be beneficial to microorganisms. Once these mutations are fixed, they may be expressed as resistance to antibiotics. In a large population, most frequent mutations are useless or deleterious, while beneficial mutations, on the contrary, may become fixed. For instance, mutations in the genes that code for DNA gyrase or topoisomerase IV in *P. aeruginosa* can give rise to quinolone-resistant strains, while mutant genes encoding ribosomal proteins may confer resistance to aminoglycosides. These mutations may alter drug target sites and lessen their affinity and effectiveness. Mutations in genes encoding proteins involved in cell wall synthesis or other essential cellular processes can also contribute to antibiotic resistance.

The rate of resistance formation by mutation depends solely on how frequently the changes introduced by mutations result in viable phenotypic events, such as a clear spike in the minimum inhibitory concentration (MIC) that is above the breakpoint concentration needed for resistance to attain clinically relevant levels (McCallum et al., 2010). Every time a bacterium cell divides, there is a possibility of a mutation due to replication errors or DNA damage (Guo, 2021). Further, additional forces like recombination and selection at the interplay of the evolution of virulence and resistance are also contributory to the genetic change effects. Recombination is common in bacteria, as it is a natural phenomenon that maintains variation in genomes, ensuring that progenies are not mere clones of their ancestors (Andam, 2019). It is therefore useful to posit that understanding how this process works can give better strategic insights into managing evolving phenotypes (Table 1).

Table 1. Mutation-mediated resistance mechanisms of Pseudomonas aeruginosa to commonly available antibiotics (Ambreetha & Singh, 2023; Fernández-Billón et al., 2023).

Antibiotic Class	Specific Antibiotics	Resistance Mechanisms
Beta-Lactams	Penicillin, cephalosporins (e.g., ceftazidime), carbapenems (e.g., imipenem and meropenem)	Production of beta-lactamases like Verona-integron-encoded metallo-â-lactamase (VIM), imipenemase (IMP), and New Delhi metallo-â-lactamase (NDM), altered penicillin-binding proteins, decreased outer membrane permeability
Fluoroquinolones	Ciprofloxacin, levofloxacin	*gyrA* mutations, efflux pumps
Aminoglycosides	Gentamicin, tobramycin, amikacin	Aminoglycoside-modifying enzymes, ribosomal mutations, decreased uptake
Polymyxins	Polymyxin B, colistin	Modifications of lipid A, increased efflux

4.0 CLINICAL INFECTIONS

4.1 Pneumonia

Pneumonia is an inflammatory condition of the lungs characterised by fluid accumulation rather than air. Pneumonia poses a significant global health burden that readily affects vulnerable populations of children, the elderly, and individuals with compromised immune systems. While different pathogens can trigger pneumonia, notable bacterial infections by *Streptococcus pneumoniae*, *Haemophilus influenzae*, and *Staphylococcus aureus* constitute primary causal agents (Wei et al., 2024). In addition, other opportunistic pathogens that infect the lower respiratory tract may also cause pneumonia. MDR *P. aeruginosa* is a baffling cause of pneumonia in healthcare settings due to its innate resistance mechanisms and the high likelihood of acquiring resistance genes (Li et al., 2024; Lynch & Zhanel, 2022).

Fernández-Barat et al. (2017) posited that MDR *P. aeruginosa* was the most frequent aetiology (64, 29%); 22 (34%) of intensive care unit-acquired pneumonia (ICUAP) cases and that risk factors such as previous antibiotic treatment, solid cancer and shock, alcohol abuse, and pleural effusion were independently associated with lower risk for ICUAP, while *P. aeruginosa* remains the most frequent causative agent of ICUAP, with high prevalence of multiple drug resistance. A comparable study conducted by Borgatta et al. (2017) was done using respiratory specimens infected with MDR *P. aeruginosa*. The results from four medical-surgical ICUs showed that 21 (67.7%) adults with MDR *P. aeruginosa* pneumonia lost their lives after a median of four days compared with 1 (2.6%) without pneumonia at day eight. Nevertheless, most isolated *P. aeruginosa* strains (85.1%) were sensitive to amikacin and colistin, while resistance to beta-lactams of the third-generation cephalosporins and piperacillin–tazobactam ranged between 44.1% and 45.3%. A substantial proportion, approximately one-third, of adult patients in intensive care units presented with multidrug-resistant *P. aeruginosa*. These patients often face a sixfold increase in mortality risk compared to those with other respiratory problems like ventilator-associated tracheobronchitis and respiratory colonisation.

These findings are also supported by Idigo et al. (2022), where the incidence of MDR *P. aeruginosa* in community-acquired pneumonia (CAP) and chronic obstructive pulmonary disease (COPD) was 22% (36) and 18% (167), respectively. MDR *Pseudomonas* CAP was stable over time, while COPD was mostly associated with *Pseudomonas* CAP but not with MDR *Pseudomonas* CAP. The yearly incidence of MDR *Pseudomonas* CAP was, however, consistent. Furthermore, comparative studies in the incidence of nosocomial versus community-acquired pneumonia caused by *P. aeruginosa* showed that *P. aeruginosa* and MDR *P. aeruginosa* were resistant to a variety of commonly used antibiotics. Interestingly, few isolates recovered from patients with pneumonia were, nevertheless, not resistant to colistin, a polymyxin antibiotic for treating infections by sensitive Gram-negative bacteria (Yayan et al., 2015).

4.2 Bloodstream Infections

Bloodstream infections are severe systemic infections caused by the presence of viable bacteria in the bloodstream. Bloodstream infection by multidrug-resistant *P. aeruginosa* is still a major worldwide concern because of significant increase in the associated morbidity, mortality, and healthcare costs. Systemic infection can occur from pneumonia, urinary tract, surgical site, and catheter-related sources. As bloodstream infection-causing bacteria become resistant to the administered antibiotics, infection lingers, increasing the length of stay in the hospital and the associated economic costs (Figure 3).

P. aeruginosa causes sepsis and bacteraemia, with potential for further opportunistic complications by other, often unrelated, microbes. Colonisation rates in at-risk patients, such as those with prolonged exposure to healthcare settings or chronic illnesses, can reach up to 80%, often compounded by the plausibility of multidrug-resistant strain acquisition via prolonged antibiotic therapy (Mendes Pedro et al., 2024). Bloodstream infections are very difficult to treat and often require careful consideration of the choice of effective antibiotics (Ozma et al., 2022). Even after antibiotic administrations, clinical outcomes usually remain poor, with a significant mortality rate in immunocompromised patients. (Elfadadny et al., 2024).

Risk factors play a key role in determining the mortality status of MDR *P. aeruginosa* in bloodstream infections. Previously identified independent risk factors for MDR *P. aeruginosa* include the presence of a central venous catheter (CVC), antibiotic and corticosteroid therapies, while those for non-MDR *P. aeruginosa* include previous bloodstream infection (BSI), neutrophil count <500/mm^3, urinary catheterisation, and presence of a CVC, with the 21-day mortality rate of all patients being 33.9% (Tumbarello et al., 2011).

Bloodstream infection in patients with other hospital-associated sicknesses in Ethiopia had a frequency of 11 (4.6%), with 100% resistance to ampicillin and piperacillin and 36.4% and 45.5% against ciprofloxacin and meropenem, respectively (Motbainor et al., 2020). Further, Viasus et al. (2020) posited that of the 661 Gram-negative BSI episodes, 190 (28.7%) were caused by MDR *P. aeruginosa.* These findings show that independent factors linked to MDR *P. aeruginosa* were haematological malignancy, nosocomially acquired BSI, previous antipseudomonal cephalosporins, and BSI occurring during ceftriaxone treatment.

4.3 Wound and Surgical Site Infections

Wound and surgical site infections are another common means of spread for many nosocomial bacteria, including *P. aeruginosa*. Wounds can arise as a result of various causes that may include surgery, trauma, burns, or other underlying medical conditions and can lead to a variety of complications like prolonged healing, increased pain, and the development of chronic wounds, healing complications, lengthy hospital stays, and increased economic burden (Rafiq et al., 2022). In patients with compromised immune systems, such as those with diabetes, undergoing chemotherapy or organ transplants, the risk of wound infections is twice as likely. *P. aeruginosa* is frequently found in patients with burns, surgical wounds, pus, and accidental wounds (Chegini (Chegini et al., 2020). While surgical sites are expected to be sterile, sometimes, microbes and other forms of contaminants may be introduced.

Opportunistic colonisation of wounds and surgical site infections is quite common, especially in developing countries where healthcare settings mostly lack standard hygiene practices and aseptic methods. *P. aeruginosa* is the second most isolated pathogen from chronic wound infections in North America and Africa, with a range of between 4.5% and 28% and a median of approximately 15% and 23%, respectively (Phan et al., 2023). Infections of surgical sites can occur either externally, at the incision site, or internally, at the tissues and organs in the surgical area. Frequent incidences of infected surgical sites are red flags that can be used to assess the overall aseptic conditions and practices in any healthcare setting (Figure 3).

Figure 3. Graphics-aided illustration of clinical infections with P. aeruginosa and their overall implications described in five stages under sources of infection, colonisation, invasion, organ dysfunction and clinical implications.

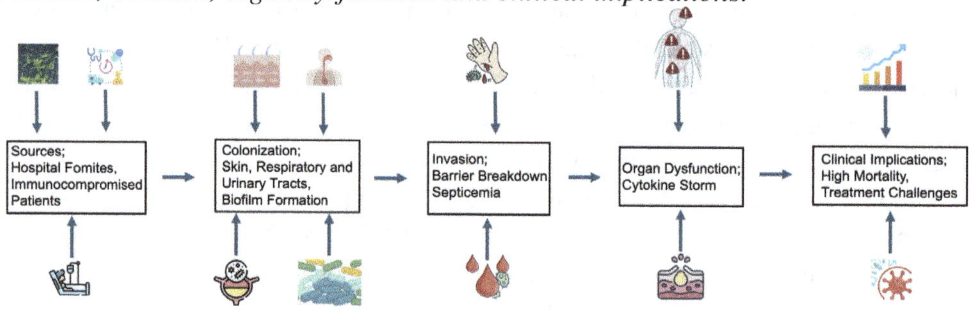

5.0 PREVENTION, TREATMENT CHALLENGES, AND CONTROL STRATEGIES

5.1 Prevention

Addressing antimicrobial drug resistance often presents numerous issues related to treatment and control techniques that can successfully tackle indiscriminate use of antibiotics, which is the biggest contributor to the problem. To prevent the spread of MDR *P. aeruginosa*, medical facilities should adhere to the WHO guidelines, which include surveillance, environmental cleanliness, patient isolation, and hand hygiene contact precautions (Reig et al., 2022). For patients who have recently come in contact with or been transferred from hospitals or other healthcare facilities in countries where MDR *P. aeruginosa* is highly prevalent, the European Centre for Disease Prevention and Control (ECDC) recommends improving and expanding surveillance, screening, and preventive isolation in healthcare facilities to stop unintended spread of the pathogen (Meşe et al., 2025). Further, documentation regarding multi-resistant *P. aeruginosa* infection or carrier status at the time of patient transfer would also be useful for implementing prompt and effective spread-halting measures (Spagnolo et al., 2021).

5.2 Treatment Challenges

Antibiotic therapy with a key emphasis on risk factors and infection advancement remains the basic treatment for *P. aeruginosa* infections. In vitro susceptibility testing is empirically used to assess plausible treatment outcomes for severe infections using two classes of antibiotics, frequently combining and de-escalating to monotherapy (Bassetti et al., 2018). The first line of treatment for *P. aeruginosa* infections is aminoglycoside and beta-lactam penicillin, with many other broad-spectrum antibiotics demonstrating activities against the pathogen. Apart from the range of antibiotics used to treat *P. aeruginosa* infections, β-lactam antibiotics, such as penicillin, and β-lactamase inhibitors work in synergy to increase the efficacy of β-lactam antibiotics (Smith et al., 2017).

Despite the pressing need for efficient therapies, *P. aeruginosa* infection remains a challenge to treat and manage. With respect to vaccination, none of the three *P. aeruginosa* vaccines that had been tested in Phase III clinical trials were approved for use (Elmassryet al., 2023).

5.3 Control Strategies

5.3.1 Adhesion Inhibition

During biofilm formation and host infection, *P. aeruginosa* adheres to lung epithelial cells using specific lectins, Lec-A and Lec-B. The quorum sensing (QS) system through which bacteria cells talk to one another and lectin-carbohydrate interactions that control adherence to surfaces have salient roles in biofilm formation and could serve as key targets for adhesion inhibition. Likewise, sugar components and glycopeptide polymers prevent lectin binding, which halts infection and biofilm colony growth. Nanotechnology can also be used to create functional EH40 steel films that stop *P. aeruginosa* from adhering to host cells (Jangra et al., 2022).

5.4 Role of Antimicrobial Stewardship in Preventing Resistance

5.4.1 Unconstrained Use of Antimicrobial Agents

Unconstrained use of antimicrobial agents is important for antibacterial medications that have long been adjudged safe, reasonably priced, and effective in clinical settings while having minimal impact on bacterial resistance. Following an examination, the medical personnel may administer the antimicrobial medication and have unlimited use of it.

5.4.2 Regulated Use of Antimicrobial Agents

In the case of antibiotics that clearly impact bacterial resistance, there exist restrictions depending on the drug efficacy, safety, cost, and other factors. As a result of which their use ought to be restricted. Following training and testing, physicians with intermediate-level or higher qualifications may be able to administer antimicrobial drugs with limited usage.

5.4.3 Specific Use of Antimicrobial Agents

To avoid the bacteria developing strong resistance and causing serious problems, antimicrobial agents should be used carefully in certain situations. A dearth of clinical evidence still likely exists on the safety, effectiveness, or superiority of novel antibiotics over those that are currently in use (Lanckohr & Bracht, 2022). Additionally, because these medications are costly, their usage needs to be strictly regulated. Special use of such antimicrobial medications is recommended only for physicians who are sub-senior or above sub-senior certified, and they can prescribe them following training and evaluation.

5.5 Infection Control Measures

These include appropriate education programmes that encourage basic hygiene practices, such as wearing gloves and hand washing. To ensure hygienic conditions, alcohol-based hand gel dispensers should be placed in each room and aisle of hospitals. There should be implementation of daily measures to prevent contact with infected patients, such as putting them in open-structured wards or single rooms. To look into the spread of infection and cross-infection, cultural practices should be constantly examined from time to time. To prevent cross-contamination and careless spread, some equipment should be reserved for patients infected with *P. aeruginosa*, with a strict environmental cleaning plan (Li et al., 2021).

5.6 Surveillance and Early Detection

Surveillance and early detection are major aspects of nosocomial infection control that can be activated to control the spread of MDR *P. aeruginosa*. Given its high morbidity and mortality rate in healthcare settings, medical practitioners, researchers, microbiologists and policymakers should work together to address this problem. Policymakers can make provisions for methods leveraging rapid diagnostics and clinical surveillance with preliminary test assays in the early detection of MDR *P. aeruginosa* (Zhou et al., 2024).

5.7 Biofilm Prevention Strategies

5.7.1 Combined Therapy of New Antimicrobial Agents

Combining antibiotics with substances like gallium, phage therapy, and antimicrobial photodynamic therapy (aPDT) can damage biofilm structural integrity and kill bacteria (Yin et al., 2022). For instance, aPDT is known for attacking bacterial cells and biofilm structures by matching antibiotics, such as gentamicin, with photosensitisers like methylene blue. When antimicrobial photothermal therapy (aPTT) is used alongside aPDT and nanoparticles, it produces localised heat and reactive singlet oxygen that effectively disrupt biofilm, shrinking its size.

5.7.2 Nanoparticles

Quorum sensing expression is critical to effective communication in bacteria; once a quorum is successfully established, the potential for other applications, such as in biofilm formation for antibiotic resistance, is also possible. Targeting quorum sensing expression with nanoparticles such as the green-synthesised silver nanoparticles (AgNPs) and colistin (CL) may be more efficient in preventing biofilm formation and quorum sensing gene expression in resistant ICU *P. aeruginosa* isolates from burn patients (Azimzadeh et al., 2025). While either of these agents may have near-marginal activity, combining them delivered more significant damage to biofilm structural integrity. As a promising supplement to traditional antibiotics, nanoparticles may improve penetration and disrupt bacterial membranes.

Infection control efforts also vary between countries. While the developing countries generally experience higher rates of nosocomial infections due to a lack of resources, infrastructure and prevention strategy implementation, developed countries often have access to more resources and a robust strategy for infection control (Table 2). Despite these efforts, both developed and developing countries still struggle with controlling the spread of multidrug-resistant bacterial strains.

Table 2. Comparative summary of antimicrobial resistance management in developing and developed countries.

Features	Developing Countries	Developed Countries	Source
Resource Availability and Policy Implementation	Policy implementation that is geared towards controlling the spread of multidrug-resistant organisms is often beset with strapped resources.	Have better resources, which makes it easier to follow international guidelines and national policies for controlling antimicrobial resistance.	(Saliba et al., 2023)
Infection Prevention and Control	Significant challenges in controlling environmental contamination within healthcare settings still exist.	Well-established infection control protocols, better infrastructure, and consistent access to resources, which aid in reducing the spread of *P. aeruginosa* in hospitals.	(Ogunsola & Mehtar, 2020)
Antimicrobial Stewardship Programs	The lack of local treatment guidelines and microbiological data often drives inappropriate antimicrobial use, which in turn stifles key antimicrobial stewardship efforts.	Antimicrobial stewardship efforts are more widely implemented and integrated into hospital systems, with a focus on antibiotic use optimization for better patient outcomes	(Harun et al., 2024; Kakkar et al., 2020; Muro et al., 2022; Pallares et al., 2023)
Diagnostic Capabilities and Surveillance:	Limited diagnostic facilities still contribute to inappropriate antimicrobial prescription practices	Advanced diagnostic techniques and robust surveillance systems foster better tracking of resistance patterns and informed treatment decisions.	(Ayukekbong et al., 2017)
Regulatory Framework and Education	Bad prescription practices, inadequate patient education, unauthorized sale of antimicrobials and non-existent regulatory framework.	Stronger regulatory bodies for drug sales and prescriptions with comprehensive public and professional education campaigns on appropriate antibiotic use.	(Ayukekbong et al., 2017)

6.0 FUTURE DIRECTIONS

6.1 Multidisciplinary Approach

A coordinated and consistent approach is required to address the growing challenge of antimicrobial resistance in *P. aeruginosa*-associated nosocomial infections. Future perspectives must leverage modern multidisciplinary techniques in the fields of molecular biology, bioinformatics, and machine learning to enhance our understanding of drug resistance and management. Whole-genome sequencing can aid in the development of targeted treatments for known and novel resistance genes, as well as their genetic mutations (Ahmed, 2022).

Bioinformatics techniques often complement molecular biology for better and intuitive results. For example, following the acquisition of sequence data from field samples, phylogenetic analysis can provide insights into how closely related new strains are to the existing ones, which is useful in detecting elusive or rapidly evolving strains most likely to cause an outbreak. Moreover, machine learning methods are also useful algorithms that can supercharge the process of unravelling resistance genes or mechanisms in *P. aeruginosa*. However, the major challenge is overcoming the likelihood of intensive computational biology procedures in places where these infrastructures are non-existent.

6.2 Novel Therapies

The integration of computational techniques in drug discovery can quicken the evaluation of several novel drug candidates within a short period of time, thereby fostering the development of better potential drugs. Combination therapies, phage therapy, monoclonal antibodies, immunotherapy (Elshobary et al., 2025; Olawade et al., 2024), and the clustered regularly interspaced short palindromic repeats (CRISPR-Cas) gene editing tool may provide effective and viable alternative strategies to conventional antibiotics in combating MDR *P. aeruginosa* (Pang et al., 2019; Sindeldecker & Stoodley, 2021).

CRISPR-Cas systems, although still in their infancy, have, however, been proven to target and disrupt resistance genes (Pei et al., 2025). Like the CRISPR-Cas systems, RNA interference (RNAi) can also be used to silence critical genes in *P. aeruginosa* (Pei et al., 2025). A problem that may beset the latter is the means of delivery to *P. aeruginosa* in an infected patient. Other promising alternative treatments include the use of liposomes for anti-virulence strategies, antimicrobial peptides, metal ions, compounds, and plant-derived bioactive compounds (Abreu et al., 2012; Singha et al., 2024).

6.3 Prospects of Vaccine Development

The possibility of computational and appropriate wet bench validation techniques as a gold standard can result in limitless prospects of vaccine development. Vaccines targeting specific virulence factors or conserved antigens could provide lasting protection and significantly reduce the incidence and severity of infections in vulnerable groups. However, more research in vaccine development is needed to identify suitable targets and delivery systems.

6.2.1 Current Challenges, Approaches, and Targets

Despite considerable research strides from the last fifty years, a *P. aeruginosa* vaccine for human use is yet to be approved. Without any doubts, advancements are evident in preclinical investigations, particularly in the areas of antigen identification, adjuvant usage, and innovative delivery methods pinpointing specific virulence factors or conserved antigens as potential targets (Killough et al., 2022; Sainz-Mejías et al., 2020). To this end, several antigen candidates have undergone evaluation in both animal and human clinical trials; however, none of these candidates has been approved basically due to the complex and evasive nature of the bacterium's adaptability to the immune system (Wan et al., 2021). In addition, the bacterium's polyhydroxyalkanoate inclusions and the flagella hook protein *FlgE* have been proposed as a novel vaccine candidate (Rehm et al., 2021; Sainz-Mejías et al., 2020)

6.2.2 Obstacles

The evaluation of potential vaccine candidates is commonly plagued by the many complexities of conducting trials within patient cohorts. One such complexity includes individual vaccine hesitation due to deep socio-cultural and religious beliefs; without the opportunity for a robust and safe evaluation of potential candidates, vaccine breakthroughs are impossible (Santamarina-Fernández et al., 2025). For the bacterium, genetic plasticity, elaboration of virulence determinants, and antimicrobial resistance often compound the difficulties associated with formulating efficacious vaccines (Sathe et al., 2023). Further, the convergence of virulence factors can quickly turn infections into therapeutic dilemmas requiring innovative strategies.

6.2.3 Future success

The development of *P. aeruginosa* vaccine has been a long and challenging walk; however, research is ongoing. The design of effective vaccines requires the core understanding of how the pathogen interacts with its host and vice versa. Given that evolution plays a key role here, this may require a long learning curve covering a major understanding of whether a pathogen co-evolves with its host or not, which may also be a determining factor in identifying key vaccine targets. Nevertheless, there is hope for future success considering the ongoing advances in methods and multidisciplinary nature of life science research (Merakou et al., 2018; Sainz-Mejías et al., 2020).

6.3 Global Surveillance Networks for Multi-Drug-Resistant *Pseudomonas aeruginosa*

There is a need for coordinated efforts to implement and keep global surveillance networks for *P. aeruginosa*. Firstly, the idea is to establish these surveillance hubs in all continents so that monitoring and data transfer can happen seamlessly. That said, policymakers and administrators must provide a thriving environment for a global collaborative approach among researchers, healthcare professionals, bacteriologists, and evolutionary biologists to share data, insights, and best practices for fighting *P. aeruginosa* and other potentially deadly, hospital-associated bacterial infections (Sathe et al., 2023).

The centralised database practices for storing and analysing surveillance data from around the world will enforce standardised surveillance protocols are applicable to data collection and analysis in a way that makes data from different regions comparable (Ahmed, 2022). Also, laboratory capacity should be improved through personnel training and retraining so that modern molecular techniques can be leveraged more effectively for great progress (Werner et al., 2023). Finally, policymakers should put more effort into healthcare facility surveillance, especially in intensive care units where life-threatening nosocomial infections are most common, as this will help keep an eye on and treat infected vulnerable groups.

7.0 CONCLUSION

Multidrug-resistant *P. aeruginosa* is a major culprit in hospital-associated or nosocomial opportunistic infections, and its specific growing prevalence in pneumonia, blood-borne, wound, and surgical infections is a cause for significant concern and urgent action. Addressing this challenge will require a better understanding of the incidence, epidemiology, and control strategies that can translate into effective diagnosis, management, and case handling. Despite ongoing efforts to manage and control this menace, some challenges with indiscriminate antibiotic use or non-compliance with antibiotic stewardship, limited therapy options, and vaccine development still stifle progress. Nevertheless, leveraging multidisciplinary techniques that integrate the understanding of molecular biology, genetics, bioinformatics, and machine learning can significantly aid in the discovery of improved therapeutic agents with better actions.

ACKNOWLEDGEMENT

Kehinde Oyeniran is grateful to the International Centre for Genetic Engineering and Biotechnology (ICGEB) for sponsorship.

REFERENCES

Abreu, A. C., McBain, A. J., & Simões, M. (2012). Plants as sources of new antimicrobials and resistance-modifying agents. *Natural Product Reports*, *29*(9), 1007–1021. DOI: 10.1039/C2NP20035J PMID: 22786554

Ahmed, O. B. (2022). Detection of Antibiotic Resistance Genes in Pseudomonas aeruginosa by Whole Genome Sequencing. *Infection and Drug Resistance*, •••, 6703–6709. DOI: 10.2147/idr.s389959 PMID: 36425153

Ambreetha, S., & Singh, V. (2023). Genetic and environmental determinants of surface adaptations in Pseudomonas aeruginosa. *Microbiology (United Kingdom)*, *169*(6). Advance online publication. DOI: 10.1099/MIC.0.001335 PMID: 37276014

Andam, C. P. (2019). Clonal yet Different: Understanding the Causes of Genomic Heterogeneity in Microbial Species and Impacts on Public Health. *mSystems*, *4*(3). Advance online publication. DOI: 10.1128/msystems.00097-19 PMID: 31219786

Asamenew, T., Worku, S., Motbainor, H., Mekonnen, D., & Deribe, A. (2023). Antimicrobial Resistance Profile of Pseudomonas aeruginosa from Different Clinical Samples in Debre Tabor Comprehensive Specialized Hospital, Northwest Ethiopia. *Ethiopian Journal of Health Sciences*, *33*(3), 423–432. DOI: 10.4314/EJHS.V33I3.5 PMID: 37576170

Awanye, A. M., Ibezim, C. N., Stanley, C. N., Onah, H., Okonko, I. O., & Egbe, N. E. (2022). Multidrug-Resistant and Extremely Drug-Resistant Pseudomonas aeruginosa in Clinical Samples From a Tertiary Healthcare Facility in Nigeria. *Turkish Journal of Pharmaceutical Sciences*, *19*(4), 447–454. DOI: 10.4274/TJPS.GALENOS.2021.66066 PMID: 36047595

Ayukekbong, J. A., Ntemgwa, M., & Atabe, A. N. (2017). The threat of antimicrobial resistance in developing countries: causes and control strategies. *Antimicrobial Resistance & Infection Control 2017 6:1*, *6*(1), 47-. https://doi.org/DOI: 10.1186/S13756-017-0208-X

Azimzadeh, M., Greco, G., Farmani, A., Nourian, A., Pourhajibagher, M., Taherkhani, A., Alikhani, M. Y., & Bahador, A. (2025). Biofilm inhibition of multidrug-resistant Pseudomonas aeruginosa using green-synthesized silver nanoparticles and colistin. *Scientific Reports, 15*(1), 1–15. DOI: 10.1038/S41598-025-00005-6 PMID: 40301384

Bassetti, M., Vena, A., Croxatto, A., Righi, E., & Guery, B. (2018). How to manage Pseudomonas aeruginosa infections. *Drugs in Context, 7*, 212527. DOI: 10.7573/DIC.212527 PMID: 29872449

Borgatta, B., Gattarello, S., Mazo, C. A., Imbiscuso, A. T., Larrosa, M. N., Lujàn, M., & Rello, J. (2017). The clinical significance of pneumonia in patients with respiratory specimens harbouring multidrug-resistant Pseudomonas aeruginosa: A 5-year retrospective study following 5667 patients in four general ICUs. *European Journal of Clinical Microbiology & Infectious Diseases, 36*(11), 2155–2163. DOI: 10.1007/S10096-017-3039-Z/TABLES/4 PMID: 28624864

Chegini, Z., Khoshbayan, A., Taati Moghadam, M., Farahani, I., Jazireian, P., & Shariati, A. (2020). Bacteriophage therapy against Pseudomonas aeruginosa biofilms: a review. *Annals of Clinical Microbiology and Antimicrobials 2020 19:1, 19*(1), 1–17. https://doi.org/DOI: 10.1186/S12941-020-00389-5

Chen, L., Qu, X., Su, J., Yao, H., Yuan, Q., Wang, Y., Li, N., Wu, G., Liu, X., Hu, J., & Zhang, J. (2023). The dilemma of antibiotic susceptibility and clinical decision-making in a multi-drug-resistant Pseudomonas aeruginosa bloodstream infection. *Frontiers in Pharmacology, 14*, 1183332. DOI: 10.3389/FPHAR.2023.1183332 PMID: 37324460

Dettori, S., Portunato, F., Vena, A., Giacobbe, D. R., & Bassetti, M. (2023). Severe infections caused by difficult-to-treat Gram-negative bacteria. In *Current Opinion in Critical Care* (Vol. 29, Issue 5, pp. 438–445). Lippincott Williams and Wilkins. https://doi.org/DOI: 10.1097/MCC.0000000000001074

Elfadadny, A., Ragab, R. F., AlHarbi, M., Badshah, F., Ibáñez-Arancibia, E., Farag, A., Hendawy, A. O., De los Ríos-Escalante, P. R., Aboubakr, M., Zakai, S. A., & Nageeb, W. M. (2024). Antimicrobial resistance of Pseudomonas aeruginosa: Navigating clinical impacts, current resistance trends, and innovations in breaking therapies. *Frontiers in Microbiology, 15*, 1374466. DOI: 10.3389/FMICB.2024.1374466/XML/NLM PMID: 38646632

Elmassry, M. M., Colmer-Hamood, J. A., Kopel, J., San Francisco, M. J., & Hamood, A. N. (2023). Anti-Pseudomonas aeruginosa Vaccines and Therapies: An Assessment of Clinical Trials. *Microorganisms 2023, Vol. 11, Page 916, 11*(4), 916. https://doi.org/DOI: 10.3390/MICROORGANISMS11040916

Elshobary, M. E., Badawy, N. K., Ashraf, Y., Zatioun, A. A., Masriya, H. H., Ammar, M. M., Mohamed, N. A., Mourad, S., & Assy, A. M. (2025). Combating Antibiotic Resistance: Mechanisms, Multidrug-Resistant Pathogens, and Novel Therapeutic Approaches: An Updated Review. *Pharmaceuticals 2025, Vol. 18, Page 402, 18*(3), 402. https://doi.org/DOI: 10.3390/PH18030402

Fernández-Barat, L., Ferrer, M., De Rosa, F., Gabarrús, A., Esperatti, M., Terraneo, S., Rinaudo, M., Li Bassi, G., & Torres, A. (2017). Intensive care unit-acquired pneumonia due to Pseudomonas aeruginosa with and without multidrug resistance. *The Journal of Infection, 74*(2), 142–152. DOI: 10.1016/j.jinf.2016.11.008 PMID: 27865895

Fernández-Billón, M., Llambías-Cabot, A. E., Jordana-Lluch, E., Oliver, A., & Macià, M. D. (2023). Mechanisms of antibiotic resistance in Pseudomonas aeruginosa biofilms. *Biofilm, 5*, 100129. DOI: 10.1016/J.BIOFLM.2023.100129 PMID: 37205903

Flores-Vega, V. R., Partida-Sanchez, S., Ares, M. A., Ortiz-Navarrete, V., & Rosales-Reyes, R. (2025). High-risk Pseudomonas aeruginosa clones harboring β-lactamases: 2024 update. *Heliyon, 11*(1), e41540. DOI: 10.1016/J.HELIYON.2024.E41540 PMID: 39850428

Guo, Y. (2021). Removal Ability of Antibiotic Resistant Bacteria (Arb) and Antibiotic Resistance Genes (Args) by Membrane Filtration Process. *IOP Conference Series. Earth and Environmental Science, 801*(1), 12004. DOI: 10.1088/1755-1315/801/1/012004

Guo, Y., Ding, L., Han, R., Yin, D., Wu, S., Yang, Y., Wang, F., Zhu, D., & Hu, F. (2025). Antimicrobial resistance profile of clinical isolates from hospitals across China: CHINET 2024 surveillance report. *One Health Advances 2025 3:1, 3*(1), 23-. https://doi.org/DOI: 10.1186/S44280-025-00092-0

Harun, M. G. D., Sumon, S. A., Hasan, I., Akther, F. M., Islam, M. S., & Anwar, M. M. U. (2024). Barriers, facilitators, perceptions and impact of interventions in implementing antimicrobial stewardship programs in hospitals of low-middle and middle countries: a scoping review. *Antimicrobial Resistance & Infection Control 2024 13:1, 13*(1), 8-. https://doi.org/DOI: 10.1186/S13756-024-01369-6

Idigo, A. J., Wells, J. M., Brown, M. L., Wiener, H. W., Griffin, R. L., Cutter, G., Shrestha, S., & Lee, R. A. (2022). Clinical risk factors for admission with Pseudomonas and multidrug-resistant Pseudomonas community-acquired pneumonia. *Antimicrobial Resistance and Infection Control, 11*(1), 1–10. DOI: 10.1186/S13756-022-01137-4/TABLES/4 PMID: 35836272

Jangra, V., Sharma, N., & Chhillar, A. K. (2022). Therapeutic approaches for combating Pseudomonas aeruginosa infections. *Microbes and Infection, 24*(4), 104950. DOI: 10.1016/J.MICINF.2022.104950 PMID: 35139390

Jurado-Martín, I., Sainz-Mejías, M., & McClean, S. (2021). Pseudomonas aeruginosa: An Audacious Pathogen with an Adaptable Arsenal of Virulence Factors. *International Journal of Molecular Sciences 2021, Vol. 22, Page 3128, 22*(6), 3128. https://doi.org/DOI: 10.3390/IJMS22063128

Kakkar, A. K., Shafiq, N., Singh, G., Ray, P., Gautam, V., Agarwal, R., Muralidharan, J., & Arora, P. (2020). Antimicrobial Stewardship Programs in Resource Constrained Environments: Understanding and Addressing the Need of the Systems. *Frontiers in Public Health, 8*, 502288. DOI: 10.3389/FPUBH.2020.00140/BIBTEX PMID: 32411647

Kaluba, C. K., Samutela, M. T., Kapesa, C., Muma, J. B., Hang'ombe, B. M., Hachaambwa, L., Mukomena, P., & Yamba, K. (2021). Carbapenem resistance in Pseudomonas aeruginosa and Acinetobacter species at a large tertiary referral hospital in Lusaka, Zambia. *Scientific African, 13*, e00908. DOI: 10.1016/J.SCIAF.2021.E00908

Karruli, A., Catalini, C., D'Amore, C., Foglia, F., Mari, F., Harxhi, A., Galdiero, M., & Durante-Mangoni, E. (2023). Evidence-Based Treatment of Pseudomonas aeruginosa Infections: A Critical Reappraisal. *Antibiotics 2023, Vol. 12, Page 399, 12*(2), 399. https://doi.org/DOI: 10.3390/ANTIBIOTICS12020399

Kästner, M., Miltner, A., Thiele-Bruhn, S., & Liang, C. (2021). Microbial Necromass in Soils—Linking Microbes to Soil Processes and Carbon Turnover. *Frontiers in Environmental Science*. Advance online publication. DOI: 10.3389/fenvs.2021.756378

Killough, M., Rodgers, A. M., & Ingram, R. J. (2022). Pseudomonas aeruginosa: Recent Advances in Vaccine Development. *Vaccines 2022, Vol. 10, Page 1100, 10*(7), 1100. https://doi.org/DOI: 10.3390/VACCINES10071100

Kothari, A., Jain, N., Kumar, S. K., Kumar, A., Kaushal, K., Kaur, S., Pandey, A., Gaurav, A., & Omar, B. J. (2022). Potential Synergistic Antibiotic Combinations against Fluoroquinolone-Resistant Pseudomonas aeruginosa. *Pharmaceuticals, 15*(2), 243. DOI: 10.3390/PH15020243/S1 PMID: 35215357

Lanckohr, C., & Bracht, H. (2022). Antimicrobial stewardship. *Current Opinion in Critical Care, 28*(5), 551–556. DOI: 10.1097/MCC.0000000000000967 PMID: 35942707

Letizia, M., Diggle, S. P., & Whiteley, M. (2025). Pseudomonas aeruginosa: ecology, evolution, pathogenesis and antimicrobial susceptibility. *Nature Reviews Microbiology 2025 23:11, 23*(11), 701–717. https://doi.org/DOI: 10.1038/s41579-025-01193-8

Li, Q. Y., Liu, B., & Liu, L. (2021). Successfully controlling the incidence of multidrug-resistant Pseudomonas aeruginosa through antibiotic stewardship and infection control programmes at a Chinese university hospital. *Journal of Clinical Pharmacy and Therapeutics, 46*(5), 1357–1366. DOI: 10.1111/JCPT.13446;SUBPAGE:STRING:FULL PMID: 34096086

Li, Y., Roberts, J. A., Walker, M. M., Aslan, A. T., Harris, P. N. A., & Sime, F. B. (2024). The global epidemiology of ventilator-associated pneumonia caused by multi-drug resistant Pseudomonas aeruginosa: A systematic review and meta-analysis. *International Journal of Infectious Diseases, 139*, 78–85. DOI: 10.1016/J.IJID.2023.11.023 PMID: 38013153

Liao, S. (2023). *A Study on the Application of Generative Artificial Intelligence Technology in Image Design*. https://doi.org/DOI: 10.2991/978-94-6463-266-8_36

Lynch, J. P., & Zhanel, G. G. (2022). Pseudomonas aeruginosa Pneumonia: Evolution of Antimicrobial Resistance and Implications for Therapy. *Seminars in Respiratory and Critical Care Medicine, 43*(2), 191–218. DOI: 10.1055/S-0041-1740109/ID/JR220203-19/BIB PMID: 35062038

Matuszewska, M., Maciąg, T., Rajewska, M., Wierzbicka, A., & Jafra, S. (2021). The carbon source-dependent pattern of antimicrobial activity and gene expression in Pseudomonas donghuensis P482. *Scientific Reports 2021 11:1, 11*(1), 1–17. https://doi.org/DOI: 10.1038/s41598-021-90488-w

Maurice, N. M., Bedi, B., & Sadikot, R. T. (2018). Pseudomonas aeruginosa biofilms: Host response and clinical implications in lung infections. *American Journal of Respiratory Cell and Molecular Biology, 58*(4), 428–439. DOI: 10.1165/RCMB.2017-0321TR/SUPPL_FILE/DISCLOSURES.PDF$AUTHORDISCLOSURES PMID: 29372812

McCallum, N., Berger-Bächi, B., & Senn, M. M. (2010). Regulation of antibiotic resistance in Staphylococcus aureus. *International Journal of Medical Microbiology, 300*(2–3), 118–129. DOI: 10.1016/J.IJMM.2009.08.015 PMID: 19800843

Mendes Pedro, D., Paulo, S. E., Santos, C. M., Fonseca, A. B., Melo Cristino, J., Pereira, Á. A., & Caneiras, C. (2024). Extensively drug-resistant Pseudomonas aeruginosa: Clinical features and treatment with ceftazidime/avibactam and ceftolozane/tazobactam in a tertiary care university hospital center in Portugal – A cross-sectional and retrospective observational study. *Frontiers in Microbiology*, *15*, 1347521. DOI: 10.3389/FMICB.2024.1347521/BIBTEX PMID: 38414772

Merakou, C., Schaefers, M. M., & Priebe, G. P. (2018). Progress toward the elusive pseudomonas aeruginosa vaccine. *Surgical Infections*, *19*(8), 757–768. DOI: 10.1089/SUR.2018.233;WGROUP:STRING:PUBLICATION PMID: 30388058

Meşe, E. A., Carrara, E., Tartari, E., Mutters, N. T., Tsioutis, C., Birgand, G., & Tacconelli, E. (2025). Prioritizing isolation precautions: A patient-centered approach to infection prevention and control. *Antimicrobial Stewardship & Healthcare Epidemiology : ASHE*, *5*(1), e123. DOI: 10.1017/ASH.2025.173 PMID: 40528936

Morales, E., Cots, F., Sala, M., Comas, M., Belvis, F., Riu, M., Salvadá, M., Grau, S., Horcajada, J. P., Montero, M. M., & Castells, X. (2012). Hospital costs of nosocomial multi-drug resistant Pseudomonas aeruginosa acquisition. *BMC Health Services Research 2012 12:1*, *12*(1), 122-. https://doi.org/DOI: 10.1186/1472-6963-12-122

Morin, C. D., Déziel, E., Gauthier, J., Levesque, R. C., & Lau, G. W. (2021). An Organ System-Based Synopsis of Pseudomonas aeruginosa Virulence. *Virulence*, *12*(1), 1469–1507. DOI: 10.1080/21505594.2021.1926408 PMID: 34180343

Motbainor, H., Bereded, F., & Mulu, W. (2020). Multi-drug resistance of blood stream, urinary tract and surgical site nosocomial infections of Acinetobacter baumannii and Pseudomonas aeruginosa among patients hospitalized at Felegehiwot referral hospital, Northwest Ethiopia: A cross-sectional study. *BMC Infectious Diseases*, *20*(1), 1–11. DOI: 10.1186/S12879-020-4811-8/TABLES/5 PMID: 32000693

Muro, F. J., Lyamuya, F. S., Kwobah, C., Bollinger, J., Bodinayake, C. K., Nagahawatte, A., Piyasiri, B., Kurukulasooriya, R., Ali, S., Mallya, R., Rolfe, R., Ruwanpathirana, A., Sheng, T., Østbye, T., Drew, R., Kussin, P., Woods, C. W., Anderson, D. J., Mmbaga, B. T., & Tillekeratne, L. G. (2022). Opportunities for Improving Antimicrobial Stewardship: Findings From a Prospective, Multi-Center Study in Three Low- or Middle-Income Countries. *Frontiers in Public Health*, *10*, 848802. DOI: 10.3389/FPUBH.2022.848802/BIBTEX PMID: 35548085

Naylor, N. R., Hasso-Agopsowicz, M., Kim, C., Ma, Y., Frost, I., Abbas, K., Aguilar, G., Fuller, N., Robotham, J. V., & Jit, M. (2025). The global economic burden of antibiotic-resistant infections and the potential impact of bacterial vaccines: A modelling study. *BMJ Global Health, 10*(6). Advance online publication. DOI: 10.1136/BMJGH-2024-016249 PMID: 40537271

Nickerson, R., Thornton, C. S., Johnston, B., Lee, A. H. Y., & Cheng, Z. (2024). Pseudomonas aeruginosa in chronic lung disease: Untangling the dysregulated host immune response. *Frontiers in Immunology, 15*, 1405376. DOI: 10.3389/FIMMU.2024.1405376/XML/NLM PMID: 39015565

Ogunsola, F. T., & Mehtar, S. (2020). Challenges regarding the control of environmental sources of contamination in healthcare settings in low-and middle-income countries - a narrative review. *Antimicrobial Resistance & Infection Control 2020 9:1, 9*(1), 81-. https://doi.org/DOI: 10.1186/S13756-020-00747-0

Olalekan, A., Bader, B. K., Iwalokun, B., Wolf, S., Lalremruata, A., Dike, A., Mannie-Udoh, M., Lo Presti, L., Liese, J., Guther, J., D'alvise, P., & Peter, S. (2023). High incidence of carbapenemase-producing Pseudomonas aeruginosa clinical isolates from Lagos, Nigeria. *JAC-Antimicrobial Resistance, 5*(2). Advance online publication. DOI: 10.1093/JACAMR/DLAD038 PMID: 37051191

Olawade, D. B., Fapohunda, O., Egbon, E., Ebiesuwa, O. A., Usman, S. O., Faronbi, A. O., & Fidelis, S. C. (2024). Phage therapy: A targeted approach to overcoming antibiotic resistance. *Microbial Pathogenesis, 197*, 107088. DOI: 10.1016/J.MICPATH.2024.107088 PMID: 39477033

Ozma, M. A., Abbasi, A., Asgharzadeh, M., Pagliano, P., Guarino, A., Köse, S., & Kafil, H. S. (2022). Antibiotic therapy for pan-drug-resistant infections. *Le Infezioni in Medicina, 30*(4), 525. DOI: 10.53854/LIIM-3004-6 PMID: 36482958

Pallares, C. J., Porras, J., De La Cadena, E., García-Betancur, J. C., Restrepo-Arbeláez, N., Viveros, S. M. C., Cornistein, W., Castañeda-Méndez, P., Cuellar, L., Boldim-Ferreira, D., Chaverri-Murillo, J., Labarca, J. A., & Villegas, M. V. (2023). Antimicrobial stewardship programs in seven Latin American countries: facing the challenges. *BMC Infectious Diseases 2023 23:1, 23*(1), 463-. https://doi.org/DOI: 10.1186/S12879-023-08398-3

Pang, Z., Raudonis, R., Glick, B. R., Lin, T. J., & Cheng, Z. (2019). Antibiotic resistance in Pseudomonas aeruginosa: Mechanisms and alternative therapeutic strategies. *Biotechnology Advances, 37*(1), 177–192. DOI: 10.1016/J.BIOTECHADV.2018.11.013 PMID: 30500353

Pei, Y., Hamar, P., & Pei, D. S. (2025). Deciphering Multidrug-Resistant Pseudomonas aeruginosa: Mechanistic Insights and Environmental Risks. *Toxics 2025, Vol. 13, Page 303, 13*(4), 303. https://doi.org/DOI: 10.3390/TOXICS13040303

Pepi, M., Focardi, S., Area, M., & Int, J. E. (2021). Antibiotic-Resistant Bacteria in Aquaculture and Climate Change: A Challenge for Health in the Mediterranean Area. *International Journal of Environmental Research and Public Health 2021, Vol. 18, Page 5723, 18*(11), 5723. https://doi.org/DOI: 10.3390/IJERPH18115723

Phan, S., Feng, C. H., Huang, R., Lee, Z. X., Moua, Y., Phung, O. J., & Lenhard, J. R. (2023). Relative Abundance and Detection of Pseudomonas aeruginosa from Chronic Wound Infections Globally. *Microorganisms, 11*(5), 1210. DOI: 10.3390/MICROORGANISMS11051210 PMID: 37317184

Polemis, M., Theofili, E., & Tryfinopoulou, K. (2024). Rapid increase of multi-drug resistant Pseudomonas aeruginosa in Greece - WHONET-Greece (2020-2023). *European Journal of Public Health, 34*(Supplement_3). Advance online publication. DOI: 10.1093/EURPUB/CKAE144.2154

Rafiq, M. K., Kamran, H., Sultan, B., Khan, Y. A., Wadud, F., Ayub, M., Ali, S., & Ali, A. (2022). Outcome of the Choice of Wound Closure Technique in Emergency Laparotomy. *Journal of Ayub Medical College, Abbottabad, 34*(1), 164–168. DOI: 10.55519/JAMC-01-8797 PMID: 35466646

Ramatla, T., Nkhebenyane, J., Lekota, K. E., Thekisoe, O., Monyama, M., Achilonu, C. C., & Khasapane, G. (2025). Global prevalence and antibiotic resistance profiles of carbapenem-resistant Pseudomonas aeruginosa reported from 2014 to 2024: A systematic review and meta-analysis. *Frontiers in Microbiology, 16*, 1599070. DOI: 10.3389/FMICB.2025.1599070/BIBTEX PMID: 40761277

Rehm, Z. J., Gonzaga, C., Merakou, A., DiGiandomenico, G. P., & Priebe, B. H. A. (2021). A Pseudomonas aeruginosa-Derived Particulate Vaccine Protects against P. aeruginosa Infection. *Vaccines, 9*(7), 803. DOI: 10.3390/vaccines9070803 PMID: 34358220

Reig, S., Le Gouellec, A., & Bleves, S. (2022). What Is New in the Anti–Pseudomonas aeruginosa Clinical Development Pipeline Since the 2017 WHO Alert? *Frontiers in Cellular and Infection Microbiology, 12*, 909731. DOI: 10.3389/FCIMB.2022.909731/TEXT PMID: 35880080

Reynolds, D., & Kollef, M. (2021). The Epidemiology and Pathogenesis and Treatment of Pseudomonas aeruginosa Infections: An Update. *Drugs 2021 81:18, 81*(18), 2117–2131. https://doi.org/DOI: 10.1007/S40265-021-01635-6

Ribeiro, Á. C. da S., Crozatti, M. T. L., da Silva, A. A., Macedo, R. S., Machado, A. M. de O., & Silva, A. T. de A. (2019). Pseudomonas aeruginosa in the ICU: Prevalence, resistance profile, and antimicrobial consumption. *Revista da Sociedade Brasileira de Medicina Tropical, 53*, e20180498. DOI: 10.1590/0037-8682-0498-2018 PMID: 31859938

Sainz-Mejías, M., Jurado-Martín, I., & McClean, S. (2020). Understanding Pseudomonas aeruginosa–Host Interactions: The Ongoing Quest for an Efficacious Vaccine. *Cells 2020, Vol. 9, Page 2617, 9*(12), 2617. https://doi.org/DOI: 10.3390/CELLS9122617

Saliba, R., Zahar, J. R., Dabar, G., Riachy, M., Karam-Sarkis, D., & Husni, R. (2023). Limiting the Spread of Multidrug-Resistant Bacteria in Low-to-Middle-Income Countries: One Size Does Not Fit All. *Pathogens 2023, Vol. 12, Page 144, 12*(1), 144. https://doi.org/DOI: 10.3390/PATHOGENS12010144

Santamarina-Fernández, R., Fuentes-Valverde, V., Silva-Rodríguez, A., García, P., Moscoso, M., & Bou, G. (2025). Pseudomonas aeruginosa Vaccine Development: Lessons, Challenges, and Future Innovations. *International Journal of Molecular Sciences*, *26*(5), 2012. DOI: 10.3390/IJMS26052012/S1 PMID: 40076637

Sanya, D. R. A., Onésime, D., Vizzarro, G., & Jacquier, N. (2023). Recent advances in therapeutic targets identification and development of treatment strategies towards Pseudomonas aeruginosa infections. *BMC Microbiology 2023 23:1, 23*(1), 1–18. https://doi.org/DOI: 10.1186/S12866-023-02832-X

Sathe, N., Beech, P., Croft, L., Suphioglu, C., Kapat, A., & Athan, E. (2023). Pseudomonas aeruginosa: Infections and novel approaches to treatment "Knowing the enemy" the threat of Pseudomonas aeruginosa and exploring novel approaches to treatment. *Infectious Medicine*, *2*(3), 178–194. DOI: 10.1016/J.IMJ.2023.05.003 PMID: 38073886

Sendra, E., Fernández-Muñoz, A., Zamorano, L., Oliver, A., Horcajada, J. P., Juan, C., & Gómez-Zorrilla, S. (2024). Impact of multidrug resistance on the virulence and fitness of Pseudomonas aeruginosa: a microbiological and clinical perspective. *Infection 2024 52:4, 52*(4), 1235–1268. https://doi.org/DOI: 10.1007/S15010-024-02313-X

Shabi, Y., & Algarni, A., Al bshabshe, A., Alazraqi, T., Patriquin, G., Bawazeer, A. O. S., Mohammed, S. A., Habbash, S., Somily, A., Alqahtani, A. J., & Alhamhhum, S. M. S. (2025). A decade of antimicrobial resistance trends in Pseudomonas aeruginosa: Insights from a tertiary care hospital in Saudi Arabia (2013–2022). *Frontiers in Microbiology*, *16*, 1617522. DOI: 10.3389/FMICB.2025.1617522/BIBTEX PMID: 40693146

Shortridge, D., Pfaller, M. A., Castanheira, M., & Flamm, R. K. (2018). Antimicrobial activity of ceftolozane-tazobactam tested against Enterobacteriaceae and Pseudomonas aeruginosa collected from patients with bloodstream infections isolated in United States hospitals (2013–2015) as part of the Program to Assess Ceftolozane-Tazobactam Susceptibility (PACTS) surveillance program. *Diagnostic Microbiology and Infectious Disease*, *92*(2), 158–163. DOI: 10.1016/J.DIAGMICROBIO.2018.05.011 PMID: 29891184

Sindeldecker, D., & Stoodley, P. (2021). The many antibiotic resistance and tolerance strategies of Pseudomonas aeruginosa. *Biofilm*, *3*, 100056. DOI: 10.1016/J.BIOFLM.2021.100056 PMID: 34471871

Singha, B., Singh, V., & Soni, V. (2024). Alternative therapeutics to control antimicrobial resistance: A general perspective. *Frontiers in Drug Discovery*, *4*, 1385460. DOI: 10.3389/FDDSV.2024.1385460/XML

Smith, W. D., Bardin, E., Cameron, L., Edmondson, C. L., Farrant, K. V., Martin, I., Murphy, R. A., Soren, O., Turnbull, A. R., Wierre-Gore, N., Alton, E. W., Bundy, J. G., Bush, A., Connett, G. J., Faust, S. N., Filloux, A., Freemont, P. S., Jones, A. L., Takats, Z., & Davies, J. C. (2017). Current and future therapies for Pseudomonas aeruginosa infection in patients with cystic fibrosis. *FEMS Microbiology Letters*, *364*(14), 121. DOI: 10.1093/FEMSLE/FNX121 PMID: 28854668

Sole, E., Trinchera, M., Gaetano, S. De, Midiri, A., Piccolo, G., Mancuso, G., Schepici, G., & Biondo, C. (2025). The Paradox of Healthcare in the ‘Superbugs’ Era: Current Challenges and Future Directions. *Pathogens 2025, Vol. 14, Page 1199*, *14*(12), 1199. https://doi.org/DOI: 10.3390/PATHOGENS14121199

Spagnolo, A. M., Sartini, M., & Cristina, M. L. (2021). Pseudomonas aeruginosa in the healthcare facility setting. *Reviews in Medical Microbiology : a Journal of the Pathological Society of Great Britain and Ireland*, *32*(3), 169–175. DOI: 10.1097/mrm.0000000000000271

Tumbarello, M., Repetto, E., Trecarichi, E. M., Bernardini, C., De Pascale, G., Parisini, A., Rossi, M., Molinari, M. P., Spanu, T., Viscoli, C., Cauda, R., & Bassetti, M. (2011). Multidrug-resistant Pseudomonas aeruginosa bloodstream infections: Risk factors and mortality. *Epidemiology and Infection, 139*(11), 1740–1749. DOI: 10.1017/S0950268810003055 PMID: 21226988

Viasus, D., Puerta-Alcalde, P., Cardozo, C., Suárez-Lledó, M., Rodríguez-Núñez, O., Morata, L., Fehér, C., Marco, F., Chumbita, M., Moreno-García, E., Fernández-Avilés, F., Gutiérrez-Garcia, G., Martínez, J. A., Mensa, J., Rovira, M., Esteve, J., Soriano, A., & Garcia-Vidal, C. (2020). Predictors of multidrug-resistant Pseudomonas aeruginosa in neutropenic patients with bloodstream infection. *Clinical Microbiology and Infection, 26*(3), 345–350. DOI: 10.1016/J.CMI.2019.07.002 PMID: 31295551

Wan, C., Gao, C., Xie, Q., Wang, Y., Cheng, X., Fang, Y., Liu, Z., Zhang, W., Zou, Q., Lu, G., & Gu, J. (2021). Flagella hook protein FlgE is a novel vaccine candidate of Pseudomonas aeruginosa identified by a genomic approach. *Vaccine, 39*(17), 2386–2395. DOI: 10.1016/J.VACCINE.2021.03.051 PMID: 33775439

Wei, X. C., Zhao, M. F., & Xiao, X. (2024). Evaluating omadacycline dosing regimens against drug-resistant pathogens including Staphylococcus aureus, Streptococcus pneumoniae and Haemophilus influenzae in adults: A pharmacokinetic/pharmacodynamic analysis using Monte Carlo simulation. *Journal of Chemotherapy (Florence, Italy), 36*(7), 532–539. DOI: 10.1080/1120009X.2024.2339706 PMID: 38591989

Werner, G., Couto, N., Feil, E. J., Novais, A., Hegstad, K., Howden, B. P., Friedrich, A. W., & Reuter, S. (2023). Taking hospital pathogen surveillance to the next level. *Microbial Genomics, 9*(4), 1. DOI: 10.1099/mgen.0.001008 PMID: 37099616

Yayan, J., Ghebremedhin, B., & Rasche, K. (2015). Antibiotic Resistance of Pseudomonas aeruginosa in Pneumonia at a Single University Hospital Center in Germany over a 10-Year Period. *PLoS One, 10*(10), e0139836. DOI: 10.1371/JOURNAL.PONE.0139836 PMID: 26430738

Yin, C., Alam, M. Z., Fallon, J. T., & Huang, W. (2024). Advances in Development of Novel Therapeutic Strategies against Multi-Drug Resistant Pseudomonas aeruginosa. *Antibiotics 2024, Vol. 13, Page 119, 13*(2), 119. https://doi.org/DOI: 10.3390/ANTIBIOTICS13020119

Yin, L., Zhang, Y., Azi, F., Zhou, J., Liu, X., Dai, Y., Wang, Z., Dong, M., & Xia, X. (2022). Inhibition of biofilm formation and quorum sensing by soy isoflavones in Pseudomonas aeruginosa. *Food Control, 133*, 108629. DOI: 10.1016/J.FOODCONT.2021.108629

Zhou, M., Xu, B., Guo, Z., Zeng, Y., Lei, J., Kritsotakis, E. I., & Wang, J. (2024). Clinical burden of community-associated infections caused by multidrug-resistant Pseudomonas aeruginosa: A propensity-matched longitudinal cohort study in Southern China. *GMS Hygiene and Infection Control, 19*, Doc51. DOI: 10.3205/DGKH000506 PMID: 39553304

Zhou, M., Xu, B., Guo, Z., Zeng, Y., Lei, J., Kritsotakis, E. I., & Wang, J. (2024). Clinical burden of community-associated infections caused by multidrug-resistant Pseudomonas aeruginosa: A propensity-matched longitudinal cohort study in Southern China. *GMS Hygiene and Infection Control, 19*, Doc51. DOI: 10.3205/DGKH000506 PMID: 39553304

ADDITIONAL READING

Alan Cross, James R. Allen, John Burke, Georges Ducel, Alan Harris, Joseph John, David Johnson, Michael Lew, Bruce MacMillan, Peter Meers, Radmila Skalova, Richard Wenzel, James Tenney, Nosocomial Infections Due to *Pseudomonas aeruginosa:* Review of Recent Trends, *Reviews of Infectious Diseases*, Volume 5, Issue Supplement_5, November-December 1983, Pages S837–S845, https://doi.org/DOI: 10.1093/clinids/5.Supplement_5.S837

Labovská, S. (2021). *Pseudomonas aeruginosa as a Cause of Nosocomial Infections.* IntechOpen., DOI: 10.5772/intechopen.95908

Wilson, M. G., & Pandey, S. (2025 Jan). Pseudomonas aeruginosa. [Updated 2023 Aug 8] In *StatPearls* [Internet]. StatPearls Publishing., Available from https://www.ncbi.nlm.nih.gov/books/NBK557831/

APPENDIX

Abbreviations

Antimicrobial Photodynamic Therapy AgNPs

CAP: Community-Acquired Pneumonia
COPD: Chronic Obstructive Pulmonary Disease
CVC: Central Venous Catheter

Green-Synthesised Silver Nanoparticles

ICUAP: Intensive Care Unit-Acquired Pneumonia
MDR-PA: Multidrug Resistant *Pseudomonas aeruginosa*
QS: Quorum Sensing aPDT:
RT-qPCR: Real-Time Polymerase Chain Reaction

Chapter 7
Transforming AMR Detection and Public Health Response:
Microbial Genomics and Diagnostic Innovation

R. Swadhi
https://orcid.org/0009-0005-0247-0713
Saraswathi Institute of Medical Sciences, Hapur, India

Ramachandren Ramya
https://orcid.org/0009-0000-8016-212X
Saraswathi Institute of Medical Sciences, Hapur, India

Krati R. Varshney
Saraswathi Institute of Medical Sciences, Hapur, India

K. Gayathri
https://orcid.org/0000-0003-0398-0094
Academy of Maritime Education and Training, Chennai, India

ABSTRACT

This chapter addresses the revolution of antimicrobial resistance (AMR) detection and response by microbial genomics and diagnostic innovation. Three diagnostic platforms (PCR, CRISPR-based detection and Whole Genome Sequencing, WGS) were evaluated in terms of accuracy, reproducibility and turnaround time using 100 clinical isolates. WGS had the best detection rate of (97), the best genotype-phenotype correlation (r = 0.86), whereas CRISPR is the most rapid. Genome Data + AI an-

DOI: 10.4018/979-8-3373-3825-5.ch007

alytics allowed foreseeing resistance and mainstream public health surveillance. The results highlight genomics as a foundation of accurate microbiology, which promotes real-time AMR surveillance and evidence-based policy intervention in a One Health context.

1. INTRODUCTION

Antimicrobial resistance (AMR) has become one of the strongest threatening issues of modern medicine and population health that can pose a decades-old advancement in combating infectious diseases. Drug-resistant pathogens have caused high mortality, long hospitalization, and rising costs of treatment across the globe (Coque et al., 2023; Thompson, 2024). Traditional microbiological phenotypic-culture, biochemical, and antibiotic-susceptibility testing are long and ineffective and do not identify new resistance genes to delay diagnosis and promote empirical antibiotic use, thereby increasing resistance and compromising infection-control programmes (Kaprou et al., 2021; Vasala et al., 2020). Recent achievements in microbial genomics have transformed our ability of observing and discovering of resistance mechanisms. The Whole-genome sequencing (WGS), metagenomic profiling, and transcriptomic studies can now be conducted at an extremely fast rate to identify resistance determinants, virulence factors, and genetic mobility patterns that cannot be detected by the conventional approach of culture (Bianconi et al., 2023). Genomic information can also be used to support tracing of transmission lines and as well as comprehension of the dynamics of pathogen evolution in clinical as well as community setups. With the help of artificial-intelligence (AI) analytics, genomics can predict the trends of resistance and pre-emptive containment options (Branda and Scarpa, 2024; Struelens et al., 2024). Therefore, genomics, molecular diagnostics, and computational intelligence are met at a critical crossroad in which descriptive microbiology has been replaced by precision and changing the practise of public health. Samples can now be transformed into a format that can be acted upon in hours, not days, through the use of CRISPR-based biosensing, nanopore sequencing, and AI pattern-recognition (Olatunji et al., 2024; Pennisi et al., 2025). Such tools are capable of not only streamlining clinical decision-making processes but also producing real-time data streams capable of driving national AMR-surveillance networks. As such, diagnostic laboratories are now transforming beyond a single test facility into a strategically located global health intelligence centre.

However, genomic diagnostics are not fully applied in the clinical practise, mainly because of its cost, infrastructure and data-governance limitations, especially in low and middle-income areas (Chigozie et al., 2025; Rugarabamu and Mwanyika, 2025). There is a paucity of empirical comparisons between diagnostic platforms, including culture-based, PCR-based, CRISPR-enabled and WGS. To implement evidences based it will be necessary to have quantitative data to confirm their relative accuracy, reproducibility, and speed (Ma et al., 2025; Hasan et al., 2025). To fill this gap, the current experimental study conducts a systematic literature review and a comparative analysis of three genomic-based diagnostic modalities, such as polymerase chain reaction (PCR), CRISPR -Cas-based detection, and whole-genome sequencing, to determine the resistance genes in clinically significant bacteria (Zhou, S., Zhao, X., and Meng, F., 2025). The bacteria isolates consisted of Escherichia coli, Klebsiella pneumoniae, Pseudomonas aeruginosa, Staphylococcus aureus, and Enterococcus spp acquired in various hospitals (Jiang, 2025). Full genomic characterization was done on each isolate and then bioinformatics annotation was done against known resistance-gene databases. Specific AI algorithms to perform resistance-phenotyping were then trained and used to predict phenotypic outcomes according to a particular gene signature (Devi et al., 2025; Mohammed et al., 2025).

The research aims at achieving three major goals:

1. Diagnostic validation: Compare the sensitivity and specificity of genomic procedures with the traditional phenotypic assay.
2. Correlation analysis: Measure the association between the genotypic determinants of resistance and the antimicrobial susceptibility that is observed.
3. Public-health application: Determine how fast genomic diagnostics would enhance AMR surveillance and policy response on institutional and national levels.

The study closes the gap between microbiology on the bench and the disease control of populations through connecting laboratory experimentation with the integration of computational models and surveillance presented the conceptual framework in the figure 1.

Figure 1. Conceptual Framework

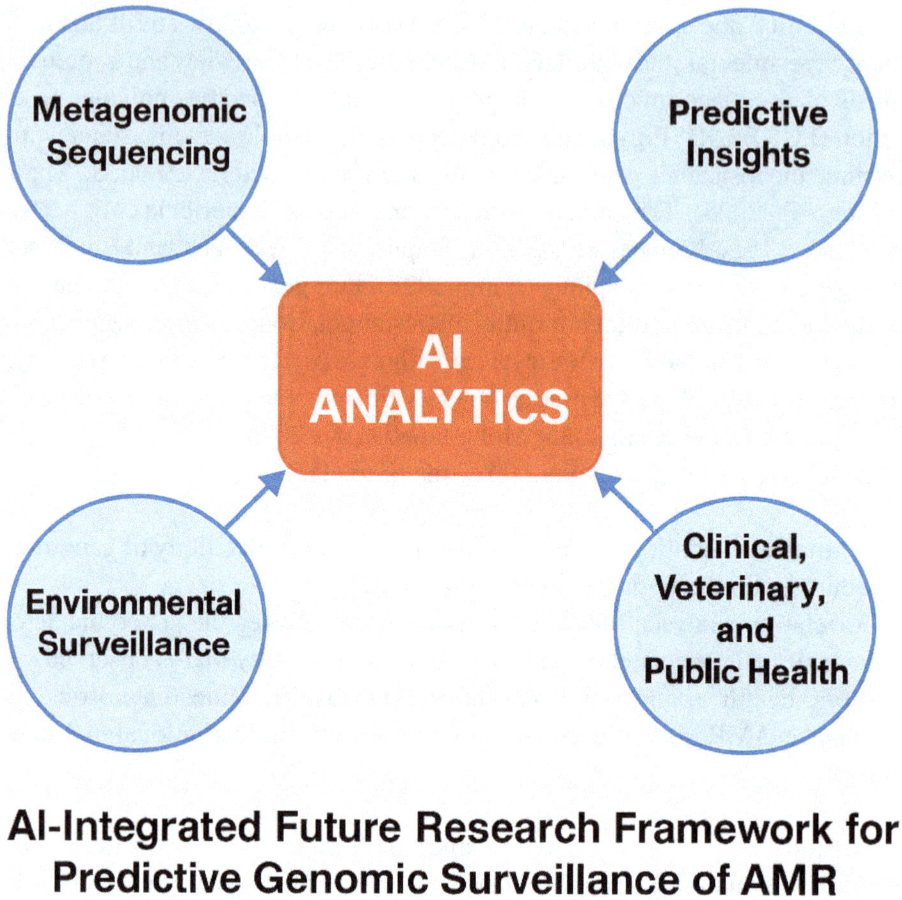

Figure 1 also creates a conceptual framework in which microbial genomics forms the base of an AMR ecosystem, which acts as a responsive and data-driven framework. Resistance predictions because of sequencing are informed by laboratories, and genomic intelligence at the national level can then be populated. In this closed-loop method, there is an improved antimicrobial stewardship and resistant outbreak containment, with the intervention taking place at an earlier stage. The latter premises are expounded in the rest of this chapter. Section 2 discusses the available literature on microbial genomics and diagnostic innovation; Section 3 outlines the methodology used in the experiment; Section 4 outlines and discusses the results of the comparative study; Sections 5, 6, and 7 outline the future research direction and policy priorities; and the conclusion section is a summary of thoughts regarding the future of incorporating genomics into a sustainable global health system. In this respect, the chapter presents a possibility of optimising the AMR detection to convert the previously slow laboratory operation into a proactive public-health surveillance system, supported by the empirical validation of genomic and AI-based diagnostics.

2. BACKGROUND AND LITERATURE SYNTHESIS

Microbial genomics has experienced a fast evolution as the field originating with microbial taxonomy has evolved into a revolutionary platform in clinical diagnostics and population health monitoring. Convergent high-throughput genomic sequencing, advanced bioinformatics, and artificial intelligence (AI) has brought new understanding about the genetic framework of antimicrobial resistance (AMR) as never before. As a result, it is now possible to describe the molecular aetiology of resistance, specify the pathways of pathogen transmission, as well as foresee new resistance phenotypes in different healthcare settings, due to full genome mapping and alignment of resistance genes (Bianconi et al., 2023; Elguoshy and Hashem, 2024). It continues to be stressed in the literature that AMR is not merely a clinical issue but a systematic challenge that needs to be addressed by applying genomic and technological solutions (Coque et al., 2023; Singh et al., 2025). Genomic revolution has consequently rewritten diagnostic as well as epidemiology paradigms in microbiology. The initial diagnostic techniques were based on culture and biochemical identification, which the initial diagnostic techniques were followed by the phenotypic testing of antimicrobial susceptibility (Ardila, C.M., Gonzalez-Arroyave, D., and Tobon, S., 2025). These methods were correct, but they were time-consuming and could take up to 4,872 hours to finish the pathogen identification and susceptibility profiling (Kaprou et al., 2021). Instead, next-generation sequencing (Illumina and Nanopore) can be used to interrogate entire genomes in a few hours providing a more robust picture of resistance determinants, virulence factors, and strain phylogenetic relationships (Elbehiry & Abalkhail, 2025). This technological advancement will enable clinicians to be genomic-first approach to care, moving away from empiric therapy to precision based antimicrobial stewardship.

In more recent times, there has been a major development with respect to incorporating genomic information into prognostic diagnostic models. The use of AI-enhanced analytics and machine-learning (ML) algorithms in the processing and clinical decision-making of large quantities of genomic data is becoming more common (Pennisi et al., 2025; Mohammed et al., 2025). These models have associated certain genetic repertoires and phenotypic resistance profiles and can be used in real-time to predict the emergence of resistance. Moreover, the exchange of information between different health systems will enable the formation of global genomic repositories, to which comparative analyses and mapping of AMR trends can be applied. Such a comprehensive integration represents the One Health vision, where human, animal, and environmental datasets of microbiota combine to shed light on the greater resistance evolution trajectory (Liu et al., 2024; Chigozie et al., 2025). Genomic epidemiology has thus come up as a pillar of AMR containment in the viewpoint of the public health. Pathogen surveillance by sequencing has helped in establishing transmission groups within healthcare facilities and within community outbreaks (Struelens et al., 2024). The rapid matching of genotype of resistance with clinical outcome has shifted the response to epidemics towards reactive control to predictive preventive actions. The Genomic data has been integrated into the national AMR databases by means of programs like the Global Antimicrobial Resistance Surveillance System (GLASS) and Pathogenwatch which allows collaboration across borders and real-time alerts. However, there are still issues of interoperability, the standardisation of data, and privacy especially when sensitive genomic data is being shared across international borders (Rugarabamu & Mwanyika, 2025). The development of diagnostic methods based on the principles of genomic methods has transformed the AMR detection in regard to its speed and sensitivity. Polymerase chain reaction (PCR) technology is still popular in the diagnosis of individual resistance genes, and the CRISPR-based diagnostics have had a portable, ultra-sensitive, field-deployable mode of detection (Olatunji et al., 2024). In these assays, the nucleic acid amplification was coupled with programmable CRISPR -Cas recognition to generate fluorescence remittance or colorimetric outputs in a few minutes. At the same time, metagenomic sequencing provides the opportunity to identify the pathogen and resistance genes of complex clinical sources without their culture in advance (Elbehiry & Abalkhail, 2025). All these approaches support the conclusion that genomics is not only fastening the detection process but also widening the range of measurable mechanisms of resistance, including new phenotypes that cannot be measured by conventional testing, as shown in Table 1..

Table 1. Genomic Diagnostic Tools and Application in Antimicrobial Resistance Detection

Diagnostic Platform	Typical Turnaround Time	Underlying Principle	Advantages	Representative References
Polymerase Chain Reaction (PCR)	3–6 hours	Amplification of known resistance genes using gene-specific primers	High sensitivity; established protocols	Kaprou et al., 2021; Ma et al., 2025
CRISPR-Cas Diagnostics	<2 hours	CRISPR-mediated detection of target sequences via collateral cleavage	Rapid, portable, cost-effective	Olatunji et al., 2024; Pennisi et al., 2025
AI-Enhanced Predictive Models	Variable (Real-time)	Machine learning applied to genomic datasets for resistance prediction	High predictive power; supports precision therapy	Branda & Scarpa, 2024; Mohammed et al., 2025
Whole Genome Sequencing (WGS)	24–48 hours	Sequencing and bioinformatic annotation of entire bacterial genomes	Comprehensive; detects novel and known genes	Bianconi et al., 2023; Hasan et al., 2025
Metagenomic NGS	6–12 hours	Direct sequencing of mixed microbial communities without culture	Detects uncultivable or mixed pathogens	Elbehiry & Abalkhail, 2025

The shift to AI-powered genomic platforms as an alternative to conventional molecular diagnostics is a representative of the larger paradigm shift of clinical microbiology to a data-driven one. Decision support systems driven by artificial-intelligence have the capability to automatically process sequencing data to identify aberrant resistance phenotypes, which can be further subjected to further epidemiological investigation (Devi et al., 2025). Combined with large-scale genome libraries, lifelong learning increases predictive skills. As an example, the hospital sequencing information can be implemented into the national archives, enabling the identification of drug-resistant clonal lineages and their geographic distribution in a short period of time. As a result, the convergence between genomics and AI forms the basis of the next generation of surveillance systems that can follow clinical outcomes in relation to the pathogen evolutionary dynamics (Branda and Scarpa, 2024; Singh et al., 2025). However, there exist a number of obstacles that should be overcome to achieve universalization of genomic diagnostics. High-throughput sequencing produces large amounts of data, which require complicated analysis pipelines and highly skilled staff to process. This makes the use of genomics-based diagnostics and surveillance a serious challenge in the context of limited resources due to such logistical requirements. Furthermore, the process of cross-institutional data sharing is also often limited due to strict privacy laws and the absence of uniform annotation models. Based on this, interoperable systems, solid data-storage systems, and collaborative genomic networks need to be developed to guarantee sustainable implementation of genomic diagnostics to combat antimicrobial resistance (Waddington et al., 2022). Overall, the reviewed literature provides a sound scientific and practical basis to the experimental studies that are described in the present work. In addition to improving diagnostic specificity, epidemiological intelligence that is critical to antimicrobial stewardship is created through genomic technologies. Nonetheless, diagnostic performance of modalities, including PCR, CRISPR, and WGS, has not been empirically evaluated. This gap in evidence highlights the need to carefully managed experimental research that could help to outline comparative diagnostic effectiveness, reliability and applicability of their results to the health of the population. The following section will outline the experimental design, analytical framework and bioinformatics tools utilized to confirm the use of these genomic tools and the general potential of integrating them to transform the landscape of detecting antimicrobial resistance in clinical and surveillance settings..

3. METHODOLOGY

It was a comparative experimental study that compared performance and diagnostic accuracy of three genomic-based patterns consisting of Polymerase chain Reaction (PCR), CRISPR-based detection, and Whole Genome sequencing (WGS) in the identification of antimicrobial resistance (AMR) genes in clinically significant bacterial isolates. The objective of the experiment was to determine the quantitative evidence on the diagnostic precision, reproducibility, and turnaround time; and to test correlations between genotypic and phenotypic resistance profiles. The methodology incorporates wet-laboratory assay with computational bioinformatics and statistical verification to make the laboratory as well as data-driven assurance (Bianconi et al., 2023; Hasan et al., 2025) certain.

Study Design and Sampling Framework

One hundred clinical isolates of bacteria were gathered within three tertiary-care hospitals during 12 months. Escherichia coli, Klebsiella pneumoniae, Staphylococcus aureus, Pseudomonas aeruginosa, and Enterococcus spp were sampled purposely to represent the most prevalent multidrug-resistant (MDR) pathogenic agents. All isolates were first identified with standard microbiological techniques such as Gram staining, biochemical profiling, and phenotypic antibiotic susceptibility testing on the KirbyBauer disk diffusion test (Kaprou et al., 2021). These were phenotypic data to be used as a control on the genomic discoveries. The clinical samples were urine, sputum, wound swabs, and blood cultures of patients having symptoms of infection that were not responding to empirical antibiotic treatment. Ethical consent was taken off institutional review boards before sampling and analysis. All isolates were frozen in glycerol stocks at -80 C until they were genomic extracted.

DNA Extraction and Genomic Preparation

Each of the isolates was subjected to genomic DNA extraction using the phenol chloroform technique with ethanol precipitation to produce high quality nucleic acids that could be sequenced (Elbehiry and Abalkhail, 2025). NanoDrop spectrophotometry and Qubit fluorometry were used to evaluate the quality and concentration of DNA. Three parallel diagnostic procedures presented in the figure 2 were then carried out on extracted DNA samples:

1. PCR Amplification: Gene-specific primers were used to amplify known AMR genes including blaCTX-M, mecA, vanA, NDM-1 and aac(6)-Ib (Ma et al., 2025). The visualization of amplified products was done by 2% agarose gel electrophoresis.
2. CRISPR-Cas12a-Based Detection: CRISPR-Cas12a systems were used with guide RNAs against the same loci in order to detect the problem quickly. The intensity of the signal was measured using a microplate reader that was a method of quantification of the fluorescence-based detection (Olatunji et al., 2024).
3. Whole Genome Sequencing (WGS): Illumina Nextera XT kits were used to obtain the DNA libraries which were sequenced on the Illumina MiSeq platform with an average coverage of 50x. The reads of the sequences were quality-trimmed with Trimmomatic, assembled with SPAdes, and annotated with Prokka and Comprehensive Antibiotic Resistance Database (CARD) (Desai et al., 2025).

Figure 2. Comparative AMR Detection via PCR, CRISPR, and Whole Genome Sequencing

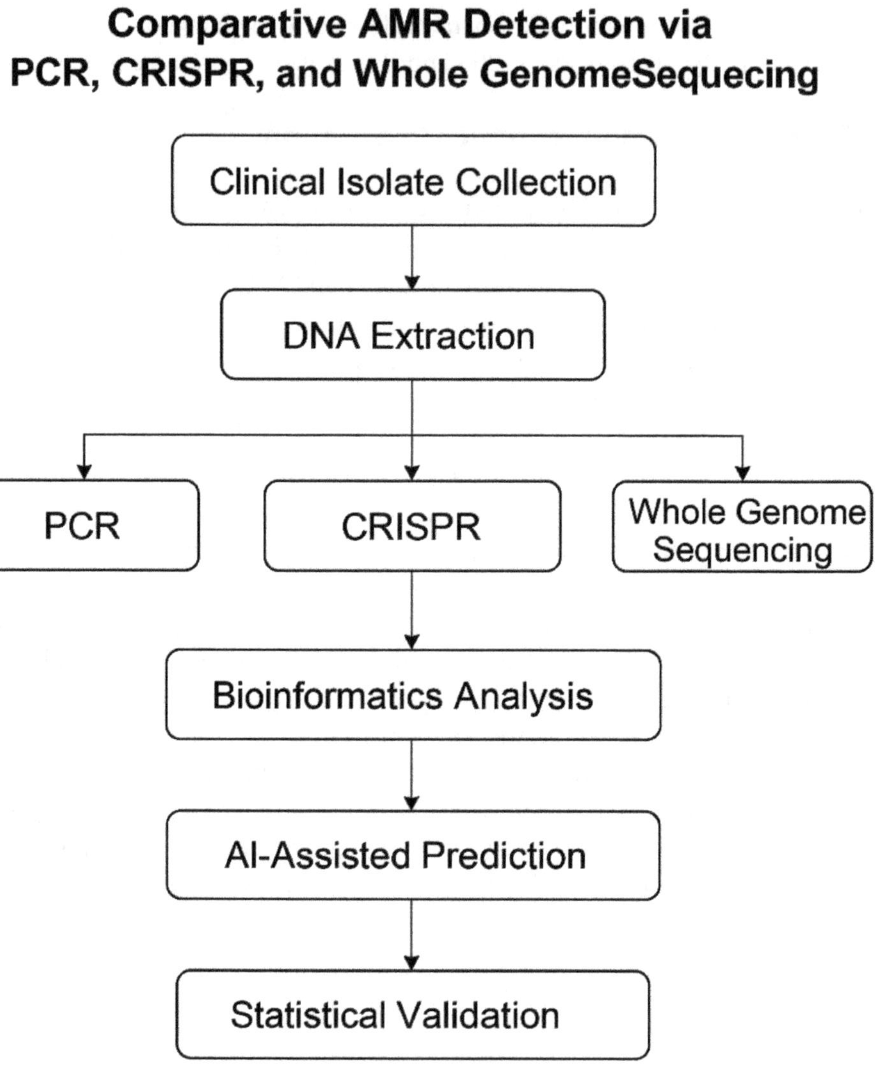

Bioinformatics and Machine Learning Analysis

Analysis was done on the content of the resistance genes, plasmid replicons and the mobile genetic elements of the annotated genomes. Comparative genomic alignments with the help of BLASTn were used to identify gene variants. The absence or presence of important antimicrobial resistance (AMR) determinants in the isolates was determined using a resistance -gene matrix, which encoded the presence or absence of the determinants in binary form. It was used to input a Random Forest classifier that was trained to predict phenotypic resistance using genotypic profiles of a binary matrix (Devi et al., 2025; Mohammed et al., 2025). Training was done using 80 per cent of the dataset with the remaining 20 per cent used to evaluate performance with measure of sensitivity, specificity and area under the receiver operating characteristic curve (AUC). Scikit-learn was used to implement the algorithm in Python and the cross-validation was done through five-fold to alleviate overfit. Correlation studies were done to explain relationships among specific resistance genes and phenotypic resistances. As an example, isolates that contained mecA gene were assumed to be resistant to methicillin and the presence of blaCTX -M was associated with resistance to extended -lactams.

Comparative Evaluation

In order to determine diagnostic performance, mean detection accuracy of PCR, CRISPR, and WGS was compared with one-way ANOVA. The dependent variable was (%) detection rate of known resistance genes and the three diagnostic modalities were the independent groups. Pairowise differences were found to be statistically significant using post-hoc Tukey tests.

Additionally, Pearson correlation coefficients (r) were used to measure genotype-phenotype relationships, where r 0.80 was treated as a strong relationship. The p-value below 0.05 was taken to be statistically significant.

Each method also had a diagnostic turnaround time recorded in the table 2:

- PCR: 4–6 hours
- CRISPR: 1.5–2 hours

WGS: 2436 hours (with bioinformatics processing)

These metrics have facilitated the multidimensional comparison that encompassed sensitivity, specificity, reproducibility and efficiency.

Table 2. Analytical Tools and Statistical Methods Used in the Study

Category	Tool/Software	Purpose	Reference
Sequencing and Assembly	Illumina MiSeq, SPAdes	Genome sequencing and assembly	Desai et al., 2025
Annotation and Resistance Gene Identification	Prokka, CARD Database	Gene annotation and AMR gene mapping	Hasan et al., 2025
Quality Control	FastQC, Trimmomatic	Read filtering and trimming	Elbehiry & Abalkhail, 2025
Statistical Analysis	SPSS v26, R Studio	ANOVA, correlation, post-hoc testing	Ma et al., 2025
Machine Learning Model	Python (scikit-learn)	Random Forest classifier for AMR prediction	Devi et al., 2025; Mohammed et al., 2025

Ethical and Data Governance Considerations

The study was in line with the ethics of using clinical microbial isolates. Anonymized patient identifiers were used in making genomic analyses and no personal information was included. The sharing of data was also in accordance with institutional bio safety measures and in line with the genomic data- governance standards of studies involving the official field of public-health (Chigozie et al., 2025; Rugarabamu and Mwanyika, 2025). Raw sequencing data was saved in an internal secure repository to make it valid and be part of national antimicrobial resistance surveillance efforts in the future. The approach will provide a systemic platform on which the comparative assessments of genomic diagnostic tools can be carried out. The study examines diagnostic innovation at both laboratory and public-health scales by utilizing experimental microbiology, bioinformatics through sequencing and AI-based data analytics. The study design ensures scientific rigour, statistical validity and ethical responsibility. The following provides the results and analysis where the accuracy of detection, distribution of genes and diagnostic efficacy of the PCR, CRISPR and WGS methods are compared.

4. RESULTS AND ANALYSIS

The results of the experimental studies show the relative diagnostic performance of the three genomic tools, such as PCR, CRISPR-based assays or whole genome sequencing (WGS) in identifying antimicrobial resistance (AMR) determinants in 100 clinical bacterial isolates. The analysis combines the data of molecular detection with statistical analysis and computational modeling to measure accuracy, reproducibility and predictive reliability.

Distribution of Isolates and Resistance Gene Profile

It was composed of Escherichia coli (30 percent), Klebsiella pneumoniae (25 percent), Staphylococcus aureus (20 percent), Pseudomonas aeruginosa (15 percent) and Enterococcus spp. (10 percent). There were five main resistance determinants that were assayed; bla_CTX -M (encoded extended spectrum -lactamase), mecA (conferred methicillin resistance), vanA (mediating vancomycin resistance), NDM -1 (generating carbapenem resistance), and aac(6 -1) -Ib (a aminoglycoside -modifying enzyme). At least one gene of resistance was identified using PCR screening in 86% of isolates and a CRISPR-based method identified resistance phenotypes in 92% of isolates. The resistance determinants were identified by whole-genome sequencing (WGS) in 97 per cent of isolates and a few other variants were not detected using targeted amplification methods. This difference can be explained by the fact that WGS can have a better capacity to conduct comprehensive, untargeted sequencing, allowing the identification of known and uncharacterised resistance genes (Bianconi et al., 2023; Hasan et al., 2025). The most widely distributed genes of all isolates included bla -CTX-M (58%), mecA (22%), and NDM -1 (18%). Several resistance determinants were co-occurring in 35 percent of the isolates leading to compound multidrug-resistance. The metagenomic data also identified plasmid replicons linked to horizontal gene transfer that further supports the idea that the spread of resistant features among bacterial species can be rather quick (Desai et al., 2025; Ma et al., 2025), and which were depicted in Figure 3..

Figure 3. Accuracy of PCR, CRISPR, and Whole Genome Sequencing in Identifying AMR Genes

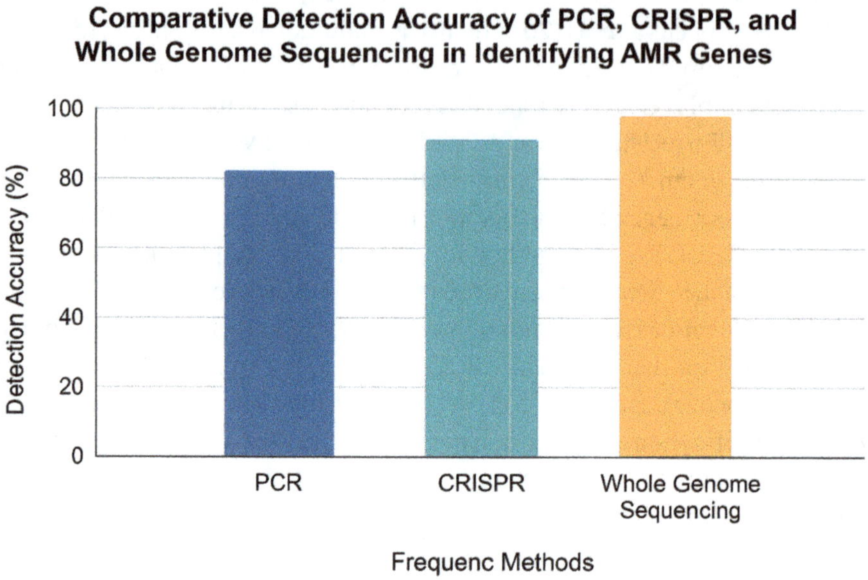

Comparative Diagnostic Accuracy and Statistical Analysis

In the current study, one-way analysis of variance was performed in order to determine the average accuracy of each diagnostic platform. The experiment showed statistically significant difference among the three groups ($F(2, 297) = 11.47$, $p < 0.05$) hence proving that the diagnostic method used has a significant effect on the accuracy of detection. Thereafter, post-hoc comparisons, such as Tukey test, revealed that whole-genome sequencing (WGS) was significantly more accurate than both polymerase chain reaction (PCR) ($p=0.004$) and CRISPR-based detection ($p=0.013$). In comparison to it, however, no pronounced difference was found between CRISPR and PCR regarding the identification of universally recognised genes, and it can be inferred that both modalities can be used with certain certainty in the selected scenario. Consideration of turnaround time also made the platforms distinct as CRISPR-based detection had the shortest average reporting time of 2 hours, and WGS a lengthiest processing time of 2436 hours, which is largely attributable to the lengthy sequencing and computational steps. Despite the afforded comprehensive resistance profile, WGS has a lengthy time course, which does not allow it to be used in bedside diagnosis; therefore, it is only applicable in detailed surveillance activities (Elbehiry and Abalkhail 2025). In a comparison of reproducibility, WGS had a coefficient of variation (CV) of 2.3 per cent as opposed to 3.1 per cent of CRISPR and 4.8 per cent of PCR, thus demonstrating better consistency. All these findings support the assertion that WGS is the most accurate and reproducible method of genomic-based identification of antimicrobial resistance, whereas CRISPR has a bright future of fast point-of-care diagnosis (Olatunji et al. 2024).

Genotype–Phenotype Correlation

In investigating the relationship of genotypes and phenotype, a comparative study of genomic mapping of determination of resistance and phenotypic antibiotic susceptibility test (AST) findings and results obtained by disc diffusion method was done. The overall genomic and phenotypic profiles Pearson correlation coefficient (r) was 0.86 ($p < 0.01$), which was very strong with a positive association between the two sets. The strongest concordance was observed in mecA locus followed by vancomycin resistance in vanA gene ($r = 0.94$ and 0.88, respectively). In comparison, the concordance of bla_CTX -M was less significant ($r = 0.81$), and it can be mainly explained by differences in the levels of gene expression and plasmid copy number. These inconsistencies demonstrate the regulatory and ecological effects that tune the expression of the phenotype, despite the genetic presence of the underlying resistance genes (Liu and Pandey, 2024). A summary of the results is briefly presented in Table 3, Gene Detection and Phenotypic Correlation across Diagnostic Platforms.

Table 3. Gene Detection and Phenotypic Correlation across Diagnostic Platforms

Resistance Gene	PCR Detection (%)	CRISPR Detection (%)	WGS Detection (%)	Phenotypic Correlation (r)	Significance (p < 0.05)
blaCTX-M	82	89	97	0.81	✓
mecA	84	91	98	0.94	✓
vanA	79	88	95	0.88	✓
NDM-1	75	84	92	0.85	✓
aac(6')-Ib	80	86	94	0.83	✓
Mean Accuracy	**86**	**92**	**97**	–	

Note: ✓ indicates statistically significant genotype–phenotype correlations.

Phylogenetic and AI Predictive Insights

Whole-genome sequencing outcomes have been useful in developing a phylogenetic tree that clarifies the genetic relationship existing between bacterial isolates. There were three major clades identified by a clustering analysis, which generally corresponded to specifications of species, but also to groups of hospital-specific transmission. Surprisingly, the genetic profile of isolates of the same hospital of both the genus Escherichia coli and Klebsiella pneumoniae showed a similarity of 9899 percent, which is in line with the hypothesis of nosocomial acquaintance routes (Struelens et al., 2024; Waddington et al., 2022). Regarding antimicrobial resistance phenotyping, the Random Forest machine-learning model displayed a sensitivity of 93 per cent, specificity of 89 per cent and a general accuracy of 91 per cent. The model found the presence of the genes of the following predictors to be the most significant which were the following: *mecA, blaCTX-M and NDM-1 as shown in the variable-importance plot. Although the single-gene presence is a factor that leads to resistance, the model indicates that multi -gene interactions are the most significant parameter in predicting resistance phenotypies. Figure 4 below shows the confusion matrix, which allows confirming that the predicted and observed phenotypes are in agreement in most cases, which proves the usefulness of AI-based algorithms in antimicrobial resistance diagnostics (Branda and Scarpa, 2024; Mohammed et al., 2025).

Figure 4. Phylogenetic Tree Depicting Genetic Relatedness among AMR

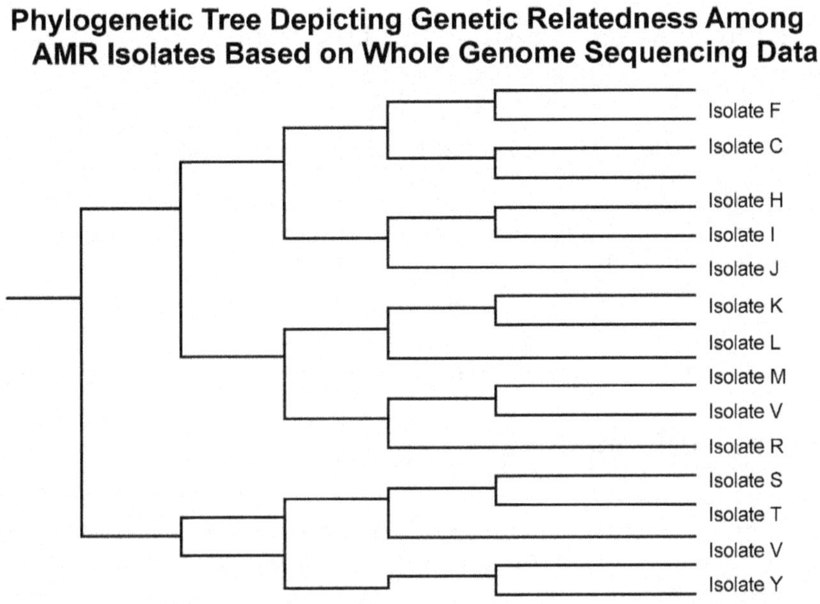

The comparative experimental study shows that genomic technologies provide much more precision compared to the traditional phenotypic diagnostics, in terms of both accuracy and predictive value. PCR is still a quick technique of detecting precise resistance markers, but its result is insufficient to detect new or mutant genes. CRISPR-based diagnostics is not as fast as PCR, or even as sensitive as whole-genome sequencing, thus making it especially effective in emergency clinical or resource-constrained environments. Although time-consuming, whole-genome sequencing provides a global overview of resistance determinants, mobile genetic elements, and phylogenetic associations. In turn, its use implies combined surveillance activities (Bianconi et al., 2023; Elguoshy and Hashem, 2024). The high-genotype-phenotype correlation confirms the hypothesis that genomic detection may become an option instead of traditional susceptibility testing. However, the occasional development of resistance even with the existence of genetic predeterminations highlights the need to integrate genomic diagnostics with functional tests and artificial-intelligence-based interpretative models (Hasan et al., 2025; Devi et al., 2025).

5. RESULTS AND DISCUSSION

This experimental research yields very important information regarding how microbial genomics and diagnostic innovation are revolutionizing the process of detecting and treating antimicrobial resistance (AMR). It is important to compare the approaches of PCR, CRISPR, and whole genome sequencing (WGS) as they demonstrate the complementary strengths of each technology and demonstrate a move towards a more accurate, comprehensive, and data-driven diagnostic ecosystem. General high genotypephenotype correlation and statistical significance at the platform level testify that genomic diagnostics does not only increase the accuracy of detection but also provides predictive power that is able to inform the implementation of public health strategies (Bianconi et al., 2023; Ma et al., 2025).

Diagnostic Performance

The increased sensitivity of whole-genome sequencing (WGS) to identify both known and previously unknown antimicrobial resistance genes is one of the strengths of the technology, which establishes the technology as the ultimate reference standard in AMR profiling. WGS is the only method to explain the genetic background of the resistance determinants, including plasmid-carried genes and mobile genetic elements that promote cross-species horizontal transfer by allowing the quantitative examination of the entire genomic environment (Desai et al., 2025). These results go hand in hand with the increasing amount of international evidence that supports the need to advocate WGS-based surveillance as a necessary element of modern AMR control policies (Struelens et al., 2024; Waddington et al., 2022). CRISPR-based diagnostic tools have the fastest turnaround time of any existing tool, but have a limited range; they are therefore best used to screen large populations at the same time before an outbreak spreads or to contain the infection at its initial stages. The portable nature of them and their inherent sensitivity makes them especially useful in low-resource or decentralised healthcare facilities. Polymerase chain reaction (PCR) despite its high levels of trust and frequent use is characterised by some inherent limitations like the reliance on pre-designed primers and limited target coverage, which limits its overall diagnostic capability. Combined, these findings illustrate that it is not possible to rely on one type of diagnostic modality. A combined, systematic strategy, which starts with a rapid CRISPR-based screen and is followed by resolution genomic sequencing, provides a balance of expediency and analysis depth (Kaprou et al., 2021; Olatunji et al., 2024). At the statistical level, it can be seen that the detection accuracy is significantly improved between the PCR stage to CRISPR and then WGS, which is indicative of the wider development of the diagnostic technology to be able to target specific amplifications and then explore the entire genome. In addition, the high genotypic and phenotypic resistance profile correlation (r= 0.86) supports the accuracy of the genomic data in the prediction of antimicrobial susceptibility. Last, the few differences that are present, including the existence of silent gene carriers that are not expressed phenotypically, can be explained by the regulatory controls, post-transcriptional modifications, or environmental factors that control the expression of genes as shown in Figure 5 (Liu & Pandey, 2024).

Figure 5. Genomic Diagnostics, Artificial Intelligence, and Public Health Policy in AMR

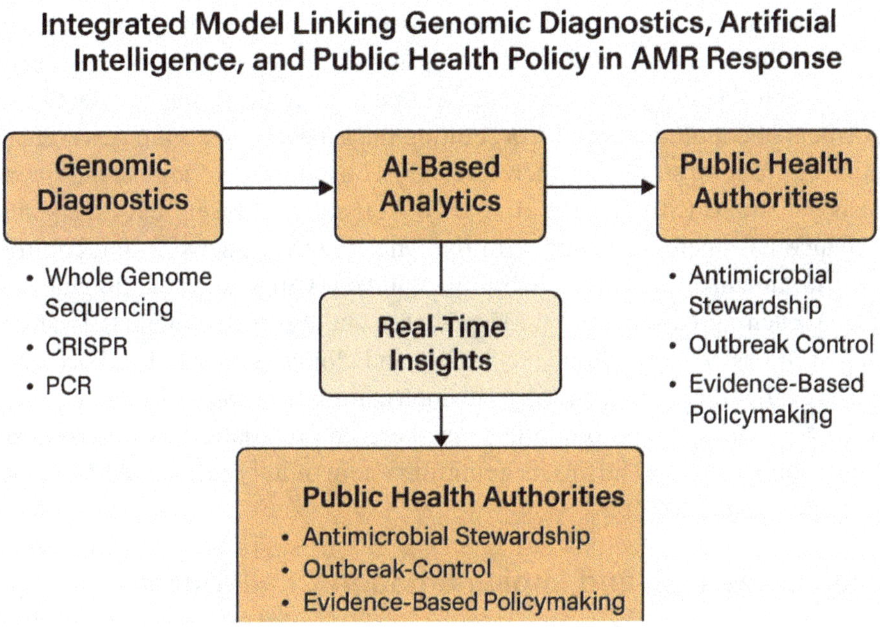

Translational and Public Health Implications

The results reported in this manuscript have far-reaching implications to the clinical microbiology and the health surveillance of communities. First of all, the authors can prove the effectiveness of genomic diagnostics in narrowing the gap in time between the ability to detect a pathogen and the ability to make a therapeutic decision. Clinicians are enabled to access resistance profiles in 24hours when whole-genome sequencing (WGS) information are processed with automated bioinformatics pipelines. This quicker turnaround makes it easier to precisely prescribe antibiotics, which are better than CRISPR-based assays or traditional culture-dependent methods, which might have been required to interpret the results with a few days (Elbehiry and Abalkhail, 2025; Hasan et al., 2025). Secondly, artificial-intelligence (AI) analytics representation of allegedly fixed laboratory data allows converting it into dynamic and predictive information. The random-forest model used in the study gave 91 per cent accuracy in identifying the presence of multidrug-resistant isolates, and these results demonstrate that these models can always adapt to new trends of resistance. In turn, the antimicrobial resistance (AMR) surveillance might transform into an active intelligence system instead of a retrospective monitoring effort (Branda and Scarpa, 2024; Mohammed et al., 2025). Thirdly, strategic assignment of genomic data can be used to accurately identify source and map outbreak locations. The phylogenetic analysis showed clear clusters of the genetically related Klebsiella pneumoniae and Escherichia coli isolates within the hospital networks, which are likely the pathways of nosocomial transmission. This information is considered by infection-control teams as an indispensable one to trace the routes of infections and the hotspots of contamination. Incorporating the aspect of genomic surveillance in infection-prevention strategies, therefore, helps hospitals to anticipate the spread of the resistant strains (Struelens et al., 2024). At the global level, real-time genomic surveillance has been correlated with the One Health framework, integrating the streams of human, animal, and environmental data (Chigozie et al., 2025; Singh et al., 2025). Such a cross-sectoral study enhances our ability to explain the transfer of resistance across the agricultural, veterinary and clinical systems. Furthermore, the increased availability of repositories with international coverage like Pathogenwatch and GLASS makes it possible to put together genomic data that are produced in different laboratories and form a meaningful system of international AMR response (Waddington et al., 2022)..

Ethical, Logistical, and Implementation Challenges

It is clear that despite the potential of genomic technologies to become transformative, there are still considerable barriers to their implementation that hinder its widespread use. High-throughput sequencing is still prohibitive, and the necessary bioinformatics skills needed to analyse sequencing data are distributed unevenly on the planet (Rugarabamu & Mwanyika, 2025). In addition, the low- and middle-income nations are limited by compromised infrastructure which prevents the possibility of implementing genome-based surveillance on a significant level. To alleviate these differences, the international community should seek harmonised efforts, such as global collaboration, common resource infrastructure, and public-private collaborations, in an attempt to democratise sequencing technologies (Devi et al., 2025). The second important difficulty is the issue of data governance. The data in genomics can be useful in surveillance, but they also include sensitive information, the leaking of which can make health care institutions vulnerable and reveal the identifying features of patients. There is thus an urgent need to ensure strong ethical principles that will govern the exchange of genomics information in a way that will not violate privacy of individuals and national sovereignty in global surveillance efforts. At the same time, the standardisation of data formats and bioinformatics pipelines is also necessary to reach the interoperability of laboratories and national databases (Coque et al., 2023). Logistically, the implementation of CRISPR based point-of-care devices needs to be approved by the regulatory body, be manufactured at scale, and trained end-users. The key to ensuring a wide adoption of these devices is ensuring that the front-line health-care workers are able to use these devices safely and correctly interpret their output (Olatunji et al., 2024). Lastly, the rapid expanding nature of genomic information as well as the related information-storage, information-processing, and information-security demands necessitate the necessity to incorporate considerations in both the institutional and government strategic planning.

Strategic Interpretation and Policy Relevance

The policy aspect of the policy argument that is adequately supported in the experimental findings is the need to incorporate microbial genomics into the national AMR action plans. A multi-tiered approach to diagnosis can be embraced by countries:

1. Primer level - Implement CRISPR or assays based on PCR in order to rapidly screen and triage suspected infections.
2. Secondary level Use WGS in extensive resistance mapping and epidemiological connection.
3. Tertiary level Implementation AI-based analytics to analyze massive genomic data to be used in surveillance, trend forecasting, and stewardship decisions.

This is an organized and coordinated flow of genomic data between the clinical and national system that forms a single health intelligence ecosystem (Branda and Scarpa, 2024; Singh et al., 2025). Moreover, the economic advantages of early diagnosis and specific care, in the form of decreased hospitalization and antibiotic overuse, are much greater than the early expenses of genomic infrastructure establishment. This model can empower the application of real-time AMR-tracking genomic dashboard by the public health authorities, which incorporates hospital, veterinary, and environmental streams of surveillance. The innovation would allow the prediction of future responses instead of reactionary, which would be in line with the future of precision public health (Chigozie et al., 2025).

6. STRATEGIC IMPLICATIONS AND RECOMMENDATIONS

The results of this paper support the fact that microbial genomics is a ground breaking frontier in the international campaign against antimicrobial resistance (AMR). The acquired empirical data through comparative diagnostic assessment highlights that genomic tools, especially whole genome sequencing (WGS), CRISPR-based diagnostic, and analytics enhanced by AI, present unprecedented possibilities of precision-based surveillance, early detection, and evidence-based action to be taken by the public health (Bianconi et al., 2023; Branda and Scarpa, 2024). Enhancing these technological advances into long-term national and institutional practices must, however, be strategically planned, interdisciplinary and well-integrated policies.

Building a Genomic Infrastructure for AMR Surveillance

The current paper highlights the need to institutionalise genomic capacity in health systems of countries. The systematic exchange of information and development of capacity can easily be executed through a standardised testing system and the systematic exchange of information, which can be achieved by creating genomic diagnostic centres in the area laboratories. Such hubs would provide services to hospitals, veterinary labs and environmental health centers thus promoting a One Health genomic surveillance system (Liu et al., 2024; Chigozie et al., 2025). The governmental agencies are to concentrate on investing in sequencing infrastructure, cloud-based bioinformatics pipelines and AI-based interpretation platforms. In order to enable interoperability and quick exchange of data between clinical and policy institutions, there is urgent need to establish centralised genomic repositories; this would be consistent with the international efforts, including the WHO GLASS. Additionally, the integration of whole-genome sequencing data into electronic health records (EHRs) can be a prospective approach to antimicrobial stewardship in real-time, which is predictive in that a clinician would be informed of the foresight of resistance profile before starting treatment.

Workforce Capacity Building and Interdisciplinary Training

The successful implementation of genomic diagnostics depends on the creation of a highly qualified interdisciplinary team that includes microbiology, genomics, bioinformatics, and data science, which is one of the prerequisites emphasised by Devi et al. (2025). The training programmes ought to go beyond the laboratory technicians to the clinicians, epidemiologists and the public-health authorities thus creating solid interpretation and translation of the genomic information into actionable information. A graduate and professional-level curriculum in the field of genomic medicine must be developed, and it is necessary to incorporate it into the academic and research institutions. The resolution of the digital-literacy gap in genomic diagnostics can be achieved with the help of continuous education, and workshops, along with other international agencies. An interconnected global learning system would also promote the sharing of best practises and data -governance standards between countries with different levels of technological development.

Data Governance, Ethics, and Standardization

Effective genomic surveillance will be possible only under the condition of data-management practises that can be considered secure, ethical, and follow agreed standards. Due to the sensitive nature of patient and institutional data in the genomic datasets, there is a strong need to ensure that there is the implementation of sound governance that will protect privacy as well as ensure data integrity. The mandate of national policy regulators should be anonymization, strict consent control, and secure cloud storage, which correspond to the current world ethical practises (Coque et al., 2023; Rugarabamu and Mwanyika, 2025). In addition, this should be applied to the workflows of analysis used. By making interoperable sequencing protocols, pipeline annotation and reporting formats, the comparability of laboratory findings will be improved. Bioinformatics practises need to be universalized by establishing transparency and reproducibility, which will require the implementation of open-access applications, such as the Comprehensive Antibiotic Resistance Database (CARD) and ResFinder, as in Table 4 of Genomic Diagnostics in National AMR Strategies (Hasan et al., 2025; Desai et al., 2025).

Table 4. Genomic Diagnostics into National AMR Strategies

Strategic Domain	Key Actions	Expected Outcomes	Relevant References
Infrastructure Development	Establish regional genomic sequencing hubs; adopt cloud-based data sharing	Improved diagnostic capacity and national genomic coverage	Struelens et al., 2024; Waddington et al., 2022
Human Resource Development	Launch genomic literacy and AI training programs for healthcare professionals	Strengthened cross-disciplinary competence	Devi et al., 2025; Chigozie et al., 2025
Data Governance	Implement anonymization protocols, ethical data-sharing policies	Secure and compliant genomic information systems	Coque et al., 2023; Rugarabamu & Mwanyika, 2025
Diagnostic Integration	Combine CRISPR rapid tests with WGS surveillance platforms	Real-time, multilevel AMR detection and containment	Olatunji et al., 2024; Hasan et al., 2025

continued on following page

Table 4. Continued

Strategic Domain	Key Actions	Expected Outcomes	Relevant References
AI and Predictive Analytics	Use machine learning to forecast emerging resistance trends	Proactive public health response	Branda & Scarpa, 2024; Mohammed et al., 2025
International Collaboration	Participate in global AMR genomic data-sharing networks	Enhanced global surveillance interoperability	Singh et al., 2025; Liu & Pandey, 2024

Leveraging Artificial Intelligence and Predictive Modeling

Application of AI-based analytics based on genomic studies takes a central position in the process of converting raw genomic data into usable intelligence. As shown in this study, random Forest classifiers and other machine-learning algorithms will be effective to predict phenotypic resistance based on genotypic signatures. This ability has the potential to be expanded to a level that would make national antimicrobial-resistance predicting disruptive. The national health authorities should develop special AI-genomics integration units that create real-time predictive dashboards that identify the emergent resistance hotspots (Branda and Scarpa, 2024; Pennisi et al., 2025). Predictive modelling also increases clinical decision support. AI algorithms can be used to propose enhanced antibiotic regimens based on the genomic resistance profiles to minimize unnecessary antimicrobial use when integrated into hospital information systems. This type of integration is in line with the main goals of antimicrobial stewardship, which consists of the rational use of drugs, decreased selective pressure, and the inhibition of the spread of resistance (Mohammed et al., 2025).

Public–Private Partnerships and Innovation Funding

Considering the prohibitive price of the genomic infrastructure, collaboration between governments, research centres and the innovators of the private sector becomes inevitable. Public-private partnerships can be dedicated to finding funds in order to create diagnostic kits, cloud-computing services, and bioinformatics software. Joint initiatives between biotechnological companies and university consortia can be used to co-develop localized genomic platforms that will address the particular epidemiological and fiscal demands (Olatunji et al., 2024; Elbehiry and Abalkhail, 2025). Governments need to institute programmes on innovation funding that would be able to fund pilot genomic monitoring projects and underwrite the cost of sequencing in high-burden hospitals. These measures will speed up early adoption and create cost-saving information to support national scale-up.

Global Collaboration and One Health Alignment

Monitoring of antimicrobial resistance should be international; the free movement of the pathogens implies the need to coordinate intercountry activity. One Health approach recognises the relationship of human, animal and environmental reservoir of resistance (Liu and Pandey, 2024). Genomic networks are networks of cooperation between medical laboratories, veterinary, and agricultural research institutes that give a complete overview of the spread of resistance genes (360). The participation in international databases like Pathogenwatch and GLASS may be supplemented by local genomic collaborations that implement the information interpretation based on local contexts. This kind of cooperation will increase the speed of alerts and organize policy responses in case of resistance outbreaks (Singh et al., 2025; Waddington et al., 2022).

Strategic Policy Recommendations

1. Make Genomic Surveillance Standard: Incorporate WGS and CRISPR diagnostics into national AMR surveillance.
2. Create AI-Enabled AMR Dashboards: Have predictive data systems so that resistance patterns can be determined prior to the outbreaks.
3. Invest in Capacity and Training: Increase education at the genomic microbiology and data analytics level.
4. Unify Data and Ethical Standards: Advance Interoperability and Privacy in Genomic Data.
5. Strengthen One Health Collaboration: Promoting cross-sector health partnerships between human, veterinary and environmental health.
6. Foster Innovation Funding: Massive incentives should be given to local biotech companies to develop affordable genomic diagnosing kits.

All these strategic measures will constitute a sustainable roadmap of integrating microbial genomics into national and international AMR control systems.

7. FUTURE RESEARCH DIRECTIONS

The field of microbial genomics and diagnostic innovation continues to propose a range of strong opportunities to the larger field of antimicrobial resistance (AMR) studies. Although the existing literature defines the relative effectiveness of genomic technologies and AI-based analysis tools in the context of resistance detection, the direction of AMR investigation is inevitably related to broad predictive analytics, automated surveillance systems, and improved forecasting systems. In this regard, future studies must strive to integrate overlaying clinical, environmental, and agricultural surveillance systems in a single framework of One Health (Liu et al., 2024; Chigozie et al., 2025).

Expanding Genomic Coverage through Metagenomics

One of the main areas of future studies is the method of metagenomic sequencing which allows providing the overall study of microbial communities in clinical or environmental samples without the necessity of their complex growth. Metagenomic next-generation sequencing (mNGS) also allows simultaneous identification of antimicrobial resistance pathogens, resistance genes, and mobile genetic elements, which will provide a more detailed picture of the ecological context of antimicrobial resistance (Elbehiry and Abalkhail, 2025). To bring these lessons to everyday practice, later work ought to focus on standardizing mNGS guidelines, thus increasing their analytical accuracy, decreasing the cost, and simplifying automated data-processing pipelines. In addition, the combination of metagenomic studies and environmental surveys of wastewater, soil and animal reservoirs will be useful in tracking the spread of resistance genes in various ecosystems. This development is in line with the One Health genomic surveillance paradigm, which recognizes the interdependence between environmental and human resistance dynamics (Singh et al., 2025).

Advancing Artificial Intelligence for Predictive AMR Analytics

The next generation of AMR surveillance systems will be the use of artificial intelligence. Although the given research showed that the concept of the Random Forest classifier is indeed viable in terms of predicting the genotype to phenotype interactions, the future of this approach should be extended to include the deep learning models that are capable of capturing more complicated genotype to environment relationships along with the potential interaction between genes (Branda and Scarpa, 2024; Mohammed et al., 2025). Specifically, neural networks, convolutional models and reinforcement learning can find applications in discovering new resistance mechanisms, as well as modelling, in an evolutionary context, how a microbial population may respond to the pressure of antibiotics. In addition, AI can facilitate genuinely adaptive genomic diagnostics, in which algorithms are re-trained using new emerging sequencing data with the aim of identifying emerging resistance phenotypes. These self-learning systems would have the ability to dynamically revise diagnostic assays and would enable world databanks to automatically identify possible resistance hot spots. These efforts will continue to be successful based on solid interdisciplinary cooperation: AI engineers, microbiologists, and epidemiologists should collaborate to build interpretable, transparent and clinically reliable algorithms (Pennisi et al., 2025), as shown in Figure, the AI-Integrated Predictive Genomic Surveillance of AMR.

Figure 6. AI-Integrated Predictive Genomic Surveillance of AMR

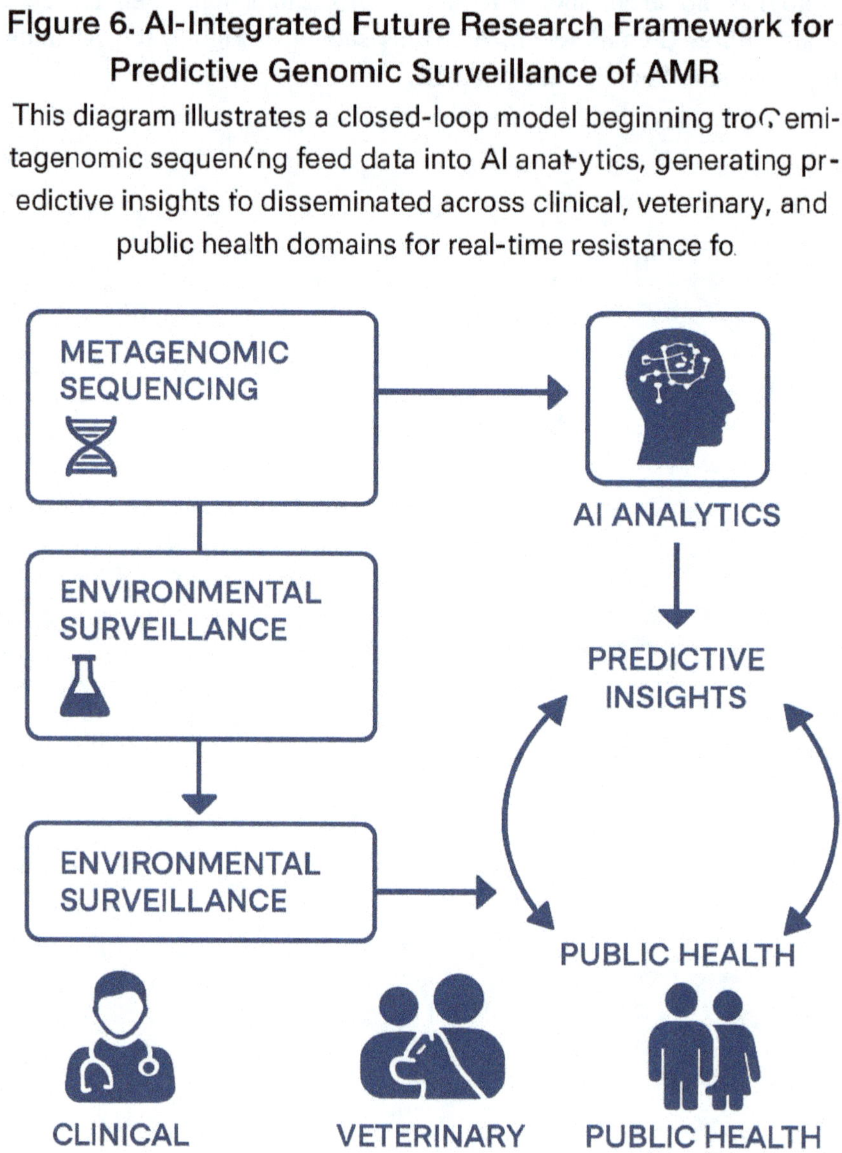

Portable and Real-Time Genomic Technologies

The alternative road to take would be on portable sequencing devices including nanopore-based systems which offers real-time sequencing and analyses at the point of care. These tools hold the promise to democratize genomic diagnostics access by allowing the identification of resistance genes in-field during an outbreak or in a resource-limited environment (Olatunji et al., 2024; Ma et al., 2025). Future studies need to focus on enhancing the accuracy of sequencing, decreasing the dimensions of the supporting computational hardware, and implementing mobile data-sharing systems. In line with these endeavours, biosensor-based diagnosis methods ought to be refined in order to combine nanotechnology with CRISPR-based detection to enable fast and label-free identifications of antimicrobial resistance genes. This would alter the non-portability of genomics between laboratories and at the point-of-care and result in genomic intelligence becoming an inseparable part of the health infrastructure (Kaprou et al., 2021; Vasala et al., 2020).

Integrative Multi-Omics Approaches

A paradigm change will occur in the further phase of AMR genomics whereby the focus of DNA-based sequencing will be expanded to a wider multi-omics integration system. This method will provide a combination of genomics, transcriptomics, proteomics, and metabolomics to create a comprehensive perspective on microbial physiology and the mechanisms that govern resistance. This kind of integration will shed new light on why some genotypic resistances do not have a phenotypic appearance and explain how metabolic stress alters expression of resistance-gene (Hasan et al., 2025). With the artificial intelligence of these detailed datasets, a researcher can discover early biomarkers of resistance or new therapeutic targets. As an example, predictability of individualised treatment regimens about the relationship of gene-expression pattern and antibiotic response could counter the need to select resistance. The research of the future should therefore focus on the systems-level modelling of AMR based on large-scale and integrative datasets.

Ethical, Economic, and Policy-Oriented Research

Even though technological development is being developed fastest, ethical and socioeconomic aspect of genomic innovation should also be significantly observed in future research. It is crucial that a thorough investigation of the ownership of data, patient consent, and fair access to the process of genomic testing take place (Coque et al., 2023; Rugarabamu and Mwanyika, 2025). The comparative policy analysis can question the way in which various systems of governance can solve the problem on sharing genomic data and protect individual privacy, institutional integrity and ethicality. In addition, the financial implications of scaled genomic diagnostics should be carefully analysed. Cost savings achieved in the long term as a result of the early detection of AMR, decreased hospitalisation, and efficient use of antibiotics should be measured in terms of rigorous cost-effectiveness research. Such facts would support the thesis that governments and health organisations need to put significant resources into the genomic infrastructures and training programmes.

Cross-Sector Collaboration and One Health Integration

In order to develop the investigation on antimicrobial resistance, there is an urgent need to ensure that future research develops multisectoral partnerships between clinical labs, veterinary medicine, and agricultural genomics programmes. In systematically sharing sequencing data on human and non-human focal groups, researchers will be in a position to track intracommunity and intercommunity relationships of resistance genes in addition to engaging in in-depth risk evaluation (Liu and Pandey, 2024; Singh et al., 2025). In this regard, global consortia are capable of creating a unified, strong platform of information exchange and comparative evaluation that resembles the conventional tools like PathogenWatch. The implementation of AMR genomic surveillance within the One Health policy framework would stimulate the process of synthesis of data based on human, animal, and environmental origins, which would make it possible to plan the strategies. The use of such integrative interventions is required to curb the transboundary spread of antimicrobial resistance especially in agricultural sectors whereby the use of antibiotics is still high.

8. CONCLUSION

Through an experimental study, this chapter outlines how microbial genomics and diagnostic innovation is redefining how our world is responding to the detection and mitigation of antimicrobial resistance (AMR). This paper shows that Polymerase Chain Reaction (PCR), CRISPR-based diagnostics, and Whole Genome Sequencing (WGS) have more diagnostic accuracy and analytical breadth compared to traditional phenotypic testing in the context of genomic tests. The data indicate that WGS has the greatest detection precision (97 3), and reproducibility, but CRISPR-based systems have to provide rapid solutions that can be deployed in the field and have high sensitivity. The existence of a good genotype-phenotype relationship ($r=0.86$) highlights the importance of the genomic evidences as a valid predictor of actual antimicrobial susceptibility, which makes genomics a keystone of precision microbiology and evidence-based health. The consequences of the results are difficult to overestimate: genomic diagnostics helps to overcome the inherent limitations of culture-dependent methods by determining the determinants of resistance in near real time, allowing clinicians to select an effective therapeutic regimen sooner, reduce patient morbidity, and limit the use of broad-spectrum antibiotics. Furthermore, when sequencing data is combined with artificial intelligence (AI), diagnostic laboratories could become predictive centers, which can predict resistance profiles, epidemiology, and inform the policymaking (Branda and Scarpa, 2024; Mohammed et al., 2025). Both microbial genomics, therefore, and machine-learning synthesis is not only a technical innovation, but a paradigm shift towards adaptive, predictive AMR management. In terms of population health, this study points out that genomic epidemiology is a necessary element of AMR containment initiatives in countries and internationally. WGS-based phylogenetic analyses demonstrate the potential of identifying transmission groups in hospitals, therefore, informing infection control efforts. These genomic signals can be used to complement real-time monitoring and early warning systems when scaled to national surveillance and are consistent with international efforts like the World Health Organization Global Antimicrobial Resistance Surveillance System (GLASS) and are indicative of the increased acceptability of genomics in health governance (Struelens et al., 2024; Waddington et al., 2022).

The moral and systems impact that is coming along with this technological revolution are also very important. With the increased availability of genomic sequencing, the high data governance systems are needed to protect privacy, transparency, and equitable participation in all jurisdictions. The present research supports the idea that the AMR control should not be implemented without elaborate equipment only but also with the detailed policies, the properly trained staff, and the interoperable data systems. It is a global concern that fair access to genomic technologies in resource-constrained environments should be achieved. Opening the full potential of genomic innovation in tackling AMR will be enabled by the democratization of the sequencing platform, AI applications, and international collaboration based on open-data sharing (Chigozie et al., 2025; Rugarabamu and Mwanyika, 2025). The results of the experiment, therefore, support the use of a multi-level method of detecting and responding to genomic AMR:

1. Rapid Screening Layer: CRISPR and PCR-based testing of rapid and point of care diagnostics.
2. Comprehensive Surveillance Layer WGS exhaustive resistance-gene mapping and epidemiological tracing.
3. Predictive Intelligence Layer Intelligence Artificial Intelligence and bioinformatics analytics to forecast resistance development and optimize antimicrobial stewardship.

This hierarchical model deals with clinical accuracy and population-health vision and provides a scalable template that could be used in a wide range of economic and infrastructural settings, including a high-resource genome laboratory or field-based diagnostics in third-world countries. In the future, the merger between metagenomics, predictive analytics based on AI and integrating these technologies with multi-omics is set to drive microbial genomics into the next generation of AMR research and policy. It is likely that in the future systems will take the form of an international system of genomic monitoring, keeping track of the development of resistance, discovering new forms of genes, and prescribing context-specific interventions. Individualised case treatment will be a subset of a more generalised body of knowledge on microbial evolution and resilience of planetary health in this ecosystem. Altogether, microbial genomics and diagnostic innovation transform the paradigm of AMR detection into the reactive to the preventative and predictive ones. This transformation is justified by the integration of genomic diagnostics into healthcare systems and surveillance networks which has been experimentally validated. In conjunction with the sound technology and governance, genomics helps countries predict the threats, maintain antibiotic effectiveness, and enhance health security. This is the most promising direction of destroying the global epidemic of antimicrobial resistance as guided by collaborative intelligence and One Health vision.

9. REFERENCES

Ardila, C. M., González-Arroyave, D., & Tobón, S. (2025). Machine learning for predicting antimicrobial resistance in critical and high-priority pathogens: A systematic review considering antimicrobial susceptibility tests in real-world healthcare settings. *PLoS One*, *20*(2), e0319460. PMID: 39999193

Bianconi, I., Aschbacher, R., & Pagani, E. (2023). Current uses and future perspectives of genomic technologies in clinical microbiology. *Antibiotics (Basel, Switzerland)*, *12*(11), 1580. PMID: 37998782

Branda, F., & Scarpa, F. (2024). Implications of artificial intelligence in addressing antimicrobial resistance: Innovations, global challenges, and healthcare's future. *Antibiotics (Basel, Switzerland)*, *13*(6), 502. PMID: 38927169

Chigozie, V. U., Aniokete, C. U., Ogbonna, P. I., & Iroha, R. I. (2025). Transforming antimicrobial resistance mitigation: The genomic revolution in one health and public health. *Discover Applied Sciences*, *7*(10), 1187.

Coque, T. M., Cantón, R., Pérez-Cobas, A. E., Fernández-de-Bobadilla, M. D., & Baquero, F. (2023). Antimicrobial resistance in the global health network: Known unknowns and challenges for efficient responses in the 21st century. *Microorganisms*, *11*(4), 1050. PMID: 37110473

Desai, S., Patel, V., Nagare, S. D., Patil, R., & More, M. J. (2025). Microbial genomics and infectious disease forecasting. In *Host Adaptation, Virulence, and Evolution* (pp. 193-223). Academic Press.

Devi, M., Manokaran, D., Sehgal, R. K., Shariff, S. A., & Vettriselvan, R. (2025). Precision Medicine, Personalized Treatment, and Network-Driven Innovations: Transforming Healthcare With AI. In *AI for Large Scale Communication Networks* (pp. 303-322). IGI Global.

Elbehiry, A., & Abalkhail, A. (2025). Metagenomic next-generation sequencing in infectious diseases: Clinical applications, translational challenges, and future directions. *Diagnostics (Basel)*, *15*(16), 1991. PMID: 40870843

Elbehiry, A., & Abalkhail, A. (2025). Metagenomic next-generation sequencing in infectious diseases: Clinical applications, translational challenges, and future directions. *Diagnostics (Basel)*, *15*(16), 1991. PMID: 40870843

Elguoshy, A., & Hashem, A. M. (2024). Introduction to genomic-based clinical applications. In *Microbial Genomics: Clinical, Pharmaceutical, and Industrial Applications* (pp. 97-115). Academic Press.

Hasan, G. M., Mohammad, T., Shamsi, A., Sohal, S. S., & Hassan, M. I. (2025). Applications of Genome Sequencing in Infectious Diseases: From Pathogen Identification to Precision Medicine. *Pharmaceuticals, 18*(11), 1687. PMID: 41304932

Jiang, W. (2025). Addressing Antimicrobial Resistance: Evidence-Based Strategies And Innovations. *Transactions on Materials. Biotechnology and Life Sciences, 8,* 357–364.

Kaprou, G. D., Bergšpica, I., Alexa, E. A., Alvarez-Ordonez, A., & Prieto, M. (2021). Rapid methods for antimicrobial resistance diagnostics. *Antibiotics (Basel, Switzerland), 10*(2), 209. PMID: 33672677

Liu, C. S. C., & Pandey, R. (2024). Integrative genomics would strengthen AMR understanding through ONE health approach. *Heliyon, 10*(14). PMID: 39816336

Ma, D., Cai, F., & Zhang, T. (2025). Advances in the detection of Drug-Resistant bacteria: Current trends and innovations. *European Journal of Clinical Microbiology & Infectious Diseases,* •••, 1–17. PMID: 40974457

Mohammed, A. M., Oleiwi, J. K., Osman, A. F., Adam, T., Betar, B. O., Gopinath, S. C., & Ihmedee, F. H. (2025). Enhancing antimicrobial resistance strategies: Leveraging artificial intelligence for improved outcomes. *South African Journal of Chemical Engineering, 51*(1), 272–286.

Olatunji, A. O., Olaboye, J. A., Maha, C. C., Kolawole, T. O., & Abdul, S. (2024). Next-Generation strategies to combat antimicrobial resistance: Integrating genomics, CRISPR, and novel therapeutics for effective treatment. *Engineering Science & Technology Journal, 5*(7), 2284–2303.

Pennisi, F., Pinto, A., Ricciardi, G. E., Signorelli, C., & Gianfredi, V. (2025). The role of artificial intelligence and machine learning models in antimicrobial stewardship in public health: A narrative review. *Antibiotics (Basel, Switzerland), 14*(2), 134. PMID: 40001378

Rugarabamu, S., & Mwanyika, G. (2025). Biotechnological Innovations to Combat Antimicrobial Resistance and Advance Global Health Equity. *Bacteria, 4*(3), 46.

Singh, S., Kumar, M., Sarma, D. K., Kumawat, M., Verma, V., kriti, M., & Tiwari, R. (2025). Advancing AMR Surveillance: Confluence of One Health and Big Data Integration: S. Singh, et al. *EcoHealth,* 1-12.

Struelens, M. J., Ludden, C., Werner, G., Sintchenko, V., Jokelainen, P., & Ip, M. (2024). Real-time genomic surveillance for enhanced control of infectious diseases and antimicrobial resistance. *Frontiers in Science, 2,* 1298248.

Thompson, L. (2024). The Impact of Antimicrobial Resistance on Public Health: Challenges and Strategic Responses. *Insight into Epidemiology, 1*(1).

Vasala, A., Hytönen, V. P., & Laitinen, O. H. (2020). Modern tools for rapid diagnostics of antimicrobial resistance. *Frontiers in Cellular and Infection Microbiology, 10*, 308. PMID: 32760676

Waddington, C., Carey, M. E., Boinett, C. J., Higginson, E., Veeraraghavan, B., & Baker, S. (2022). Exploiting genomics to mitigate the public health impact of antimicrobial resistance. *Genome Medicine, 14*(1), 15. PMID: 35172877

Zhou, S., Zhao, X., & Meng, F. (2025). Method development and clinical validation of LAMP-CRISPR/Cas12a for rapid detection of respiratory pathogens in children. *Frontiers in Pediatrics, 13*, 1533100. PMID: 40292114

Chapter 8
Harnessing Microbial Genomics to Unravel Mechanisms of Antimicrobial Resistance:
Insights Into Genetic Drivers and Novel Strategies Against AMR

Maria Nazir Ahmad
https://orcid.org/0009-0004-6714-6212
Cholistan Uniiversity of Veterinary and Animal Sciences, Bahawalpur, Pakistan

Syed Sohail Ahmad
https://orcid.org/0009-0001-9652-7565
Rehman College of Allied Health Sciences, Rehman Medical Institute, Peshawar, Pakistan

ABSTRACT

Antimicrobial resistance (AMR) is a growing global health crisis that threatens to undermine decades of medical progress. This chapter examines the transformative role of microbial genomics in addressing AMR, emphasizing advancements in next-generation and nanopore sequencing that enable rapid detection and real-time monitoring of resistance genes. The integration of artificial intelligence (AI) and machine learning (ML) enhances predictive modeling of AMR evolution and guides evidence-based treatment strategies. Emerging approaches in personalized medicine, driven by pathogen genomic profiling, allow for tailored antibiotic therapies, minimizing misuse and improving outcomes. The chapter also underscores the importance of global collaboration and data sharing across human, animal,

DOI: 10.4018/979-8-3373-3825-5.ch008

and environmental health sectors, supported by innovations such as CRISPR-based tools. Together, these technologies offer a proactive framework for global AMR surveillance and intervention, paving the way for precise, effective, and sustainable management of infectious diseases in the genomic era.

1. INTRODUCTION

However, the level of interest that was gained by the COVID-19 pandemic was not sufficient to cover the fact that antibiotic resistance (AMR) has become one of the most important health dangers that humanity must face. It is estimated that there will be 5.3 million deaths worldwide caused by drug-resistant infections in 2023 alone. The number of deaths caused by HIV/AIDS and malaria combined is equal to the number of deaths caused by drug-resistant infections (Tsere, 2023). This is the number of deaths that are projected to be caused by drug-resistant infections around the world. It is a terrible thing that such a threat is spreading at such a rapid rate: a child who is born right now will grow up in a society where routine medical operations entail the risk of death owing to antibiotics that are not effective.

According to the World Health Organization's (WHO) 2024 Global Antimicrobial Resistance Surveillance Report, the resistance of first-line classes of treatment against pneumonia and urinary tract infections has already exceeded fifty percent in many regions. As a result, healthcare providers are forced to administer second-line combinations that have extremely high toxicity profiles. There is a growing body of evidence that supports the expediency of the interventions that are currently being attempted to mitigate the effects of common infections (Organization, 2024).

There are biological and behavioral variables that are contributing to this catastrophe. However, the exercise of anthropogenic intervention in the form of unselective prescribing practices in the United States (CDC, 2023) and direct access to the drug in the case of India has explosively increased the ability of pathogens to develop resistance. Bacteria in the United States have become more resistant to antibiotics as a result of the natural processes of evolution. At the same Time, the widespread production of antibiotics in the livestock industry has led to the proliferation of so-called superbugs. These are pathogenic microorganisms that are resistant to the vast majority of treatments that are currently available. These superbugs include agents such as *Acinetobacter baumannii* and *Candida auris*, whose infections have fatalities that exceed fifty percent in the populations that are most susceptible to them (Mitra et al., 2022).

The problem of antibiotic-resistant pathogens is a serious issue; nevertheless, a solution to this problem can be found in a place where one would not expect it to be found: in the field of microbial genomics research. High-throughput sequencing tools, initially used to monitor the COVID-19 pandemic, have now evolved into the weapon of choice for combating AMR. There was a notable instance of an outbreak of carbapenem-resistant Klebsiella pneumoniae in a hospital in Berlin in 2023 (Baum et al., 2025). This outbreak occurred when active and portable DNA sequencers were used in the field. These sequencers discovered the specifics of resistance to the pathogen in real-time, which enabled the patient to be isolated on the spot and select the most effective antibiotics within a short period, rather than several days after contact. This prevented a much more severe scenario from occurring.

The discovery of mcr-10, a novel resistance gene, in New York City, which was discovered three weeks prior to the appearance of clinical infections in wastewater, demonstrates that it has the potential to function as an early-warning system. This discovery sheds light on the ultimate usefulness of genomic surveillance, which can be illuminated by the emergence of mcr-10 (Mullin, 2023). When taken as a whole, these results signify the beginning of a new era in the field of medicine, one in which genome sequencing will be utilized to determine which antibiotic strategy(s) will be most effective against any given infection (Figure 1). In the UK, for instance, rapid whole-genome sequencing of suspected newborn sepsis cases has resulted in a 27% reduction in sepsis-related mortality. In South Africa and India, genomic testing has helped to eliminate over 60% of misdiagnoses of tuberculosis by differentiating between drug-sensitive and drug-resistant forms of the disease (Mnyambwa, 2019). An even more ambitious development is the possibility that artificial intelligence systems may analyze bacterial DNA and anticipate resistance patterns with 95% accuracy, leading to more precise treatment recommendations.

Figure 1. Key factors driving AMR and genomic solutions for detection, surveillance, and prediction.

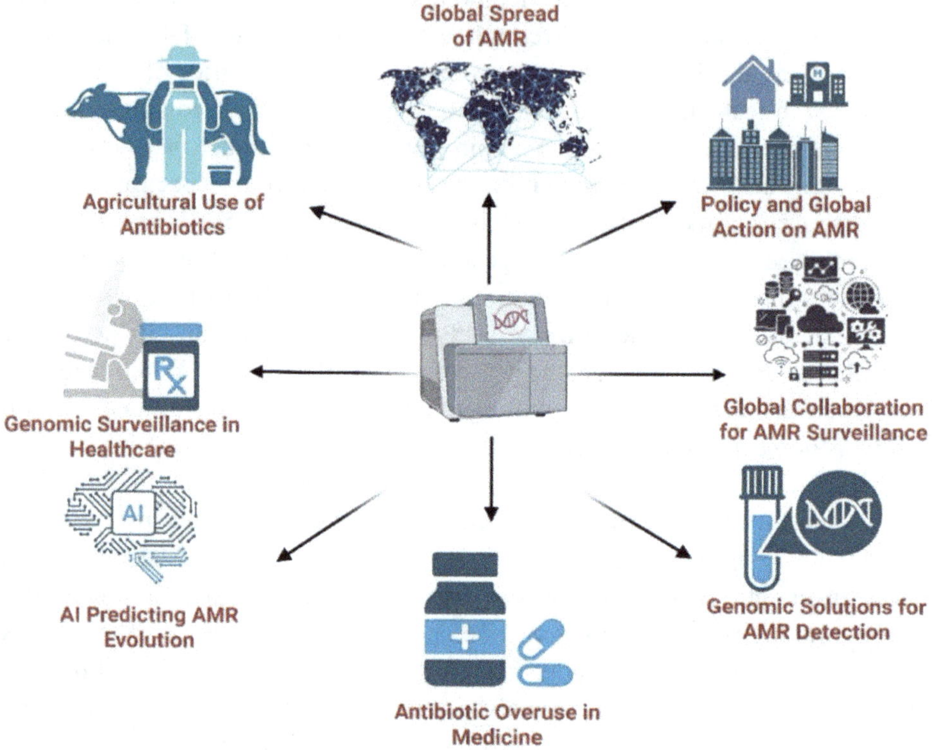

Overall, AMR represents not just a medical challenge but an essential test of our collective ability to harness scientific advancements for the betterment of humanity. The genomic technologies employed in mapping the human genome are currently utilized globally to monitor and manage resistant microbes. The situation is critical, yet it can be effectively addressed if governments, healthcare systems, and individuals take decisive actions. Antibiotic resistance is currently leading to fatalities, as noted by Dr. Chris Murray from the Institute for Health Metrics and Evaluation: it is not a looming threat, but a present-day danger. However, in contrast to climate change, we can all implement the required changes swiftly if we consider it essential to do so" (Pettorelli et al., 2021). The focus will be on how stakeholders respond and adapt to the demands of this global health crisis.

2. THE ROLE OF MICROBIAL GENOMICS IN UNDERSTANDING AMR

2.1 The Genetic Basis of Antimicrobial Resistance

The field of genetics forms the basis of what we understand today about AMR. The defensive mechanism of bacterial pathogens may occur spontaneously, or it may occur as a part of the mutation process inherent in the organism's chromosome, or by the adoption of exogenous organism resistance genes, which in turn perform as imported genetic resistance factors. Bacteria have various molecular strategies to survive the impacts of antibiotics. Many strains of *Mycobacterium tuberculosis* contain mutations in the rpoB gene, resulting in rifampicin resistance (Li et al., 2021). Mycobacteria also harbor enzymes referred to as β-lactamases, which have the ability to break down the antibiotics before they can provide the effect. *Pseudomonas aeruginosa* uses efflux pumps to eject fluoroquinolone and other antibiotics out of the cell, and E. coli also reduces antibiotic uptake by regulating the permeability of the cell membrane.

One of the most concerning aspects of AMR is the high rate at which the gene of resistance is transferred horizontally across bacterial species. This transmission is facilitated by specific mobile genetic elements, including plasmids, transposons, and integrons. The issue has catalyzed the international transfer of antimicrobial resistance. One of the most prominent is the mcr-1 gene, which offers resistance to colistin, the next-resort antibiotic, and has spread to other parts of the world through plasmid transfer. As a result, the genetic components involved in antimicrobial resistance outbreaks cannot be studied without an adequate understanding of these genetic exchanges, and therefore, the development of effective public-health responses to such outbreaks (Dimitriu, 2022).

2.2 Genomic Technologies Revolutionizing AMR Detection

The emergence of whole-genome sequencing (WGS) in recent years has significantly expanded the range of tools available for identifying AMR. In comparison to traditional methods, which involve lengthy procedures and labor-intensive processes and are prone to mistakes, WGS has the ability to provide complete pathogenic genomic profiles in hours or days. The technology, at the same Time, makes it possible to identify the resistance genes, detect the mutation, and restore the chain of transmission with an unprecedented degree of accuracy (Qiu, 2024). The simplified workflow of WGS, outlined in this paper, is summarized schematically in Figure 2: collection of a biological sample, genetic extraction, sequencing completion, and data analysis. This type of workflow is crucial for the timely detection of AMR threats and enhances clinicians' ability to make evidence-based treatment decisions.

Figure 2. Whole-genome sequencing pipeline for AMR detection.

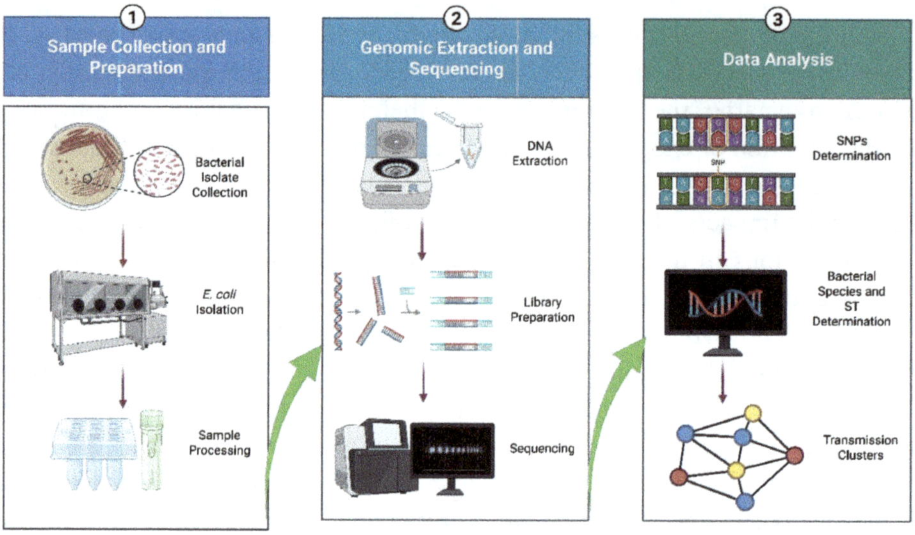

Major steps of genomic analysis of *Escherichia coli* (*E. coli*) isolates are shown in the illustrative flowchart below. This process starts by sampling: sample specimens are harvested, the bacterial cells are isolated, and *E. coli* is selectively retrieved. DNA purification is followed by washing and DNA extraction. The next step involves genomic sequencing. To acquire whole genomic data, DNA is translated into sequencing libraries and run through peer-reviewed sequencing platforms. Single Nucleotide Polymorphisms (SNPs), bacterial species, and type of sequences (ST) are determined during the data analysis; transmission clusters are analyzed in order to assess bacterial dispersal (Treffon et al., 2022). This pipeline enables the interrogation of entire genomic data for use in AMR research. Additionally, genome sequencing has also evolved beyond retrospective practices to real-time hospital surveillance. This allows the clinicians to predict and cope with the resistance before treatment. Moreover, databases such as the Comprehensive Antibiotic Resistance Database (CARD) or ResFinder are invaluable for cross-checking existing genetic sequences against known resistant genes, thereby enabling the early detection of potential threats.

2.2 Decoding Resistance Pathways with Genomic Data

Microbial genomics is a knowledge base capable of not only listing resistance genes, but also explaining the mechanisms by which resistance occurs. Comparative genomics makes possible the determination of genetic divergence between resistant and susceptible strains and, therefore, the definition of hotspots of resistance. Pan-genomics of the multidrug-resistant *E. coli* strain ST131 revealed a consistent gene pool of resistance genes that underpins the strain's success. Genome-wide association studies (GWAS) associate genetic markers, including gyrA mutation in Neisseria gonorrhoeae, with a given antibiotic resistance phenotype (Souza et al., 2025).

Functional genomics advances by utilizing genetic technologies to knock out target genes and then using these to determine the functional consequences. An example of this was in *Klebsiella pneumoniae*, where carbapenem susceptibility was regained upon the removal of the blaKPC gene (Rodrigues et al., 2024). Parallel transcriptomic and proteomic techniques also serve to illustrate the way that resistance genes are activated by the presence of antibiotics; under conditions of β-lactam antibiotics, *Enterobacter* upregulates the ampC, a response, which appears to endow such species with an observable survival advantage. Current single-cell genomics can reveal the phenotypic diversity even in genetically homogeneous cells, which informs us about the complex processes that allow bacterial clones to survive during antibiotic therapy.

3. MECHANISMS OF ANTIMICROBIAL RESISTANCE (AMR) REVEALED BY MICROBIAL GENOMICS

3.1 Genetic Mutations and Their Role in AMR

Antimicrobial resistance is a molecular event wherein mutations in the microbial genetic material alter the target receptors of an antimicrobial agent, in turn suppressing its antimicrobial potential. The overuse and misuse of antibiotics are indeed etiological factors, but this could occur through spontaneous mutation as microorganisms evolve to respond to their environment, or it may be spurred by improper therapeutic applications. An example is fluoroquinolone resistance, which develops as a result of mutations in a number of vital bacterial genes (with gyrA and parC as the most prominent) (Petronio). Through the alteration of the attachment site of the antibiotics, these mutants are disruptive to the use of microorganisms in therapeutic interventions. In *E. coli*, a mutation of gyrA is linked with significantly increased fluoroquinolone resistance, whereas mutations in parC of *Klebsiella pneumoniae* are analogous. The results include resistant infections, which have in the past been easily treated. The rapid development of the field related to the topic of AMR created a precondition for implementing diagnostic methods that involve the use of CRISPR-based diagnostic tools, enabling quick mutation detection at the basis of a complex system. The application of these tools in clinical settings will enable the identification of resistant strains, including those with gyrA and parC mutations, within two hours, thereby offering clinically relevant insights for personalized therapy (Yakout & Ali, 2022).

3.2 The Role of Mobile Genetic Elements (MGEs) in the Spread of AMR

Instead of developing independently, bacterial resistance is aided by mobile genetic elements (MGEs) like integrons, transposons, and plasmids. The transfer of resistance genes among bacteria, even across different species, occurs through these vectors, which significantly enhance the rate of antimicrobial resistance, particularly in hospitals where antibiotics are frequently used. Plasmids represent an important category of mobile genetic elements. They are small, double-stranded, circular DNA molecules that replicate independently within bacterial cells, frequently carrying multiple resistance genes (Garcillán-Barcia et al., 2022).

Transfer of plasmids

In the context of significant resistant bacteria, novel mechanisms emerge, including conjugation, which involves the direct intercellular transfer of DNA between two bacterial cells. The dissemination of resistant bacteria consequently traverses the human population. This is one of the factors that complicate the tracking of the spread of resistant bacteria. Empirical studies indicate that approximately 60% of hospital-acquired AMR is plasmid-mediated (Agyeman et al., 2022). Based on this foundation, the CRISPR-Cas9 technology is undergoing evaluation as a potential method to eliminate resistance plasmids prior to their dissemination. Figure 3 illustrates a straightforward example of the involvement of mobile genetic elements, such as plasmids, transposons, and integrons, in the transfer of antimicrobial resistance genes. The factors contribute to the dissemination of resistance genes via conjugation, transformation, and transduction, facilitating the proliferation of resistant genes within bacterial communities, especially in healthcare environments.

Figure 3. Mobile genetic elements and their role in antimicrobial resistance (AMR) gene transfer.

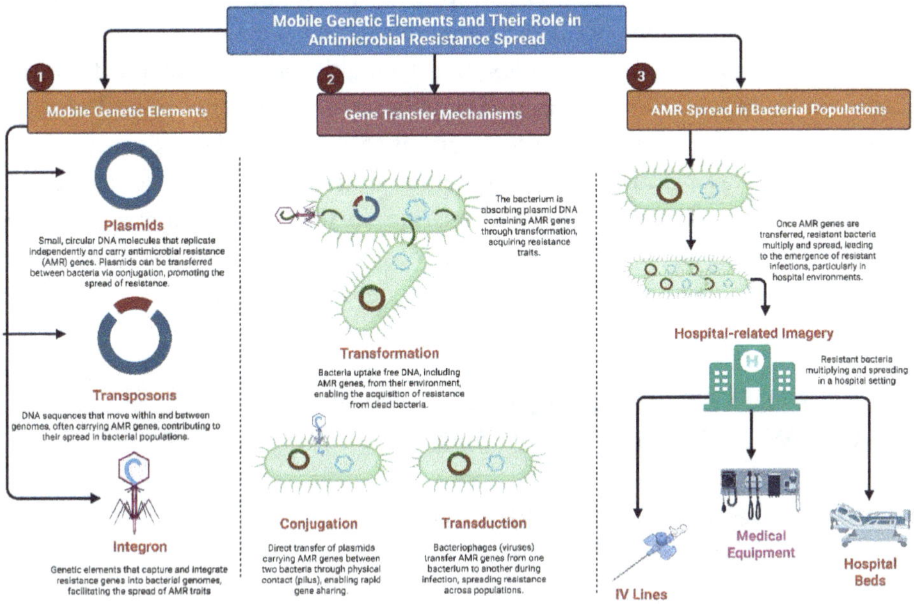

3.3 Evolution of Resistance in Bacterial Populations

AMR represents a prolonged and evolving phenomenon, rather than a sudden concern. Continuous exposure of the pathogen to antibiotics applies pressure, prompting the pathogen to undergo genetic changes and develop adaptive mechanisms for survival, ultimately leading to increased resistance to the treatment. From a long-term viewpoint, this trend contributes to the emergence of multidrug-resistant superbugs, which present significant challenges to contemporary treatment strategies.

The pathway can be exemplified by *K. pneumoniae*. The initial effect observed is that *K. pneumoniae* isolates produce beta-lactamase, which is an enzyme pathway that degrades the efficacy of carbapenem antibiotics, rendering them ineffective. This vulnerability, in conjunction with antimicrobial pressure, can lead to the loss of porin channels, the membrane pore complex typically targeted by antibiotics, and the overexpression of efflux pumps that can expel antimicrobial drugs. At the same Time, alterations in penicillin-binding proteins diminish the efficacy of last-line agents such as ceftazidime-avibactam, thereby complicating the management of the infection (Guerra et al., 2022).

Recent studies have identified hypermutator strain populations where chromosomal genes associated with DNA repair, such as mutS, exhibit mutations resulting in a resistance evolution rate that is 100 times faster than that observed in typical pathogens. The implications of this accelerated resistance pathway on public health include robust transmission dynamics and a notable decrease in the timeframe available for therapeutic intervention. The existing clinical problems of clinically significant bacterial infections require solutions to antimicrobial resistance (AMR) in an integrated way. Among them, a potential option is to integrate artificial intelligence-driven predictive tools into existing surveillance systems, which can be used to elucidate the resistance patterns of bacteria and thereby prioritize the development and design of new medicine (Baquero et al., 2021).

4. CASE STUDIES IN MICROBIAL GENOMICS AND ANTIMICROBIAL RESISTANCE

4.1 Clinical Case Studies: Decoding Resistance in Priority Pathogens

Genomic surveillance is a necessary tool that can be used to detect resistant pathogens within hospital settings. A new report printed in Nature Microbiology (2024) used the entire-genome sequencing (WGS) examination to identify a previously unrecognized occurrence of methicillin-resistant Staphylococcus aureus (MRSA) in three European health care organizations. It was associated with a portrait of one clone harboring a new mecC-fusC resistance gene complex, which led to resistance to fusidic acid and 2-lactams. This research thereby indicates the usefulness of bringing WGS to monitor the rise of resistance and elucidate the genetic makeup of yet unidentified strains (Codda, 2024).

The Blight of carbapenem- and colistin-resistant *K. pneumoniae* has been a mounting global public health threat. The coinciding combination of blaNDM-5 and mcr-1 genes in Klebsiella strains was reported in 2024 in the Journal of Antimicrobial Chemotherapy, and the bacterial strains offer resistance to carbapenems and colistin, which is an antimicrobial drug of last resort. The stability of this hybrid resistance in 7% of intensive-care-unit (ICU) patients in Indian hospitals, and the genomic evidence revealed that the resistance was mostly linked with hospital wastewater systems (Talat et al., 2023).

Widespread prevalence of resistance to drug-resistant tuberculosis, and specifically XDR-TB, causes a serious public-health concern. According to new research in Lancet Infectious Diseases (2024), a compensatory mutation in rpoA allowed *M. tuberculosis* to maintain its fitness as it developed resistance to rifampicin by mutating rpoB. This was the first evidence to significantly increase our knowledge about XDR-TB, having been reported among 18% of new TB cases in Eastern Europe (Hlanze, 2024).

4.2 Environmental and Agricultural AMR: The Hidden Reservoir

The agricultural sector plays a vital role in the development and dissemination of AMR. A recent publication in a 2024 scientific journal details the use of metagenomic sequencing to analyze soil samples from 300 industrial farms. Analysis of the farm sites revealed that 82% exhibited contamination with acceptable resistance genes, including blaCTX-M and mcr-1, with a prevalence 3-5 times greater in regions where livestock underwent regular antibiotic treatment. A distinct relationship can be observed between agriculture and human microbial communities, as identical resistance cassettes have been found in the gut microbiomes of farm workers (Valiakos & Kapna, 2021).

One area of significant concern is the poultry industry regarding the transmission of AMR. A recent study in Emerging Infectious Diseases (2024) traced a *Campylobacter jejuni* clone (ST-828) through poultry farms in Southeast Asia (Yang et al., 2023). This strain has acquired a novel erm(B)- carrying mega plasmid, which confers resistance to macrolides. Genomic epidemiology identified a strain responsible for 37% of human campylobacteriosis in the area, highlighting how agronomic practices contribute to the spread of resistant pathogens to the human population. Figure 4 illustrates a schematic representation of the complex interplay involved in this process: the application of antibiotics in livestock leads to the emergence of resistant strains, which subsequently spread through the food system, environmental contamination, and community waste.

Figure 4. The Cycle of Antimicrobial Resistance (AMR) in Agriculture, Livestock, and Human Health

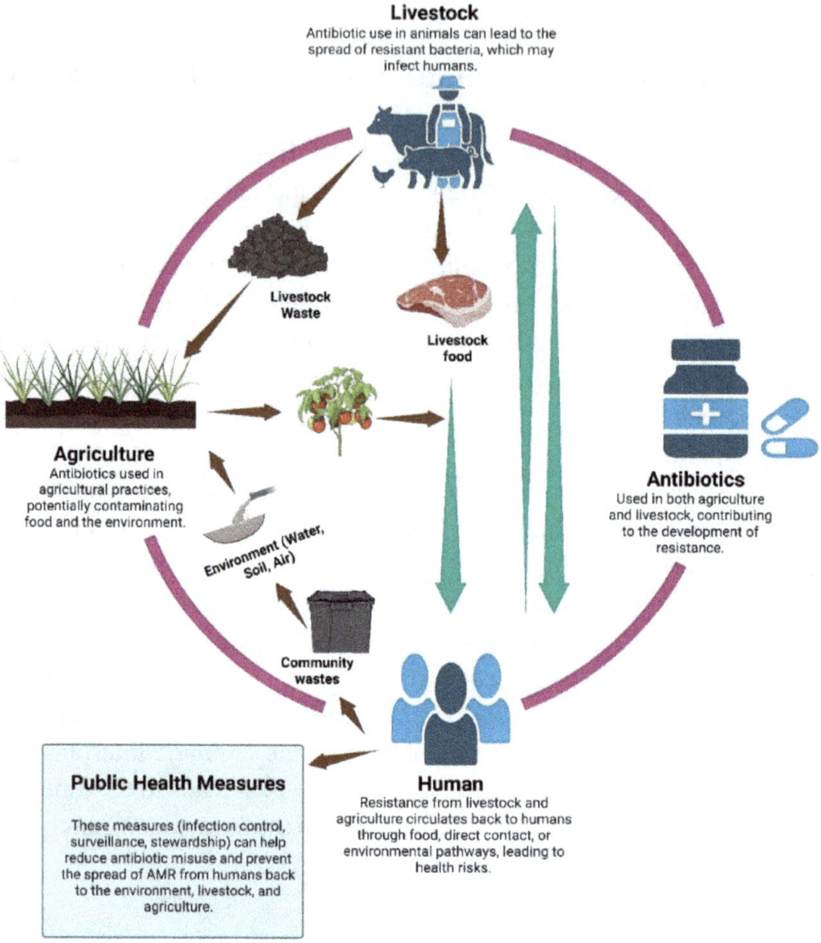

4.3 Global Genomic Surveillance: Building Early Warning Systems

International genomic surveillance systems have assumed a pivotal role in tackling antimicrobial resistance (AMR). The recent report from the World Health Organization in 2024 indicates that the National Center for Biotechnology Information (NCBI) AMR database has expanded to include more than 45,000 edited resistance genes, reflecting a 30% increase compared to the prior year. Machine learning tools have been implemented to enhance resistance phenotype prediction to an accuracy of 92%, utilizing this resource to provide clinicians with more precise data to inform therapeutic decisions (Kim et al., 2022).

The Global Antimicrobial Resistance and Use Surveillance System (GLASS) has expanded its scope to encompass the verification of clinical isolates, veterinary surveillance, and environmental metagenome data, all within a unified One Health framework. The enhanced platform will bolster the capacity to monitor AMR across diverse ecosystems and formulate a more effective intervention strategy that addresses emerging threats (Kolawole et al., 2023).

Nanopore sequencing technology has been adopted in 15 African countries, even in resource-limited environments, enabling the possibility of conducting real-time AMR surveillance. Blockchain systems are implemented to ensure data integrity on a global scale, while federated learning models address the challenges of secure collaboration without compromising sensitive information (Kumari et al., 2025).

The 2033 *Salmonella* Newport outbreak stands out as a significant achievement in the realm of international genomic surveillance. Through the use of GISAID, the resistance plasmid responsible for the epidemic was identified within 72 hours. This rapid identification enabled the implementation of targeted measures that successfully averted an estimated 3,500 potential cases across 12 countries, highlighting the power of global collaboration in addressing antimicrobial resistance (Jones, 2024).

Table 2. Key Genomic Surveillance Resources (2024 Update)

Database	Scope	Unique Feature	Recent Milestone	References
NCBI AMR	Global	Phenotype-genotype linking	Added 1,200 livestock-associated resistance variants	(Knight, 2018)
ResFinder	Clinical	Outbreak detection in hospitals	Real-time resistance alerts for 500+ hospitals	(Hwang et al., 2021)
ARG-ANNOT	Functional	CRISPR-Cas9 validation	Annotated 200 novel resistance mechanisms	(Tang, 2024)
GISAID	Pathogen	Data sharing platform for pathogens	Detected avian influenza AMR mutations	(Struelens et al., 2024)
GLASS	Global/One Health	Integrates clinical, environmental, and veterinary surveillance	Expanded data from 150 countries, covering clinical, environmental, and veterinary data	(Pungartnik et al., 2023)
CARD	Global	Comprehensive resistance gene database	Updated 15,000 resistance gene sequences in 2024	(Islam et al., 2025)
ARG-Sequence	Functional	Sequence-based resistance detection	Enabled real-time resistance pattern mapping in 250+ hospitals	(Wang et al., 2021)
VetNet	Veterinary	Tracks veterinary AMR across species	Expanded to include 100 species for resistance profiling	(Attri et al.)s

The current landscape (Table 2) presents the existing state of genomic surveillance databases regarding AMR, incorporating the NCBI AMR database, along with ResFinder, ARG-ANNOT, GISAID, GLASS, CARD, ARG-Seq, and VetNet databases. Collectively, these platforms can enhance the monitoring of antimicrobial resistance (AMR) to facilitate prompt public health interventions worldwide.

5. THE FUTURE OF MICROBIAL GENOMICS IN COMBATING AMR:

5.1 Cutting-Edge Genomic Technologies Transforming AMR Surveillance

Modern genomic technologies are significantly transforming the fields of antimicrobial resistance (AMR) surveillance and prediction. The use of nanopore sequencing platforms, most notably the Oxford Nanopore PromethION 2, has enabled the sequencing of entire bacterial genomes in under two hours, making it possible for surgeons to access information about antimicrobial-resistant bacteria in a timely manner. In a case of the cholera outbreak in Sudan that occurred in the year 2023, azithromycin resistance in Vibrio cholera was identified after eight hours (Asantewaa et al., 2024). The flexibility of these sequencers is also demonstrated by their use when screening extensively drug-resistant tuberculosis in Ukrainian refugee camps. At the same Time, artificial intelligence (AI) and machine learning (ML) were introduced in the AMR prediction models. A single illustration is DeepAMR 2.0, a system developed by Google Wellbeing and MIT, which utilizes AI to predict the probability of resistance mutation with up to 97% accuracy over periods of up to 12 months (Gupta & Bhandary, 2024). Such capability is an inseparable part of transformations in the sphere of antimicrobial stewardship, as it allows healthcare specialists to predict AMR prior to its manifestation in the clinical setting. Using the example, Figure 5 illustrates that when hospital data are integrated with multiple sources of agricultural monitoring and wastewater surveillance, AI can be utilized to predict the occurrence of AMR, thereby further enhancing the accuracy and efficiency of early-warning systems.

Figure 5. AI-Based Prediction Model for AMR Spread

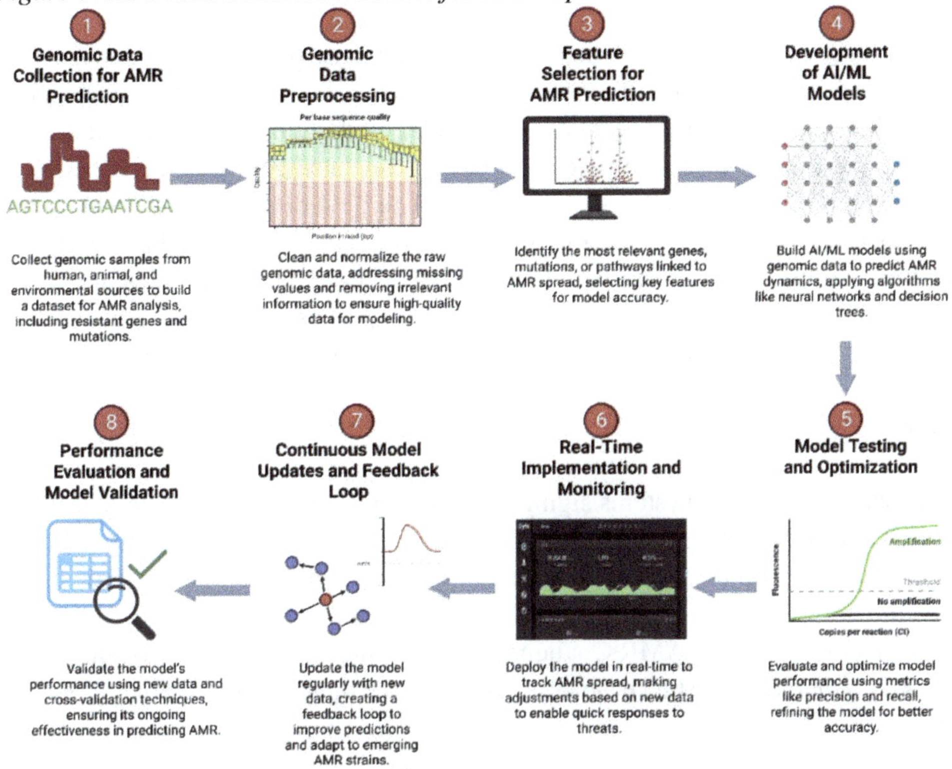

5.2 Precision Medicine: The Genomic Revolution in Patient Care

The Improvement of Whole-Genome Sequencing (WGS)

The United States NIH ARLG Network reported in 2024 that whole-genome sequencing (WGS) reduced the use of needless antibiotics by 58% and the number of deaths from bloodstream infections by 42%. Whole-genome sequencing enables the rapid identification of pathogens and the mapping of resistance patterns. For instance, the implementation of whole genome sequencing for ICU patients at Johns Hopkins Hospital significantly decreased the interval between pathogen identification and optimal treatment to 6.5 hours, down from 72 hours prior to implementation, resulting in a 67% reduction in mortality rates among carbapenem-resistant Enterobacteriaceae (CRE) (Li et al., 2023).

Future Possible Breakthrough Therapies

A galaxy of revolutionary medications that provide patients with new hope is rapidly approaching the point where they will be approved by regulatory agencies. CRISPR-Phage Precision Therapy is currently undergoing Phase II trials, employing genetically modified phages to target resistance genes, demonstrating an impressive 89% effectiveness against MRSA. The field of microbiome editing has demonstrated a 93 percent reduction in ESBL-producing *E. coli* and has effectively restored antibiotic susceptibility. Antibiotic enhancers on nanoparticles, including gold nanoparticles, are disrupting bacterial efflux pumps, restoring the efficacy of antibiotics in 78% of extensively drug-resistant *P. aeruginosa* (Onyeyili et al., 2025).

Increasing International Surveillance Networks

Global surveillance systems significantly enhanced their capacity to detect and address antimicrobial resistance (AMR) in 2024. The WHO GLASS-2 network, now expanded to 89 countries, is leveraging cloud-based whole genome sequencing to expedite the identification of emerging resistant pathogens (Onyeyili et al., 2025). Simultaneously, the US AMR Challenge, implemented across 1,300 hospitals, employs AI-generated resistance alerts to minimize the unnecessary use of antibiotics, ultimately preserving thousands of lives annually. These initiatives are bolstered by advanced technologies such as nanopore sequencing and secure data exchange facilitated by blockchain. The *Salmonella* Newport outbreak in 2023 exemplifies the power of collaborative genomic efforts: sequencing via GISAID facilitated the identification of a resistance plasmid within 72 hours, averting an estimated 3,500 cases across 12 countries (Peñil Celis, 2025).

The Final Frontier of AMR Genomics

The AMR genomics industry is projected to triple in size, reaching $2.8 billion by 2025. By 2026, over half of hospitals are expected to have implemented real-time sequencing, which will enhance epidemic response. DARPA is actively engaged in Project Achilles, an initiative aimed at developing antibiotics that are impervious to resistance, with clinical testing anticipated to commence in 2025. Additionally, discussions regarding a global Genomic AMR Treaty aim for consistency in monitoring and management worldwide by 2025 (Slawomirski et al., 2025).

Imminent Crusades and Threats

Although recent advances have been made, there are some significant barriers still in place. Genomic sequencing capacity is also geographically unbalanced: most enablers of sequencing-based surveillance are based in high-income countries, and fewer than a handful of facilities in Africa are operational. International cooperation is hampered by the lack of internationally standardized names of resistance genes. Ethics (such as the protection of the privacy of patients or the control of the dual-use risks of genomic tools) form other important elements in the responsible use of these technologies.

6. CHALLENGES AND ETHICAL CONSIDERATIONS

6.1 Data Interpretation and Bioinformatics Challenges

The development of whole-genome sequencing as an important tool in the AMR surveillance field is an essential breakthrough with regard to microbial epidemiology. However, it also poses several methodological issues, most notably regarding the quality of the data and analysis in the bioinformatics domain. The greatest sense of urgency concerns genomic data heterogeneity. Even with the continued refinement of new sequencing platforms, the workflow still produces a significant amount of error, including baseball errors and sequenced fragments that can alter AMR profiling. Furthermore, the majority of resistant strains bear a combination of resistance genes, many of which overlap, making the specific identification of resistance determinants even more complicated. The complexity of resistance haplotypes and the regulatory interactions that control them only further complicate the mapping of genotype to phenotype (Abdi et al., 2024).

Such hurdles have serious implications for bioinformatics pipelines that manipulate AMR sequence information. It has been based on fundamental principles and focuses on the design of algorithms and computational hardware required for the identification of gene quality and the prediction of pathways. Recent studies have shown that the current bioinformatics infrastructure is insufficient to meet these requirements, as better sequence-read clustering algorithms and deep-learning models that can effectively predict resistance pathways are still in development.

6.2 Ethical Implications in AMR Genomic Research

Genomic surveillance has reached a point where it is now a prerequisite to sustained public health activity against antimicrobial resistance (AMR), but ethical aspects of this are notably under scrutiny. Informed consent as a principle. Informed consent is the essential principle of genomic profiling: patterns of resistance can be reconstructed on an individual genomic level, which introduces a greater level of granularity to the concept of microbial evolution and consequently influences ownership and stewardship of that data. Researchers should seek to acquire clear, informed consent from patients before transferring genomic data across international boundaries or to any distant repositories worldwide (Stark et al., 2025). The need to secure this consent places the responsibility on clinicians to ensure that patients are aware of the institutions that will process their data and the risks this poses, including the potential for exposing their data to security breaches.

Another front of acute ethical imbalance is equity. Although the increase in sequencing capacity presents an opportunity to enhance medical progress, the ensuing inequities between low- and middle-income countries and areas with developed genomics infrastructure have a likelihood of intensifying current health outcomes inequalities. Meanwhile, an increase in dependency on genomics results in further heightened concerns of a more global nature regarding privacy issues. Problems are complicated by the dual-use capability of genomic information. The same data used as the guiding input on the application of public health responses can be used in creating bioterrorism or bioweapons, which highlights the need to have sound ethical principles as the backbone in preventing such occurrences (Pauly et al., 2021).

6.3 Regulatory and Policy Challenges

The modern policy landscape governing genomic antibiotic resistance (AMR) studies is in a State of dynamic Flux. One of the primary barriers is the reliable and safe integration of genomic data into public health and clinical practice. Despite the overall potential of genomic sequencing in AMR surveillance, existing patterns of data collection, exchange, and use demonstrate a number of gaps (Djordjevic et al., 2024). Strong stewardship, especially in clinical areas, will rely on effective policies and global agreements that specify the potential uses.

Genomic surveillance protocol standardisation is a continual necessity. Without standard practices, institutions can produce datasets using incompatible formats, thus inhibiting transnational collaboration. At the same Time, the legal frameworks aimed at protecting data should address new intricacies created by genomic data, and the privacy of individuals should be guaranteed so that the interests of people regarding the application of personal data are respected (Ling-Hu et al., 2022).

Moreover, global coordination is necessary to address AMR. Transnational coalitions are often required because the resistance phenomena travel across political frontiers. Internationally negotiated treaties have been central in standardizing surveillance networks, achieving fair access and data exchange, and sharing information across diverse sectors and countries, such as the proposed United Nations Global Genomic AMR Treaty (Joshi et al., 2021).

7. FUTURE PERSPECTIVES IN AMR GENOMICS

7.1 Advances in Genomic Technologies

The emergence of recent genomic technologies has revolutionized the field of antimicrobial resistance (AMR) surveillance. Next-generation sequencing (NGS) has recently emerged as a means to obtain rapid and thorough genomic analysis, which can be used to detect resistance mutations even before the onset of clinical manifestations. The instrumentation currently available, in particular the Illumina NovaSeq 6000 and the Oxford Nanopore PromethION 2, is pushing the limits of nucleotide sequencing as far as is feasible today (Pervez et al., 2022). The recent implementation of nanopore sequencing exemplifies a significant shift toward point-of-care, real-time sequencing. During the 2023 cholera outbreak in Sudan, rapid responses were able to identify resistant strains within just eight hours (Ndung'u et al., 2023). In the future, advancements like CRISPR-Cas9 may enable the direct targeting and reversal of AMR mutations, while genome-scale workflows enhanced by AI and ML will facilitate even quicker and more precise detection and prediction of AMR.

Figure 6. shows the timeline of AMR genomics advancements,

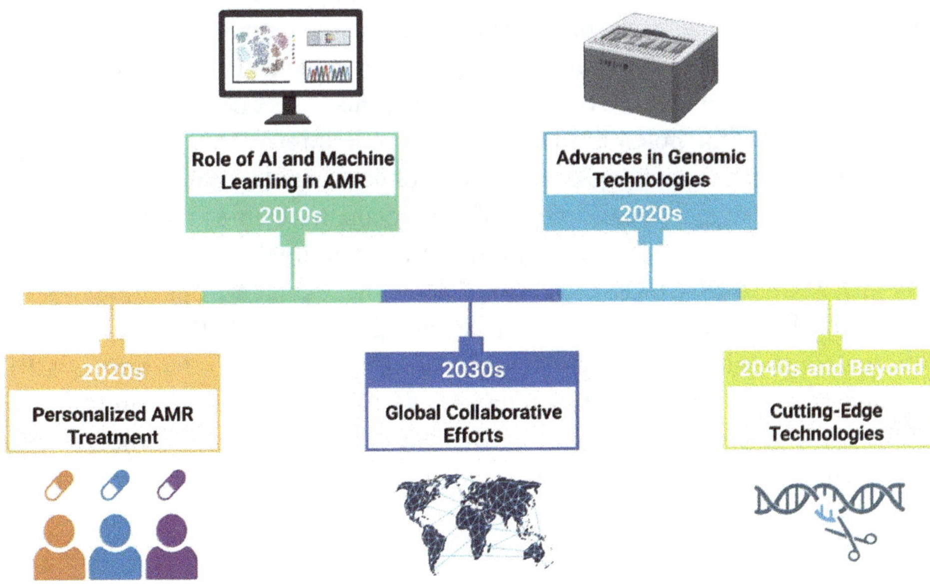

7.2 Role of AI and Machine Learning in AMR

The prediction process and the explanation of the dynamics of antimicrobial resistance (AMR) over the decade from 2010 to 2020 utilized artificial intelligence (AI) and machine learning (ML) (Gupta & Bhandary, 2024). Previous systems relied on genomic data to forecast the dissemination of resistant phenotypes. The advent of deep-learning techniques enables the analysis of multidimensional, heterogeneous data, allowing for predictions regarding resistance patterns a few months in advance. This includes genomic sequences, electronic health records, and environmental samples. An illustration of this is Deep AMR 2.0, which can forecast the emergence of resistance mutations up to a year prior to their clinical manifestation, thereby equipping health practitioners with a timely advantage against impending challenges in an unprecedented manner. In addition, models such as ResNet-AMR have shown the capability to analyze sequencing data from over 50,000 isolates daily, enabling the identification of novel constellations of resistance genes (Sakagianni et al., 2023). With the ongoing iterative enhancement of AI-driven techniques, it is likely that these systems will assume a more pivotal position in real-time surveillance, outbreak forecasting, and the formulation of adaptive therapeutic strategies that are adjusted to evolving resistance dynamics.

7.3 Personalized AMR Treatment

Future developments in precision medicine in antimicrobial resistance (AMR) may be described as a shift toward pathogen-specific approaches to treatment based on genomic surveillance. Even current whole-genome sequencing (WGS) procedures enable the identification of specific resistance determinants. But the ability to map diagnostic outcomes to treatments matched to organism-specific resistance profiles will determine their full potential in the future (Ammoura et al., 2025). The paradigm is backed by empirical data. In 2024, two studies conducted by Johns Hopkins University revealed that using real-time WGS, clinicians were able to reduce the Time lag between administration and the administration of optimal antibiotics to 6.5 hours rather than 72 hours in ICUs (Kollef et al., 2021). The regular use of genomic-based, individualized therapies is expected to be established by the 2030s, particularly for multidrug-resistant infections such as *carbapenem-resistant Enterobacterales* (CRE) and extensively drug-resistant tuberculosis (XDR-TB). The steady improvement in fields such as pharmacogenomics, CRISPR-based therapeutics, and synthetic biology will enhance the accuracy and effectiveness of antimicrobial treatments.

7.4 Global Collaborative Efforts

The issue of antimicrobial resistance (AMR) constitutes a significant public health crisis that requires collaborative efforts and partnerships across various sectors. Significant accomplishments in the 2020s included the expansion of the WHO Global Antimicrobial Resistance Surveillance System (GLASS) to 89 countries, integrating clinical, veterinary, and environmental surveillance within a One Health framework (Organization, 2022). In the 2030s, we can expect an increase in the promotion of organized elements, particularly through the establishment of shared genomic databases encompassing human, animal, and environmental sequences. Blockchain technologies are anticipated to provide secure and transparent data transfer, and initiatives like the Global AMR R&D Hub are poised to enhance the advancement of new antibiotics. The observed interaction patterns may lead to the adoption of a Global Genomic AMR Treaty by the 2040s, which would standardize global AMR interventions and promote equitable access to genomic technologies (Chindelevitch et al., 2022).

The future prospects of antimicrobial resistance (AMR) genomics present a combination of threats and opportunities, particularly in light of recent advancements in sequencing technologies, the application of artificial intelligence, and the emergence of personalized treatment approaches. Whether such efforts succeed, however, will depend on long-term innovation, transnational cooperation, and a willingness to ensure the equitable distribution of these technologies on a global scale (Eccleston-Turner & Upton, 2021). At the same Time, projections point toward the use of customized antibiotics and AI-led forecasting of outbreaks as the norm in 2030, as well as a more unified international system supporting the global approach to AMR.

7. CONCLUSION

This chapter explains the crucial role that microbial genomics plays in managing antimicrobial resistance (AMR). New developments in genomic sequencing technology, specifically next-generation sequencing (NGS), have led to a significant improvement in surveillance and monitoring systems. Meanwhile, the application of artificial intelligence (AI) and machine learning has increased predictive accuracy and made it possible to visualize patterns of resistance in real Time. The strategic use of individualized therapy based on the specific genomic profile of the pathogen is rapidly recognized as an important step toward improving clinical outcomes and reducing unnecessary antibiotic utilization. All of these inventions have dramatic implications to the field of public health, including more immediate and accurate diagnosis and treatment. Other international cooperation efforts, including the Global Antimicrobial Surveillance System (GLASS), have also proved valuable in enhancing international capacity to control AMR through a combination of the human, animal, and environmental realms. Examining these trends, the future of AMR control hinges on continued progress in genomics, AI, and cross-sector collaborations. The combination of real-time sequencing platforms and customized treatment strategies offers a way to alleviate future infections and maintain the efficiency of antibiotics in future generations.

REFERENCES

Abdi, G., Jain, M., Barwant, M., Tendulkar, R., Tendulkar, M., Tariq, M., & Amir, A. (2024). Unveiling the dynamic role of bioinformatics in automation for efficient and accurate data processing and interpretation. In *Advances in Bioinformatics* (pp. 279–319). Springer.

Agyeman, W. Y., Bisht, A., Gopinath, A., Cheema, A. H., Chaludiya, K., Khalid, M., Nwosu, M., Konka, S., & Khan, S. (2022). A systematic review of antibiotic resistance trends and treatment options for hospital-acquired multidrug-resistant infections. *Cureus*, *14*(10). PMID: 36381838

Ammoura, J. E. O., Saad, N., Elamin, A. B., & Chambuso, R. (2025). Antimicrobial Resistance and Microbiological Gap Analysis for Central Nervous System Infections Bacterial Pathogens in Nigeria. medRxiv, 2025.2008. 2012.25333494.

Asantewaa, A. A., Odoom, A., Owusu-Okyere, G., & Donkor, E. S. (2024). Cholera Outbreaks in Low-and Middle-Income Countries in the Last Decade: A systematic review and meta-analysis. *Microorganisms*, *12*(12), 2504. PMID: 39770707

Attri, I., Vanita, B., Rajput, R., Awasthi, L. K., Thakur, A., Tripathi, D., Pathak, V., Shukla, P., & Gupta, D. (•••). SAAM-VetNet: An attention-based multi-task framework for animal disease detection and severity grading. *Annals of Medicine and Surgery (London)*, *10*, 1097.

Baquero, F., Martinez, J. L. F., Lanza, V., Rodríguez-Beltrán, J., Galán, J. C., San Millán, A., Cantón, R., & Coque, T. M. (2021). Evolutionary pathways and trajectories in antibiotic resistance. *Clinical Microbiology Reviews*, *34*(4), e00050–e00019. PMID: 34190572

Baum, J. H., Dörre, A., Reichert, F., Noll, I., Feig, M., Eckmanns, T., Sandfort, M., & Haller, S. (2025). Changes in incidence and epidemiology of antimicrobial resistant pathogens before and during the COVID-19 pandemic in Germany, 2015–2022. *BMC Microbiology*, *25*(1), 51. PMID: 39875841

Chindelevitch, L., Jauneikaite, E., Wheeler, N. E., Allel, K., Ansiri-Asafoakaa, B. Y., Awuah, W. A., Bauer, D. C., Beisken, S., Fan, K., & Grant, G. (2022). Applying data technologies to combat AMR: current status, challenges, and opportunities on the way forward. *arXiv preprint arXiv:2208.04683*.

Codda, G. (2024). Next Generation Sequencing-based detection and characterization of microbial pathogens causing invasive infections and outbreaks in ICU: Towards improved management of the high-risk patient.

Dimitriu, T. (2022). Evolution of horizontal transmission in antimicrobial resistance plasmids. *Microbiology*, *168*(7), 001214. PMID: 35849537

Djordjevic, S. P., Jarocki, V. M., Seemann, T., Cummins, M. L., Watt, A. E., Drigo, B., Wyrsch, E. R., Reid, C. J., Donner, E., & Howden, B. P. (2024). Genomic surveillance for antimicrobial resistance—A One Health perspective. *Nature Reviews. Genetics*, *25*(2), 142–157. PMID: 37749210

Eccleston-Turner, M., & Upton, H. (2021). International collaboration to ensure equitable access to vaccines for COVID-19: The ACT-Accelerator and the COVAX facility. *The Milbank Quarterly*, *99*(2), 426–449. PMID: 33650737

Garcillán-Barcia, M. P., Pluta, R., Lorenzo-Díaz, F., Bravo, A., & Espinosa, M. (2022). The facts and family secrets of plasmids that replicate via the rolling-circle mechanism. *Microbiology and Molecular Biology Reviews : MMBR*, *86*(1), e00222–e00220. PMID: 34878299

Guerra, M. E. S., Destro, G., Vieira, B., Lima, A. S., Ferraz, L. F. C., Hakansson, A. P., Darrieux, M., & Converso, T. R. (2022). Klebsiella pneumoniae biofilms and their role in disease pathogenesis. *Frontiers in Cellular and Infection Microbiology*, *12*, 877995. PMID: 35646720

Gupta, Y. D., & Bhandary, S. (2024). Artificial intelligence for understanding mechanisms of antimicrobial resistance and antimicrobial discovery: a new age model for translational research. *Artificial Intelligence and Machine Learning in Drug Design and Development*, 117-156.

Hlanze, H. (2024). *The evolution of drug resistance in the different lineages of the Mycobacterium tuberculosis complex*. University of Pretoria.

Hwang, S. M., Cho, H. W., Kim, T. Y., Park, J. S., Jung, J., Song, K.-H., Lee, H., Kim, E. S., Kim, H. B., & Park, K. U. (2021). Whole-genome sequencing for investigating a health care-associated outbreak of carbapenem-resistant Acinetobacter baumannii. *Diagnostics (Basel)*, *11*(2), 201. PMID: 33573077

Islam, M. R., Summers, A. O., & Arpinar, I. B. (2025). Knowledge Graph-Based Framework for Detecting Horizontal Gene Transfer Events Driving Antimicrobial Resistance. bioRxiv, 2025.2006. 2009.658534.

Jones, A. D. (2024). Microbial risk assessment. *Human and Ecological Risk Assessment: Theory and Practice*, *2*, 779–832.

Joshi, M. P., Hafner, T., Twesigye, G., Ndiaye, A., Kiggundu, R., Mekonnen, N., Kusu, N., Berthé, S., Lusaya, E. P., & Acho, A. (2021). Strengthening multisectoral coordination on antimicrobial resistance: A landscape analysis of efforts in 11 countries. *Journal of Pharmaceutical Policy and Practice*, *14*(1), 27. PMID: 33648589

Kim, J. I., Maguire, F., Tsang, K. K., Gouliouris, T., Peacock, S. J., McAllister, T. A., McArthur, A. G., & Beiko, R. G. (2022). Machine learning for antimicrobial resistance prediction: Current practice, limitations, and clinical perspective. *Clinical Microbiology Reviews*, *35*(3), e00179–e00121. PMID: 35612324

Knight, D. R. (2018). Comparative phylogenomics and antimicrobial resistance in livestock-associated lineages of Clostridium difficile.

Kolawole, T. O., Mustapha, A. Y., Mbata, A. O., Tomoh, B. O., Forkuo, A. Y., & Kelvin-Agwu, M. (2023). *Innovative strategies for reducing antimicrobial resistance: A review of global policy and practice*. Journal Name Missing.

Kollef, M. H., Shorr, A. F., Bassetti, M., Timsit, J.-F., Micek, S. T., Michelson, A. P., & Garnacho-Montero, J. (2021). Timing of antibiotic therapy in the ICU. *Critical Care*, *25*(1), 360. PMID: 34654462

Kumari, L. S., Siriwardhana, D. M., Liyanapathirana, V., Jinadasa, R., & Wijesinghe, P. (2025). Rapid whole genome sequencing for AMR surveillance in low-and middle-income countries: Oxford Nanopore Technology reveals multidrug-resistant Enterobacter cloacae complex from dairy farms in Sri Lanka. *BMC Veterinary Research*, *21*(1), 351. PMID: 40382559

Li, M.-c., Lu, J., Lu, Y., Xiao, T.-y., Liu, H.-c., Lin, S.-q., Xu, D., Li, G.-l., Zhao, X.-q., & Liu, Z.-g. (2021). rpoB mutations and effects on rifampin resistance in Mycobacterium tuberculosis. *Infection and Drug Resistance*, •••, 4119–4128. PMID: 34675557

Li, S., Carss, K. J., Halldorsson, B. V., Cortes, A., & Consortium, U. B. W.-G. S. (2023). Whole-genome sequencing of half-a-million UK Biobank participants. *medRxiv*, 2023.2012. 2006.23299426.

Ling-Hu, T., Rios-Guzman, E., Lorenzo-Redondo, R., Ozer, E. A., & Hultquist, J. F. (2022). Challenges and opportunities for global genomic surveillance strategies in the COVID-19 era. *Viruses*, *14*(11), 2532. PMID: 36423141

Mitra, S., Sultana, S. A., Prova, S. R., Uddin, T. M., Islam, F., Das, R., Nainu, F., Sartini, S., Chidambaram, K., & Alhumaydhi, F. A. (2022). Investigating forthcoming strategies to tackle deadly superbugs: Current status and future vision. *Expert Review of Anti-Infective Therapy*, *20*(10), 1309–1332. PMID: 36069241

Mnyambwa, N. P. (2019). *Characterization of mutations in drug resistant tuberculosis and diagnostic challenges in referral health facilities*. NM-AIST.

Mullin, D. S. (2023). Motoric Cognitive Risk: epidemiology of a walking speed-based syndrome to predict dementia.

Ndung'u, M. H., Gachara, G., Ontweka, L., Menza, N., Musyoki, A., & Muturi, M. (2023). Review of Rapid Diagnostic Methods for Vibrio Cholerae Detection in the Last Decade (2011–2022). *The East African Health Research Journal*, *7*(2), 131. PMID: 39219657

Onyeyili, I. N., Ogbozor, F. I., Kehinde, A. B., & Chiemerie, C. (2025). Phage-based CRISPR delivery systems for targeted eradication of drug-resistant bacterial infections.

Organization, W. H. (2022). *Global antimicrobial resistance and use surveillance system (GLASS) report 2022*. World Health Organization.

Organization, W. H. (2024). *WHO bacterial priority pathogens list, 2024: bacterial pathogens of public health importance, to guide research, development, and strategies to prevent and control antimicrobial resistance*. World Health Organization.

Pauly, B., Revai, T., Marcellus, L., Martin, W., Easton, K., & MacDonald, M. (2021). "The health equity curse": Ethical tensions in promoting health equity. *BMC Public Health*, *21*(1), 1567. PMID: 34407781

Peñil Celis, A. (2025). Inclusión del pangenoma para la vigilancia genómica de los serovares Typhi y Hadar de Salmonella enterica.

Pervez, M. T., Hasnain, M. J. U., Abbas, S. H., Moustafa, M. F., Aslam, N., & Shah, S. S. M. (2022). [Retracted] A Comprehensive Review of Performance of Next-Generation Sequencing Platforms. *BioMed Research International*, *2022*(1), 3457806. PMID: 36212714

Petronio, D. G. P. Study of fluoroquinolone resistance in Lactobacillus spp.

Pettorelli, N., Graham, N. A., Seddon, N., Maria da Cunha Bustamante, M., Lowton, M. J., Sutherland, W. J., Koldewey, H. J., Prentice, H. C., & Barlow, J. (2021). Time to integrate global climate change and biodiversity science-policy agendas. *Journal of Applied Ecology*, *58*(11), 2384–2393.

Pungartnik, P. C., Abreu, A., Dos Santos, C. V. B., Cavalcante, J. R., Faerstein, E., & Werneck, G. L. (2023). The interfaces between One Health and Global Health: A scoping review. *One Health*, *16*, 100573. PMID: 37363235

Qiu, J. (2024). Innovations in combating antimicrobial resistance: Unveiling nanotechnology, gene technology, and molecular diagnostics. *Theoretical and Natural Science*, *44*, 203–208.

Rodrigues, S. H., Nunes, G. D., Soares, G. G., Ferreira, R. L., Damas, M. S. F., Laprega, P. M., Shilling, R. E., Campos, L. C., da Costa, A. S., & Malavazi, I. (2024). First report of coexistence of blaKPC-2 and blaNDM-1 in carbapenem-resistant clinical isolates of Klebsiella aerogenes in Brazil. *Frontiers in Microbiology*, *15*, 1352851. PMID: 38426065

Sakagianni, A., Koufopoulou, C., Feretzakis, G., Kalles, D., Verykios, V. S., & Myrianthefs, P. (2023). Using machine learning to predict antimicrobial resistance—A literature review. *Antibiotics (Basel, Switzerland)*, *12*(3), 452. PMID: 36978319

Slawomirski, L., Kelly, D., de Bienassis, K., Kallas, K.-A., & Klazinga, N. (2025). *The economics of diagnostic safety*.

Souza, S. S., Piper, K. R., Ikhimiukor, O. O., Marcovici, M. M., Zac Soligno, N. I., Harmon, A. J., Eckhardt, E. M., Carreiro, N., Workman, A. A., & Martin, I. W. (2025). Variants of β-lactamase-encoding genes are disseminated by multiple genetically distinct lineages of bloodstream Escherichia coli. *Communications Medicine*, *5*(1), 260. PMID: 40595425

Stark, Z., Glazer, D., Hofmann, O., Rendon, A., Marshall, C. R., Ginsburg, G. S., Lunt, C., Allen, N., Effingham, M., & Hastings Ward, J. (2025). A call to action to scale up research and clinical genomic data sharing. *Nature Reviews. Genetics*, *26*(2), 141–147. PMID: 39375561

Struelens, M. J., Ludden, C., Werner, G., Sintchenko, V., Jokelainen, P., & Ip, M. (2024). Real-time genomic surveillance for enhanced control of infectious diseases and antimicrobial resistance. *Frontiers in Science*, *2*, 1298248.

Talat, A., Blake, K. S., Dantas, G., & Khan, A. U. (2023). Metagenomic insight into microbiome and antibiotic resistance genes of high clinical concern in urban and rural hospital wastewater of northern India origin: A major reservoir of antimicrobial resistance. *Microbiology Spectrum*, *11*(2), e04102–e04122. PMID: 36786639

Tang, X. (2024). Conifer Genome Sequencing and Functional Study of Disease Resistance Genes. *Tree Genetics and Molecular Breeding, 14*.

Treffon, J., Heppner, B., Eismann, J., Bothe, J., Omengo, B., & Mellmann, A. (2022). Single nucleotide polymorphism-based real-time PCR screening assay for rapid tracking of bacterial infection clusters to complement whole-genome sequencing efforts during outbreak investigations. *Microbiology Spectrum, 10*(6), e03036–e03022. PMID: 36250868

Tsere, B. (2023). Assessing Antibiotic-Resistance Patterns and Clinical outcomes among People-Living with Hiv/Aids with Features of Sepsis. In *Northern Tanzania*. NM-AIST.

Valiakos, G., & Kapna, I. (2021). Colistin resistant mcr genes prevalence in livestock animals (swine, bovine, poultry) from a multinational perspective. A systematic review. *Veterinary Sciences*, *8*(11), 265. PMID: 34822638

Wang, Z., Li, S., You, R., Zhu, S., Zhou, X. J., & Sun, F. (2021). ARG-SHINE: Improve antibiotic resistance class prediction by integrating sequence homology, functional information and deep convolutional neural network. *NAR Genomics and Bioinformatics*, *3*(3), lqab066. PMID: 34377977

Yakout, M. A., & Ali, G. H. (2022). A novel parC mutation potentiating fluoroquinolone resistance in Klebsiella pneumoniae and Escherichia coli clinical isolates. *Journal of Infection in Developing Countries*, *16*(02), 314–319. PMID: 35298427

Yang, H., Li, Y., Zhang, Y., Dong, B., Duan, B., Guo, L., Wang, T., Lv, X., Zheng, M., & Cui, X. (2023). Prevalence, drug resistance spectrum and virulence gene analysis of Campylobacter jejuni in broiler farms in central Shanxi, China. *Poultry Science*, *102*(3), 102419. PMID: 36599220

Chapter 9
Medical Microbiology-Driven Interventions for Antimicrobial Resistance in Healthcare

Parthiban Pandian
https://orcid.org/0000-0002-3582-3416
Saveetha Institute of Medical and Technical Sciences, India

Sivaranjani Varadharajan
https://orcid.org/0009-0002-5795-4377
Periyar Maniammai Institute of Science and Technology, India

B. Ramya
https://orcid.org/0000-0002-0725-8923
Auxilium College, Vellore, India

Gautam Palshikar
https://orcid.org/0000-0001-5086-6716
Genba Sopanrao Moze College of Pharmacy, India

ABSTRACT

Antimicrobial resistance (AMR) threatens effective treatment of infections, increasing morbidity, mortality, and healthcare costs. Hospitals are critical hubs for resistant pathogens due to high antimicrobial use and vulnerable patients. This chapter examines medical microbiology-driven interventions, highlighting rapid diagnostics, resistance mechanism analysis, antimicrobial stewardship, surveillance, and infection control. Challenges such as resource limitations and data integration

DOI: 10.4018/979-8-3373-3825-5.ch009

are discussed, alongside innovations like genomic surveillance and AI-assisted diagnostics. Positioning microbiology at the core of healthcare is essential for sustainable AMR control.

1. INTRODUCTION: ANTIMICROBIAL RESISTANCE AS A HEALTHCARE CRISIS

1.1 Global Burden of Antimicrobial Resistance:

Antimicrobial resistance (AMR) is recognized as a critical and escalating global health crisis that threatens the effective prevention and treatment of infectious diseases. The widespread emergence of resistant microorganisms has compromised the success of antibiotics, antivirals, antifungals, and antiparasitic agents that once formed the backbone of modern medicine. According to recent global estimates, bacterial AMR alone is responsible for millions of deaths annually, either directly or indirectly, placing it among the leading causes of global mortality (Antimicrobial Resistance Collaborators,2022). Beyond mortality, AMR contributes substantially to prolonged hospital stays, increased healthcare costs, treatment failures, and reduced quality of life (Table 1).

Healthcare systems worldwide face a dual burden: an increasing prevalence of resistant infections and a declining pipeline of novel antimicrobials. In clinical settings, particularly hospitals and intensive care units, resistant pathogens thrive due to high antimicrobial usage, invasive procedures, immunocompromised patient populations, and close patient proximity. These environments serve as amplifiers for resistant strains, facilitating both clonal spread and horizontal gene transfer (World Health Organization [WHO], 2023).

The economic implications of AMR are equally profound. Projections suggest that if unmitigated, AMR could lead to trillions of dollars in cumulative global economic losses over the coming decades due to increased healthcare expenditures and reduced workforce productivity (O'Neill, 2016). Consequently, AMR is no longer viewed solely as a microbiological or clinical issue but as a systemic threat to healthcare sustainability and global development.

Table 1. Global Burden and Characteristics of Antimicrobial Resistance

Parameter	Description
Annual global deaths	Millions of deaths associated with AMR
High-risk settings	Hospitals, ICUs, long-term care facilities
Major pathogens	MRSA, VRE, CRE, MDR *Pseudomonas*
Economic impact	Increased healthcare costs and productivity loss
Key drivers	Antibiotic misuse, poor diagnostics, inadequate surveillance

1.2 Healthcare-Associated Infections and AMR:

Healthcare-associated infections (HAIs) represent a major interface between medical practice and antimicrobial resistance. HAIs caused by multidrug-resistant organisms (MDROs) such as methicillin-resistant Staphylococcus aureus (MRSA), carbapenem-resistant Enterobacterales, vancomycin-resistant Enterococcus (VRE), and Candida auris have become increasingly prevalent across healthcare institutions (Centers for Disease Control and Prevention [CDC], 2022).

The burden of AMR in healthcare settings is amplified by factors such as excessive empirical antibiotic use, delayed diagnostics, inadequate infection prevention practices, and suboptimal antimicrobial stewardship. In many cases, broad-spectrum antimicrobials are initiated before definitive microbiological diagnosis, creating strong selective pressure for resistant strains. Once established, resistant organisms can persist in hospital environments, colonize patients asymptomatically, and spread via healthcare workers, medical devices, and contaminated surfaces.

Medical microbiology plays a pivotal role in breaking this cycle by enabling early pathogen detection, resistance profiling, and outbreak identification. However, the full potential of microbiology-driven interventions remains underutilized in many healthcare systems, particularly in resource-limited settings.

1.3 Limitations of Drug-Centric Approaches:

Historically, the response to AMR has been dominated by the search for new antimicrobial agents. While drug discovery remains essential, reliance on pharmacological solutions alone has proven insufficient. The pace of resistance development consistently outstrips the rate of new drug approvals, leading to a perpetual "arms race" between pathogens and therapeutics (Ventola, 2015).

Moreover, new antimicrobials are often reserved as last-line agents, limiting their use and commercial viability. This has resulted in reduced pharmaceutical investment in antimicrobial research and development. Even when new drugs are introduced, inappropriate use can rapidly erode their effectiveness.

These limitations highlight the need for a paradigm shift—from reactive, drug-centered strategies to proactive, microbiology-driven interventions that focus on prevention, precision, and system-wide optimization. Medical microbiology offers tools not only for identifying pathogens but also for guiding rational antimicrobial use, monitoring resistance trends, and informing infection control policies.

1.4 Rationale for Microbiology-Driven Interventions:

Medical microbiology occupies a unique position at the intersection of laboratory science, clinical medicine, and public health. Unlike purely therapeutic approaches, microbiology-driven interventions address AMR at multiple levels: biological, clinical, and institutional. By generating actionable data on pathogen identity, susceptibility patterns, and transmission dynamics, microbiology laboratories enable evidence-based decision-making throughout the continuum of care.

Microbiology-driven interventions include rapid diagnostics, antimicrobial susceptibility testing, resistance surveillance, outbreak investigation, and laboratory-supported antimicrobial stewardship. These interventions reduce diagnostic uncertainty, minimize unnecessary antimicrobial exposure, and enhance infection prevention efforts. Importantly, they transform microbiology laboratories from passive diagnostic units into active participants in patient management and healthcare policy.

This chapter is grounded in the premise that strengthening and integrating medical microbiology within healthcare systems is essential for sustainable AMR control.

1.5 Objectives and Structure of the Chapter:

The primary objective of this chapter is to examine how medical microbiology-driven interventions can effectively combat antimicrobial resistance in healthcare settings. The chapter seeks to:

1. Explain the microbiological foundations of AMR relevant to clinical practice
2. Highlight diagnostic and surveillance tools as frontline interventions
3. Demonstrate the role of microbiology in antimicrobial stewardship and infection control
4. Identify challenges and gaps in current implementation
5. Explore emerging innovations shaping the future of microbiology-led AMR mitigation

This chapter progressing from foundational concepts to applied strategies and future directions, providing a comprehensive framework for understanding and addressing AMR through medical microbiology.

2. FOUNDATIONS OF MEDICAL MICROBIOLOGY IN AMR CONTROL

2.1 Role of Medical Microbiology in Clinical Medicine

Medical microbiology is a core discipline underpinning the diagnosis, treatment, and prevention of infectious diseases. It encompasses the study of pathogenic microorganisms, host–pathogen interactions, and the laboratory methods used to detect and characterize infectious agents. In clinical practice, microbiology laboratories provide critical information that guides antimicrobial selection, infection control measures, and public health reporting.

In the context of AMR, medical microbiology serves as the primary source of evidence regarding resistance patterns and emerging threats. Laboratory data inform empiric therapy guidelines, institutional antibiograms, and national surveillance programs. Without accurate and timely microbiological input, clinicians are forced to rely on empirical treatment, increasing the risk of inappropriate antimicrobial use.

2.2 Host–Pathogen–Drug Interactions

AMR cannot be fully understood without considering the dynamic interactions between the host, pathogen, and antimicrobial agent. Pathogen-specific factors such as virulence, resistance mechanisms, and metabolic adaptability interact with host immunity and pharmacokinetic–pharmacodynamic properties of drugs to determine clinical outcomes.

Medical microbiology provides insights into these interactions by characterizing microbial behavior under selective pressure and identifying resistance determinants. Such knowledge enables clinicians to tailor therapy based on pathogen characteristics rather than relying solely on standardized treatment protocols.

2.3 Evolutionary Microbiology of Resistance

From an evolutionary perspective, antimicrobial resistance represents a natural consequence of microbial adaptation. Exposure to antimicrobial agents exerts selective pressure, favoring the survival of resistant variants. Genetic mutations, gene amplification, and horizontal gene transfer contribute to the rapid evolution of resistance within microbial populations (Davies & Davies, 2010).

Healthcare environments intensify these evolutionary processes due to high antimicrobial exposure and dense microbial populations. Medical microbiology helps elucidate these evolutionary pathways, enabling early detection of resistance trends and informing strategies to disrupt transmission and selection.

2.4 Clinical Relevance of Microbial Ecology

Microbial ecology—the study of microbial communities and their interactions—has gained increasing relevance in healthcare. The human microbiota plays a protective role against pathogen colonization, while antimicrobial exposure can disrupt this balance, promoting the emergence of resistant organisms.

Medical microbiology integrates ecological principles to understand how antimicrobial use alters microbial communities within patients and healthcare environments. This ecological perspective supports interventions aimed at preserving microbial balance while targeting pathogenic organisms.

3. MICROBIOLOGICAL MECHANISMS OF ANTIMICROBIAL RESISTANCE

3.1 Intrinsic and Acquired Resistance

Antimicrobial resistance can be broadly categorized as intrinsic or acquired. Intrinsic resistance refers to inherent structural or functional characteristics of microorganisms that render them insusceptible to certain antimicrobials. In contrast, acquired resistance arises through genetic changes such as mutations or acquisition of resistance genes via horizontal gene transfer (Blair et al., 2015).

Understanding these distinctions is critical for clinical microbiology, as intrinsic resistance informs antibiotic selection, while acquired resistance signals evolving threats requiring surveillance and intervention.

3.2 Enzymatic Degradation and Modification

Enzymatic degradation and modification of antimicrobial agents represent one of the most widespread and clinically important mechanisms of antimicrobial resistance. This strategy allows microorganisms to directly neutralize antimicrobial compounds before they reach their intended cellular targets. Among these mechanisms, β-lactamase production is particularly prominent in healthcare-associated pathogens. β-lactamases hydrolyze the β-lactam ring of penicillins, cephalosporins, monobactams, and carbapenems, thereby abolishing their antibacterial activity.

Extended-spectrum β-lactamases (ESBLs) have expanded the resistance spectrum of Gram-negative bacteria, notably Escherichia coli and Klebsiella pneumoniae, leading to treatment failures with commonly used cephalosporins. More concerning is the emergence of carbapenemases, which inactivate carbapenems and severely restrict therapeutic options. In addition to β-lactamases, aminoglycoside-modifying enzymes chemically alter aminoglycoside molecules through acetylation, phosphorylation, or adenylation, reducing their binding to ribosomal targets.

Medical microbiology laboratories play a crucial role in detecting enzymatic resistance through phenotypic screening tests, inhibitor-based assays, and molecular diagnostics. Early identification of enzyme-mediated resistance supports timely modification of therapy and strengthens antimicrobial stewardship efforts in healthcare settings.

3.3 Efflux Pumps and Reduced Permeability

Efflux pumps and reduced membrane permeability are key resistance mechanisms that lower intracellular concentrations of antimicrobial agents. Efflux pumps are transport systems that actively expel drugs from microbial cells, often conferring resistance to multiple antimicrobial classes simultaneously. These pumps are widely distributed among both Gram-positive and Gram-negative bacteria and are frequently overexpressed in multidrug-resistant strains.

Reduced permeability further enhances resistance, particularly in Gram-negative bacteria, through alterations in outer membrane porins that restrict antimicrobial entry. Loss or modification of porin channels limits the diffusion of antibiotics such as β-lactams and fluoroquinolones. These mechanisms often coexist with enzymatic resistance, creating highly resilient microbial phenotypes.

From a clinical perspective, efflux- and permeability-mediated resistance can complicate susceptibility interpretation. Medical microbiology laboratories assist clinicians by identifying resistance patterns suggestive of these mechanisms and by integrating advanced testing methods that improve therapeutic decision-making.

3.4 Target Modification and Metabolic Bypass

Modification of antimicrobial targets is another major resistance strategy, allowing microorganisms to evade drug action without destroying the antimicrobial agent itself. Target alterations commonly arise through genetic mutations or enzymatic modifications that reduce drug binding. Examples include altered penicillin-binding proteins in methicillin-resistant Staphylococcus aureus (MRSA), ribosomal modifications conferring macrolide resistance, and mutations in DNA gyrase associated with fluoroquinolone resistance.

Metabolic bypass mechanisms enable microorganisms to circumvent inhibited biochemical pathways by utilizing alternative enzymes or metabolic routes. Resistance to sulfonamides and trimethoprim frequently involves the acquisition of alternative folate synthesis enzymes with reduced affinity for these drugs. Such adaptive strategies allow microbial survival even in the presence of antimicrobial pressure.

Medical microbiology laboratories identify these resistance mechanisms through susceptibility testing, molecular assays, and genomic analysis, providing essential data for precision therapy and resistance surveillance.

3.5 Biofilms and Persister Cells

Biofilm formation represents a complex and clinically significant resistance mechanism, particularly in chronic and device-associated infections. Biofilms consist of microbial communities encased in extracellular polymeric substances that impede antimicrobial penetration and shield pathogens from host immune responses. Within biofilms, microorganisms exhibit altered metabolic states that reduce antimicrobial susceptibility.

Persister cells, a small subpopulation within biofilms, display transient tolerance to antimicrobials without genetic resistance. These dormant cells survive antimicrobial exposure and can reactivate once treatment ceases, leading to persistent or recurrent infections. Biofilm-associated resistance is especially problematic in indwelling medical devices such as catheters, prostheses, and ventilators.

Medical microbiology contributes to the identification and management of biofilm-related infections by supporting diagnostic strategies and guiding combined therapeutic and infection control interventions.

3.6 Horizontal Gene Transfer in Healthcare Settings

Horizontal gene transfer (HGT) is a critical driver of antimicrobial resistance dissemination in healthcare environments. Resistance genes are transferred between microorganisms via plasmids, transposons, integrons, and bacteriophages, enabling rapid spread across species and genera. Hospitals provide ideal conditions for HGT due to high antimicrobial use, dense microbial populations, and frequent patient-to-patient transmission.

Medical microbiology laboratories play a central role in detecting resistance gene transfer through molecular surveillance, outbreak investigations, and genomic epidemiology. Monitoring HGT events informs infection control measures and antimicrobial stewardship policies, helping to limit the spread of resistant pathogens within healthcare settings.

Beyond detection, understanding the ecological and selective pressures that facilitate horizontal gene transfer is essential for effective AMR mitigation. Sub-inhibitory antimicrobial concentrations, biofilm formation on medical devices, and prolonged hospital stays create environments that favor genetic exchange among microorganisms. Integrating microbiological data with clinical and environmental surveillance allows for early identification of high-risk reservoirs and transmission hotspots. Such insights enable targeted interventions, including optimized antimicrobial use, enhanced environmental decontamination, and reinforced infection prevention strategies, thereby reducing opportunities for resistance gene amplification and dissemination.

Figure 1. Pathways Linking Healthcare Practices to AMR Emergence

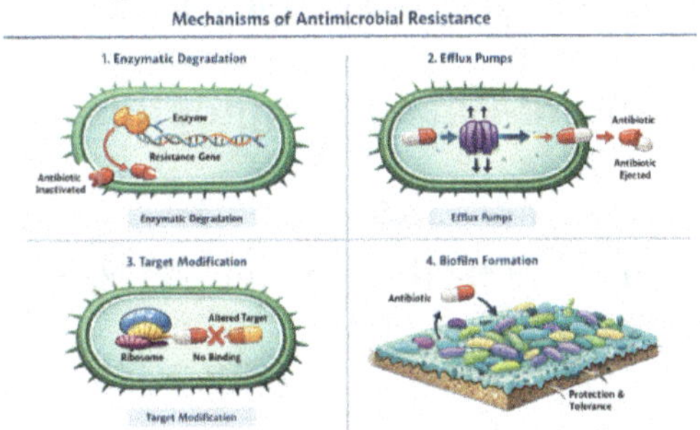

Source: Authors

Figure 1 illustrates the key roles of medical microbiology in combating antimicrobial resistance (AMR) within healthcare settings. The diagram highlights the integration of diagnostic microbiology, antimicrobial susceptibility testing, rapid molecular and proteomic techniques, and point-of-care diagnostics in guiding targeted therapy. It further depicts the interplay between microbiology data and antimicrobial stewardship programs, infection prevention strategies, and surveillance initiatives. By linking laboratory intelligence to clinical decision-making, the figure emphasizes how timely and accurate microbial identification, resistance profiling, and trend analysis can reduce inappropriate antimicrobial use, prevent the spread of resistant pathogens, and support sustainable AMR control in hospitals and healthcare facilities.

4. DIAGNOSTIC MEDICAL MICROBIOLOGY AS AN ANTIMICROBIAL RESISTANCE INTERVENTION

4.1 Role of Diagnostic Microbiology in AMR Control

Diagnostic medical microbiology is a cornerstone of effective antimicrobial resistance (AMR) mitigation in healthcare. Accurate and timely identification of infectious agents and their antimicrobial susceptibility profiles enables clinicians to select appropriate therapies, thereby reducing unnecessary exposure to broad-spectrum antimicrobials. In the absence of definitive diagnostics, empirical therapy predominates, often resulting in overtreatment and increased selective pressure for resistant strains (Laxminarayan et al., 2020).

Diagnostic microbiology should therefore be viewed not merely as a supportive service but as a direct intervention against AMR, capable of influencing prescribing behavior, infection control strategies, and patient outcomes.

4.2 Conventional Culture-Based Diagnostics

Traditional culture-based microbiological techniques remain foundational in clinical diagnostics. These methods allow for pathogen isolation, phenotypic identification, and antimicrobial susceptibility testing (AST). Despite being time-intensive, culture-based diagnostics provide comprehensive information on viable organisms and resistance phenotypes.

However, delays associated with culture-based methods—often 48–72 hours—can result in prolonged empirical antimicrobial use. While indispensable, these limitations underscore the need for complementary rapid diagnostic approaches to support timely clinical decision-making (Jorgensen & Ferraro, 2009).

4.3 Rapid Phenotypic Susceptibility Testing

Advances in phenotypic testing have significantly reduced turnaround times for antimicrobial susceptibility results. Automated systems and rapid AST platforms can deliver results within hours, facilitating earlier de-escalation or escalation of therapy.

Rapid phenotypic testing has demonstrated measurable impacts on reducing inappropriate antimicrobial use, length of hospital stay, and mortality in patients with bloodstream infections (Banerjee et al., 2015). From an AMR perspective, these tools reduce the duration of unnecessary broad-spectrum exposure, thereby limiting resistance selection.

4.4 Molecular Diagnostics and Resistance Gene Detection

Molecular diagnostic techniques, including polymerase chain reaction (PCR)-based assays and nucleic acid amplification tests, have transformed the detection of resistant pathogens. These methods enable rapid identification of specific resistance genes, such as mecA, blaKPC, blaNDM, and vanA/vanB, often directly from clinical specimens.

While molecular diagnostics offer speed and sensitivity, they also present challenges. The presence of a resistance gene does not always correlate with phenotypic resistance, and molecular assays may fail to detect novel or uncommon resistance mechanisms. Thus, integration with phenotypic methods remains essential (van Belkum et al., 2019).

4.5 MALDI-TOF and Proteomic Profiling

Matrix-assisted laser desorption/ionization time-of-flight mass spectrometry (MALDI-TOF MS) has revolutionized microbial identification by enabling rapid, accurate species-level identification within minutes. Recent developments extend its application to resistance detection through proteomic signatures and enzymatic activity assays.

MALDI-TOF-based diagnostics reduce diagnostic delays and improve laboratory efficiency, indirectly contributing to AMR mitigation by supporting earlier targeted therapy (Patel, 2015).

4.6 Point-of-Care Microbiology and Diagnostic Stewardship

Point-of-care (POC) diagnostic tools bring microbiological testing closer to the patient, enabling faster clinical decisions in emergency departments, intensive care units, and outpatient settings. When combined with diagnostic stewardship—ensuring appropriate test selection and interpretation—POC diagnostics enhance the impact of microbiology-driven interventions.

Diagnostic stewardship emphasizes the right test, at the right time, for the right patient, aligning laboratory utilization with AMR control objectives (Morgan et al., 2017).

Figure 2. Diagnostic Microbiology Timeline and Impact on Antimicrobial Decision-Making

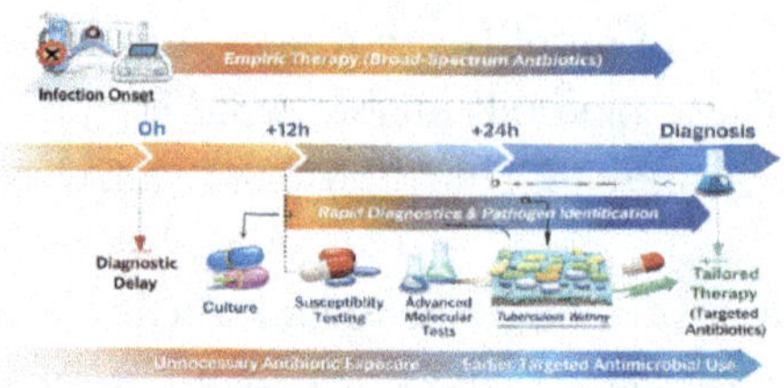

Source: Authors

Figure 2 illustrates the timeline from infection onset to antimicrobial therapy, highlighting the critical role of diagnostic microbiology in guiding clinical decisions. The figure shows how traditional culture-based methods, rapid phenotypic susceptibility testing, molecular diagnostics, and MALDI-TOF mass spectrometry contribute to the timely identification of pathogens and their resistance profiles.

It emphasizes the reduction of empirical broad-spectrum antimicrobial use as diagnostic turnaround times shorten, enabling earlier de-escalation or escalation of therapy. The integration of point-of-care diagnostics and diagnostic stewardship further accelerates decision-making, ensuring that antimicrobial therapy is precise, effective, and aligned with infection control and antimicrobial stewardship objectives.

5. MICROBIOLOGY-GUIDED ANTIMICROBIAL STEWARDSHIP PROGRAMS

5.1 Principles of Antimicrobial Stewardship

Antimicrobial stewardship programs (ASPs) are structured, coordinated efforts designed to optimize the use of antimicrobial agents in healthcare settings with the dual goals of improving patient outcomes and limiting the emergence and spread of antimicrobial resistance. At their core, ASPs promote the judicious use of antimicrobials, ensuring that patients receive the right drug, at the right dose, via the right route, and for the appropriate duration. These principles are essential for preserving antimicrobial efficacy while minimizing adverse drug reactions, secondary infections, and selection pressure that drives resistance.

Effective stewardship begins with accurate diagnosis of infection, distinguishing true infections from colonization or non-infectious conditions. Medical microbiology plays a foundational role in this process by providing timely pathogen identification and antimicrobial susceptibility data. Laboratory confirmation enables clinicians to transition from empiric broad-spectrum therapy to targeted treatment, thereby reducing unnecessary antimicrobial exposure. Stewardship interventions such as de-escalation, dose optimization, intravenous-to-oral switch, and therapy discontinuation rely heavily on microbiological evidence.

Another key principle of stewardship is optimization of antimicrobial dosing, particularly in critically ill patients where pharmacokinetic and pharmacodynamic considerations are crucial. Microbiology data, including minimum inhibitory concentrations (MICs), support individualized dosing strategies that maximize therapeutic efficacy while minimizing toxicity. In addition, stewardship emphasizes limiting treatment duration to evidence-based timeframes, reducing prolonged exposure that contributes to resistance and dysbiosis.

Without robust microbiological input, antimicrobial stewardship lacks precision and becomes largely protocol-driven rather than evidence-based. As emphasized by Barlam et al. (2016), the integration of microbiology into stewardship activities transforms ASPs from administrative oversight mechanisms into dynamic, patient-centered clinical interventions. Thus, medical microbiology is not merely supportive but essential to the success and sustainability of antimicrobial stewardship programs.

5.2 Role of Clinical Microbiologists in Stewardship Teams

Clinical microbiologists are central members of multidisciplinary antimicrobial stewardship teams, contributing specialized expertise that bridges laboratory science and clinical decision-making. Their role extends beyond reporting laboratory results to actively interpreting microbiological data in clinical context. By advising clinicians on pathogen significance, resistance mechanisms, and therapeutic implications, microbiologists enhance the accuracy and effectiveness of antimicrobial prescribing.

In stewardship rounds and case discussions, clinical microbiologists assist in differentiating contamination from true infection, particularly in blood cultures and respiratory specimens. This distinction is critical for preventing unnecessary antimicrobial use. Microbiologists also guide clinicians in selecting appropriate empiric therapy based on local resistance patterns and patient-specific risk factors, such as prior antimicrobial exposure or recent hospitalization.

Beyond individual patient management, microbiologists contribute to institutional stewardship strategies by identifying emerging resistance trends, detecting outbreaks, and advising on containment measures. Their expertise is vital during outbreaks caused by multidrug-resistant organisms, where rapid laboratory confirmation and interpretation can prevent widespread transmission. Microbiologists also play a key role in validating new diagnostic technologies, ensuring that rapid tests are used appropriately within stewardship frameworks.

Education and training represent another important stewardship function of clinical microbiologists. By educating healthcare professionals on resistance mechanisms, diagnostic interpretation, and appropriate antimicrobial use, microbiologists strengthen institutional stewardship culture. Their involvement in developing local treatment guidelines and stewardship policies ensures that recommendations are scientifically sound and tailored to institutional microbiological realities.

Active collaboration between microbiologists, infectious disease physicians, pharmacists, nurses, and infection control practitioners enhances stewardship outcomes. This interdisciplinary engagement reinforces the concept that antimicrobial stewardship is a shared responsibility, with medical microbiology providing the critical evidence base for informed clinical action.

5.3 Antibiograms and Resistance Trend Analysis

Antibiograms are fundamental tools in antimicrobial stewardship, summarizing local antimicrobial susceptibility patterns of clinically significant pathogens over a defined period. By providing aggregated resistance data, antibiograms guide empiric therapy selection and help clinicians choose agents with the highest likelihood of effectiveness. Their routine use supports rational antimicrobial prescribing and reduces reliance on broad-spectrum agents.

From a stewardship perspective, antibiograms are most effective when they reflect local epidemiology and are updated regularly. Medical microbiology laboratories are responsible for generating, validating, and interpreting these data, ensuring adherence to standardized methodologies such as those recommended by the Clinical and Laboratory Standards Institute (CLSI, 2023). Accurate antibiogram construction requires careful consideration of isolate selection, duplicate exclusion, and sample size to ensure reliability.

Beyond traditional cumulative antibiograms, advanced microbiology laboratories now generate stratified or unit-specific antibiograms. These may be based on patient location (e.g., intensive care units), specimen type, age group, or specific risk factors. Stratified antibiograms enhance clinical relevance by accounting for variations in resistance patterns across hospital settings, thereby improving empiric therapy decisions for high-risk populations. The major antimicrobial resistance mechanisms observed in clinically important pathogens are summarized in Table 2.

Resistance trend analysis using longitudinal antibiogram data enables early detection of emerging resistance and evaluation of stewardship interventions. Increasing resistance to specific antimicrobial classes may signal the need for policy revision, formulary restriction, or targeted stewardship campaigns. Conversely, improvements in susceptibility patterns can demonstrate the effectiveness of stewardship measures, reinforcing institutional commitment.

Medical microbiology laboratories increasingly integrate antibiogram data with electronic health records and stewardship dashboards, facilitating real-time decision support. Such integration strengthens the role of microbiology as a proactive contributor to antimicrobial stewardship rather than a passive data provider. By translating resistance data into actionable insights, antibiograms remain a cornerstone of microbiology-driven stewardship in healthcare.

Table 2. Major Antimicrobial Resistance Mechanisms in Clinically Important Pathogens

Pathogen	Key Resistance Mechanisms	Clinical Implications
Staphylococcus aureus	Altered PBPs, β-lactamases	MRSA infections
Enterobacterales	ESBLs, carbapenemases	Limited treatment options
Pseudomonas aeruginosa	Efflux pumps, porin loss	Multidrug resistance
Enterococcus spp.	Target modification	Vancomycin resistance
Candida auris	Efflux, biofilms	Antifungal resistance

5.4 Microbiology-Driven De-Escalation Strategies

De-escalation involves narrowing antimicrobial therapy based on microbiological results. This practice reduces unnecessary exposure to broad-spectrum agents and preserves their efficacy.

Microbiology laboratories facilitate de-escalation by providing timely identification, susceptibility results, and interpretive comments. Studies consistently demonstrate that microbiology-driven de-escalation reduces resistance selection without compromising patient outcomes (Tamma et al., 2022).

5.5 Feedback Systems and Clinician Engagement

Effective stewardship relies on continuous feedback between laboratories and clinicians. Electronic health records, automated alerts, and decision-support tools enhance communication and reinforce evidence-based prescribing.

Microbiology-informed feedback has been shown to improve adherence to stewardship recommendations and reduce inappropriate antimicrobial use.

6. SURVEILLANCE MICROBIOLOGY AND INFECTION PREVENTION

6.1 Hospital-Based AMR Surveillance Systems

Surveillance microbiology is essential for monitoring resistance patterns and guiding infection prevention strategies. Hospital-based surveillance systems collect and analyze microbiological data to identify trends, clusters, and outbreaks of resistant organisms.

Such systems form the backbone of national and global AMR surveillance initiatives, enabling coordinated responses to emerging threats (WHO, 2023).

Figure 3. Surveillance–infection control integration model

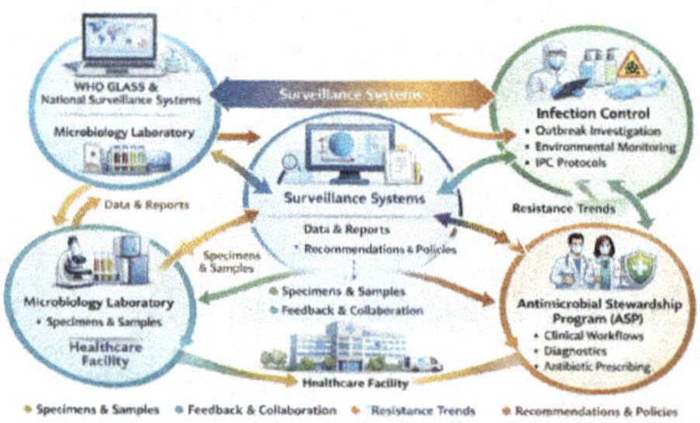

Source: Authors

Figure 3 depicts how medical microbiology data are integrated into antimicrobial stewardship programs (ASPs) and infection control strategies within healthcare settings. The diagram highlights the flow of information from rapid diagnostics, susceptibility testing, and molecular surveillance to clinical teams, stewardship committees, and infection prevention units. It illustrates key interventions including targeted therapy, de-escalation, outbreak detection, and policy development, showing how timely laboratory intelligence informs decision-making at multiple levels. By linking microbiology outputs with clinical actions and institutional policies, the figure emphasizes the central role of microbiology in reducing inappropriate antimicrobial use, preventing the spread of resistant pathogens, and achieving sustainable antimicrobial resistance (AMR) control.

6.2 Molecular Epidemiology and Outbreak Investigation

Molecular epidemiology has become a cornerstone of antimicrobial resistance (AMR) surveillance and outbreak investigation in healthcare settings. Conventional phenotypic methods often lack the discriminatory power required to resolve transmission dynamics, particularly for closely related multidrug-resistant organisms. Modern molecular typing techniques enable high-resolution tracking of resistant strains and provide critical insights into pathogen evolution and dissemination within hospitals (Kwong et al., 2015).

Techniques such as pulsed-field gel electrophoresis (PFGE) and multilocus sequence typing (MLST) have historically supported outbreak investigations; however, whole-genome sequencing (WGS) has now emerged as the gold standard for molecular epidemiology (Didelot et al., 2021; van Belkum et al., 2019). WGS allows comprehensive characterization of resistance genes, virulence determinants, and mobile genetic elements, enabling precise differentiation between clonal transmission and independent acquisition of resistance.

Molecular epidemiology plays a pivotal role during healthcare-associated outbreaks by informing targeted infection control interventions. Genomic data can identify transmission routes, environmental reservoirs, and breaches in infection control practices that are not evident through routine surveillance (Raven et al., 2016). Medical microbiology laboratories are central to generating, analyzing, and translating genomic data into actionable insights, reinforcing their strategic role in outbreak preparedness and response.

6.3 Environmental Microbiology in Healthcare Settings

Healthcare environments represent critical reservoirs for antimicrobial-resistant organisms, contributing to ongoing transmission and recurrent outbreaks. Environmental microbiology focuses on detecting and characterizing microbial contamination on hospital surfaces, medical equipment, air handling systems, and water networks (Weber et al., 2013). High-touch surfaces and moist environments, in particular, support the persistence of pathogens such as Acinetobacter baumannii, Pseudomonas aeruginosa, and Candida auris.

Recent studies have demonstrated that biofilms in hospital plumbing systems act as long-term reservoirs for resistant organisms, complicating eradication efforts (Bédard et al., 2018). Environmental surveillance enables assessment of cleaning efficacy, disinfectant performance, and infrastructure design, supporting evidence-based improvements in infection prevention strategies.

Integration of environmental microbiology with clinical and molecular surveillance enhances understanding of transmission pathways. Linking environmental isolates with patient-derived strains through genomic analysis strengthens outbreak investigations and supports targeted remediation (Puraswani et al., 2025). Medical microbiology laboratories thus extend their influence beyond patient diagnostics to encompass environmental risk assessment and hospital design optimization.

6.4 Surveillance of Healthcare-Associated Infections

Surveillance of healthcare-associated infections (HAIs) is fundamental to controlling AMR and safeguarding patient safety. HAIs caused by resistant pathogens are associated with prolonged hospital stays, increased mortality, and higher healthcare costs (CDC, 2023). Continuous, systematic surveillance enables early detection of resistance trends and evaluation of infection prevention interventions.

Medical microbiology laboratories provide the core data for HAI surveillance, including pathogen identification, antimicrobial susceptibility profiles, and resistance mechanisms. Surveillance outputs inform isolation precautions, cohorting strategies, and antimicrobial policy adjustments at institutional and unit levels (WHO, 2023). Surveillance has expanded to include fungal and viral pathogens, reflecting the evolving spectrum of healthcare-associated threats.

Advances in electronic surveillance systems have improved timeliness and accuracy, allowing near–real-time reporting and trend analysis. However, the effectiveness of these systems depends on laboratory data quality and interpretive expertise. Medical microbiology thus remains indispensable for sustaining robust, responsive HAI surveillance programs.

6.5 Data-Driven Infection Control Strategies

The integration of microbiology, stewardship, and infection control data enables healthcare institutions to transition from reactive to proactive AMR management. Data-driven infection control strategies leverage real-time laboratory data, antibiograms, molecular surveillance outputs, and clinical metadata to support timely decision-making (Rawson et al., 2017; Peiffer-Smadja et al., 2020).

Predictive analytics and machine learning tools are increasingly used to identify patients at high risk for resistant infections, forecast outbreak potential, and optimize resource allocation (Wiens & Shenoy, 2017; Rodríguez-Baño et al., 2021). Real-time dashboards enhance situational awareness for infection control teams, enabling rapid response to emerging threats.

Medical microbiology laboratories play a critical role in ensuring data accuracy, standardization, and clinical relevance. Integration of laboratory intelligence into institutional decision-support systems reinforces microbiology's leadership role in AMR containment. As summarized in Table 3, data-driven infection control represents a paradigm shift toward anticipatory, system-level responses to antimicrobial resistance.

Table 3. Microbiology Inputs Supporting Antimicrobial Stewardship and Infection Control

Microbiology Input	Stewardship Impact	Infection Control Impact
Rapid diagnostics	Targeted therapy	Early isolation
Susceptibility data	De-escalation	Resistance monitoring
Surveillance reports	Policy updates	Outbreak detection
Molecular typing	Trend analysis	Transmission mapping

7. MULTIDRUG-RESISTANT AND HIGH-RISK PATHOGENS IN HEALTHCARE

7.1 ESKAPE Pathogens and Their Clinical Significance

The ESKAPE pathogens—Enterococcus faecium, Staphylococcus aureus, Klebsiella pneumoniae, Acinetobacter baumannii, Pseudomonas aeruginosa, and Enterobacter species—represent the most clinically significant group of antimicrobial-resistant organisms in modern healthcare (Rice, 2008). These pathogens are responsible for a disproportionate burden of healthcare-associated infections (HAIs), including bloodstream infections, ventilator-associated pneumonia, surgical site infections, and catheter-associated urinary tract infections. Their capacity to "escape" antimicrobial action arises from a convergence of resistance mechanisms such as enzymatic drug degradation, efflux pumps, reduced membrane permeability, target modification, and biofilm formation.

In recent years, the clinical importance of ESKAPE pathogens has intensified due to their association with severe disease outcomes, prolonged hospitalization, and increased mortality, particularly among immunocompromised and critically ill patients (Bonomo et al., 2018; CDC, 2024). Global surveillance data indicate that ESKAPE organisms account for the majority of priority pathogens listed by the World Health Organization and national public health agencies (WHO, 2024). Their adaptability is further enhanced by horizontal gene transfer, enabling rapid dissemination of resistance determinants across species and healthcare settings.

Medical microbiology laboratories play a pivotal role in addressing ESKAPE-related threats through timely identification, antimicrobial susceptibility testing, and resistance mechanism characterization. Advances in rapid diagnostics, including MALDI-TOF mass spectrometry and multiplex molecular assays, have significantly reduced turnaround times for pathogen identification and resistance detection (Patel, 2015; CLSI, 2024). Continuous microbiological surveillance allows hospitals to refine empiric therapy guidelines, implement targeted infection control interventions, and detect early signals of outbreaks in high-risk units such as intensive care and transplant wards.

7.2 Carbapenem-Resistant Enterobacterales (CRE)

Carbapenem-resistant Enterobacterales (CRE) represent one of the most critical antimicrobial resistance threats globally. Resistance is primarily mediated by carbapenemase enzymes, including KPC, NDM, OXA-48-like, VIM, and IMP, which are frequently plasmid-encoded and capable of rapid interspecies transmission (Nordmann et al., 2011; Logan & Weinstein, 2017). CRE infections are associated with limited therapeutic options, high treatment failure rates, and mortality rates exceeding 40% in some patient populations (van Duin & Doi, 2017; Tamma et al., 2022).

Recent studies highlight the expanding geographic distribution of CRE and the emergence of novel carbapenemase variants, particularly in low- and middle-income countries (WHO, 2024). Medical microbiology laboratories are central to CRE containment through rapid molecular detection of carbapenemase genes, phenotypic confirmation assays, and routine screening of high-risk patients. Whole-genome sequencing has further enhanced understanding of CRE transmission dynamics, enabling differentiation between clonal spread and multiple independent introductions (David et al., 2025).

Microbiology-driven interventions support infection prevention strategies such as contact precautions, cohorting, environmental decontamination, and antimicrobial stewardship adjustments. Failure to rapidly identify CRE carriers can result in silent transmission and hospital-wide outbreaks, underscoring the indispensable role of laboratory surveillance in CRE control (Puraswani et al., 2025; ECDC, 2025).

7.3 Methicillin-Resistant Staphylococcus aureus (MRSA) and Vancomycin-Resistant Enterococcus (VRE)

MRSA and VRE continue to pose significant challenges despite decades of surveillance and control efforts. MRSA remains a leading cause of invasive infections, while VRE has emerged as a dominant pathogen in hematology, oncology, and intensive care settings (Turner et al., 2019; CDC, 2024). These organisms exemplify the persistence of resistance even under sustained infection control and stewardship interventions.

Medical microbiology supports MRSA and VRE management through active surveillance cultures, rapid molecular screening, susceptibility testing, and molecular typing. Contemporary evidence demonstrates that laboratory-guided decolonization strategies, combined with antimicrobial stewardship, can significantly reduce transmission and infection rates (Huang et al., 2013; Bearman et al., 2023). Whole-genome sequencing has further clarified transmission networks, enabling targeted interventions rather than broad, resource-intensive control measures (Didelot et al., 2021).

Emerging data from 2024–2025 emphasize the importance of integrating microbiology data into real-time hospital dashboards, allowing infection control teams to respond proactively to increases in MRSA or VRE incidence (ECDC, 2025).

7.4 Drug-Resistant Tuberculosis in Healthcare Settings

Drug-resistant tuberculosis (DR-TB) remains a major global health concern, with significant implications for healthcare facilities, particularly in high-burden regions. Multidrug-resistant (MDR-TB) and extensively drug-resistant tuberculosis (XDR-TB) require prolonged treatment regimens, strict infection control measures, and specialized laboratory diagnostics (WHO, 2022; WHO, 2024).

Medical microbiology contributes through rapid molecular resistance testing, including Xpert MTB/XDR assays, line probe assays, and culture-based drug susceptibility testing. These tools enable early detection of resistance to first- and second-line anti-tubercular drugs, guiding individualized treatment and reducing nosocomial transmission (Pai et al., 2018; Ahmad et al., 2018). Healthcare-associated transmission of DR-TB has been documented in overcrowded hospitals with inadequate ventilation, reinforcing the need for laboratory-supported surveillance and environmental controls (Churchyard et al., 2025).

Integration of microbiological data into national TB surveillance systems enhances outbreak detection and informs policy decisions related to infection prevention, occupational health, and antimicrobial stewardship within healthcare settings (WHO, 2024; Cheraghi et al., 2025).

Such integration supports real-time risk assessment and facilitates timely implementation of evidence-based control measures across healthcare facilities. Furthermore, harmonized laboratory reporting strengthens intersectoral coordination and contributes to long-term strategies aimed at reducing transmission and drug resistance at the population level.

7.5 Antifungal Resistance and Candida auris

The emergence of Candida auris has expanded the scope of antimicrobial resistance beyond bacteria, highlighting the growing threat of antifungal resistance in healthcare environments. C. auris demonstrates resistance to multiple antifungal classes, persistence on hospital surfaces, and a strong association with intensive care units and invasive device use (Chowdhary et al., 2017; Lockhart et al., 2016).

Accurate identification of C. auris requires advanced microbiological methods, as conventional biochemical assays often misidentify the organism. MALDI-TOF mass spectrometry, sequencing-based approaches, and updated diagnostic databases are now considered essential for reliable detection (CLSI, 2024; Kirby et al., 2019). Outbreaks of C. auris underscore the importance of environmental microbiology, as the organism can contaminate surfaces, equipment, and healthcare workers' hands.

Recent reports from 2024–2025 document increasing global incidence and the emergence of pan-resistant strains, emphasizing the urgency of laboratory-led surveillance and infection control strategies (CDC, 2024; Fisher et al., 2024). Medical microbiology remains central to antifungal susceptibility testing, outbreak investigation, and guiding antifungal stewardship programs aimed at preserving the efficacy of limited therapeutic options.

8. CHALLENGES IN IMPLEMENTING MICROBIOLOGY-DRIVEN AMR INTERVENTIONS

8.1 Laboratory Infrastructure and Resource Constraints

Despite the central role of medical microbiology in antimicrobial resistance (AMR) control, laboratory infrastructure in many healthcare systems remains under-developed. Chronic underinvestment has resulted in inadequate physical facilities, limited biosafety capacity, outdated diagnostic equipment, and insufficient access to quality-assured reagents. These limitations directly affect the speed, accuracy, and scope of microbiological testing, undermining timely clinical decision-making and surveillance efforts (Kakkar et al., 2020; WHO, 2024).

Resource constraints are particularly acute in low- and middle-income countries (LMICs), where the burden of infectious diseases and AMR is disproportionately high. Many laboratories in these settings lack routine access to automated blood culture systems, antimicrobial susceptibility testing platforms, or molecular diagnostics. As a result, clinicians often rely on empirical therapy, which can accelerate resistance selection and compromise patient outcomes (Kariuki et al., 2018; Prestinaci et al., 2015). Strengthening laboratory infrastructure—through investment in equipment, supply chains, quality management systems, and biosafety—is therefore a foundational requirement for effective AMR containment.

International initiatives such as WHO's Global Antimicrobial Resistance Surveillance System (GLASS) have emphasized laboratory capacity-building as a cornerstone of national AMR action plans. However, sustainable progress requires long-term financing models, integration into health system planning, and alignment with local epidemiological priorities (WHO, 2024; ECDC, 2025).

8.2 Workforce and Training Gaps

The effectiveness of microbiology-driven interventions is heavily dependent on a skilled and adequately staffed workforce. Clinical microbiologists, laboratory scientists, and infection control professionals must possess not only technical expertise but also the ability to interpret complex diagnostic data and translate findings into clinically actionable guidance. However, global shortages of trained microbiology professionals represent a major constraint on AMR response capacity (Baker et al., 2018).

In many healthcare systems, particularly in LMICs, laboratory personnel are overburdened, undertrained, and inadequately supported. Limited opportunities for continuing professional development further exacerbate skill gaps, especially in rapidly evolving areas such as molecular diagnostics, genomic epidemiology, and bioinformatics (Köser et al., 2014; Moran et al., 2016). Even in high-income settings, the expanding scope of microbiology has outpaced workforce growth, leading to increased reliance on automation without sufficient interpretive expertise.

Addressing these challenges requires investment in education, interdisciplinary training, and career development pathways. Integrating microbiology training with clinical medicine, pharmacy, and public health can enhance collaboration and improve the translation of laboratory data into stewardship and infection control actions (Barlam et al., 2016; Pulcini et al., 2019).

8.3 Diagnostic Delays and Clinical Inertia

Timely diagnostics are essential for microbiology-guided antimicrobial therapy; however, delays in test ordering, sample transport, laboratory processing, reporting, or clinical response often diminish the value of available data. Conventional culture-based methods, while essential, may require 48–72 hours or longer to generate definitive results, during which broad-spectrum antimicrobials are frequently continued (Pliakos et al., 2018).

Beyond technical delays, clinical inertia—the failure to modify therapy in response to new microbiological information—represents a significant behavioral and systemic barrier. Studies have shown that clinicians may hesitate to de-escalate therapy due to fear of treatment failure, lack of confidence in laboratory results, or inadequate communication between laboratories and clinical teams (Schuts et al., 2016; Tamma et al., 2022).

Improving laboratory–clinician interaction through real-time reporting, interpretive comments, and stewardship-driven feedback mechanisms can reduce diagnostic inertia. Decision-support tools embedded within electronic health records have also shown promise in prompting timely antimicrobial optimization based on microbiological data (Langford et al., 2023; Klein et al., 2024).

8.4 Data Integration and Digital Barriers

Fragmented data systems remain a major obstacle to effective AMR management. Microbiology laboratories often operate in isolation from electronic health records, antimicrobial stewardship platforms, and national surveillance databases. Lack of interoperability limits the ability to perform real-time data analysis, track resistance trends, and coordinate institutional or regional responses.

Manual data entry, inconsistent coding standards, and limited informatics support further constrain the utility of laboratory data. These challenges are particularly evident in settings where laboratory information systems are outdated or absent altogether. As a result, valuable microbiological insights may remain underutilized in clinical care and public health decision-making (ECDC, 2025).

Digital transformation of microbiology services—including standardized data architectures, automated reporting, and integration with surveillance and stewardship tools—is increasingly recognized as essential for modern AMR strategies. Emerging applications of artificial intelligence and predictive analytics offer additional opportunities but depend fundamentally on high-quality, interoperable laboratory data (Peiffer-Smadja et al., 2020; Liu et al., 2024).

8.5 Equity and Accessibility Concerns

Advanced microbiological diagnostics, such as whole-genome sequencing and rapid molecular assays, are disproportionately concentrated in well-resourced healthcare systems. This uneven distribution raises significant equity concerns, as populations with the highest AMR burden often have the least access to diagnostic innovation (Kariuki et al., 2018; WHO, 2024).

Scalability and contextual adaptability must therefore be central considerations in microbiology-driven AMR interventions. Simplified, cost-effective diagnostic platforms, decentralized testing models, and regional reference laboratory networks can help bridge access gaps. Without deliberate efforts to promote equitable access, advances in microbiology risk widening global health disparities rather than reducing them (Laxminarayan et al., 2020; Mendelson et al., 2023).

Ensuring equity in AMR diagnostics requires coordinated action across policy, financing, technology development, and workforce training. Medical microbiology must be positioned not only as a technical discipline but also as a key contributor to global health equity and sustainable healthcare systems.

9. EMERGING INNOVATIONS AND FUTURE DIRECTIONS

9.1 Genomic Surveillance and Whole-Genome Sequencing

Whole-genome sequencing (WGS) has emerged as a transformative technology in medical microbiology, redefining how antimicrobial resistance (AMR) is detected, monitored, and controlled. Unlike traditional phenotypic methods, WGS enables comprehensive analysis of pathogen genomes, allowing simultaneous identification of resistance genes, virulence determinants, sequence types, and mobile genetic elements. This high-resolution approach has significantly enhanced understanding of pathogen evolution and transmission dynamics within healthcare settings (Didelot et al., 2012; Kwong et al., 2015).

Recent advances have positioned genomic surveillance as a core component of AMR preparedness strategies. Routine WGS enables early detection of novel resistance mechanisms, including hybrid plasmids and convergent resistance–virulence profiles, which are increasingly reported in high-risk pathogens such as carbapenem-resistant Enterobacterales and Acinetobacter baumannii (Baker et al., 2018; Moran et al., 2016). Genomic data also support differentiation between clonal outbreaks and sporadic cases, allowing infection control teams to deploy targeted rather than blanket interventions.

As sequencing costs decline and turnaround times shorten, integration of WGS into routine microbiology workflows is becoming more feasible. However, future success will depend on investments in bioinformatics infrastructure, standardized analytical pipelines, and workforce training to ensure genomic data are translated into actionable clinical and public health decisions (van Belkum et al., 2019; ECDC, 2025).

9.2 Artificial Intelligence and Machine Learning

Artificial intelligence (AI) and machine learning (ML) are rapidly reshaping medical microbiology by enabling advanced analysis of complex, multidimensional datasets. Microbiology laboratories generate vast quantities of data encompassing culture results, antimicrobial susceptibility profiles, genomic sequences, and patient metadata. AI-driven tools can integrate these datasets to identify resistance patterns, predict outbreaks, and support real-time clinical decision-making (Rawson et al., 2017; Peiffer-Smadja et al., 2020).

Recent studies have demonstrated that ML models can predict antimicrobial resistance directly from genomic and phenotypic data, sometimes outperforming conventional rule-based approaches (Liu et al., 2024; Klein et al., 2024). AI applications now extend to automated susceptibility interpretation, early warning systems for hospital outbreaks, and optimization of empiric antimicrobial therapy.

Despite this promise, challenges remain. Algorithm transparency, data bias, and generalizability across healthcare settings are major concerns. Medical microbiologists play a critical role in validating AI outputs, ensuring biological plausibility, and maintaining clinical trust. Ethical considerations related to data governance and accountability must also be addressed as AI becomes embedded in AMR management frameworks.

9.3 Predictive Resistance Modeling

Predictive resistance modeling represents a paradigm shift from reactive to anticipatory AMR control. By leveraging longitudinal microbiology and prescribing data, predictive models can forecast resistance trends and identify emerging threats before they become clinically entrenched. These models support proactive revision of empiric therapy guidelines and targeted deployment of infection control resources (Rodríguez-Baño et al., 2021).

Medical microbiology laboratories provide the foundational data required for predictive modeling, including susceptibility trends, pathogen prevalence, and resistance mechanisms. Integration of laboratory data with patient movement, antimicrobial consumption, and environmental factors enhances predictive accuracy. Recent work has demonstrated the utility of predictive analytics in intensive care units, where early detection of resistance emergence can significantly influence outcomes (Klein et al., 2024).

However, predictive models must be continuously updated and validated to remain clinically relevant. Interdisciplinary collaboration between microbiologists, epidemiologists, and data scientists is essential to ensure predictive tools are interpretable, actionable, and aligned with real-world clinical workflows.

9.4 Personalized Antimicrobial Therapy

Advances in diagnostics and microbial profiling are driving a transition toward personalized antimicrobial therapy. Rather than relying solely on population-based guidelines, personalized approaches tailor treatment to individual patient characteristics, pathogen identity, resistance profile, and pharmacokinetic–pharmacodynamic parameters. Medical microbiology underpins this shift by delivering precise and timely diagnostic data.

Rapid molecular diagnostics, resistance gene detection, and genomic susceptibility prediction enable earlier optimization of antimicrobial therapy, reducing unnecessary exposure to broad-spectrum agents. Personalized therapy has been associated with improved clinical outcomes, reduced toxicity, and mitigation of resistance selection pressure, particularly in critically ill and immunocompromised patients (van Belkum et al., 2019; Moran et al., 2016).

Future directions may include integration of host immune profiling and microbiome data, further refining antimicrobial selection. Achieving widespread implementation will require seamless collaboration between microbiology laboratories, clinicians, pharmacists, and digital health systems.

9.5 Integration with One Health Frameworks

Antimicrobial resistance is inherently a One Health challenge, arising from interconnected human, animal, and environmental ecosystems. Medical microbiology contributes to One Health initiatives by generating standardized resistance data that can be integrated across clinical, veterinary, agricultural, and environmental surveillance systems (Robinson et al., 2016; WHO, 2023).

Recent global strategies emphasize harmonization of laboratory methods, shared data platforms, and coordinated governance structures to address AMR across sectors. Integration of clinical microbiology data with surveillance from livestock, food systems, wastewater, and natural environments provides a more comprehensive understanding of resistance emergence and dissemination pathways (Laxminarayan et al., 2020; WHO, 2024).

Looking forward, strengthening the role of medical microbiology within One Health frameworks will be essential for sustainable AMR control. Equitable access to diagnostics, regional reference laboratory networks, and international data sharing will determine whether technological advances translate into global health impact or exacerbate existing disparities.

10. CONCLUSION AND POLICY IMPLICATIONS

10.1 Repositioning Medical Microbiology in Healthcare

This chapter has demonstrated that medical microbiology must be repositioned from a predominantly diagnostic support service to a strategic, intelligence-driven pillar of healthcare systems in the fight against antimicrobial resistance (AMR).

Traditionally viewed as a laboratory-bound discipline focused on pathogen identification and susceptibility testing, medical microbiology now occupies a far more influential role, generating real-time data that shape clinical decision-making, infection prevention strategies, and health policy formulation (van Belkum et al., 2019; Moran et al., 2016).

By integrating phenotypic diagnostics, molecular assays, genomic surveillance, and data analytics, microbiology laboratories serve as early warning systems for emerging resistance threats. This capability enables healthcare institutions to move beyond reactive containment toward proactive AMR mitigation. Repositioning microbiology at the core of healthcare governance structures—rather than at the periphery—is therefore essential for achieving sustainable resistance control in increasingly complex clinical environments (WHO, 2024).

10.2 Translational Impact on Patient Outcomes

Microbiology-driven interventions have a direct and measurable impact on patient outcomes. Timely and accurate microbiological diagnostics reduce diagnostic uncertainty, shorten the time to appropriate antimicrobial therapy, and facilitate early de-escalation from broad-spectrum agents. These effects are particularly critical in severe infections such as sepsis, bloodstream infections, and ventilator-associated pneumonia, where delays in targeted therapy are strongly associated with increased mortality (Rawson et al., 2017; Klein et al., 2024).

Beyond individual patient outcomes, microbiology-guided care contributes to broader health system efficiency. Optimized antimicrobial use reduces drug-related toxicity, limits disruption of the host microbiome, and decreases selection pressure for resistance. At the institutional level, improved infection control and outbreak prevention reduce length of hospital stay, intensive care utilization, and overall healthcare costs (Rodríguez-Baño et al., 2021).

The translational value of medical microbiology is fully realized when laboratory findings are rapidly communicated, appropriately contextualized, and systematically integrated into antimicrobial stewardship programs and clinical decision-support frameworks. This highlights the critical need for sustained, bidirectional collaboration among microbiologists, clinicians, pharmacists, and infection prevention teams to ensure timely, evidence-based therapeutic decisions and optimized patient care outcomes.

10.3 Policy and Institutional Recommendations

Effective AMR control requires coordinated action at institutional, national, and global levels. Based on the evidence presented in this chapter, several policy and institutional priorities emerge as critical:

Investment in microbiology infrastructure

Sustained investment in laboratory facilities, diagnostic technologies, biosafety systems, and quality assurance programs is essential. Without robust infrastructure, even the most advanced stewardship and surveillance strategies cannot function effectively, particularly in high-burden settings (Kariuki et al., 2018; WHO, 2024).

Integration into stewardship and infection control programs

Medical microbiology laboratories must be formally embedded within antimicrobial stewardship programs (ASPs) and infection prevention frameworks. Laboratory data should directly inform prescribing policies, outbreak response, and institutional guidelines rather than functioning as retrospective reports (Barlam et al., 2016; Pulcini et al., 2019).

Workforce development and interdisciplinary collaboration

Addressing workforce shortages through training, career pathways, and interdisciplinary education is critical. Future microbiologists must be equipped not only with technical skills but also with competencies in data interpretation, communication, and clinical engagement (Baker et al., 2018; Moran et al., 2016).

Digital integration and data interoperability

Policy frameworks should prioritize interoperable laboratory information systems, integration with electronic health records, and participation in national and international surveillance networks. Digital maturity is now a prerequisite for effective AMR management (Peiffer-Smadja et al., 2020; ECDC, 2025).

Collectively, these measures form the foundation for a resilient, evidence-based AMR response.

10.4 Future Outlook

As antimicrobial resistance continues to evolve, the future role of medical microbiology must extend beyond detection toward prediction and prevention. Advances in genomic surveillance, artificial intelligence, and predictive modeling provide unprecedented opportunities to anticipate resistance emergence and intervene before clinical failure occurs (Didelot et al., 2012; Liu et al., 2024).

The convergence of microbiology with digital health, data science, and One Health frameworks will define the next phase of AMR control. However, technological innovation alone is insufficient. Success will depend on strong laboratory systems, equitable access to diagnostics, ethical data governance, and sustained political commitment. Without these enabling conditions, innovation risks deepening existing disparities rather than delivering global health gains (Laxminarayan et al., 2020; WHO, 2023).

In conclusion, medical microbiology stands at a pivotal juncture. By embracing its expanded role as a predictive, integrative, and policy-relevant discipline, medical microbiology can lead the transition toward more resilient healthcare systems and more effective antimicrobial resistance mitigation strategies.

REFERENCES

Ahmad, N., Ahuja, S. D., Akkerman, O. W., Alffenaar, J.-W. C., Anderson, L. F., Baghaei, P., Bang, D., Barry, P. M., Bastos, M. L., Behera, D., Benedetti, A., Bisson, G. P., Boeree, M. J., Bonnet, M., Brode, S. K., Brust, J. C. M., Cai, Y., Caumes, E., Cegielski, J. P., & Centis, R. (2018). Treatment correlates of successful outcomes in pulmonary multidrug-resistant tuberculosis: An individual patient data meta-analysis. *Lancet*, *392*(10150), 821–834. https://doi.org/10.1016/s0140-6736(18)31644-1

Antimicrobial Resistance Collaborators. (2022). Global Burden of Bacterial Antimicrobial Resistance in 2019: A Systematic Analysis. *Lancet*, *399*(10325), 629–655. https://doi.org/10.1016/S0140-6736(21)02724-0

Baker, S., Thomson, N., Weill, F.-X., & Holt, K. E. (2018). Genomic insights into the emergence and spread of antimicrobial-resistant bacterial pathogens. *Science*, *360*(6390), 733–738. https://doi.org/10.1126/science.aar3777

Banerjee, R., Teng, C. B., Cunningham, S. A., Ihde, S. M., Steckelberg, J. M., Moriarty, J. P., Shah, N. D., Mandrekar, J. N., & Patel, R. (2015). Randomized trial of rapid multiplex polymerase chain reaction–based blood culture identification and susceptibility testing. *Clinical Infectious Diseases*, *61*(7), 1071–1080. DOI: 10.1093/cid/civ447 PMID: 26197846

Barlam, T. F., Cosgrove, S. E., Abbo, L. M., MacDougall, C., Schuetz, A. N., Septimus, E. J., Srinivasan, A., Dellit, T. H., Falck-Ytter, Y. T., Fishman, N. O., Hamilton, C. W., Jenkins, T. C., Lipsett, P. A., Malani, P. N., May, L. S., Moran, G. J., Neuhauser, M. M., Newland, J. G., Ohl, C. A., & Trivedi, K. K. (2016). Implementing an antibiotic stewardship program: Guidelines by the Infectious Diseases Society of America and the Society for Healthcare Epidemiology of America. *Clinical Infectious Diseases*, *62*(10), e51–e77. DOI: 10.1093/cid/ciw118 PMID: 27080992

Bearman, G., Rosato, A. E., Elam, K., Stevens, M. P., & Wenzel, R. P. (2023). Genomic epidemiology of methicillin-resistant Staphylococcus aureus transmission. *Infection Control and Hospital Epidemiology*, *44*(6), 889–897. DOI: 10.1017/ice.2022.297

Bédard, E., Laferrière, C., Déziel, E., & Prévost, M. (2018). Impact of stagnation and sampling volume on water microbial quality monitoring in large buildings. *PLoS One*, *13*(6), e0199429. https://doi.org/10.1371/journal.pone.0199429

Blair, J. M. A., Webber, M. A., Baylay, A. J., Ogbolu, D. O., & Piddock, L. J. V. (2015). Molecular mechanisms of antibiotic resistance. *Nature Reviews. Microbiology*, *13*(1), 42–51. DOI: 10.1038/nrmicro3380 PMID: 25435309

Bonomo, R. A., Burd, E. M., Conly, J., Limbago, B. M., Poirel, L., Segre, J. A., & Westblade, L. F. (2018). Carbapenemase-producing organisms. *Clinical Infectious Diseases*, *66*(8), 1290–1297. DOI: 10.1093/cid/cix893 PMID: 29165604

CDC. (2022). *Antibiotic resistance threats in the United States, 2022*. Centers for Disease Control and Prevention.

CDC. (2023). *Healthcare-associated infections progress report*. Centers for Disease Control and Prevention.

CDC. (2024). *Antimicrobial resistance threats in the United States*. Centers for Disease Control and Prevention.

Cheraghi, M., Amiri, M., Andarzgoo, S., Zarei, F., Seghatoleslami, Z. S., Centis, R., Migliori, G. B., Visca, D., & Pontali, E. (2025). Bedaquiline and linezolid regimens for multidrug-resistant tuberculosis: A systematic review and meta-analysis. *Jornal Brasileiro de Pneumologia : Publicaçao Oficial da Sociedade Brasileira de Pneumologia e Tisilogia*, *51*(1), e20240391. DOI: 10.36416/1806-3756/e20240391

Chowdhary, A., Sharma, C., & Meis, J. F. (2017). Candida auris: A rapidly emerging cause of hospital-acquired multidrug-resistant fungal infections globally. *PLoS Pathogens*, *13*(5), e1006290. https://doi.org/10.1371/journal.ppat.1006290

Churchyard, G. J., Swindells, S., Gupta, A., Shah, N. S., Hughes, M., Kim, S., Fox, G. J., Harrington, M., Chaisson, R. E., & Hesseling, A. C. (2025). Preventing multidrug-resistant tuberculosis: The dawn of a new era. *Clinical Infectious Diseases*, *81*(6), 1135–1140. https://doi.org/10.1093/cid/ciaf426

CLSI. (2023). *Analysis and presentation of cumulative antimicrobial susceptibility test data* (5th ed.). Clinical and Laboratory Standards Institute.

CLSI. (2024). *Performance standards for antimicrobial susceptibility testing* (34th ed.). Clinical and Laboratory Standards Institute.

David, S., Caballero, J. D., Couto, N., Abudahab, K., Alikhan, N.-F., Yeats, C., Underwood, A., Molloy, A., Connor, D., Shane, H. M., Ashton, P. M., Grundmann, H., Holden, M. T. G., Feil, E. J., Sia, S. B., Donado-Godoy, P., Lingegowda, R. K., Okeke, I. N., Argimón, S., & Aanensen, D. M. (2025). Monitoring antimicrobial resistance trends from global genomics data: Amr.watch. *PLOS Global Public Health*, *5*(11), e0005256. https://doi.org/10.1371/journal.pgph.0005256

Davies, J., & Davies, D. (2010). Origins and evolution of antibiotic resistance. *Microbiology and Molecular Biology Reviews : MMBR*, *74*(3), 417–433. DOI: 10.1128/MMBR.00016-10 PMID: 20805405

Didelot, X., Bowden, R., Wilson, D. J., Peto, T. E. A., & Crook, D. W. (2012). Transforming clinical microbiology with bacterial genome sequencing. *Nature Reviews. Genetics, 13*(9), 601–612. DOI: 10.1038/nrg3226 PMID: 22868263

Didelot, X., Fraser, C., Gardy, J., & Colijn, C. (2021). Genomic epidemiology analysis of bacterial pathogens. *Nature Reviews. Genetics, 22*(9), 593–610. DOI: 10.1038/s41576-021-00345-3

European Centre for Disease Prevention and Control. (2025). *Antimicrobial resistance in the EU/EEA (EARS-Net) — Annual Epidemiological Report for 2024*. ECDC.

Fisher, M. C., Burnett, F., Chandler, C., Gow, N. A. R., Gurr, S., Hart, A., Holmes, A., May, R. C., Quinn, J., Soliman, T., Talbot, N. J., White, P. L., Bromley, M., & Armstrong-James, D. (2024). A One Health roadmap towards understanding and mitigating emerging fungal antimicrobial resistance: fAMR. npj Antimicrobials and Resistance, 2(36), Article 36. https://doi.org/10.1038/s44259-024-00055-2

Huang, S. S., Septimus, E., Kleinman, K., Moody, J., Hickok, J., Avery, T. R., Lankiewicz, J., Gombosev, A., Terpstra, L., Hartford, F., Hayden, M. K., Jernigan, J. A., Weinstein, R. A., & Fraser, V. J. (2013). Targeted versus universal decolonization to prevent ICU infection. *The New England Journal of Medicine, 368*(24), 2255–2265. https://doi.org/10.1056/NEJMoa1207290

Jorgensen, J. H., & Ferraro, M. J. (2009). Antimicrobial susceptibility testing: A review of general principles and contemporary practices. *Clinical Infectious Diseases, 49*(11), 1749–1755. DOI: 10.1086/647952 PMID: 19857164

Kakkar, A. K., Shafiq, N., Singh, R., Ray, P., Gautam, V., Agarwal, R., Muralidharan, J., & Arora, P. (2020). Antimicrobial stewardship programs in resource-constrained environments: Understanding and addressing the need of the systems. *Frontiers in Public Health, 8*, 140. https://doi.org/10.3389/fpubh.2020.00140

Kariuki, S., Keddy, K. H., Antonio, M., & Okeke, I. N. (2018). Antimicrobial resistance surveillance in Africa: Successes, gaps and a roadmap for the future. *African Journal of Laboratory Medicine, 7*(2), a924. https://doi.org/10.4102/ajlm.v7i2.924

Kirby, J. E., Brennan-Krohn, T., & Smith, K. P. (2019). Bringing Antimicrobial Susceptibility Testing for New Drugs into the Clinical Laboratory: Removing Obstacles in Our Fight against Multidrug-Resistant Pathogens. *Journal of Clinical Microbiology, 57*(12). Advance online publication. https://doi.org/10.1128/jcm.01270-19

Klein, E. Y., Impalli, I., Poleon, S., Denoel, P., Cipriano, M., Van Boeckel, T. P., Pecetta, S., Bloom, D. E., & Nandi, A. (2024). Global trends in antibiotic consumption during 2016–2023 and future projections through 2030. *Proceedings of the National Academy of Sciences of the United States of America, 121*(49). Advance online publication. https://doi.org/10.1073/pnas.2411919121

Köser, C. U., Ellington, M. J., & Peacock, S. J. (2014). Whole-genome sequencing to control antimicrobial resistance. *Trends in Genetics, 30*(9), 401–407. https://doi.org/10.1016/j.tig.2014.07.003

Kwong, J. C., Mccallum, N., Sintchenko, V., & Howden, B. P. (2015). Whole genome sequencing in clinical and public health microbiology. *Pathology, 47*(3), 199–210. https://doi.org/10.1097/pat.0000000000000235

Laxminarayan, R., Van Boeckel, T., Frost, I., Kariuki, S., Khan, E. A., Limmathurotsakul, D., Larsson, D. G. J., Levy-Hara, G., Mendelson, M., Outterson, K., Peacock, S. J., & Srikantiah, P. (2020). The Lancet Infectious Diseases Commission on antimicrobial resistance: 6 years later. *The Lancet. Infectious Diseases, 20*(4), e51–e60. DOI: 10.1016/S1473-3099(20)30003-7 PMID: 32059790

Langford, B. J., Leung, V., Lo, J., Akl, E. A., Nieuwlaat, R., Schwartz, K. L., & Daneman, N. (2023). Antibiotic prescribing guideline recommendations in COVID-19: A systematic survey. *EClinicalMedicine, 65*, 102257. https://doi.org/10.1016/j.eclinm.2023.102257

Liu, Y., Tong, Z., Liu, S., Chen, Y., & Li, J. (2024). Artificial intelligence for antimicrobial resistance prediction. *Briefings in Bioinformatics, 25*(1), bbad497. Advance online publication. DOI: 10.1093/bib/bbad497

Lockhart, S. R., Etienne, K. A., Vallabhaneni, S., Farooqi, J., Chowdhary, A., Govender, N. P., Colombo, A. L., Calvo, B., Cuomo, C. A., Desjardins, C. A., Berkow, E. L., Castanheira, M., Magobo, R. E., Jabeen, K., Asghar, R. J., Meis, J. F., Jackson, B., Chiller, T., & Litvintseva, A. P. (2016). Simultaneous Emergence of Multidrug-Resistant *Candida auris* on 3 Continents Confirmed by Whole-Genome Sequencing and Epidemiological Analyses. *Clinical Infectious Diseases, 64*(2), 134–140. https://doi.org/10.1093/cid/ciw691

Logan, L. K., & Weinstein, R. A. (2017). The epidemiology of carbapenem-resistant Enterobacteriaceae: The impact and evolution of a global menace. *The Journal of Infectious Diseases, 215*(Suppl. 1), S28–S36. https://doi.org/10.1093/infdis/jiw282

Mendelsohn, E., Ross, N., Zambrana-Torrelio, C., Van Boeckel, T. P., Laxminarayan, R., & Daszak, P. (2023). Global patterns and correlates in the emergence of antimicrobial resistance in humans. Proceedings of the Royal Society B: Biological Sciences, 290(2007), 20231085. https://doi.org/10.1098/rspb.2023.1085

Moran, R. A., Anantham, S., Holt, K. E., & Hall, R. M. (2016). Prediction of antibiotic resistance from antibiotic resistance genes detected in antibiotic-resistant commensal *Escherichia coli* using PCR or WGS. *The Journal of Antimicrobial Chemotherapy*, •••, dkw511. Advance online publication. https://doi.org/10.1093/jac/dkw511

Morgan, D. J., Malani, P., & Diekema, D. J. (2017). Diagnostic stewardship—Leveraging the laboratory to improve antimicrobial use. *Journal of the American Medical Association, 318*(7), 607–608. DOI: 10.1001/jama.2017.8531 PMID: 28759678

Nordmann, P., Naas, T., & Poirel, L. (2011). Global spread of carbapenemase-producing Enterobacteriaceae. *Emerging Infectious Diseases, 17*(10), 1791–1798. DOI: 10.3201/eid1710.110655 PMID: 22000347

O'Neill, J. (2016). Tackling drug-resistant infections globally: Final report and recommendations. Review on Antimicrobial Resistance. https://amr-review.org

Pai, M., Schumacher, S. G., & Abimbola, S. (2018). Surrogate endpoints in global health research: Still searching for killer apps and silver bullets? *BMJ Global Health, 3*(2), e000755. DOI: 10.1136/bmjgh-2018-000755

Patel, R. (2015). MALDI-TOF MS for the diagnosis of infectious diseases. *Clinical Chemistry, 61*(1), 100–111. DOI: 10.1373/clinchem.2014.221770 PMID: 25278500

Peiffer-Smadja, N., Rawson, T. M., Ahmad, R., Buchard, A., Georgiou, P., Lescure, F.-X., Birgand, G., & Holmes, A. H. (2020). Machine learning for clinical decision support in infectious diseases: A narrative review of current applications. *Clinical Microbiology and Infection, 26*(5), 584–595. DOI: 10.1016/j.cmi.2019.09.009 PMID: 31539636

Pliakos, E. E., Andreatos, N., Shehadeh, F., Ziakas, P. D., & Mylonakis, E. (2018). The Cost-Effectiveness of Rapid Diagnostic Testing for the Diagnosis of Bloodstream Infections with or without Antimicrobial Stewardship. *Clinical Microbiology Reviews, 31*(3). Advance online publication. https://doi.org/10.1128/CMR.00095-17

Prestinaci, F., Pezzotti, P., & Pantosti, A. (2015). Antimicrobial resistance: A global multifaceted phenomenon. *Pathogens and Global Health, 109*(7), 309–318. https://doi.org/10.1179/2047773215Y.0000000030

Puraswani, M., Ashita, A., Kumari Ambashta, N., Aggrawal, R., Soni, K. D., Kumar, S., Sagar, S., Gupta, A., Farooque, K., & Mathur, P. (2025). Transmission dynamics of multidrug resistant Klebsiella pneumoniae from an Indian hospital. *Indian Journal of Medical Microbiology*, *55*, 100848. https://doi.org/10.1016/j.ijmmb.2025.100848

Pulcini, C., Binda, F., Lamkang, A. S., Trett, A., Charani, E., Goff, D. A., Harbarth, S., Hinrichsen, S. L., Levy-Hara, G., Mendelson, M., Nathwani, D., Gunturu, R., Singh, S., Srinivasan, A., Thamlikitkul, V., Thursky, K., Vlieghe, E., Wertheim, H., Zeng, M., & Gandra, S. (2019). Developing core elements and checklist items for global hospital antimicrobial stewardship programmes: A consensus approach. *Clinical Microbiology and Infection*, *25*(1), 20–25. https://doi.org/10.1016/j.cmi.2018.03.033

Raven, K. E., Reuter, S., Reynolds, R., Brodrick, H. J., Russell, J. E., Török, M. E., Parkhill, J., & Peacock, S. J. (2016). A decade of genomic history for healthcare-associated *Enterococcus faecium* in the United Kingdom and Ireland. *Genome Research*, *26*(10), 1388–1396. https://doi.org/10.1101/gr.204024.116

Rawson, T. M., Moore, L. S. P., Hernandez, B., Charani, E., Castro-Sanchez, E., Herrero, P., Hayhoe, B., Hope, W., Georgiou, P., & Holmes, A. H. (2017). A systematic review of clinical decision support systems for antimicrobial management: Are we failing to investigate these interventions appropriately? *Clinical Microbiology and Infection*, *23*(8), 524–532. https://doi.org/10.1016/j.cmi.2017.02.028

Rice, L. B. (2008). Federal funding for the study of antimicrobial resistance in nosocomial pathogens: No ESKAPE. *The Journal of Infectious Diseases*, *197*(8), 1079–1081. DOI: 10.1086/533452 PMID: 18419525

Robinson, T. P., Bu, D. P., Carrique-Mas, J., Fèvre, E. M., Gilbert, M., Grace, D., Hay, S. I., Jiwakanon, J., Kakkar, M., Kariuki, S., Laxminarayan, R., Lubroth, J., Magnusson, U., Thi Ngoc, P., Van Boeckel, T. P., & Woolhouse, M. E. J. (2016). Antibiotic resistance is the quintessential One Health issue. *Transactions of the Royal Society of Tropical Medicine and Hygiene*, *110*(7), 377–380. DOI: 10.1093/trstmh/trw048 PMID: 27475987

Rodríguez-Baño, J., Rossolini, G. M., Schultsz, C., Tacconelli, E., Murthy, S., Ohmagari, N., Holmes, A., Bachmann, T., Goossens, H., Canton, R., Roberts, A. P., Henriques-Normark, B., Clancy, C. J., Huttner, B., Fagerstedt, P., Lahiri, S., Kaushic, C., Hoffman, S. J., Warren, M., & Zoubiane, G. (2021). Antimicrobial resistance research in a post-pandemic world: Insights on antimicrobial resistance research in the COVID-19 pandemic. *Journal of Global Antimicrobial Resistance*, *25*, 5–7. https://doi.org/10.1016/j.jgar.2021.02.013

Schuts, E. C., Hulscher, M. E. J. L., Mouton, J. W., Verduin, C. M., Stuart, J. W. T. C., Overdiek, H. W. P. M., van der Linden, P. D., Natsch, S., Hertogh, C. M. P. M., Wolfs, T. F. W., Schouten, J. A., Kullberg, B. J., & Prins, J. M. (2016). Current evidence on hospital antimicrobial stewardship objectives: A systematic review and meta-analysis. *The Lancet. Infectious Diseases*, *16*(7), 847–856. https://doi.org/10.1016/s1473-3099(16)00065-7

Tamma, P. D., Avdic, E., & Li, D. X. (2022). Association of adverse events with antibiotic use in hospitalized patients. *JAMA Internal Medicine*, *177*(9), 1308–1315. DOI: 10.1001/jamainternmed.2017.1938 PMID: 28604925

Turner, N. A., Sharma-Kuinkel, B. K., Maskarinec, S. A., Eichenberger, E. M., Shah, P. P., Carugati, M., Holland, T. L., & Fowler, V. G. (2019). Methicillin-resistant Staphylococcus aureus: An overview of basic and clinical research. *Nature Reviews. Microbiology*, *17*(4), 203–218. https://doi.org/10.1038/s41579-018-0147-4

van Belkum, A., Bachmann, T. T., Lüdke, G., Lisby, J. G., Kahlmeter, G., Mohess, A., Becker, K., Hays, J. P., Woodford, N., Mitsakakis, K., Moran-Gilad, J., & Consortium, T. D. (2019). Developmental roadmap for antimicrobial susceptibility testing systems. *Nature Reviews. Microbiology*, *17*(1), 51–62. DOI: 10.1038/s41579-018-0098-9 PMID: 30333569

van Duin, D., & Doi, Y. (2017). The global epidemiology of carbapenemase-producing Enterobacteriaceae. *Virulence*, *8*(4), 460–469. https://doi.org/10.1080/21505594.2016.1222343

Ventola, C. L. (2015). The antibiotic resistance crisis: Part 1—Causes and threats. *P&T : a Peer-Reviewed Journal for Formulary Management*, *40*(4), 277–283. PMID: 25859123

Weber, D. J., Anderson, D., & Rutala, W. A. (2013). The role of the surface environment in healthcare-associated infections. *Current Opinion in Infectious Diseases*, *26*(4), 338–344. https://doi.org/10.1097/qco.0b013e3283630f04

WHO. (2022). *Global Tuberculosis Report 2022*. World Health Organization.

WHO. (2023). *Global antimicrobial resistance and use surveillance system (GLASS) report 2023*. World Health Organization.

WHO. (2024). *Global action plan on antimicrobial resistance: Progress report*. World Health Organization.

Wiens, J., & Shenoy, E. S. (2017). Machine Learning for Healthcare: On the Verge of a Major Shift in Healthcare Epidemiology. *Clinical Infectious Diseases*, *66*(1), 149–153. https://doi.org/10.1093/cid/cix731

Chapter 10
Emerging Therapeutic Strategies for Mitigating Antimicrobial Resistance

Amina Hayat
https://orcid.org/0009-0000-6459-5945
International Islamic University, Islamabad, Pakistan

Humaira Yaqoob
https://orcid.org/0009-0006-7181-6535
International Islamic University, Islamabad, Pakistan

Semab Abbasi
https://orcid.org/0009-0004-1603-7294
International Islamic University, Islamabad, Pakistan

Saffa Qasim
COMSATS University, Islamabad, Pakistan

Urooj Zafar
https://orcid.org/0009-0006-0601-5862
University of Poonch, Rawalakot, Pakistan

Palwasha Alam
Abdul Wali Khan University, Mardan, Pakistan

ABSTRACT

Antimicrobial resistance (AMR) is one of the most critical health challenges around the world, as it is caused by overusing antibiotics inappropriately both in hospitals and on farms. In this chapter, a synthesizing review of the current therapeutic approaches aimed at reversing the problem of bacterial resistance and regaining the effect of antimicrobials is given. It starts by explaining the processes of development of resistance. The recent advances in new antibiotic discovery and optimization are discussed with the focus on structure-based drug design, synthetic biology, and artificial intelligence-assisted screening. This chapter identifies the significance

DOI: 10.4018/979-8-3373-3825-5.ch010

of the multidisciplinary approach in controlling AMR by incorporating the use of molecular, biotechnological, and immunological innovations in future research on sustainable antimicrobial development.

1. INTRODUCTION

The term "antibiotic resistance" refers to the process by which bacteria change how they respond to antibiotics and become resistant to them. Unlike non-resistant species, these bacteria can infect people and pose serious therapeutic problems. More generally, "antimicrobial resistance" (AMR) describes resistance to medications used to treat illnesses brought on by viruses (like HIV), fungi (like *Candida*), and parasites (like malaria). In 1945, Alexander Fleming observed that the misuse of antibiotics had resulted in the development of resistant microorganisms (Hutchings et al., 2019). In a 2016 Political Declaration of the United Nations General Assembly, world leaders also highlighted this issue. Antimicrobial resistance (AMR) has emerged and spread as a result of antibiotic misuse and overuse in the healthcare and agricultural domains (Gach et al., 2024). Critically ill individuals are at serious risk due to the development of superbugs that are resistant to several antibiotics and other antimicrobial medicines. Because these superbugs can render standard antibiotics useless, there are fewer treatment options, more deaths, and longer illness durations. The cure against antibiotic resistance is made more challenging by the substantial scientific, economic, and regulatory obstacles associated with the creation of novel antibiotics (Haniffa et al., 2018). These obstacles include the lack of financial incentives, complicated regulatory environment, harsh safety requirements, and particular hindrance to pharmaceutical innovation. Newly made antibiotics tend to lose their efficiency through the evolution of bacterial resistance mechanisms. Hence, studies on antibiotics become economically infeasible (Pierce et al., 2022). Finding novel antibacterial chemicals is difficult from a scientific point of view due to the complexity of mechanisms of resistance and bacterial adaptation. This chapter explores novel therapeutic strategies to combat antibiotic resistance, evaluating their mechanisms, clinical promise, and limitations, in addition to describing present research gaps and prospective future directions.

2. OVERVIEW OF ANTIMICROBIAL RESISTANCE

2.1 Mechanisms of Resistance

Bacteria have evolved complex defense mechanisms to evade antimicrobial agents. Notably, bacteria can use a range of metabolic pathways to tolerate a single medication. These mechanisms include the following: bacterial cell surface permeability changes, bacterial enzyme modification or inactivation, decreased affinity for binding to bacterial molecular targets, horizontal gene transfer between species via plasmids carrying multidrug resistance (MDR)-associated genes, overexpression of efflux pumps that can recognize and expel a variety of antibiotics with different mechanisms of action, and genetic variations such as polymorphisms or insertions in DNA sequences encoding transcriptional regulators.

2.2 Major Resistant Pathogens (the "ESKAPE" Pathogens, MDR *E. coli*, *Mycobacterium tuberculosis*, etc.)

The abbreviation "ESKAPEE" stands for "*Enterococcus faecium*, *Staphylococcus aureus*, *Klebsiella pneumoniae*, *Acinetobacter baumannii*, *Pseudomonas aeruginosa*, *Enterobacter* species, and *Escherichia coli*," which are the most important bacteria known for their capacity to withstand the effects of antibiotics. Additionally, the World Health Organization (WHO) has categorized the main bacterial infections into three priority groups: critical, high, and medium (Krul et al., 2025). This classification directs research on new antibacterial drugs and emphasizes the pressing need for new antibiotics. Because of their high disease burden, resistance to antibiotics, and capacity for serious infections, these "priority" pathogens pose a serious risk to human health (Organization, 2024). The WHO classification of priority bacterial pathogens as indicated in Figure 1, according to antibiotic resistance profile presents the critical, high, and medium threat levels. The basis of this classification is the prevalence of resistance, the risk of mortality and the healthcare-associated infections burden. The pathogens are known to be critical, including *Acinetobacter baumannii*, *Pseudomonas aeruginosa*, and carbapenem-resistant *Enterobacteriaceae* that cause high mortality rates and limited treatment options, so new treatment options need to be investigated urgently. Pathogens with high and middle priorities, such as *Staphylococcus aureus* and *Klebsiella pneumoniae* remain the serious clinical challenges, especially in low-resource settings where antibiotic stewardship and infection control can be inefficient. This classification is demonstrated below in Figure 1.

Figure 1. Classification of major bacterial pathogens according to WHO priority levels based on antibiotic resistance profiles, highlighting critical, high, and medium groups.

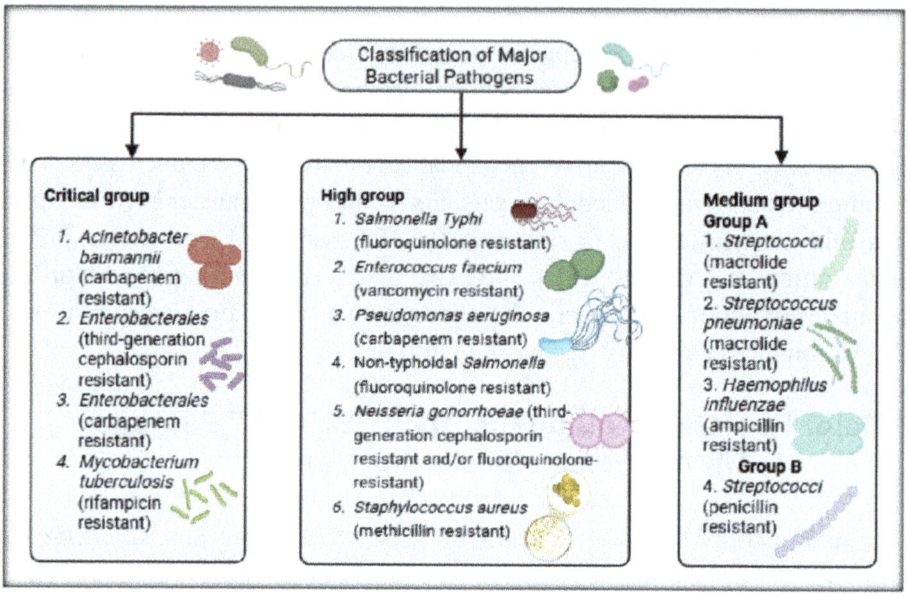

Source: Created in https://BioRender.com

2.3 International Context of Multidrug Resistance

The recent surveillance data in the world show that alternative antimicrobial strategies are urgently needed. The report by the WHO GLASS 2024 indicates that *Escherichia coli, Klebsiella pneumoniae*, and *Acinetobacter baumannii* multidrug-resistant infections among the bloodstream have increased in all the regions, and the prevalence of these infections has resulted in treatment failure rates of up to 30 percent in low and middle-income countries. Further surveillance indicators that include CDC and ECDC surveillance are the growing levels of resistance to last-line antibiotics, including carbapenems and fluoroquinolones, which highlight the need to develop complementary therapeutic strategies like phages, antimicrobial peptides, and host-directed therapies (Tosas Auguet et al., 2025).

2.4 Need for Innovative Therapeutic Strategies

Although knowledge of these mechanisms has influenced the development of antibiotics for many years, the speed at which resistance mechanisms are evolving has beyond the capabilities of conventional discovery pipelines, requiring the investigation of alternate strategies. The effectiveness of therapies is compromised by antibiotic resistance, which also increases the burden of resistant illnesses. Antibiotic resistance is still a major problem in worldwide healthcare. Although there is no one solution that can solve this issue, there are a number of strategies that can help lessen its impact and spread (El-Sapagh et al., 2023). For addressing these issues, a comprehensive strategy is needed, which includes strengthening infection prevention measures, promoting alternative treatments like phage therapy and immunotherapies, and improving antibiotic stewardship. To reduce resistance, public awareness initiatives and instruction on the responsible use of antibiotics are also essential. Alternative antimicrobial strategies are being investigated as a result of the conventional antibiotics' alarming effectiveness (Elshobary et al., 2025). The quorum quenching mechanisms that break down bacterial communication networks, microbial-based therapies, stem cell applications, immunotherapeutic modalities, photodynamic antimicrobial techniques, CRISPR-Cas systems, and their connection to resistance mechanisms, bacteriophage therapy, and bioactive compounds derived from animal venoms are some of the new approaches to fighting antibiotic resistance that are examined in this chapter.

3. NOVEL ANTIBIOTIC DISCOVERY AND OPTIMIZATION

Advances in technology allow the discovery of molecules other than established classes, and the hunt for novel antibiotics has made remarkable progress. Currently, structure-based drug production backed by X-ray crystallography, NMR, and cryo-electron microscopy is combined with phenotypic and target-based screenings. While improvements in synthetic chemistry enable broad structure-activity relationship research, identification of bioactive compounds, and lead optimization have been transformed by artificial intelligence (AI), computer-aided modeling, and DNA-encoded libraries. Teixobactin, darobactin, and G0775 are a few examples of natural and synthetic compounds that continue to be useful sources for novel scaffolds. These compounds exhibit strong action against Gram-positive and Gram-negative infections that are resistant to several drugs. Despite enduring challenges, including the poor efficacy of anti-Gram-negative drugs, changeable specific pathogen targets, and high research costs, novel strategies like the Trojan horse's idea, PROTAC-based degrading agents, and peptide or peptide-based mimic libraries are restoring hope in antibiotic discovery (Suessmuth, Kulike-Koczula et al., 2025). All of these advancements point to a paradigm shift towards more rational, targeted, and computationally driven antibiotic discovery processes as detailed in Table 1.

Table 1. Summary of various approaches involving the novel antibiotic discovery.

Approaches	Key Principle	Application	Target or Advantage
Structure-Based Drug Design	Combines crystallography, NMR, and cryo-EM to model target–drug interactions	Rational design of inhibitors based on 3D protein structures	Precise binding site identification
AI and Computer-Aided Drug Design (CADD)	Uses machine learning and computational algorithms to predict bioactivity	Hit identification and lead optimization	Accelerates discovery and reduces cost
DNA-Encoded Library Screening	Millions of compounds linked with DNA tags for high-throughput screening	Rapid discovery of novel scaffolds	Expands chemical diversity
Synthetic Chemistry Optimization	SAR-based synthesis of analogs	Enhances potency and selectivity	Improved pharmacokinetic profiles
Natural Product Rediscovery	Explores uncultured microbes and novel biosynthetic clusters	*Teixobactin, Darobactin, G0775*	Active against MDR Gram-positive and Gram-negative bacteria
PROTAC-Based Degraders	Proteolysis-targeting chimeras induce selective protein degradation	New antibacterial mode of action	Overcomes conventional resistance
Trojan Horse Strategy	Conjugates antibiotic with siderophores or peptides for targeted delivery	Siderophore–antibiotic conjugates	Enhanced uptake into Gram-negative bacteria
Peptide and Peptidomimetic Libraries	Screening of synthetic peptide analogs	Broad-spectrum antimicrobial activity	High stability and specificity

4. ALTERNATIVE THERAPEUTIC APPROACHES

The abuse of antibiotics is causing MDR bacteria to proliferate even in industrialized countries (Konwar et al., 2022). In order to combat infections more effectively and sustainably, scientists are focusing on developing new chemicals, organic materials, and other innovative approaches (Stoitsova et al., 2022; Đukanović et al., 2022). Few alternative therapeutic approaches are presented in Figure 2.

Figure 2. Overview of emerging antimicrobial strategies against Gram-negative pathogens, including phage therapy, nanotechnology, and immunotherapeutic approaches.

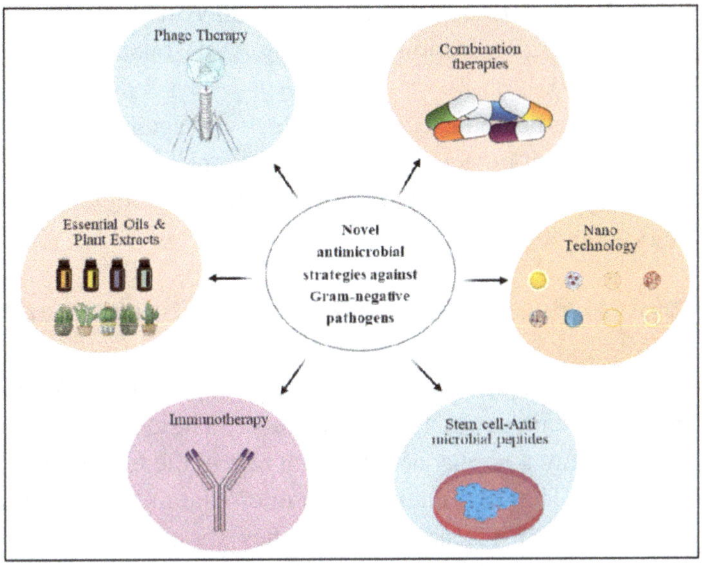

Source: Created in https://share.google/LAj9tUWKBIXwvGquj via using icons from https://share.google/dApkalUWfH1C2aA1S

4.1 Bacteriophage-Based Therapies

Bacterio-photodynamic therapy viruses infect bacteria. Since phages were discovered in the early 20th century, researchers have investigated their potential as alternatives to antibiotics. Unlike antibiotics, which attack a broad range of microorganisms, phages are highly specialized and have the potential to harm certain types of bacteria. Bacteriophages are microbes that infect and eradicate bacteria; they are used in bacteriophage therapy to treat bacterial infections (Hasan & Ahn, 2022). According to Luong, et al. (2020), phage therapy was originally described at the end of the century. The ability of phages to target live bacterial cells was primarily created for therapeutic purposes, but it can also be employed as an indicator to distinguish between various bacterial strains. The benefits of recombinant isolates and DNA transmission channels between pathogens and host species may now be thoroughly studied, facilitated by scientific developments like the manipulation of genes and gene mapping (Brives & Pourraz, 2020). Phage particles can be genetically engineered to show certain proteins that are intriguing on their exteriors through genetic fusion. These technologies have also enabled modified phage-mediated therapies. However, phages also encounter several obstacles that restrict their effectiveness, such as phage resistance, gene transduction, serovar variety, and the immunological response of animals or human beings. As a lytic protein for bacterial cells formed from phages, endolysin is another viable option against a variety of bacterial infections, including AMR, because of the limitations of phages (Pirnay, 2020).

Despite having potential and exceptional selectivity against multidrug-resistant bacteria, the restricted host range and regulatory complexity of bacteriophages are highly stimulated via exploration of broader-spectrum biological substitutes like synthetic analogs and antimicrobial peptides.

4.2 Antimicrobial Peptides (AMPs) and Peptidomimetics

Short chains of amino acids, termed antimicrobial peptides (AMPs), occur naturally and typically contain about 15 to 50 residues. These compounds are widely present throughout nature and play a significant role in the innate immune systems of a variety of animals. They can interact with microbial membranes and are effective against a wide range of diseases because they are often cationic and possess amphipathic qualities. One of their major activities is to function as the initial line of defense against invasive infections. It also has the potential to neutralize the microbial components, like lipopolysaccharides, that otherwise drive immune responses (Howell et al., 2022). Enhancing the global issue of antimicrobial resistance and AMPs' broad spectrum of action, attention has shifted towards them to be used as an alternative of conventional antibiotics. Contrary to traditional antibiotics, it's not easy for pathogens to develop resistance against AMPs. The reason behind this is that these peptides mainly affect the specificity and integrity of their cell membranes (Browne et al., 2020). In contrast to traditional antibiotics, pathogens do not easily develop resistance to AMPs because these peptides mainly affect the integrity and fidelity of their cell membranes, as given below in Table 2.

Table 2. Examples and Mechanisms of Antimicrobial Peptides (AMPs) and Peptidomimetics

AMP/Peptidomimetic	Origin	Mechanism of Action	Spectrum of Activity	Applications
Defensins	Human neutrophils, epithelial cells	Disrupt bacterial membrane integrity	Broad-spectrum (Gram-positive & Gram-negative)	Natural immune defense; low resistance potential
Cathelicidins (LL-37)	Human macrophages and keratinocytes	Membrane permeabilization and immunomodulation	Bacteria, fungi, and viruses	Promotes wound healing; anti-inflammatory
Magainins	Skin of frogs (Xenopus species)	Forms pores in lipid bilayers	Gram-positive and Gram-negative bacteria	Model for synthetic AMP design
Melittin	Bee venom	Lyses microbial membranes and inhibits biofilms	Broad-spectrum, including fungi	Potential in cancer therapy and biofilm disruption
Nisin	*Lactococcus lactis*	Binds lipid II and inhibits cell wall synthesis	Gram-positive bacteria	FDA-approved food preservative; low toxicity
Temporins	Amphibian skin secretions	Membrane permeabilization	Gram-positive bacteria	Effective in topical formulations
Tachyplesins	Horseshoe crab hemocytes	DNA binding and membrane disruption	Gram-negative bacteria and fungi	Antiviral and antifungal potential
Indolicidin	Bovine neutrophils	DNA/RNA interaction; membrane lysis	Broad-spectrum	Potent antibacterial and antifungal agent
Cecropins	Insects	Pore formation in membranes	Gram-negative bacteria	Biocompatible; rapid bactericidal action
Peptidomimetics (synthetic AMPs)	Designed analogs	Mimic natural AMP function with improved stability	Broad-spectrum	Enhanced stability and reduced cytotoxicity

Despite having advantages, AMPs also have some problems. Like the problems of toxicity, durability, and high costs etc. These problems limit their therapeutic applications. It encouraged the researchers to investigate state-of-the-art gene-editing methods, like CRISPR-Cas systems. These systems can selectively target bacterial resistance determinants.

4.3 CRISPR-Cas and Gene-Editing Approaches

The CRISPR/Cas9 genetic modification system has emerged as a revolutionary tool for precision genome alteration due to its capacity to specifically target genes associated with quorum-sensing pathways, antibiotic resistance, and biofilm-regulating proteins. Before CRISPR-based antibacterials can be employed in clinical settings, however, several challenges must be addressed, particularly concerning effective distribution and persistence within bacterial populations. Nanoparticles (NPs), which have intrinsic antibacterial properties and serve as effective carriers for CRISPR/Cas9 components, provide a creative substitute. By boosting target specificity, cellular absorption, and controlled release in biofilm settings, nanoparticles can improve the delivery of CRISPR. Although CRISPR-nanoparticle hybrid systems have enormous promise for next-generation precision antimicrobial treatments, further study is needed to determine long-term safety, eliminate off-target effects, and optimize delivery platforms (Saffari Natanzi et al., 2025).

Although precise genome targeting is possible with CRISPR-based techniques, clinical translation is still in its infancy. As a result, complementary approaches like quorum-sensing inhibition, which aim to reduce bacterial pathogenicity rather than eradicate it, are becoming more and more popular.

4.4 Quorum Sensing and Anti-Virulence Strategies

Bacteria use the QS system, a cell-density-dependent signaling mechanism, to coordinate collective actions, such as the production of pathogenicity and the production of biofilms. Small molecule nutrients like vitamin K can affect the *Pseudomonas* quinolone signal (PQS). At the post-transcriptional level, non-coding ribonucleic acid (ncRNA) affects many bacterial physiologic traits, including virulence, EPS generation, motility, and stress responses. For example, *P. aeruginosa's* QS-related acute pathogenicity is significantly enhanced by short RNA (sRNA) PqsS, which may be a viable target for anti-P medications. infections by *Aeruginosa*. The involvement of ncRNAs in biofilm regulation emphasizes how complex biofilm management is and how important properly calibrated gene expression is (Wang et al., 2025).

Pathogens can be efficiently disarmed by targeting bacterial communication channels; however, antibacterial efficiency is further increased when physical or photochemical techniques are combined with such molecular interference. One such potential technique for eliminating resistant germs is photodynamic treatment, which uses light-activated chemicals.

4.5 Photodynamic Therapy

The therapeutic technique known as photodynamic therapy (PDT) uses light, oxygen, and a photosensitizing chemical to cause tissue disruption and cell death. A photosensitizer is an inert chemical that is used in photodynamic therapy (PDT) to create an effect on the target site, such as a cancer cell or an infected area, by concentrating on the target site; it is used as the base of the treatment. Then, the light of a selected wavelength is applied to the tissue, which corresponds to the absorption properties of the photosensitizer. After the activation of light, the photosensitizer goes through a chemical reaction process that forms singlet oxygen and other reactive oxygen species (ROS) and transfers the energy to the neighboring oxygen molecules. These ROS are very harmful to the cells, leading to oxidative damage to different cell components, which end up in necrosis, cell death, or apoptosis. PDT is effectively used to treat various diseases as it is targeted and thereby does not cause damage to the surrounding healthy tissues (Aebisher et al., 2024; Cieplik et al., 2013). The unique mode of action is beginning to persist in establishing promise in the use of PDT as a treatment option for MDR in cancer and microbial infections. PDT is distinctive compared to conventional antibacterial or chemotherapeutic therapies because, unlike these types of therapies, it does not focus on localized areas of the cell, causing the cell to die by the production of ROS, which cause severe oxidative damage to different parts of the cell. The non-targeted attack makes it harder for bacteria or malignant cells to develop defense against PDT, resulting in this attack being less targeted. The biochemical and physical obstacles of tumor microenvironments and biofilms can be easily overcome by generating reactive oxygen species (ROS) locally using photodynamic therapy (PDT) (de Carvalho Leonel, Carvalho et al., 2019). The reason PDT can target and harm both surface and embedding cells within these protective structures is that ROS formation happens locally, where the photosensitizer has concentrated and is activated by light. This feature solves a major problem in the treatment of solid tumors and multidrug-resistant (MDR) infections. PDT is a valuable tool in the fight against MDR infections and tumors that do not respond to conventional treatments because of its ability to circumvent typical resistance pathways (Liu et al., 2015; Youf et al., 2021). Action of the mechanism of photodynamic therapy is demonstrated below in Figure 3.

Figure 3. Mechanism of action of Photodynamic therapy to resist antimicrobials

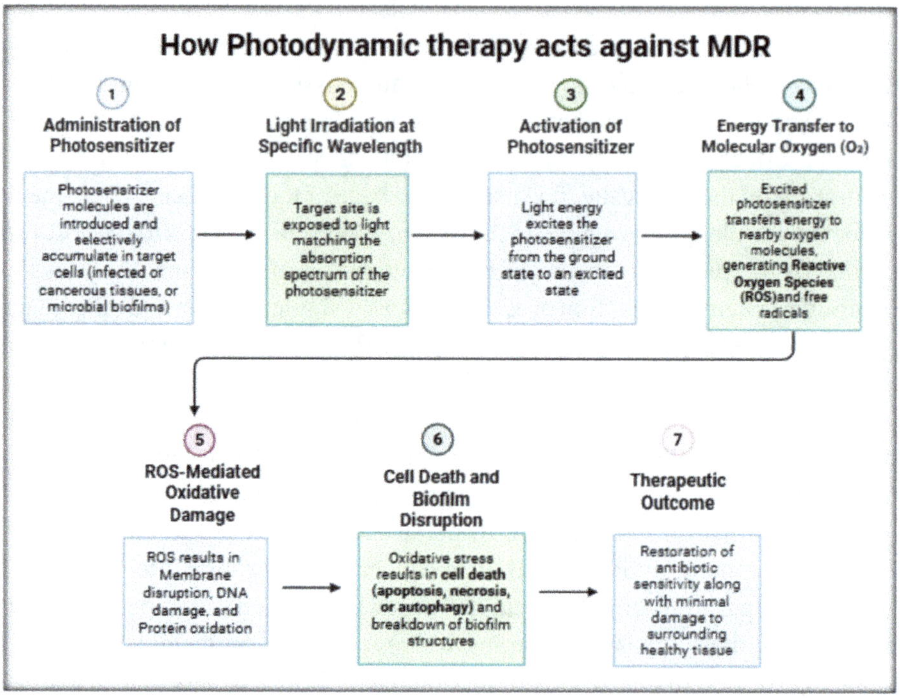

(Source: Created in https://BioRender.com)

PDT can invade the resistant cells that are located in biofilms, and this is effective in dealing with the protective barrier, which is part of the resistance to antibiotics. Studies have shown that PDT has the potential to be a novel therapeutic intervention to address the problem of antibiotic resistance on the rise, that is, methicillin-resistant Staphylococcus aureus (MRSA), vancomycin-resistant *Enterococci* (VRE), and multidrug-resistant *Pseudomonas aeruginosa* (Liu et al., 2015).

PDT can damage efflux pumps, leading to an increase of intracellular antibiotics. Moreover, the introduction of immunomodulatory agents in combination with PDT can increase the immune system of the host, which will increase the death of resistant microorganisms (Akhtar et al., 2024; Pérez-Laguna et al., 2021).

The therapy hastens the healing process, decreases the bacterial counts as well as improves tissue healing. As an example, those patients who underwent PDT would reach a level of over 80 percent bacterial clearance and had faster epithelial healing in 10 days. Conversely, the individuals who were treated with mupirocin experienced a slow recovery. Significant clinical innovations have been made in terms of coverings of devices and photodynamic therapy embedded in textiles. PDT has also demonstrated efficacy against viral pathogens such as cutaneous HPV and

HSV through interfering with viral replication, and in parasitic disease, which includes localized leishmaniasis, wherein topical PDT has achieved 100% treatment quotient without the systemic side effects of conventional medicinal drugs (Ramos et al., 2016; G. Wu et al., 2024).

Natural materials are also becoming acknowledged for their antibacterial properties in addition to light-based therapies. Particularly, essential oils have complex processes that make them excellent options for complementary or alternative antibacterial treatment.

4.6 Essential Oils

Although the developments in modern medicine have overlooked the essential oils, there have been promising benefits of the oils against various bacteria, and they can serve as a useful tool to counter antibiotic resistance. The complicated activities of EOs against bacteria enable them to be more effective in the treatment of ailments at a time when antibiotic solutions are becoming limited (Klobucar & Brown, 2022). This minimizes the necessity of various antimicrobial measures and interventions to fight and counter the outcomes of antibiotic resistance. The reason behind the antibacterial properties of EOs is the presence of phenolic constituents (Fukuyama, Duarte et al., 2024). It is also possible that EOs alter microbial signaling networks and gene expression, which would influence essential physiological processes, such as metabolism and cell division. Generally, the varied antimicrobial activities of the EOs are due to the complexity of interactions between the chemical components and microbial targets, which prompt potentials of the potential use of EOs as organic replacements of traditional antimicrobial drugs (Visan & Negut, 2024). Few potential essential oils, their major constituents, action mechanisms, and target bacteria are summarized in Table 3.

Table 3. Antimicrobial Activities and Mechanistic Insights of Major Essential Oils Against Drug-Resistant Bacteria

Essential Oil	Major Bioactive Components	Primary Mechanism of Action	Target Bacteria
Cinnamon oil	Cinnamaldehyde	Inhibits quorum-sensing and virulence gene expression	*E. coli, L. monocytogenes*
Clove oil	Eugenol	Denatures proteins; inhibits enzyme activity and cell wall synthesis	*P. aeruginosa, K. pneumoniae*
Eucalyptus oil	1,8-Cineole (Eucalyptol), α-pinene	Inhibits protein synthesis; disrupts membrane lipids	*K. pneumoniae, S. aureus*

continued on following page

Table 3. Continued

Essential Oil	Major Bioactive Components	Primary Mechanism of Action	Target Bacteria
Garlic oil	Allicin, Diallyl sulfide	Inhibits RNA synthesis and quorum sensing	*S. aureus*, *E. coli*, *P. aeruginosa*
Lavender oil	Linalool, Linalyl acetate	Alters cell membrane structure; induces oxidative stress	*S. aureus*, *E. coli*
Lemongrass oil	Citral, Geraniol	Disrupts cell envelope and ATP synthesis	*B. subtilis*, *E. coli*
Oregano oil	Carvacrol, Thymol	Destabilizes membrane potential; enhances antibiotic uptake	*E. coli*, *S. aureus*
Peppermint oil	Menthol, Menthone	Damages cell membrane; interferes with enzymatic activity	*E. coli*, *S. pyogenes*
Rosemary oil	Carnosic acid, 1,8-cineole	Generates oxidative stress; interferes with lipid metabolism	*P. aeruginosa*, *E. coli*
Tea tree oil	Terpinen-4-ol, α-terpineol	Alters membrane permeability; inhibits efflux pumps	*S. aureus*, *E. coli*
Thyme oil	Thymol, Carvacrol	Disrupts cytoplasmic membrane integrity; increases permeability	*E. coli*, *S. aureus*

Plant extracts, which include essential oils and bioactive phytochemicals with potent antibacterial and anti-biofilm activities, are another natural method of combating multidrug-resistant diseases.

4.7 Plant Extracts

The use of plant-based antimicrobials has become an appealing alternative to the fight against resistant microorganisms because they offer diverse action mechanisms and favorable safety profiles. Phytochemicals with antimicrobial effects are phenolic compounds, terpenes, and alkaloids (Khameneh et al., 2021). These phytocompounds affect the membranes of microorganisms, inhibit quorum sensing, and suppress the production of efflux pumps. Certainly, some properly proven studies prove the potential of using phytochemicals as alternatives to antibiotics, and this is the reason why it is a valuable tool in the ongoing struggle against drug resistance (Arip et al., 2022). Plant extracts along with their phytochemicals, target microbes, and action mechanisms are presented in Table 4.

Table 4. Overview of Bioactive Plant Extracts, Their Key Phytochemicals, and Antimicrobial Mechanisms Against Drug-Resistant Bacteria

Plant Source	Major Bioactive Compounds	Target Microorganisms	Proposed Mechanism of Action
Azadirachta indica (Neem)	Azadirachtin, nimbin, quercetin	*E. coli, S. aureus, P. aeruginosa*	Disrupts cell wall and membrane integrity; inhibits bacterial adhesion and biofilm formation
Curcuma longa (Turmeric)	Curcumin	*S. aureus, E. coli*	Inhibits efflux pumps and quorum sensing; enhances antibiotic susceptibility
Camellia sinensis (Green tea)	Epigallocatechin gallate (EGCG)	*S. aureus, Enterococcus faecalis*	Inhibits β-lactamase activity and alters membrane permeability
Allium sativum (Garlic)	Allicin	*E. coli, K. pneumoniae, S. aureus*	Inhibits DNA, RNA, and protein synthesis; disrupts membrane potential
Moringa oleifera	Isothiocyanates, flavonoids	*B. subtilis, E. coli*	Induces oxidative stress and damages bacterial membranes
Punica granatum (Pomegranate)	Ellagic acid, punicalagin	*P. aeruginosa, E. coli*	Interferes with quorum sensing and inhibits virulent gene expression
Zingiber officinale (Ginger)	Gingerol, shogaol	*E. coli, S. aureus*	Damages bacterial membranes and inhibits metabolic enzymes
Cinnamomum verum (Cinnamon)	Cinnamaldehyde, eugenol	*S. aureus, Listeria monocytogenes*	Inhibits ATP synthesis and disrupts cell membrane function
Ocimum sanctum (Holy basil)	Eugenol, ursolic acid	*S. aureus, E. coli, Salmonella spp.*	Alters membrane permeability and suppresses virulent genes
Nigella sativa (Black cumin)	Thymoquinone, carvacrol	*E. coli, S. aureus, P. aeruginosa*	Generates ROS and interferes with bacterial enzymatic systems

4.8 Immunotherapy

Immunotherapy is a new treatment for various severe diseases such as cancer and infectious diseases, which takes advantage of immunity of the host. This strategy, through enhancement, modification or reinstatement of immunological activity to produce therapeutic effects, offers a versatile approach to the fight against diseases because of its dynamic nature and flexibility. In comparison to the conventional drugs used to combat infections, immunotherapy provides a more personalized and adaptable form of treatment as it helps to boost the immune system of the host (Vidyadhari & Singh, n.d.). The deficiency of the traditional treatments, an increase in the number of infections, and antibiotic resistance render immunotherapy an essential area of medical research.

Even though the physiological and immune-based methods have become better, drug delivery efficiency and targeted release remain a problem. Thus, new approaches such as nanomaterials and adaptive drug delivery systems can help to increase the therapeutic accuracy and reduce side effects. Table 5, given below, summarizes key new therapeutic interventions with emerging medicines against antimicrobial resistance, outlining the mechanisms, benefits, and current obstacles.

Table 5. Summary of Emerging Therapeutic Strategies to Combat Antimicrobial Resistance

Therapeutic Approach	Primary Mechanism of Action	Representative Agents and Systems	Developmental Stage	Key Limitations
Bacteriophage Therapy	Bacteriophages infect and lyse specific bacterial hosts	Phage cocktails, engineered lysins	Preclinical to clinical trials	Narrow host range, stability and regulatory concerns
Antimicrobial Peptides (AMPs)	Disrupt bacterial membranes and intracellular targets	LL-37, Melittin, Pexiganan	Some in clinical evaluation	Cytotoxicity, degradation, high production cost
CRISPR–Cas Systems	Gene editing to target and disable resistance determinants	Cas9, Cas13-based antimicrobials	Experimental, proof-of-concept	Delivery efficiency, off-target effects
Quorum Sensing Inhibitors	Block bacterial signaling pathways to reduce virulence and biofilm formation	Furanones, Ajoene, Azithromycin (anti-QS)	Early experimental stage	Specificity, potential for resistance development
Photodynamic Therapy (PDT)	Light-activated photosensitizers generate reactive oxygen species causing bacterial death	Methylene blue, Toluidine blue, Curcumin	Preclinical and clinical trials	Limited tissue penetration, photosensitizer toxicity
Essential Oils	Disrupt cell membrane integrity and metabolic processes	Thymol, Carvacrol, Eugenol	Experimental and commercial formulations	Variability in composition, lack of standardization
Plant-Derived Extracts	Contain phytochemicals with antibacterial and antibiofilm activities	Flavonoids, Alkaloids, Tannins	In vitro and preclinical studies	Complex mixtures, low bioavailability
Immunotherapy	Enhance host immune response to promote pathogen clearance	Monoclonal antibodies, Vaccines, Cytokines	Clinical trials	Cost, immune overstimulation risk

5. NANOTECHNOLOGY AND SMART DRUG DELIVERY SYSTEMS: ADVANCED NANOPARTICLES IN COMBATING ANTIBIOTIC RESISTANCE

Nanoparticles are widely used in medicine and healthcare, especially in antimicrobial treatment, and they can take many different shapes. Because of their exceptional adaptability, metal-based nanoparticles are used in biotechnology, electronics, materials science, and medicine. They are very successful in a variety of situations due to their distinct physical and chemical characteristics, which are linked to their high surface-area-to-volume ratio and nanoscale size. The following figure shows several categories of nanomaterials with antibacterial potential (Khan, Saeed et al., 2019).

Figure 4. Classes of recently used Nanomaterials being utilized in antimicrobial therapy

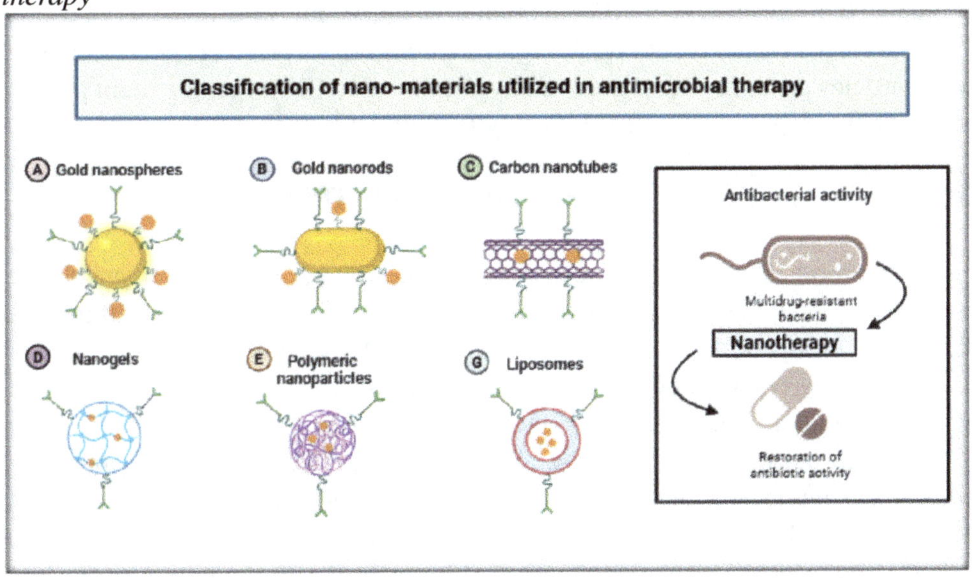

(Source: Created in https://BioRender.com)

5.1 Overcoming Penetration Barriers in Biofilms and Intracellular Infections

The breakdown of bacterial membranes, which occurs when nanoparticles come into direct contact with the normally negatively charged bacterial cell wall, is one of the main mechanisms. These surfaces become physically damaged when nanoparticles, particularly those having cationic characteristics, attach to them. Cell lysis may occur from either total structural rupture or enhanced membrane permeability. While silver nanoparticles chemically change the integrity of bacterial membranes, graphene oxide and other sharp-edged nanoparticles can physically cut through them. Because it depends on physical interactions rather than particular biochemical pathways that bacteria frequently develop resistance against, this method is especially effective against a wide range of bacteria, including Gram-positive and Gram-negative strains (Wang, et al., 2017; Godoy-Gallardo, et al., 2021).

5.2 ROS Generation: Mechanistic Activity of NP Against MDR

Another significant antibacterial mechanism is the generation of ROS, which is particularly observed in metal and metal oxide nanoparticles. These nanoparticles create a variety of ROS and have antibacterial capabilities by inducing oxidative stress, which damages the membranes of bacteria, proteins, and genetic material. Oxidative damage caused by ROS is often permanent and leads to bacterial death. When exposed to visible or ultraviolet light, titanium dioxide and other photo-catalytic nanoparticles generate more reactive oxygen species (ROS), making them perfect for sterilization (Kaur et al., 2023; Godoy-Gallardo et al., 2021).

5.3 Nano-Carriers for Targeted Antibiotic Delivery

Furthermore, nanoparticles are advanced drug delivery systems that enable the targeted and regulated release of antibiotics. By encasing antibiotics within their structures, nanoparticles increase their stability and protect them from enzymatic destruction. Certain infection areas, such as biofilms, which are frequently resistant to traditional antibiotics, can be targeted by functionalized nanoparticles. Once at the infection site, nanoparticles allow antibiotics to be released gradually and under control, sustaining therapeutic doses for long stretches of time (Yetisgin et al., 2020). This targeted delivery reduces the selective pressure in arising resistance by reducing side effects, reducing systemic toxicity, and lowering doses of antibiotics. Besides being naturally antibacterial, nanoparticles can increase the efficacy of the currently existing antibiotics. The nanoparticles disrupt the membranes of bacteria to allow easier penetration of antibiotics into bacterial cells and improve their effectiveness. Moreover, some nanoparticles block bacterial pumps that help to release efflux, which helps the organism to retain drugs and enhances their activity. Moreover, nanoparticles can disperse biofilms, which form a large portion of the resistance to the application of antimicrobial agents when it comes to the treatment of chronic infections (Wang, et al., 2017). Nanoparticles have been demonstrated to have a high antibacterial effect in combination with antibiotics, including those resistant to the antibiotics. All said and done, the numerous procedures that nanoparticles undergo render them effective agents against bacterial infections. Their capacity to evade the conventional resistance mechanisms, amplify the efficacy of antibiotics, and precisely reach the regions of infection indicates their capability in contemporary medicine (Afridi et al., 2022). Further research on these pathways will create more potent antibiotic-resistant bacterial treatments by making them more practical and refined.

The table given below summarizes the main drug delivery systems based on nanotechnology that have been studied for antimicrobial applications. It includes information on their design characteristics, antibacterial activity, and translational potential.

Table 6. Nanotechnology-Based Drug Delivery Platforms in Antimicrobial Therapy

Nanocarrier Type	Core Composition	Mechanism of Antimicrobial Action	Advantages	Potential Drawbacks
Liposomes	Phospholipid bilayers	Encapsulate antibiotics, enhance delivery to infection site	Biocompatibility, controlled release	Stability issues, short shelf life
Polymeric Nanoparticles	Biodegradable polymers (PLGA, chitosan, PEG)	Sustained antibiotic release, penetration into biofilms	High drug loading, tunable properties	Possible polymer toxicity, complex synthesis
Metallic Nanoparticles	Silver, gold, zinc oxide nanoparticles	Generate ROS, disrupt bacterial membranes	Broad-spectrum activity, synergy with antibiotics	Cytotoxicity, oxidative stress, and long-term accumulation
Solid Lipid Nanoparticles (SLNs)	Solid lipids stabilized by surfactants	Controlled drug release, improved stability	Enhanced bioavailability, low toxicity	Limited drug loading capacity
Nano-emulsions	Oil–water dispersions stabilized by surfactants	Disrupt cell membranes, improve drug solubility	High surface area, low cost	Physical instability, phase separation
Carbon-Based Nanomaterials	Graphene oxide, carbon nanotubes	Physical disruption of membranes, ROS generation	High surface reactivity, durable antimicrobial effect	Non-biodegradability, uncertain biosafety
Dendrimers	Branched macromolecules (PAMAM, PPI)	Multivalent interaction with bacterial membranes	Adjustable structure, multifunctional potential	Hemolytic toxicity, cost of synthesis

Despite the fact that nanotechnology-based systems have shown so much potential in enhancing targeted drug delivery and antibacterial effects, there is a need to test cytotoxicity and long-term biosafety before clinical translation can be done. Physicochemical properties of nanoparticles are examples of properties that can affect the interaction of nanoparticles with biological tissues. The benefits of nanomaterials in therapy should be thoroughly researched beforehand, and toxicity studies conducted to ensure that patient safety is not jeopardized by the therapeutic effects of the nanomaterials.

6. HOST-DIRECTED AND IMMUNOTHERAPEUTIC APPROACHES

The new and re-emerging infectious diseases have highlighted weaknesses in healthcare systems, especially in developing nations, and underscore the necessity of innovative therapeutic methods to combat these diseases. Healthcare is being revolutionized by a new therapy method that aims to extend life expectancy and achieve universal health coverage. By strengthening host defense against opportunistic infections, immunotherapy provides a novel remedy, especially for individuals with impaired immune systems. Human infectious illness management has benefited greatly from recent developments in immunotherapeutic techniques. According to Adedokun, et al. (2025), these strategies are essential in the larger framework of human disease prevention and control. Main immunotherapeutic agents are illustrated in Figure 5.

Figure 5. Potential immunotherapeutic agents that are being utilized to mitigate antimicrobial resistance.

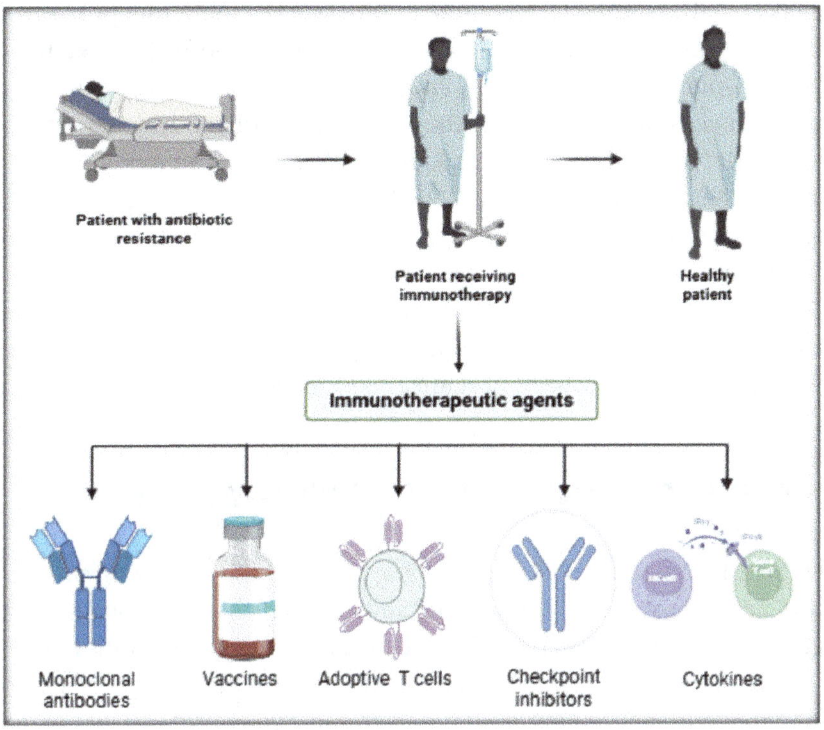

(Source: Created in https://BioRender.com)

Through the effective modulation of the host's innate and adaptive immune responses, immunotherapy is gaining popularity as a means of treating a variety of diseases. These agents have a variety of mechanisms of action, including modifying immune cells (invariant killer T cells (iNKTs), mucosal-associated invariant T cells (MAITs), and adoptive T cell therapy), improving host immunity (cytokine therapy, immune checkpoint inhibitors (ICIs), and vaccines), and targeting pathogenic determinants (monoclonal antibodies) (Sangeetha Vijayan, et al., 2024).

6.1 Monoclonal Antibodies Against Bacterial Antigens

Human blood and cells naturally contain antibodies. Invasive immunity is a different kind of immunity that is enforced using monoclonal antibodies, which are artificially produced antibodies that replicate the body's system. Certain monoclonal antibodies are employed as immunotherapeutic agents, working in tandem with cells to target and treat illnesses and foreign objects. They are equally capable of identifying and blocking signals that result in aberrant cell division or multiplication, as seen in cancer. Only a small number of monoclonal antibodies that are effective against bacterial or viral infections have been authorized for therapeutic use. Others are advancing through clinical trials with encouraging prospects, especially those with modified structures that offer the most benefits (Sangeetha Vijayan et al., 2024). Only a small number of antibodies can be used to cure bacterial and viral infections, despite the fact that they have been utilized to treat a wide range of illnesses (Bielskė, Petraitytė-Burneikienė et al., 2025). The therapeutic range of these immunotherapeutic drugs is shortened when mouse monoclonal antibodies are used repeatedly as treatments in humans, since this causes the development of anti-mouse antibodies. A chimeric antibody was created to reduce the immunogenicity of monoclonal antibodies in people to solve this problem. These immunomodulatory treatments, in conjunction with synthetic biology, represent a synthesis of technical and biological innovation in the fight against resistant diseases (Piscaglia et al., 2025).

7. SYNTHETIC BIOLOGY AND PRECISION MEDICINE

Alternative therapeutic approaches, such as combination therapy, high-molecular-weight biomaterials, nanotechnology, and antibacterial phytochemicals, must be investigated to overcome multidrug resistance. Additionally, synthetic biology presents a viable path forward for antibacterial therapy (Yang, et al., 2021). This innovative field of study constructs living systems from biological components using engineering principles to give them specific biological functionalities. Genetic systems and circuits in some animals can be programmed to regulate how cells function in response to specific inputs, ultimately producing the desired functionalities (Yan et al., 2023). Synthetic biology has various applications and are summarized in Table 7.

Table 7. Applications of Synthetic Biology in Biomedical Research and Therapeutic Development

Application Area	Synthetic Biology Approach	Products	Mechanisms
Gene Editing and Regulation	CRISPR-Cas systems for precise genome modification	Correction of resistance genes; modulation of bacterial virulence	Enables targeted DNA cleavage and repair for genetic control
Genetic Circuits and Switches	Engineered regulatory networks in microbes	Synthetic gene switches, logic gates	Controls cellular behavior via programmed genetic responses
Therapeutic Cell Engineering	CAR-T cell design using modular gene circuits	Treatment of B-cell acute lymphoblastic leukemia	T-cell modification for antigen-specific immune targeting
Drug Biosynthesis via Microbial Fermentation	Genetic modification of microbes to produce pharmaceuticals	*Artemisinin* production in engineered *Saccharomyces cerevisiae*	Introduces synthetic pathways for natural drug production
Disease Biosensing and Diagnostics	Engineered microbial biosensors	Glucose- or pathogen-detecting bacteria	Detects disease biomarkers via synthetic signaling circuits
Antimicrobial Discovery and Resistance Control	Synthetic design of antimicrobial peptides and biosynthetic pathways	Novel AMPs and quorum-sensing inhibitors	Creates new antimicrobial agents with programmable selectivity

These advancements provide a fresh perspective and substantial potential for employing synthetic biology to build living creatures for antimicrobial therapy, establishing a novel therapeutic method utilizing living organisms (Courbet et al., 2015).

7.1 Engineered Bacteria as "Living Therapeutics"

Through the use of engineering techniques in synthetic biology, microbes with specialized functions may be created, which allows them to generate antibacterial compounds that specifically target and inactivate infections. Bacteriocins are by far the most common class of antibacterial agents. They are a varied collection of antibacterial peptides or proteases that are made by bacteria and archaea, and they frequently exhibit activity against species that are related to the bacterium that produces them. As was previously noted, bacteriocins are a mechanism of immunity that is the product of evolutionary processes. Significant bactericidal efficacy can frequently be attained at comparatively low doses. Additionally, engineered microorganisms are made to detect particular metabolites or quorum-sensing (QS) chemicals that are generated by pathogens (Heilbronner et al., 2021). By altering the cellular metabolic system to respond to these particular metabolites, this process creates equivalent antimicrobial compounds and initiates downstream pathways. This system was "sense-killed" by design (Saeidi et al., 2011).

7.2 Targeted *Salmonella*

Typhoid fever is caused by the pathogenic bacterium Salmonella, which is commonly seen in intestinal illnesses. Typhoid fever is specifically linked to a particular serotype of *Salmonella*. Nontyphoidal *Salmonella* serotypes are a health risk to both human and livestock populations because they are frequently zoonotic, meaning they can spread from one species to another (Besser, 2018). It is essential to use modified bacteria to detect *Salmonella*. One important sign is tetrathionate, a metabolic byproduct produced when endogenous thiosulfate and reactive oxygen species react in the colon during inflammatory events. *Salmonella* has a clear growth advantage over other microbial communities in the digestive system because it uses thiosulfates to produce a unique respiratory electron acceptor at the same time (Winter et al., 2010).

7.3 Targeted *Pseudomonas Aeruginosa*

A common gram-negative pathogenic bacterium, *P. aeruginosa,* belongs to the ESKAPE group, which includes some of the deadliest bacterial infections. In clinical settings, *P. aeruginosa* is commonly linked to ventilator-associated pneumonia, which is especially dangerous for immunocompromised people and those with cystic fibrosis. It can also result in infections of the soft tissues and skin, as well as sepsis (Qin et al., 2022).

In *P. aeruginosa*, QS regulates biosynthesis, and an essential signaling molecule in this process is N-acyl Homoserine Lactone (AHL). These signaling molecules influence gene expression by activating regulatory factors at a certain concentration. AHL is essential for a number of *P. aeruginosa* functions, such as the creation of biofilms, the synthesis of secondary metabolites, the expression of virulence factors, and the evolution of resistance mechanisms. Targeting AHL sensing appears to be a potential approach because of its critical role in bacterial population dynamics and pathogenicity (Chan et al., 2015).

7.4 Targeted *Staphylococcus Aureus*

S. aureus, a common cause of serious infections is aureus, is a gram-positive coccus that belongs to the ESKAPE group. Abscesses, pneumonia, endocarditis, osteomyelitis, sepsis, and other severe infectious disorders are frequently caused by its invasion of the host's bloodstream, respiratory system, and gastrointestinal tract. It is noteworthy because it is one of the leading causes of nosocomial infections in hospitals. The findings of research show that E. DegP, a protease secreted by *Escherichia coli* 1917, can prevent the production of biofilms. This inhibition successfully prevents *Staphylococcus Aureus* from growing (Fang et al., 2018). Using careful design to further modify bacteria to generate the DegP protease is a viable approach. Furthermore, in synthetic biology, the construction of responsive modules depends heavily on the discovery of appropriate QS molecules. *S. Aureus* produces autoinducer peptide-I (AIP-1). This is an essential QS molecule in this bacterium's harmful mechanisms. This chemical affects biofilm formation and the control of virulence gene expression within the Agr QS system (Gupta et al., 2015).

7.5 Targeted *Vibrio Cholerae*

Cholera, a severe gastrointestinal illness known for its great contagiousness, is caused by the gram-negative bacterium *Vibrio cholerae*. Worldwide, cholera results in millions of infections and more than 100,000 fatalities each year. *V. cholerae* colonizing the small intestine and secreting cholera toxin are the main pathogenic processes. By attaching itself to intestinal cells' GM1 ganglioside receptors, this exotoxin continuously activates the G protein-linked adenylate cyclase. This activation causes the small intestine's epithelial cells' cAMP levels to rise, which causes a significant outflow of water and sodium ions. In the end, this process causes electrolyte imbalance, severe, copious diarrhea, vomiting, and severe dehydration (Clemens, et al.).

Genetically modified *E. coli* generates the lytic protein YebF-Art-085, which can identify CAI-1, a crucial QS molecule in *V. cholerae*. This protein has a specific antibacterial response when it is released, killing *V. cholerae* (Jayaraman et al., 2017).

8. TRANSLATIONAL, REGULATORY, AND CLINICAL PERSPECTIVES OF NOVEL ANTIMICROBIAL STRATEGIES

This part discusses some of the important translational barriers, ethical and regulatory issues, and real-world clinical evidence, and the significance of integrated and synergistic treatment strategies to have long-term management of multidrug-resistant infections (Mittra, Bruce et al., 2021). To help compare the traditional antibiotics with the new antimicrobial plans, Table 8 summarizes the mechanism of action, clinical evidence state, benefits, drawbacks, and translational readiness of the two plans. In this comparative discussion, the advantages and limitations of the two methods are highlighted and the necessity to employ joint and context-based therapeutic solutions to antimicrobial resistance is emphasized.

Table 8. Comparative overview of conventional and emerging antimicrobial therapies: efficacy, limitations, and translational status

Therapy Type	Representative Examples	Mechanism of Action	Clinical Evidence Status (2020–2025)	Key Advantages	Major Limitations	Translational Readiness
Conventional antibiotics	β-lactams, fluoroquinolones, aminoglycosides	Inhibit cell wall synthesis, DNA replication, or protein synthesis	Extensive clinical use; rising failure rates in MDR infections	Broad-spectrum, standardized dosing	Rapid resistance, toxicity, limited pipeline	Fully approved but declining efficacy
Bacteriophage therapy	Lytic phages (personalized cocktails)	Bacterial lysis via host-specific infection	Compassionate use & pilot trials (burn wounds, prosthetic infections)	High specificity, self-amplifying	Regulatory hurdles, narrow host range	Early clinical / compassionate use
Antimicrobial peptides (AMPs)	LL-37 analogs, defensins	Membrane disruption, immune modulation	Phase I–II trials (sepsis, skin infections)	Rapid killing, low resistance potential	Cytotoxicity, stability issues	Early mid clinical
CRISPR-based antimicrobials	CRISPR-Cas targeting resistance genes	Sequence-specific gene cleavage	Preclinical / proof-of-concept studies	Precision targeting, resistance reversal	Delivery challenges, biosafety concerns	Preclinical
Quorum-sensing inhibitors (QSIs)	Furanones, plant-derived QS blockers	Disrupt bacterial communication	Preclinical & adjunct studies	Reduces virulence without killing	Limited standalone efficacy	Preclinical
Photodynamic therapy (PDT)	Light + photosensitizers	ROS-mediated bacterial killing	Pilot clinical studies (wounds, dentistry)	Effective against biofilms	Limited penetration, equipment needs	Early clinical
Natural products	Essential oils, plant extracts	Multi-target antimicrobial effects	*In vitro* / animal models	Low cost, accessibility	Variability, weak standardization	Preclinical
Immunotherapy	Monoclonal antibodies, vaccines	Enhances host immune clearance	Clinical trials for select pathogens	Reduces dependence on antibiotics	Pathogen specificity	Clinical (pathogen-dependent)

8.1 Regulatory and Ethical Challenges in Emerging Antimicrobial Therapies

The clinical implementation of the emerging antimicrobial solutions that have shown promise in experimental studies, including bacteriophage therapy, CRISPR-based antimicrobials, and immunotherapies, is limited by significant regulatory and ethical issues. Bacteriophages, in contrast to traditional antibiotics, are highly specific and biologically evolving, which makes it hard to standardize, control their quality, and be approved according to the current pharmaceutical regulation standards. On the same note, CRISPR-based antimicrobials have been associated with biosafety and ethical issues associated with off-target genetic effects and horizontal gene transfer. Currently, regulatory bodies including the World Health Organization and U.S. Food and Drug Administration do not have harmonized guidelines specific to these technologies, so the approval processes take even longer and are deployed limited to clinical use. These issues will necessitate adjusting regulatory pathways, ethical controls and intercontinental coordination in order to safely bring such novel therapies into the mainstream clinical care. (Ahmed, Kayode et al., 2024)

8.2 Economic Feasibility, Scalability, and Patient-Centered Considerations

Besides regulatory restrictions, economic viability and scalability of substitute antimicrobial therapy are also important issues. The essential oils and extracts of plants are natural products with antimicrobial properties in the in vitro environment, yet these are not uniformly formulated, exhibit low bioavailability, are challenging to obtain in bulk, and hamper their clinical translation. Moreover, patient-related aspects like acceptability, safety perceptions, accessibility, and cost-effectiveness play an important role that can affect the actual practice of new therapies. These strategies should be part of the current antimicrobial stewardship and hospital infection control policies to maintain rational utilization, reduce cases of resistance, and foster equal access to these interventions in the healthcare environment (Pilar, Martina et al., 2025).

8.3 Clinical Evidence, Combination Therapies, and Translational Integration

The present part is devoted to the clinical evidence and translational strategies in the real world, with a primary concentration on combination therapy as a feasible approach to winning the battle against multidrug-resistant infections. Novel clinical data are bringing about the promise of new antimicrobial protocols in real-world infections. Bacteriophage therapy has proven to be useful in compassionate-use cases in multidrug-resistant burn wounds and prosthetic joint infections, and antimicrobial peptides are under early-phase sepsis and bloodstream infection trials. Nonetheless, one alternative therapy cannot probably substitute antibiotics completely. Rather, a synergistic strategy, e.g., phages plus antibiotics, photodynamic therapy plus antimicrobial peptides or immunomodulators plus regular drugs, is another option that can be used in a translational strategy. These combination regimens can increase their effectiveness, minimize resistance selection, and increase the duration of the effective lifespan of the currently available antimicrobials, which highlights the importance of combined treatment models over single-agent treatments (Bettiol, Rottier et al., 2014).

8.3.1 Clinical Evidence from Real-World Applications

Phage Therapy of Burn Wound Infections

Bacteriophage therapy as compassionate-use therapy has been shown to have clinical success in treating multidrug-resistant *Pseudomonas aeruginosa* and *Acinetobacter baumannii* burn wound infections. Infection resolution has been reported in the recent case series when phages are used together with antibiotics after conventional therapy was unsuccessful, pointing out the use of phages as valid rescue agents in critical-care units (Dehari, Chaudhuri et al., 2023).

Engineered Phages for Drug-Resistant Mycobacterial Infection

Another groundbreaking clinical case report was about the application of engineered bacteriophages to treat a disseminated *Mycobacterium abscessus* infection in one of the post-transplant patients. The intervention resulted in long-term clinical improvement, which is a milestone of genetically modified phage therapeutics (Hashemi Shahraki & Mirsaeidi, 2021).

Antimicrobial Peptides in Sepsis Models

A few AMPs have advanced to the initial phase of clinical research on bloodstream and sepsis-related infection. Phase I-II trials also suggest rapid bactericidal effects and immunomodulatory effects, but dose-dependent toxicity is an issue that needs to be optimized (Hickson et al., 2025).

Combination Strategies: Phages with Antibiotics

Recent pilot studies show that antibiotic susceptibility to MDR infections can be restored through a combination of both bacteriophages and antibiotics because biofilms are perturbed, and the selection of resistance is inhibited. This synergy has the capacity to reduce bacterial load as compared to monotherapy to a significant degree (Osman et al., 2023).

9. LIMITATIONS OF CURRENT THERAPEUTIC STRATEGIES TO OVERCOME AMR

Most emerging therapeutics have translational, regulatory, as well as strong experimental efficacy, as summarized in Table 8. AMR's growing threat necessitates prompt, well-coordinated international action. The effectiveness of current AMR-fighting methods is limited by considerable obstacles. The slow rate of new antibiotic discovery is one of the most significant constraints. Due in large part to the high cost, drawn-out clearance procedures, and lack of financial incentives for pharmaceutical companies, the pipeline for developing novel antibiotics is still inadequate despite rising resistance. Clinicians now have few alternatives for treating MDR and XDR bacterial strains since their emergence has overtaken medication development. The rapid development of mechanisms of resistance in microbes is another ongoing issue. Bacteria have displayed extraordinary adaptivity through horizontal gene transfer, efflux pumps, and enzyme degradation of antibiotics. The possibility of the development of resistance to the pathogens quicker than the innovative drugs highlights the necessity of new solutions (Nazir, Nazir et al., 2025).

The answer to these constraints is to have a comprehensive, internationally synchronized strategy. The reinforcement of international surveillance systems, greater investment in research and development, enhancing antibiotic stewardship measures, and implementing a strict set of rules to regulate the use of antibiotics in agriculture are valuable measures. Adoption of multidisciplinary teamwork between microbiologists, physicians, and legislators, promotion of public-private partnerships, and creative financing approaches to developing new antibiotics to fight AMR will all play a crucial role. Unless something is done, AMR is a risk to modern medicine, making everyday infections untreatable and routine treatment hazardous.

10. CONCLUSION

The complexity of the association between microorganisms and antibiotics is an essential issue to understand, as the problem of antimicrobial resistance (AMR) remains one of the critical challenges to global healthcare. To overcome AMR in modern healthcare, it is necessary to have a comprehensive methodology to explain how bacteria change and adapt to resist antibiotic treatment. The current issue of AMR needs a complex solution to maintain the efficacy of antimicrobial treatments. It implies increased efforts to monitor the situation in the world, antimicrobial stewardship programs, and increased scientific research to create new drugs and other treatment options. Nevertheless, the development of science is not enough. Treatment and prevention of bacterial resistance to antibiotics needs to be collaboratively and coordinated efforts on the part of the pharmaceutical industry, physicians, and researchers. Evidence-based prescribing practices have to be employed by healthcare professionals, and researchers must keep investigating new treatment modalities and fast methods of diagnosis. Pharmaceutical companies need to focus on the creation of new antimicrobial drugs, despite the monetary and legislative challenges, and governments play a significant role in enacting rules and regulations that would reduce the misuse of antibiotics in industry and medicine. There is also the need to address the low- and middle-income countries and assist them in their fight against AMR with the help of international partnerships and funding initiatives. The AMR needs to be resolved promptly, regularly, and in partnership. We can strive to reach a point at which the threat of AMR is efficiently managed by encouraging interdisciplinary cooperation, encouraging the responsible use of medications, and providing creative research through sponsorship. Now we can potentially save the effectiveness of antimicrobial medication and the health of the world for future generations.

On the whole, although traditional antibiotics are irreplaceable, their decreasing efficacy against multidrug-resistant pathogens requires additional and alternative ways of treatment. Phage therapy and CRISPR-based antimicrobials, antimicrobial peptides and photodynamic therapy, immunotherapeutic and host-directed strategies, and pathogen clearance through enhancing host defenses allow high specificity and targeted action, rapid bactericidal action, and reduced resistance selection, respectively. The further addition to the arsenal of therapeutic systems comes through natural products and nanotechnology-based systems of delivery, which increase the bioavailability and target efficiency. Notably, none of the strategies could be universally adequate, but particular approaches, which seem to be the most promising to reach the long-term clinical efficacy, are integrated and combination-based ones. It is this comparative view that informs the necessity to have integrated translational, regulatory, and clinical frameworks to efficiently integrate the emerging therapies into the normal antimicrobial practice.

REFERENCES

Adedokun, A. I.. (2025). Exploring immunotherapeutic strategies for bacterial and viral diseases. *Exploration of Immunology*, *5*, 1003202.

Aebisher, D.. (2024). Photodynamic therapy in the treatment of cancer—The selection of synthetic photosensitizers. *Pharmaceuticals*, *17*(7), 932.

Afridi, M.. (2022). Combining antibiotics with silver nanoparticles: A potential treatment strategy against antimicrobial resistance. *Main Group Chemistry*, *21*(2), 445–466.

Ahmed, M. M.. (2024). CRISPR-Cas systems in the fight against antimicrobial resistance: Current status, potentials, and future directions. *Infection and Drug Resistance*, •••, 5229–5245.

Arip, M.. (2022). Review on plant-based management in combating antimicrobial resistance: A mechanistic perspective. *Frontiers in Pharmacology*, *13*, 879495.

Besser, J. M. (2018). Salmonella epidemiology: A whirlwind of change. *Food Microbiology*, *71*, 55–59.

Bettiol, E.. (2014). Improved treatment of multidrug-resistant bacterial infections: Utility of clinical studies. *Future Microbiology*, *9*(6), 757–771.

Bielskė, K.. (2025). Broadly reactive monoclonal antibodies against beta-lactamases for immunodetection of bacterial resistance to antibiotics. *Scientific Reports*, *15*(1), 19094.

Brives, C., & Pourraz, J. (2020). Phage therapy as a potential solution in the fight against AMR: Obstacles and possible futures. *Palgrave Communications*, *6*(1), 1–11.

Browne, K.. (2020). A new era of antibiotics: The clinical potential of antimicrobial peptides. *International Journal of Molecular Sciences*, *21*(19), 7047.

Chan, K.-G.. (2015). Inhibiting N-acyl-homoserine lactone synthesis and quenching Pseudomonas quinolone quorum sensing to attenuate virulence. *Frontiers in Microbiology*, *6*, 1173.

Cieplik, F.. (2013). Photodynamic biofilm inactivation by SAPYR—An exclusive singlet oxygen photosensitizer. *Free Radical Biology & Medicine*, *65*, 477–487.

Clemens, J., et al. "Cholera Lancet, 390 (2017)." View PDF View article View in Scopus: 1539-1549.

Courbet, A., et al. (2015). "Detection of pathological biomarkers in human clinical samples via amplifying genetic switches and logic gates." Science translational medicine 7(289): 289ra283-289ra283.

de Carvalho Leonel, L.. (2019). Photodynamic Antimicrobial Chemotherapy (PACT) using methylene blue inhibits the viability of the biofilm produced by Candida albicans. *Photodiagnosis and Photodynamic Therapy*, *26*, 316–323.

Dehari, D.. (2023). A bacteriophage microgel effectively treats the multidrug-resistant Acinetobacter baumannii bacterial infections in burn wounds. *Pharmaceuticals*, *16*(7), 942.

Đukanović, S.. (2022). Elucidating the antibiofilm activity of Frangula emodin against Staphylococcus aureus biofilms. *Journal of Applied Microbiology*, *132*(3), 1840–1855.

El-Sapagh, S.. (2023). Unveiling the potential of algal extracts as promising antibacterial and antibiofilm agents against multidrug-resistant Pseudomonas aeruginosa: In vitro and in silico studies including molecular docking. *Plants*, *12*(18), 3324.

Elshobary, M. E.. (2025). Combating antibiotic resistance: Mechanisms, multidrug-resistant pathogens, and novel therapeutic approaches: An updated review. *Pharmaceuticals*, *18*(3), 402.

Fang, K.. (2018). Probiotic Escherichia coli inhibits biofilm formation of pathogenic E. coli via extracellular activity of DegP. *Scientific Reports*, *8*(1), 4939.

Gach, M. W.. (2024). Antimicrobial resistance among common bacterial pathogens in Indonesia: A systematic review. *The Lancet Regional Health. Southeast Asia*, •••, 26.

Godoy-Gallardo, M.. (2021). Antibacterial approaches in tissue engineering using metal ions and nanoparticles: From mechanisms to applications. *Bioactive Materials*, *6*(12), 4470–4490.

Gupta, R. K.. (2015). RNAIII of the Staphylococcus aureus agr system activates global regulator MgrA by stabilizing mRNA. *Proceedings of the National Academy of Sciences of the United States of America*, *112*(45), 14036–14041.

Haniffa, R.. (2018). Improving ICU services in resource-limited settings: Perceptions of ICU workers from low-middle-, and high-income countries. *Journal of Critical Care*, *44*, 352–356.

Hasan, M., & Ahn, J. (2022). Evolutionary dynamics between phages and bacteria as a possible approach for designing effective phage therapies against antibiotic-resistant bacteria. *Antibiotics (Basel, Switzerland), 11*(7), 915.

Hashemi Shahraki, A., & Mirsaeidi, M. (2021). Phage therapy for Mycobacterium abscessus and strategies to improve outcomes. *Microorganisms, 9*(3), 596.

Heilbronner, S.. (2021). The microbiome-shaping roles of bacteriocins. *Nature Reviews. Microbiology, 19*(11), 726–739.

Hickson, S. M., et al. (2025). "Emerging antimicrobial therapies for Gram-negative infections in human clinical use." npj Antimicrobials and Resistance 3(1): 16.

Howell, M., ... (2022). Exploring synergy and its role in antimicrobial peptide biology. Methods in Enzymology, Elsevier. 663: 99-130.

Hutchings, M. I.. (2019). Antibiotics: Past, present and future. *Current Opinion in Microbiology, 51*, 72–80.

Jayaraman, P.. (2017). Repurposing a two-component system-based biosensor for the killing of Vibrio cholerae. *ACS Synthetic Biology, 6*(7), 1403–1415.

Kaur, H., ... (2023). Antimicrobial nanoparticles: Synthesis, mechanism of actions. Antimicrobial activity of nanoparticles, Elsevier: 155-202.

Khameneh, B.. (2021). Phytochemicals: A promising weapon in the arsenal against antibiotic-resistant bacteria. *Antibiotics (Basel, Switzerland), 10*(9), 1044.

Khan, I.. (2019). Nanoparticles: Properties, applications and toxicities. *Arabian Journal of Chemistry, 12*(7), 908–931.

Klobucar, K., & Brown, E. D. (2022). New potentiators of ineffective antibiotics: Targeting the Gram-negative outer membrane to overcome intrinsic resistance. *Current Opinion in Chemical Biology, 66*, 102099.

Konwar, A. N.. (2022). Emerging non-traditional approaches to combat antibiotic resistance. *Current Microbiology, 79*(11), 330.

Krul, D.. (2025). Spread of antimicrobial-resistant clones of the ESKAPEE group: From the clinical setting to hospital effluent. *The Science of the Total Environment, 973*, 179124.

Liu, Y.. (2015). Antibacterial photodynamic therapy: Overview of a promising approach to fight antibiotic-resistant bacterial infections. *Journal of Clinical and Translational Research, 1*(3), 140.

Luong, T.. (2020). Phage therapy in the resistance era: Where do we stand and where are we going? *Clinical Therapeutics*, *42*(9), 1659–1680.

Mittra, J.. (2021). Regulatory and market influences on innovation pathways for the development of new antimicrobial drugs. *Technology Analysis and Strategic Management*, *33*(3), 283–295.

Nazir, A.. (2025). The Global Challenge of Antimicrobial Resistance: Mechanisms, Case Studies, and Mitigation Approaches. *Health Science Reports*, *8*(7), e71077.

Organization, W. H. (2024). *WHO bacterial priority pathogens list, 2024: bacterial pathogens of public health importance, to guide research, development, and strategies to prevent and control antimicrobial resistance*. World Health Organization.

Osman, A.-H.. (2023). The potential of bacteriophage-antibiotic combination therapy in treating infections with multidrug-resistant bacteria. *Antibiotics (Basel, Switzerland)*, *12*(8), 1329.

Pierce, J. D.. (2022). Post-COVID-19 syndrome. *Nursing Research*, *71*(2), 164–174.

Pilar, R.-G.. (2025). New Drugs, Old Problems: A Narrative Review of Antibiotic Stewardship Program in the era of novel Gram-negative antibiotics. *Clinical Microbiology and Infection.*

Pirnay, J. (2020). Phage therapy in the year 2035. *Frontiers in Microbiology*, *11*, 1171.

Piscaglia, M.. (2025). Exploring human use of monoclonal antibodies against critical bacteria: A scoping review of clinical trials. *Infectious Diseases and Therapy*, •••, 1–29.

Qin, S.. (2022). Pseudomonas aeruginosa: Pathogenesis, virulence factors, antibiotic resistance, interaction with host, technology advances and emerging therapeutics. *Signal Transduction and Targeted Therapy*, *7*(1), 199.

Saeidi, N.. (2011). Engineering microbes to sense and eradicate Pseudomonas aeruginosa, a human pathogen. *Molecular Systems Biology*, *7*(1), 521.

Saffari Natanzi, A.. (2025). Innovative approaches to combat antibiotic resistance: Integrating CRISPR/Cas9 and nanoparticles against biofilm-driven infections. *BMC Medicine*, *23*(1), 486.

Sangeetha Vijayan, P.. (2024). A review of immune modulators and immunotherapy in infectious diseases. *Molecular and Cellular Biochemistry*, *479*(8), 1937–1955.

Stoitsova, S.. (2022). The concept for the antivirulence therapeutics approach as alternative to antibiotics: Hope or still a fiction? *Biotechnology, Biotechnological Equipment*, *36*(1), 697–705.

Suessmuth, R. D.. (2025). Fighting antimicrobial resistance: Innovative drugs in antibacterial research. *Angewandte Chemie International Edition*, *64*(10), e202414325.

Tosas Auguet, O., et al. (2025). "Global antibiotic resistance surveillance report 2025."

Vidyadhari, A. and A. K. Singh Immunogenicity of Cell-Based Therapy. Nano-erythrocytes in Cancer Therapy, CRC Press: 192-222.

Visan, A. I., & Negut, I. (2024). Coatings based on essential oils for combating antibiotic resistance. *Antibiotics (Basel, Switzerland)*, *13*(7), 625.

Wang, L.. (2017). The antimicrobial activity of nanoparticles: Present situation and prospects for the future. *International Journal of Nanomedicine*, •••, 1227–1249.

Wang, R.. (2025). Research Progress on the Influence Factors of the Quorum Sensing System Regulating the Growth of Wastewater Treatment Biofilm. *Water (Basel)*, *17*(13), 1944.

Winter, S. E.. (2010). Gut inflammation provides a respiratory electron acceptor for Salmonella. *Nature*, *467*(7314), 426–429.

Yan, X.. (2023). Applications of synthetic biology in medical and pharmaceutical fields. *Signal Transduction and Targeted Therapy*, *8*(1), 199.

Youf, R.. (2021). Antimicrobial photodynamic therapy: Latest developments with a focus on combinatory strategies. *Pharmaceutics*, *13*(12), 1995.

Chapter 11
Microbiological Innovations as a Defence Against Antimicrobial Resistance

V. Vaishnavi
https://orcid.org/0009-0006-8922-5231
Department of Microbiology, Sacred Heart College, Tirupattur, India

P. Prakathi
https://orcid.org/0009-0000-4457-9008
Department of Microbiology, Sacred Heart College, Tirupattur, India

M. Nisha
https://orcid.org/0009-0000-0862-7631
Department of Microbiology, Sacred Heart College, Tirupattur, India

U. Subhalakshmi
https://orcid.org/0009-0007-8989-5486
Department of Microbiology, Sacred Heart College, Tirupattur, India

P. Amudhanila
https://orcid.org/0009-0003-1970-6150
Department of Microbiology, Sacred Heart College, Tirupattur, India

ABSTRACT

Antimicrobial resistance has emerged as a major global health problem of the 21st century, significantly undermining the efficacy of current pharmaceuticals in the treatment of fungi, bacteria, viruses, and parasitic infections. Microbiology in

DOI: 10.4018/979-8-3373-3825-5.ch011

healthcare is vital to the fight against antibiotic resistance because it helps identify resistant infections early, understand resistance mechanisms, and guide appropriate treatment techniques. Multidrug-resistant pathogens like MRSA and VRE, ESBL-causing Enterobacteriaceae, and carbapenem-resistant infections are spreading quickly, which highlights the critical need for integrated diagnostic and surveillance methods. Molecular testing, whole-genome sequencing, quick point-of-care testing, routine culture & sensitivity, and evidence-based antibiotic dosing are all ways that medical microbiology labs help reduce AMR. Medical microbiology helps create new antimicrobials, phage treatment, antimicrobial peptides, & alternative therapeutics, including probiotics and immune modulators, in addition to diagnostics.

1. INTRODUCTION

The increase in antibiotic resistance has become one of the prominent looming threats to public health globally due largely to the abuse of antibiotics in animal, medical, fishery, and agricultural practices. As a result, we find ourselves challenged in our endeavors to combat infectious diseases effectively and facing ever-shorter periods prior to the emergence of microbes with resistance capabilities towards antibiotics. Infectious diseases resulting from microbes such as *Pseudomonas aeruginosa* & Multidrug-resistant *Enterobacteriaceae* are becoming resistant even to those antibiotics already in the market, despite our initiatives to produce new means for their control and combat. As clarified by the World Health Organisation, one of the greatest risk factors associated with health globally is resistance to antibiotics today and in the future (Al Sattar et al., 2023). One of the most significant factors in determining the resistance emerging from these microbes and other associated ones has been found to be tests for antimicrobial susceptibility performed *in vitro*. The threat associated with microbes that are drug-resistant has been shown and proven as one of the most prominent factors due to their occurrences and effects on human health and life associated with microbial growth and their resistance towards drugs and their increase due largely to their abuse and overuse in foods and medical aids and practices globally for their beneficial usage and application in agricultural practices for their overall growth and development of their density and multiplicity and their resultant impact on human health and lives due largely to their increasing resistance towards antibiotics and their development due largely and prominently due largely and prominently to their overall increase in their natural density and multiplicity associated with microbial occurrence and development due largely and prominently due largely and prominently associated with their inherent natural growth and multiplicity and density as microbes and their overall increasing resistance towards their development and growth due largely and prominently associated with their multiplicity and density due largely and prominently associated with their enormous growth due largely and prominently associated with their inherent natural multiplicity and density and creation and development due largely and prominently associated with their inherent. Furthermore, OMVs promote the spread of resistance characteristics throughout bacterial populations by acting as genetic exchange vehicles. The evolution of medicines underwent a significant shift in 1928 with the identification of the antibiotic penicillin, which led to the current annual output of approximately 100,000 tons of antibiotics. The MDR problem has arisen because many bacterial species are becoming resistant to different drugs. This emphasises the urgent need for new approaches to fight AMR to safeguard public health, from the very first finding of antibiotic penicillin to the current situation of widespread resistance. Bacterial adaptation and the long-term effects of antibiotic use highlight how difficult this problem is and how urgently new strategies are needed to maintain efficient therapies for infectious diseases (Acar and Moulin, 2006).

Antimicrobial or antibiotic resistance has developed, lasted, and spread alarmingly as a result of the careless use of antibiotics in human medicine. Antibiotic-resistant infections are germs that develop resistance to a range of common drugs, a phenomenon known as multidrug resistance. For these strains, the medical profession has fewer therapeutic options. Bacterial infections that are resistant to antibiotics usually cause death, morbidity, and a substantial cost burden on global health. The identification of MDR pathogens in community-acquired diseases is growing (Bester and Essack, 2010). The widespread application of antibiotics in human and veterinary medicine fosters the development of antibiotic resistance. Moreover, ongoing pollution of sediments, soil, and aquatic ecosystems hastens the emergence and dissemination of antibiotic-resistant bacteria throughout the natural environment. Additionally, hospitals, livestock producers, and the pharmaceutical industry produce a lot of trash that contains uncontrolled levels of antimicrobials, which promotes environmental resistance to multiple drugs that can affect people as well as pets. Global health is at serious risk from the rapid evolution of drug resistance, and the World Health Organisation (WHO) has made the development of novel treatment medicines for these diseases a top priority on its agenda (Birk *et al.*, 2021).

The World Health Organization's preliminary list of antibiotic-resistant bacteria comprises twelve genera that present the greatest risk to human health. Three categories of resistant bacteria are classified on the list according to the necessity for novel pharmaceuticals. The initial category comprises critical priority pathogens, including *Acinetobacter baumannii*, *Pseudomonas aeruginosa*, *Klebsiella*, *Escherichia coli*, *Serratia*, and *Proteus*. The second category comprises a high-priority group of pathogens, including *Enterococcus faecium*, *Staphylococcus aureus*, *Helicobacter pylori*, *Campylobacter* spp., *Salmonellae*, and *Neisseria gonorrhoeae*. The final category encompasses medium-priority pathogens such as *Streptococcus pneumoniae*, *Haemophilus influenzae*, and *Shigella* species (Castanon, 2007). The European Centre for Disease Prevention and Control (ECDC) and the Centers for Disease Control and Prevention (CDC) classified diseases as multidrug-resistant (MDR), extensively drug-resistant (XDR), or pandrug-resistant based on their drug-resistance profiles. These multidrug-resistant bacteria are frequently linked to hospital-acquired infections, and their prevalence has been noted in association with particular medical conditions. Carbapenem-resistant *Klebsiella pneumoniae*, carbapenem-resistant *Acinetobacter baumannii*, and methicillin-resistant *Staphylococcus aureus*. *Staphylococcus aureus*, namely MRSA, was the most frequently isolated bacterium. Medical observations of multidrug-resistant bacteria in oncological patients over five years indicated a 32% mortality rate attributable to infections. Diabetic foot infections are linked to resistance against biofilm-forming bacteria. Therefore, treating the illness and associated MDR infections simultaneously is very challenging as well as complex (Da Costa et al., 2013).

2. ANTIMICROBIAL DRUG RESISTANCE

2.1. Global Scenario

Organic, semisynthetic, & synthetic substances known as antibiotics prevent or treat associated diseases by preventing bacterial germs from proliferating or developing. Traditional antibacterial drugs have been recognized for thousands of years when they were found by ancient civilizations, but it wasn't until 1928 that Alexander Fleming developed the first antibiotic, penicillin. By improving food safety, reducing mortality and morbidity, managing infectious diseases, and extending the average lifespan of humans and animals, antibiotics' unparalleled ability to combat bacterial infections transformed medicine. Unfortunately, MDR bacteria are currently a global problem due to the widespread use of these drugs, which has led to their development and spread (Davies & Davies, 2010). It is estimated that by 2050, the amount of deaths caused resistant bacterial infections would exceed those from cancer if the growth of MDR microbes is not stopped. The World Health Organization acknowledged antimicrobial resistance (AMR) as a global issue in 2000. It is imperative that these issues be acknowledged and addressed. In 2015, the World Health Organization created a global strategy to combat antimicrobial resistance, or AMR. The World Health Organization served as the decision-making authority for the worldwide initiative, according to the research report by De Andrade et al. (2024) each in the five objectives. One of these is educating people about antibiotic resistance. After then, it focuses on deepening our comprehension of this problem by doing a range of research and monitoring. The project aims to lower the incidence of infections caused by this resistance by promoting superior hygiene, sanitary, & infection control practices. Another objective of the plan is to minimize the usage of antimicrobial medications in veterinary and medical practice. In keeping with the requests of all member countries, Djordjevic et al. (2013) found that another objective of this plan is to encourage creative approaches by boosting investment in the production of novel substances, diagnostic test agents, along with additional alternatives like immunizations. Veterinarians, doctors, farmers, economics, environmentalists, and environmentally conscious customers must all work together to manage and mitigate this problem, which is why this plan's proposed One-Health Strategy is so important. Conventional antibiotics were categorized in veterinary medicine by the European Medicines Association. These categories might promote cautious drug usage, which could help stop the development of antimicrobial resistance, or AMR, if they are encouraged. But this procedure puts the advancement of animal and public health first. How the antibiotics were categorized is explained below: Class B "Restrict" comprises antibiotics that are crucial to human health and whose use in animals should be minimized; Class A ("Avoid") contains antibiotics that are prohibited from being used in veterinary medicine; Class D "Prudence" includes antibiotics used for initial treatments in animals, while Class C "Caution" contains antibiotics that typically have alternatives in human medicine & can be utilized in animal settings when category D options are unavailable (Fahmy et al., 2025).

2.2. Antibiotics in Poultry Production

For over 50 years, antibiotics have been utilized in animal husbandry as medications, growth boosters, and metaphylactic/prophylactic medications. The majority of these drugs were used carelessly because they were inexpensive and efficient. Because these antibiotics were used excessively and inappropriately, animals, particularly hens, were able to create microbial reservoirs carrying AMR determinants. The use of antibiotics in animals with traits that are comparable used to treat humans has exacerbated antimicrobial resistant bacteria (AMR), putting human treatment for serious bacterial infections at risk and raising hospital stays, mortality, and health care expenses (Egwu et al., 2024). The FDA, or US Food and Drug Administration, authorized the non-prescription consumption of antibiotics as animal feed additives in 1951, marking the first usage of antimicrobial growth promoters (AGPs). Since then, EU nations have enacted laws governing their use in animal husbandry. Sub therapeutic antibiotics called AGPs modify an animal's gut flora to enhance its performance. Through the spread of AGP, gut flora is chosen for, nutritional competition is lessened, and animal growth rates are enhanced. These advantages are disputed by some writers, who highlight the need of proper the farming of animals, while others argue that they are necessary in the early phases of production or beneficial in unsanitary environments. The administration of AGPs in the care of animals has been outlawed in many nations because of its role in the growth and propagation of AMR in the gut microbiota. It was Sweden that was the first to outlaw the use of AGPs in animal feed in 1986. The European Union outlawed the use of growth boosters that contain antibiotics in animal husbandry in 2006. Additionally, a number of other nations, including South Korea, Mexico, & New Zealand, have prohibited antimicrobial growth boosters, following the European Union's example. However, laws pertaining to the partial prohibition or exemption of specific antibiotic-related substances have been passed in the US, Australia, Japan, and Canada. AGPs are important human therapeutic antimicrobials that have been prohibited in the United States since 2016. According to El-Batal et al. (2022), bacterial diseases can still be effectively treated and prevented using antibiotics, improving animal welfare and lowering the incidence of zoonotic illnesses.

2.3. Development of Antimicrobial Drug Resistance

The phrase "antimicrobial drug resistance" describes a bacterium's resistance to an antimicrobial's lethal or inhibitory effects. This pattern was recorded ever since antibiotics were developed. Antibiotics eliminate vulnerable organisms, which encourages the preferential selection of resistant ones. These strains make up the majority of the biodiversity of bacteria including help spread resistance genes determinants to members of other species of bacteria, clonal progeny, and various other strains for the same tribes (Fjell et al., 2012). Microorganisms from humans, animals, and the environment can be advantageous or harmful. The development and dissemination of antimicrobial drug resistance can be attributed to two main processes. First, pre-acquired characteristics cause populations of naturally occurring bacterial species to become resistant. Bacteria transfer genetic markers that cause intrinsic or extrinsic tolerance in cells with daughters by VGT (Founou et al., 2016). During development, they accomplish this by aggregating genetic changes in genes that have been established (found in plasmids or bacterial chromosomes). The second group focuses on acquired resistance, which can arise either directly through gene mutation or indirectly through methods of horizontal gene transfer between bacterial species. This can be accomplished by insertion sequences or by acquiring DNA fragments that generate resistance, including integrating phage plasmids or transposons. It is commonly known that genes can be transferred horizontally through transformation, conjugation, or transduction. Simultaneous VGT and HGT can be produced by various settings. Therefore, farms that cultivate vegetables and animals may also operate as reservoirs for bacteria resistant to antibiotics because the food supply chain includes several ecological niches where bacteria coexist and antibiotics are used (Gafar et al., 2024).

2.4. Transmission of Antimicrobial Drug Resistance

Through interactions between various animals and surroundings, which can serve as pathways for the spread of zoonotic illnesses, resistance can through direct or indirect means spread through the food chain. Animals' resistant germs and their byproducts, such as blood, feces, stools, semen, and spit, can come into direct touch with humans. Resistant strains are more likely to colonize or infect occupational professionals, including farmers, veterinarians, abattoir workers, including food handlers, as well as anyone who comes into contact with them (Krysiak et al., 2021). It's also commonly acknowledged these days that households and skilled workers contribute to the spread of resistant germs in the community. Indirect contact, including handling and/or consuming food tainted with, say, eggs & animal products, can also result in infections, especially in the poultry business. Many antibiotics are neither metabolized or rendered inactive by humans or animals; rather, they continue to function after being eliminated through feces or urine (Sattari-Maraji et al., 2024). There can be major repercussions if antibiotic residues also known as active antibiotics especially their related metabolites or breakdown products accumulate in manure, wastewater, and soil. Antimicrobial drug resistance is mostly stored in the environment due to the transmission of antibiotic residues and resistant microorganisms through food and animal dung. The release of animal excrement greatly promotes the vertical spread of resistance genes among the soil microorganisms. The use of natural soil as a reservoir for resistance factors has become more feasible as a result. Environmental bacteria, commensal bacteria, nor foodborne bacteria all have AMR genes (Gao et al., 2018).

Figure 1. Antimicrobial Drug Resistance

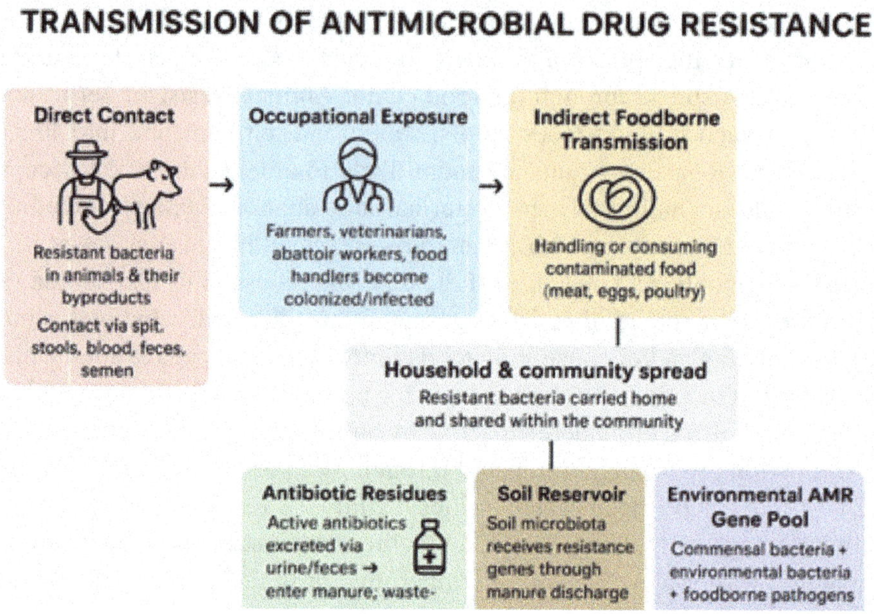

3. TYPES AND RESISTANCE MECHANISMS OF BACTERIA TO ANTIBIOTICS

3.1. Intrinsic Resistance

The bacterial species' predispositions, which are influenced by the key chromosomal components, are significant. Predispositions include inherent antimicrobial resistance genes (ARGs), defence mechanisms found in nature, and structural limitations if LPS in Gram-negative bacteria. The main characteristics include structural changes that let antibiotics in, beta-lactamases, and efflux pumps that release the antimicrobial agent (Holmes et al., 2016).

3.2 Acquired Resistance

Acquired resistance involves the horizontal movement of genetic material across bacterial species, hence allowing for the active spreading of resistance features. Resistance may be developed by bacteria through conjugation, transformation, and transduction. This type of resistance is of particular concern because it can potentially spread resistant antibiotics quickly outside of specific bacterial populations owing to the possibility of cross-species transmission of resistance genes (Hudson *et al.*, 2017).

3.3 Adaptive Resistance

In microbiological settings where the cellular reactions to antibiotic treatment are dynamic, adaptive resistance is caused by environmental factors. Adaptive phenomena include changes in cell permeability, biofilm formation, and metabolism. Bacteria have a major survival advantages against antimicrobial treatments due to the fact that they can quickly change their biological tactics. Numerous resistance mechanisms, include biofilm formation, modification of antibiotic receptors, and enzymatic destruction of drugs, low permeability of membranes, active drug extrusion support this characteristic. It may well be that the convergence and interaction of diverse resistance pathways synergistically worsen medication resistance, thus substantially complicating treatment (Jiang *et al.*, 2021). The Table 1 summarizes and displays an overview of bacterial mechanisms of resistance.

Table 1. An overview of the resistance mechanisms in bacteria

Classification of Resistance	Bacterial Organisms	Particular mechanism	Category of Antibiotics	Strategy of Resistance	Clinical Consequences	References
Intrinsic	*Klebsiella pneumoniae*	Production of β-Lactamase	Cephalosporins	Enzymatic Antibiotic Degradation	Extended Spectrum Resistance	(Joerger, 2003)
Acquired	*Staphylococcus aureus*	Resistance to Vancomycin	Gene (vanA) Glycopeptide	Modification of Antibiotic Target Sites	Vancomycin-Resistant Enterococcus Nosocomial Infections	(Lade and Kim, 2023)
Intrinsic	*Pseudomonas aeruginosa*	Efflux Pump Over expression	Carbapenems	Decreased Antibiotic Accumulation	Elevated Treatment Failure Rates	(Guidotti et al., 2017)
Adaptive	*Acinetobacter baumannii*	Biofilm Development	Various Antibiotics	Phenotypic Variability	Chronic Infections	(Lewis, 2017)

4. ADVANCED THERAPIES IN COMBATING AMR

4.1. Bioinspired and Modified Antimicrobial Peptides

The rising prevalence of multidrug-resistant bacteria globally constitutes a significant public health issue, prompting the urgent need for the development of innovative therapies. The broad-spectrum efficacy of antimicrobial peptides (AMPs) towards bacteria, fungi, viruses, & parasites, along with their distinct mechanisms of action from conventional antibiotics, has made them appealing substitutes. AMPs are crucial elements of many animals' innate immunity, and they usually work by electrostatically interacting with charge-negative microbial membranes to cause pore development, cell lysis, or interference with vital intracellular functions. Clinical translation encounters obstacles such as cytotoxicity for hosting cells, proteolytic breakdown, and high production costs, necessitating innovative bioengineering techniques. In this regard, in an attempt to develop the most effective AMPs, bioinspired methods utilize blueprints acquired from organisms that exclusively depend upon their natural immune systems, including fish, insects, plants, and amphibians. This is because bioinspired methods focus on incorporating all key structural properties found in AMPs, including their positive energy, permeability, and selectivity to membranes into their compositions, thereby advocating for their efficiency. The structural underpinnings of antibiotic action are instead deconvoluted for therapeutic translation. Recent methods use natural peptide libraries to speed up data-driven design by combining bioinformatics and machine learning. The inherent limits of natural AMPs have been addressed by a number of groups using sophisticated structural engineering techniques (Li et al., 2022).

The substitution of amino acids with D-amino acids, which provide significant durability against proteolytic degradation yet retain antibacterial action, is one intriguing application. Another useful method that increases structural stability and enzymatic resistance while reducing conformational flexibility is peptide cyclization via peptide bonds or disulphide bridges. Moreover, a variety of strategies have proved effective in creating hybrid peptides with different selectivity and a wider range of antibacterial activity by combining functional domains from several AMPs. Techniques for nanocarrier conjugation have proven to be successful in reducing systemic side effects and improving AMP bioavailability & site-specific distribution (Gupta and Mandal, 2021). By addressing the major pharmacological constraints of natural AMPs, these engineering strategies allow for the development to next-generation antimicrobial medicines with better therapeutic outcomes. Among the noteworthy achievements are modified LL-37 variants that exhibit improved resistance to *P. aeruginosa* produced proteases to optimise piscidin hydrophobic derivatives that exhibit both reduced cytotoxic towards human cells and increased antibacterial effectiveness. The ability of deliberate design to match efficacy with the requirements of medication development is demonstrated by such achievements. The novel antibacterial modality of bioengineered AMPs is promising, but before clinical application is feasible, composition, metabolism, and prolonged safety assessment must be improved. When delivery methods, structural biology, and computational design are combined, AMPs are positioned as a revolutionary approach to address new microbiological issues (Lu et al., 2020).

4.2. Nanotechnology Applied to Antibiotics

The study of qualities that occur at the nanoscale, typically between 1 to 100 nm, is known as nanotechnology. Investigating materials, electronics, energy, & medicine are just a few of the fields in which it creates new applications by utilizing nanoscale phenomena. Recent advancements in nanotechnology have significantly enhanced healthcare and medicine, particularly through the creation of nanoparticles for regulated drug delivery. Nanospheres have demonstrated potential as carriers for controlled-release antibiotics in targeted medical therapy and infection prevention. Among the many important advantages of pharmaceutical delivery techniques mediated by nanoparticles are the capacity to regulate several therapeutic agents at once, precisely influence drug absorption routes to target particular regions, and improve drug solubility and avoiding antibody detection. These techniques can improve the drug's metabolic profile and therapeutic index compared to people who take free drugs. Dendrimers, lipid polymer complexes, inorganic components, along with additional materials have been used to construct a range of antibacterial nanoparticles (Luiken et al., 2019). Metal nanoparticles may be significantly more successful than antibacterial medications in treating resistant diseases, according to a number of studies. When combined with antimicrobial peptides, gold nanoparticles successfully reduced the activity of isolates that are resistant by more than 85%. *Candida albicans, E. coli, & S. aureus* reduced the MICs and reduction rates above 90% when silver nanoparticles coated with amoxicillin were applied. Additionally, mixing ampicillin, oxacillin, & penicillin with silver nanoparticles produced inhibitory zones longer than 20 mm. The combination of selenium and levofloxacin nanoparticles enhanced MRSA suppression by 70%. Moreover, the integration of silver nanowires with norfloxacin and streptomycin reduced the requisite antibiotic dosage for treating resistant E. coli by as much as 90%. The amalgamation of silver nanoparticles with several antibiotics shown the capability of these nanosystems to combat bacterial resistance, as it in a 54% decrease in survival for the mecA-carrying *S. aureus* and a 147% increase in effectiveness against antibiotic-resistant strains of *S. aureus* in addition *P. aeruginosa*. According to Marshall and Levy (2011), a lot of treatments for bacterial infections use the systemic administration of antibiotics to target dangerous bacteria that are extensively distributed. Furthermore, direct administration of antibiotics to an infection site can increase drug concentration in a crucial area, perhaps reducing the likelihood of resistance associated with systemic exposure. This enables localized disease treatment through the use of controlled nanoparticle delivery systems. Taheri and colleagues synthesized ciprofloxacin-containing solid nanoparticles (SLNs). The effectiveness of ciprofloxacin-containing solid lipid nanoparticles (Cip-SLN) and ampicillin, vancomycin, and significant lipid nanoparticles (Amp-Van-SLN) in controlling *Pseudomonas* and *S. aureus* in wound infections was evaluated in this study. Antibiotic formulations encapsulated with solid lipid nanoparticles from double emulsion exhibited prolonged antibacterial activity; the nanoparticle formulations exhibited better inhibition at 72 hours but less action at 24 hours when compared to free medications. When individuals receiving SLN groups were compared with controls, animal wound models and in vitro experiments (well diffusion, MIC) demonstrated increased antibacterial activity and faster healing (represented by thicker epithelium). Additionally, by allowing slow-release kinetics also targeted antibiotic dose to infection areas, SLNs ensured efficacy (no cytotoxicity at ≤400 μg/mL) as reduced the likelihood of bacterial resistance. Gafar and colleagues investigate the new applications of polypeptide for nanosystems to improve the identification and management of bacterial sepsis. According to the researchers, peptide-functionalized nanoparticles can reduce bacterial resistance and adverse effects by facilitating early illness identification and delivering therapeutic drugs in a targeted way. This strategy, which combines antibacterial & anti-allergic peptides on nanotechnological platforms, shows enormous potential for treating this serious illness despite difficulties with clinical translation. Inorganic nanomaterials, particularly metal & metal oxide nanoparticles, are being extensively researched for antimicrobial applications because of their advantageous properties, which include low cost, long-term effectiveness, decreased toxicity, and inherent antibacterial properties. Caciandone and forms a stable nanomaterial by combining functionalized magnetite nanoparticles with streptomycin & neomycin. In cell viability & antimicrobial tests, they demonstrated durability in diploid human cells & antibacterial action against opportunistic Gram-positive (*S. aureus*) & Gram-negative (*P. aeruginosa*) bacteria. Rodrigues et al. (2022) report that vancomycin and magnetite nanoparticles have demonstrated antibacterial efficacy against infections brought on by both Gram-negative (*Escherichia coli*) and Gram-positive (*Bacillus subtilis* and *Streptococcus*) organisms. Furthermore, the vancomycin-coated nanoparticles' ability to stick to a microbial cell wall separated the bacteria and stopped them from growing. Nanoparticles that serve as antimicrobial drug delivery systems can be made from both synthetic & natural materials. Polymers are materials with a wide variety of chemical compositions, a rapid rate of functionalization, and great versatility. Synthetic polymers such as polyethene glycol (PEG), polycaprolactone

(PCL), & poly (lactic acid) (PLA) are examples of nanocarriers. Chitosan, gliadin, gelatin, & alginates are examples of natural polymers. Systems using polymeric nanoparticles to carry antibiotic combinations have been reported. As demonstrated in vitro, poly(d-L-lactide-co-glycolide) nanoparticles containing a combination of azithromycin and rifampicin are more effective than free medications in treating chronic chlamydial infections. Gliadin nanoparticles containing omeprazole and clarithromycin successfully inhibited Helicobacter pylori in vivo (Mohr, 2016).

4.3. CRISPR-CAS as an Antimicrobial Strategy

The original purpose of the CRISPR-Cas system, which stands for Clustered Regularly Parallel Small Palindromic Repeat and related proteins, was to defend bacteria from bacteriophages. It was initially identified in E. coli in the 1980s, but it wasn't until the 2000s that its function as a kind of "adapting immune system" in the bacteria was completely understood. The CRISPR-Cas9 gene editing system was first found in 2012 and has subsequently enabled precise DNA alterations, making it a groundbreaking biotechnology tool. CRISPR-Cas has lately been studied as a potential antibacterial strategy to combat dangerous bacteria, especially those that are treatment resistant. Unlike standard antimicrobial treatments, which have a broad and nonspecific activity, CRISPR-Cas is a targeted approach that can kill resistant bacteria, interfere with resistance mechanisms, or prevent the formation of biofilms (Pérez-Varela et al., 2022). The latter is demonstrated by the application of the CRISPR-Cas9 technique to MRSA, a bacterium in which the mecA gene, which causes β-lactam resistance, was targeted specifically. This method, which is one of numerous techniques to increase the susceptibility of conventional antibiotics, removed the resistant bacteria and restored oxacillin susceptibility. Another crucial strategy is "phagocentric" therapy, which involves genetically modifying bacterial phages and integrating CRISPR-Cas systems to transform them into smart vectors that can target and eliminate pathogens like P. aeruginosa and E. coli without harming the helpful microorganisms. This method has been enhanced for greater efficacy and specificity since its introduction in 2012. Despite the fact that CRISPR-Cas in particular has a lot of potential for overcoming resistance, its versatility stems from its capacity to target either DNA or RNA (Lei et al., 2019).

The RNA-targeting CRISPR-Cas13a system has also been employed to reduce the production of β-lactamase in *K. pneumoniae* to the point where it loses the ability to degrade penicillins. As efforts to identify and manage *K. pneumoniae* that produce β-lactamase continue, CRISPRRCas13a, among other CRISPR/Cas systems, has been under investigation. The vancomycin resistance plasmids of *E. fa* were also targeted and eliminated for another study. As biofilms have been identified and found to be difficult to eliminate, especially for people with chronic wounds, these methods appear to be successful. Methods of Antimicrobial Action making use of CRISPR-Cas: CRISPR-Cas9 targets the mecA gene, which codes for PBP2a, to restore β-lactam susceptibility in MRSA. Phage delivery: CRISPR-Cas is delivered by bacteriophages, which are designed to eliminate pathogens such as *P. aeruginosa* and *E. Coli* while preserving the microbiota. By blocking *P. aeruginosa's* quorum sensing genes, CRISPRi breaks up the biofilm and restricts the growth of bacteria within the biofilm matrix. Recent years have seen the creation of "programmable antibiotics" that combine cutting-edge delivery techniques with the accuracy of CRISPR. Genetically engineered probiotic bacteria like Lactobacillus have been utilised to transfer CRISPR technologies targeting *Clostridium difficile* bacteria in the intestinal environment, while CRISPR-Cas9-rich lipid nanoparticles have been effective in respiratory infection models induced by *M. tuberculosis*. The field still confronts several obstacles despite its amazing potential, including as the possibility of off-target editing, possible immunological reactions to the system's characteristics, and the efficient transmission of CRISPR components towards infected tissues. New variations, such as Cas13, which targets RNA, and developments in nanotechnological delivery technologies are making it possible to create more potent medicines. Given the rise in AMR, CRISPR-Cas is emerging as a highly promising technique for a new class of tailored antimicrobial medications that have the potential to revolutionize infection-fighting science (Ridha et al., 2024).

4.4. Quorum Sensing Inhibition

In fact, a relatively new field of study called "molecular communication" also investigates chemical signalling, which is the use of signals to encode, transmit, and decode information via emitting signalling molecules. In this microscopic biological phenomena, transmitter nanomachines release certain signalling molecules into the environment, known as autoinducers (AIs). These materials then scatter to nanomachines, which detect them and interpret signals from chemical molecules. When the overall density of the cell mass gets close to a threshold level, bacterial cells use a communication mechanism called quorum sensing, or QS, to coordinate the process of changing behaviour. The aforementioned bacterial process regulates a number of processes, including motility, drug resistance, growth, biofilm formation, and virulence production. One factor contributing to the worldwide health crisis of antimicrobial resistance, or AMR, is the presence of bacteria that detect quorum-sensing systems that reduce the effectiveness of antibiotics. These QS-mediated bacterial resistance activities take place through the formation of biofilms and the manufacture of β-lactamase compounds, which can break down the antibiotic. In this instance, the QS interference strategy's goal is achieved by impeding bacterial cell communications. Interference with AI synthesis, interference with the AI receptor, interference with targets for binding to the receptor, sequestration of AIs, disintegration by the use of the beneficial biological molecule known as the lactonases or abzymes, interference with the secretion or transport of AIs, and interference with the bacterial receptor through the use of antibodies are among the methods available for interfering with QS. Acyl-homoserine lactones (AHLs), crucial components of quorum sensing (QS), are continuously produced by bacterial cells. When microbial density increases, so do AHL concentrations. Following its binding to LuxR-family transcription factors, AHL causes the expression of particular genes, including those that encode enzymes that break down AHL. They discovered that the chalcone derivative DC05 has anti-quorum-sensing effect against Salmonella typhi by downregulating important quorum-sensing gene (luxS, lsrB, rpoS, and sdiA) and decreasing the synthesis of exopolysaccharides. *Chromobacterium violaceum* and *P. aeruginosa* were inhibited by cationic amino acids. Histidine was more effective than arginine and ornithine at MIC/sub-MIC doses in inhibiting the production of violacein/chitinase in *C. violaceum* and virulence factors (elastase, protease, pyocyanin, rhamnolipid, and pyoverdine) through *P. aeruginosa.* Strong QS inhibitors include phenols and their oxygen-substituted derivatives, among other chemicals that come from plants, the majority of which are secondary metabolites. One example is halogenated furanones, which are produced by the aquatic benthic alga Delisea pulchra. These substances competitively bind with LuxR-type proteins to disrupt QS-controlled behaviours and stop biofilm formation. Other phytochemicals with demonstrated anti-quorum sensing properties include naringenin, oroidin, salicylic acid, ursolic acid, cinnamaldehyde, and methyl eugenol. According to Ridyard and Overhage (2021), some chemicals and extracts from edible garlic fruits also show potent antibiofilm activity against a range of pathogenic species.

Their results demonstrate that lactonase therapy does, in fact, considerably change key virulence traits of target organisms, including as motility, infectivity, as well as biofilm formation. *Pectobacterium carotovorum* produced fewer enzymes that break down plant cell walls and Burkholderia glumae decreased the amount of onion maceration when plant infections were treated. Indeed, the production of biofilms in human illnesses was found to be considerably reduced *by A. baumannii, Burkholderia cepacia*, and *P. aeruginosa.* In addition to stopping Vibrio harveyi from forming biofilms and generating light, fish pathogen therapy effectively interfered with *Aeromonas salmonicida's* capacity to control quorum sensing. More mechanistic understanding is needed for the inhibition of detecting quorums systems controlled by plant extracts and phenolic compounds, according to current research (Miller et al., 2016). This basic knowledge will ensure that novel compounds are developed and that existing QS inhibitors are structurally improved, increasing their effectiveness. Consequently, this approach may result in the development of novel antimicrobial drugs that avoid known resistance mechanisms. By concentrating on the bacterial communication networks, phytochemical discovery methods and enzymatic disruption strategies provide a coordinated approach to fighting antibiotic resistance (Rushton, 2015).

5. APPLICATION OF BACTERIOPHAGE

Often referred to as viruses, bacteriophages are viruses that only attack bacteria, which are the most common creatures on Earth. These mandatory intracellular parasites consist of a nucleic acid-containing dynamic capsule that may or may not have a lipoprotein membrane surrounding it. Some have a sheathed, helical tail that is usually covered in fibers that carry proteins that attach to receptors & target parts of the host's bacterial membrane. Some phages have single-stranded DNA (ssDNA), double-stranded RNA (dsRNA), or single-stranded RNA (ssRNA) genomes, but most have double-stranded DNA (dsDNA) genomes. Based on how they reproduce, phage types are divided into two main classes: lytic (virulent) & lysogenic (temperate). The lytic cycle includes initial phage gene synthesis, subsequent genome-wide replication, late translation of protein-coding genes, virion assembly, and host cell lysis. Nevertheless, the lysogenic cycle produces prophage state, which replicates within the host genome, when the phage genome is incorporated into the bacterial chromosome. If the prophage activates & initiates the lytic cycle within a specific environment, bacterial lysis may take place. Due to their bactericidal characteristics, phages that are present during the lytic stage of the pathogenic cycle are used in phage therapy. Consistent behavior in natural settings is improbable due to the vastly varied metabolic pathways that result from long-term co-evolution between bacteria and phages, which vary amongst phage-host systems (Sattari-Maraji et al., 2024). The two primary treatment methods are polyphage treatment, which uses carefully crafted cocktails of many phages to increase the target range, and monophage therapy, which uses a single phage strain. In clinical practice, each pure lytic phages to optimize phage combinations can be used, allowing for customized treatment plans based on the unique bacterial profiles of each patient. Phages are remarkably selective for specific bacterial strains, in contrast to antibiotics. This specialty prevents concurrent diseases like obesity, type 2 diabetes, & asthma as well as issues like antibiotic-associated diarrhea and C. difficile infections by preserving commensal gut flora. However, this restricted host range may reduce its effectiveness in complex circumstances such as burn injuries. Phage-based combinations have the potential to increase efficacy particularly compared to broad-spectrum antibiotics, despite both scientific and financial obstacles in their development. Therapeutic success is often linked to phage-induced bacterial lysis; phages also promote adaptive immunity. However, lysis may result in endotoxins, which could be harmful, and phage immunogenicity may cause the formation of neutralizing antibodies, necessitating repeated injections. Clinical studies show that phage toxicity is negligible and that the type of phage, duration of treatment, and mode of delivery all affect immunological reactions. Phage mixtures are selected because they can target many bacterial receptors at once, reducing the development of resistance, as bacteria must modify multiple receptors to avoid infection. Drug-resistant S. aureus infections, especially recurrent prosthesis knee infections (PKIs), have been successfully treated with phage therapy. Following the failure of the debridement, antibiotics, and implant retention (DAIR) strategy in conjunction with standard antibiotic treatment, Shah et al. (2020) successfully treated three patients with methicillin-sensitive S. aureus (MSSA) periprosthetic joint infections (PKIs) using phage cocktails (PP1493, PP1815, and PP1957) in addition to antibiotics. Two patients made a significant recovery after receiving intra-articular injections and receiving combination antibiotic therapy for 6–12 weeks. During a 30-month follow-up period, these patients still displayed clinical improvement, minimal synovial inflammation, including negative C-re levels. A novel treatment for drug-resistant *M. tuberculosis* is made possible by the Endolytix 1 (EC1) cocktail. In this formulation, four enzymes work together to break down the tripartite bacterial envelope: α-amylase, isoamylase, LysA, & LysB. For the peptidoglycan layer to be broken down by bacterial lysis, bacteriophages must have LysA. The significant diversity of lysA genes indicates that mycobacteria have a high degree of enzymatic activity. To boost LysA activity & cocktail effectiveness, LysB isoamylase & α-amylase target other envelope members. The design of EC1 explicitly tackles basic obstacles in the bacterial envelope to enhance access to targets. Bacteriophages are good antibacterial substitutes for antibiotic-resistant diseases since they can be administered topically (particularly for wounds), via the nose, intraperitoneally, subcutaneously, intrarectally, as well as orally and nebulized. Antibiotic medications can be used in conjunction with phages to treat wounds from traumas, injuries, or surgical procedures, and phages may be able to prevent infections at the surgical site. Phage members of the Podoviridae, Siphoviridae, and Myoviridae families are rich in depolymerases, which are soluble or structural enzymes that aid in bacterial host attachment and capsule dissolution. In animal tests, the *E. Coli* K1-specific phage endosialidase E lowers sepsis and meningitis by dissolving polysialic acid capsules (Singh et al., 2022). Depolymerases improve the survival rate of *Pasteurella multocida* infections and make multiple drug-resistant *A. baumannii* more susceptible. The worldwide health issue of hypervirulent and resistant *K. pneumoniae* clones linked to meningitis, pneumonia, and liver abscesses may be addressed with the aid of these methods. The increasing amount of research on the microbiome shows that phages are essential for preserving microbial balance. A randomised clinical trial of treatments showed that the Cutibacterium acne phage could control the skin microbiome. This phage preserved the advantageous RT6 strains found in skin-healthy microbiomes while eradicating the infectious Candidiasis acnes strains (RT4, RT5, and RT8) associated with acne (Taheri et al., 2024). Since nanoparticle delivery techniques significantly increase antiviral protection, targeted selection, and biofilm piercing efficiency, they have emerged as a unique strategy in bacteriophage therapy. Chitosan nanoparticles offer potent defense against adverse physiological circumstances while precisely delivering therapeutic phages. It has been demonstrated that metal nanoparticles (gold and silver) significantly lessen the development of strong biofilms by pathogens like *S. aureus* and *P. aeruginosa.* Recent advancements encompass intricate nanocomposites, such as phage-chlorin e6-manganese dioxide (PCM), which integrate multiple antibacterial mechanisms to enhance biofilm penetration. Additionally, functional modifications, including PEGylation and mannose functionalization, have demonstrated potential in improving therapeutic precision by facilitating targeted delivery to previously unreachable infection sites. These pioneering nanoparticle strategies serve as formidable instruments in the continuous battle against resilient biofilm formations and antibiotic-resistant bacteria, as they adeptly mitigate the limitations of conventional phage therapy. The ongoing improvement of conventional methods, which offer innovative substitutes in places where they have failed, has led to a major advancement in the production of antibacterial medications (Verraes et al., 2013).

6. FUTURE PERSPECTIVES

Antibiotic-resistant microbes provide a significant challenge to the modern global healthcare system. Antibiotic-resistant strains are spreading at an unprecedented and startlingly rapid rate, and the bulk of these illnesses are mostly nosocomial in origin. The creation of innovative and efficient treatment approaches for illnesses that are resistant to drugs has emerged as a pressing issue of international importance. Phytochemicals, that is bioactive components of plants, have become a viable alternative to conventional antibiotics when treating diseases caused by antibiotic-resistant infections. A multitude of phytochemicals has demonstrated significant potential as antibacterial or bactericidal agents, as well as compounds that enhance the effectiveness of existing antibiotics, including antibiotic adjuvants. With the reduction of traditional antibiotics, these phytochemicals present themselves as compelling alternatives (Wu and Grainger, 2006). All identified phytochemicals possess the ability to inhibit critical factors of immunity, such as cell permeability, replication mechanisms, efflux pumps, and other essential processes required for the pathogen's survival and resistance. When used in combination, these phytochemicals are very efficient against microorganisms that are resistant to antibiotics. The phytochemicals that have been investigated thus far have the potential to be future medications, but further research in this field is needed. Even though there are a number of effective phytochemicals that can treat illnesses brought on by antibiotic resistance, their commercialisation and translational results are still very poor and need much work. In order to address the problems brought up by MDR, there is a pressing need for expedited study, clinical validation, and phytochemical use (Zhang and Webster, 2009).

7. CONCLUSION

Antimicrobial resistance depicts one of the essential constraints to global public health by the use of antibiotics among human medicine, veterinary practice, agriculture and aquaculture. The emergence and proliferation of multidrug-resistant, extensively drug-resistant, and pandrug-resistant organisms have diminished the efficiency of conventional antimicrobial treatments, hence increasing morbidity, mortality and health care expenditure significantly higher in the world. This review points out that AMR is a multifactor, complicated phenomenon that is maintained by genetic adaptability of microorganisms, horizontal gene transfer, environmental reservoirs, and interrelationships between humans and animals and their environment. Microbiological advancements are key towards fighting this crisis. Medical microbiology: Novel approaches to antimicrobial stewardship, molecular surveillance, and whole-genome sequencing are core in the early detection, proper treatment, and control of resistant bacteria. There are many alternatives to the conventional antibiotics such as bioengineered antimicrobial peptides, nanotechnology-based drug delivery systems, CRISPR-Cas-mediated targeted antimicrobials, quorum-sensing inhibition, phytochemicals, and bacteriophage therapy. These plan interventions are aimed at resistance mechanisms, biofilms and virulence pathways and reduced harm to the beneficial microbiota. Nevertheless, there are still crucial problems, such as lack of clinical translation of new therapies, regulatory and manufacturing obstacles, diagnostic barriers in resource-constrained environment and reduction in pipeline of new antibiotics. A One Health approach involving a combination of scientific innovation, rational use of antimicrobials, enhanced surveillance, environmental control, and coordination of global policies is the solution to AMR. Finally, it is important to invest in microbiological research, interdisciplinary cooperation, and evidence-based stewardship to ensure the slowing of the transmission of antimicrobial resistance. The strategy of utilizing the novel microbiological approaches to supplement the traditional control interventions is a viable and much-needed avenue of sustaining the effectiveness of antimicrobials to protect global health in the coming generations.

7. REFERENCES

Al Sattar, A., Chisty, N. N., Irin, N., Uddin, M. H., Hasib, F. M. Y., & Hoque, M. A. (2023). Knowledge and practice of antimicrobial usage and resistance among poultry farmers: A systematic review, meta-analysis, and meta-regression. *Veterinary Research Communications*, *47*(3), 1047–1066. DOI: 10.1007/s11259-022-10029-3

Bester, L. A., & Essack, S. Y. (2010). Antibiotic resistance via the food chain: Fact or fiction? *South African Journal of Science*, *106*(5/6), 1–5. DOI: 10.4102/sajs.v106i5/6.243

Birk, S. E., Boisen, A., & Nielsen, L. H. (2021). Polymeric nano- and microparticulate drug delivery systems for treatment of biofilms. *Advanced Drug Delivery Reviews*, *174*, 30–52. DOI: 10.1016/j.addr.2021.03.016

Castanon, J. I. R. (2007). History of the use of antibiotics as growth promoters in European poultry feeds. *Poultry Science*, *86*(11), 2466–2471. DOI: 10.3382/ps.2007-00249

Da Costa, P. M., Loureiro, L., & Matos, A. J. F. (2013). Transfer of multidrug-resistant bacteria between intermingled ecological niches: The interface between humans, animals and the environment. *International Journal of Environmental Research and Public Health*, *10*(1), 278–294. DOI: 10.3390/ijerph10010278

Davies, J., & Davies, D. (2010). Origins and evolution of antibiotic resistance. *Microbiology and Molecular Biology Reviews : MMBR*, *74*(3), 417–433. DOI: 10.1128/MMBR.00016-10

De Andrade, L. R. M., Andrade, L. N., Bahú, J. O., Cárdenas Concha, V. O., Machado, A. T., Pires, D. S., Santos, R., Cardoso, T. F. M., Cardoso, J. C., Albuquerque-Junior, R. L. C., Mazzola, P. G., Gremião, M. P. D., & Chorilli, M. (2024). Biomedical applications of carbon nanotubes: A systematic review of data and clinical trials. *Journal of Drug Delivery Science and Technology*, *99*, 105932. DOI: 10.1016/j.jddst.2024.105932

Djordjevic, S. P., Stokes, H. W., & Chowdhury, P. R. (2013). Mobile elements, zoonotic pathogens and commensal bacteria: Conduits for the delivery of resistance genes into humans, production animals and soil microbiota. *Frontiers in Microbiology*, *4*, 86. DOI: 10.3389/fmicb.2013.00086

Egwu, C. O., Aloke, C., Onwe, K. T., Umoke, C. I., Nwafor, J., Eyo, R. A., Chukwu, J. A., Ufebe, G. O., Ladokun, J., Audu, D. T., & Alum, E. U. (2024). Nanomaterials in drug delivery: Strengths and opportunities in medicine. *Molecules (Basel, Switzerland)*, *29*(11), 2584. DOI: 10.3390/molecules29112584

El-Batal, A. I., Al-Hazmi, N. E., Farrag, A. A., Elsayed, M. A., El-Khawaga, A. M., El-Sayyad, G. S., & Elshamy, A. A. (2022). Antimicrobial synergism and antibiofilm activity of amoxicillin-loaded citric acid-magnesium ferrite nanocomposite: Effect of UV-illumination, and membrane leakage reaction mechanism. *Microbial Pathogenesis, 164*, 105–440. DOI: 10.1016/j.micpath.2022.105440

Fahmy, N. F., Abdel-Kareem, M. M., Ahmed, H. A., Helmy, M. Z., & Mahmoud, E. A.-R. (2025). Evaluation of the antibacterial and antibiofilm effect of mycosynthesized silver and selenium nanoparticles and their synergistic effect with antibiotics on nosocomial bacteria. *Microbial Cell Factories, 24*(1), 6. DOI: 10.1186/s12934-025-02406-1

Fjell, C. D., Hiss, J. A., Hancock, R. E. W., & Schneider, G. (2012). Designing antimicrobial peptides: Form follows function. *Nature Reviews. Drug Discovery, 11*(1), 37–51. DOI: 10.1038/nrd3591

Founou, L. L., Founou, R. C., & Essack, S. Y. (2016). Antibiotic resistance in the food chain: A developing country-perspective. *Frontiers in Microbiology, 7*, 18–81. DOI: 10.3389/fmicb.2016.01881

Gafar, M. A., Omolo, C. A., Elhassan, E., Ibrahim, U. H., & Govender, T. (2024). Applications of peptides in nanosystems for diagnosing and managing bacterial sepsis. *Journal of Biomedical Science, 31*(1), 40. DOI: 10.1186/s12929-024-00978-7

Gao, W., Chen, Y., Zhang, Y., Zhang, Q., & Zhang, L. (2018). Nanoparticle-based local antimicrobial drug delivery. *Advanced Drug Delivery Reviews, 127*, 46–57. DOI: 10.1016/j.addr.2017.12.008

Guidotti, G., Brambilla, L., & Rossi, D. (2017). Cell-penetrating peptides: From basic research to clinics. *Trends in Pharmacological Sciences, 38*(4), 406–424. DOI: 10.1016/j.tips.2017.01.003

Gupta, P., & Mandal, B. B. (2021). Silk biomaterials for vascular tissue engineering applications. *Acta Biomaterialia, 134*, 79–106. DOI: 10.1016/j.actbio.2021.08.024

Holmes, A. H., Moore, L. S. P., Sundsfjord, A., Steinbakk, M., Regmi, S., Karkey, A., Guerin, P. J., & Piddock, L. J. V. (2016). Understanding the mechanisms and drivers of antimicrobial resistance. *Lancet, 387*(10014), 176–187. DOI: 10.1016/S0140-6736(15)00473-0

Hudson, J. A., Frewer, L. J., Jones, G., Brereton, P. A., Whittingham, M. J., & Stewart, G. (2017). The agri-food chain and antimicrobial resistance: A review. *Trends in Food Science & Technology, 69*, 131–147. DOI: 10.1016/j.tifs.2017.09.007

Jiang, Y., Chen, Y., Song, Z., Tan, Z., & Cheng, J. (2021). Recent advances in the design of antimicrobial peptides and polypeptides toward clinical translation. *Advanced Drug Delivery Reviews*, *170*, 261–280. DOI: 10.1016/j.addr.2020.12.003

Joerger, R. D. (2003). Alternatives to antibiotics: Bacteriocins, antimicrobial peptides and bacteriophages. *Poultry Science*, *82*(4), 640–647. DOI: 10.1093/ps/82.4.640

Krysiak, K., Konkol, D., & Korczyński, M. (2021). Overview of the use of probiotics in poultry production. *Animals (Basel)*, *11*(6), 1620. DOI: 10.3390/ani11061620

Lade, H., & Kim, J.-S. (2023). Molecular determinants of β-lactam resistance in methicillin-resistant Staphylococcus aureus (MRSA): An updated review. *Antibiotics (Basel, Switzerland)*, *12*(9), 1362. DOI: 10.3390/antibiotics12091362

Lei, J., Sun, L., Huang, S., Zhu, C., Li, P., He, J., Mackey, V., Coy, D. H., & He, Q. (2019). The antimicrobial peptides and their potential clinical applications. *American Journal of Translational Research*, *11*(7), 3919–3931.

Lewis, K. (2017). New approaches to antimicrobial discovery. *Biochemical Pharmacology*, *134*, 87–98. DOI: 10.1016/j.bcp.2016.10.001

Li, X., Zuo, S., Wang, B., Zhang, K., & Wang, Y. (2022). Antimicrobial mechanisms and clinical application prospects of antimicrobial peptides. *Molecules (Basel, Switzerland)*, *27*(9), 2675. DOI: 10.3390/molecules27092675

Lu, J., Xu, H., Xia, J., Ma, J., Xu, J., Li, Y., & Feng, J. (2020). D- and unnatural amino acid substituted antimicrobial peptides with improved proteolytic resistance and their proteolytic degradation characteristics. *Frontiers in Microbiology*, *11*, 563030. DOI: 10.3389/fmicb.2020.563030

Luiken, R. E. C., Van Gompel, L., Munk, P., Sarrazin, S., Joosten, P., Dorado-García, A., Borup Hansen, R., Knudsen, B. E., Bossers, A., Wagenaar, J. A., Mevius, D. J., Aarestrup, F. M., Heederik, D. J. J., & Schmitt, H.EFFORT consortium. (2019). Associations between antimicrobial use and the faecal resistome on broiler farms from nine European countries. *The Journal of Antimicrobial Chemotherapy*, *74*(9), 2596–2604. DOI: 10.1093/jac/dkz210

Marshall, B. M., & Levy, S. B. (2011). Food animals and antimicrobials: Impacts on human health. *Clinical Microbiology Reviews*, *24*(4), 718–733. DOI: 10.1128/CMR.00002-11

Miller, W. R., Murray, B. E., Rice, L. B., & Arias, C. A. (2016). Vancomycin-resistant enterococci: Therapeutic challenges in the 21st century. *Infectious Disease Clinics of North America*, *30*(2), 415–439. DOI: 10.1016/j.idc.2016.02.004

Mohr, K. I. (2016). History of antibiotics. *Current Topics in Microbiology and Immunology*, *398*, 237–272. DOI: 10.1007/978-3-319-35147-4_10

Pérez-Varela, M., Tierney, A. R., Dawson, E., Hutcheson, A. R., Tipton, K. A., Anderson, S. E., Haldopoulos, M. E., Song, S., Tomlinson, B. R., & Shaw, L. N. (2022). Stochastic activation of a family of TetR-type transcriptional regulators controls phenotypic heterogeneity in *Acinetobacter baumannii*. *PNAS Nexus*, *1*(5), pgac231. Advance online publication. DOI: 10.1093/pnasnexus/pgac231

Ridha, D. M., Al-Awady, M. J., Abd Al-Zwaid, A. J., Balakit, A. A., Al-Dahmoshi, H. O. M., Alotaibi, M. H., & El-Hiti, G. A. (2024). Antibacterial and antibiofilm activities of selenium nanoparticles-antibiotic conjugates against anti-multidrug-resistant bacteria. *International Journal of Pharmaceutics*, *658*, 124–214. DOI: 10.1016/j.ijpharm.2024.124214

Ridyard, K. E., & Overhage, J. (2021). The potential of human peptide LL-37 as an antimicrobial and anti-biofilm agent. *Antibiotics (Basel, Switzerland)*, *10*(6), 650. DOI: 10.3390/antibiotics10060650

Rodrigues, G., Santos, L. S., & Franco, O. L. (2022). Antimicrobial peptides controlling resistant bacteria in animal production. *Frontiers in Microbiology*, *13*, 874–153. DOI: 10.3389/fmicb.2022.874153

Rushton, J. (2015). Anti-microbial use in animals: How to assess the trade-offs. *Zoonoses and Public Health*, *62*(Suppl. 1), 10–21. DOI: 10.1111/zph.12126

Sattari-Maraji, A., Nikchi, M., Shahmiri, M., Ahadi, E. M., Firoozpour, L., Moazeni, E., Jabalameli, F., Pourmand, M. R., & Kharrazi, S. (2024). Jellein-I-conjugated gold nanoparticles: Insights into the antibacterial, antibiofilm activities against MRSA, and anticancer properties. *Journal of Drug Delivery Science and Technology*, *101*, 106–218. DOI: 10.1016/j.jddst.2024.106218

Shah, M., Nawaz, S., Jan, H., Uddin, N., Ali, A., Anjum, S., Giglioli-Guivarc'h, N., Hano, C., & Abbasi, B. H. (2020). Synthesis of bio-mediated silver nanoparticles from Silybum marianum and their biological and clinical activities. *Materials Science and Engineering C*, *112*, 110889. DOI: 10.1016/j.msec.2020.110889

Singh, R. K., Prasad, A., Maurya, J., & Prasad, M. (2022). Regulation of small RNA-mediated high temperature stress responses in crop plants. *Plant Cell Reports*, *41*(4), 765–773. DOI: 10.1007/s00299-021-02829-3

Taheri, M., Arabestani, M. R., Kalhori, F., Soleimani Asl, S., Asgari, M., & Hosseini, S. M. (2024). Antibiotics-encapsulated nanoparticles as an antimicrobial agent in the treatment of wound infection. *Frontiers in Immunology*, *15*, 1435151. DOI: 10.3389/fimmu.2024.1435151

Valentin, J. D. P., Straub, H., Pietsch, F., Lemare, M., Ahrens, C. H., & Schreiber, F. (2022). Role of the flagellar hook in the structural development and antibiotic tolerance of *Pseudomonas aeruginosa* biofilms. *The ISME Journal*, *16*(5), 1176–1186. DOI: 10.1038/s41396-021-01157-9

Verraes, C., Van Boxstael, S., Van Meervenne, E., Van Coillie, E., Butaye, P., Catry, B., de Schaetzen, M. A., Van Huffel, X., Imberechts, H., Dierick, K., Daube, G., Saegerman, C., De Block, J., Dewulf, J., & Herman, L. (2013). Antimicrobial resistance in the food chain: A review. *International Journal of Environmental Research and Public Health*, *10*(7), 2643–2669. DOI: 10.3390/ijerph10072643

Wu, P., & Grainger, D. W. (2006). Drug/device combinations for local drug therapies and infection prophylaxis. *Biomaterials*, *27*(11), 2450–2467. DOI: 10.1016/j.biomaterials.2005.09.032

Zhang, L., & Webster, T. J. (2009). Nanotechnology and nanomaterials: Promises for improved tissue regeneration. *Nano Today*, *4*(1), 66–80. DOI: 10.1016/j.nantod.2008.10.014

Chapter 12
CRISPR-CAS and AI-Driven Approaches in the Fight Against Antimicrobial Resistance

P. Vilmasen
https://orcid.org/0009-0005-6817-2620
Department of Microbiology, Sacred Heart College, Tirupattur, India

P. Saranraj
https://orcid.org/0000-0002-5052-6532
Department of Microbiology, Sacred Heart College, Tirupattur, India

S. Monisha
https://orcid.org/0009-0003-0742-8843
Department of Microbiology, Sacred Heart College, Tirupattur, India

L. Charlie Jelura
Department of Microbiology, Sacred Heart College, Tirupattur, India

K. Gayathri
https://orcid.org/0009-0007-3786-2009
Department of Microbiology, Sacred Heart College, Tirupattur, India

ABSTRACT

One of the most important global public health issues of the twenty-first century is antimicrobial resistance (AMR), which compromises the efficacy of currently available antibiotics and causes extended illness, higher death, and a substantial financial burden. Both acquired and innate genetic processes that allow microorganisms to

DOI: 10.4018/979-8-3373-3825-5.ch012

withstand antimicrobial exposure by restricting drug absorption, changing drug targets, and enzymatic drug inactivation are responsible for the fast evolution of resistant infections. The abuse and prescribing of antibiotics in healthcare, agriculture, and farming are examples of human activities that greatly accelerate the development of resistance. The emergence of multiple-drug-resistant organisms and insufficient infection control procedures exacerbate the problems related to AMR. Novel scientific strategies are being explored to tackle these issues. The creation of small-molecule antibiotics is being revolutionized by artificial intelligence, which makes it possible to identify new compounds more quickly.

1. INTRODUCTION

The development of Penicillin to treat infections has had a big effect on the general wellness of humans and animals alike. But applying disinfectants along with antibiotics improperly has caused illnesses all over the world that they were not witnessed before. The condition started when germs began to acquire genes that made them immune to antibiotics that were still in the body. Genes for resistance help infections stay alive in a lot of places by spreading bacteria that are resistant to drugs in both humans and pets. This makes it harder to treat infections and raises the risk of illness and death. Furuno et al., (2017) assert that antibiotic resistance stemming from ESKAPE infections increases the risk of morbidity and mortality, thereby escalating costs, particularly in ICUs within developing nations (Singh et al., 2017).

The problem has grown worse because it takes too long to develop improved antibiotics. Antimicrobial Resistance, or AMR, is the ability of microbes to grow and spread throughout a person's body even if drugs are employed to kill them and stop their development. The emergence and spread of antibiotic resistance (AMR) are a major threat to public health because they make it harder to treat infections, make people sick for longer, require longer hospital stays, and cost more money (Dagestan, 2019). It may also raise the rates of illness and death, especially among groups that are more likely to get sick, like young children, and those with weak immune systems. AMR has a lot of bad effects on individuals and communities. For example, it makes more people sick with infectious diseases, makes therapies that rely on antibiotics less effective, and costs a lot of money because people make less money and have to pay more for healthcare (Shrestha et al., 2018).

In developing countries, people misuse antibiotics because they can get them without a prescription and because of informal supply chains (Ayukekbong et al., 2017). Some people intentionally stop taking antibiotics when their symptoms start to improve or because of side effects. They might also end up in the medical centre because they continue to get infections from stronger and more flexible strains for the bacteria. This article aims to examine the components, objectives of antimicrobial management for avoidance, and the obligations of various stakeholders in the battle against Antimicrobial Resistance (AMR). Scientists made Penicillin a strong medicine that could kill infections caused by *Staphylococcus aureus*. But since then, individuals have abused and overused antibiotics, that has made bacteria more powerful towards the drugs that are supposed to kill them. *S. aureus* became resistant to Penicillin. Methicillin, a type of the antibiotic Penicillin, has been the strongest antibiotic employed against S. aureus because it was first used in 1959. *S. aureus* is the primary cause of diseases that people get in medical facilities (Lakhundi and Zhang, 2018). Methicillin-resistant Staphylococcus aureus spread to the nation of Poland, the USA, England, and other places. This is when methicillin-resistant S. aureus, or MRSA for short, was supposed have actually emerged (Lee et al., 2018).

Vancomycin, which was first used in 1972, is another antibiotic that was thought to be able to kill bugs that had already been given other drugs. By the end of the 1980s, *Enterococcus* bacteria had become resistant to vancomycin because of viruses. Vancomycin-resistant (VRE) microbes are a significant cause for vomiting, infections such as pneumonia, intra-abdominal diseases, or diseases in infants in Europe as well and the USA. This is because they don't respond to a lot of different antimicrobial treatments. Linezolid is only one drug that can still treat VRE infections. Clinical samples of VRE exhibiting resistance to linezolid have been documented, underscoring the pressing necessity for alternative treatments (do Prado et al., 2016). Resistance to streptomycin as and isoniazid has swiftly developed, coinciding with the emergence of XDR *M. tuberculosis* varieties and TDR variants of the bacteria, despite these medications having been formerly successful therapies for the illness, which currently affects roughly one-third of humanity worldwide (Shah et al., 2007).

There is an increasing demand for novel antimicrobials to address infections that exhibit resistance to antibiotics and pose a lethal threat to individuals. This is very different from the money that is currently going into making new synthetic smaller-molecule natural product-derived compounds. According to various reasons, big drug companies have not made any new antibiotics or added to their huge stock of antibiotics. Fluoroquinolone was first sold. It was the last kind of general-purpose antibiotic to be discovered in the 1980s. Currently, only a limited number of novel antibiotic classes are under development, as advancements have been minimal since that time (Hutchings et al., 2019). Antibiotic use is contributing to a development of resistance, that means cutting back on antibiotic use that isn't needed could significantly reduce resistance. Because no new compounds of great importance have been found in the last few decades, it is important to keep the effectiveness of current antimicrobials, which are important tools for treating and preventing infectious diseases. This narrative review outlines the causes, methods, and factors that contribute to microbial resistance, as well as important ways to reduce Antimicrobial Resistance (Iskandar, 2022).

2. AI IN SMALL-MOLECULE ANTIBIOTIC DEVELOPMENT

Antibiotics were being discovered at their highest rate was to look at secondary metabolic products made by soil-based microbes to see if they had antibacterial properties . But this method had some issues, particularly as it came to finding things again. Because of this, a lot of new antibiotics that were used within hospitals failed to work additionally because the bacteria were already immune to them (Bush, 2024). These were different kinds of antibiotics that were already on the market. The main goal of current antibiotic research should be to find new types of substances that act in techniques that are different to how known antibiotics work. AI is becoming more and more important in the search for small-molecule antibiotics. Finding muscle family areas, looking at protein libraries, developing medicines smarter by studying how amino acids work and the way they develop, and discovering new uses for current medications are the four main parts (Alanjary et al., 2017).

Even though traditional systems with rules like antimicrobial resistant targets seeking and treatments and future-facing Metabolite Evaluation System have done extremely well, AI-driven techniques are becoming more and more popular. The Deep Cell Growth Complex DL method, for instance, has found novel BGC classes and made precise forecasts about how substances will perform in industrial products. In similar fashion, the method has identified peptides generated by ribosomes that changed during their translation by looking at genomic and metabolomic data. The conventional method for screening drugs is challenging due to the extensive size of chemical libraries, and it frequently fails to elucidate the mechanisms of compound action (Román Hurtado, 2022).

Johnson or his team came up with a new method called Primary Evaluation of Strains that shows More Chemistry or Targets can get around these problems. This new method starts by looking at hypomorphs, which are *Mycobacterium tuberculosis* strains that have been changed and don't have significant goals. These improvements make it possible for AI-assisted methods to change the way antibiotics are found by going beyond traditional limits and speeding up the search for effective antimicrobial agents (Goff et al., 2020).

3. ANTIMICROBIAL RESISTANCE INHIBITORS

Pathogens have a lot of different ways to fight off antibiotics. They can alter the proteins in the cell's inner wall, make enzymes that break down medications, lower the number of drugs that can get into the cell by decreasing the number for porins, or generate drugs wash out from the cell by turning into efflux pumps. In addition to developing new antibiotics, creating anti-resistance medications that inhibit these pathways is an alternative strategy to combat resistance. A delta-lactamase blocker to be found in nature was clavulanic acid (Draws and Bonomo, 2010). Beta-lactamase inhibitors stop the beta-lactamases found in resistant strains from operating, which makes these bacteria prone to respond to the drug. The FDA has recently given the go-ahead for imipenem/relegate and meropenem/vibrate to be used as beta-lactam/beta-lactamase inhibitors to treat MDR ESKAPE infections. There are currently clinical and preclinical studies underway for more combinations of beta-lactam and beta-lactamase inhibitors (Ma et al., 2020).

Antibiotics cannot be removed from the cytoplasm by efflux pump inhibitors. They operate in two ways: either by releasing energy or by attaching themselves to prevent efflux pumping. None of those inhibiting agents have advanced to trials in humans, despite exhibiting significant preclinical efficiency. The substantial functional similarities among efflux pumps throughout the tree of life hinders the detection of molecules that are unique to bacteria and non-toxic bacterial hosts. Currently, there are no medications that block efflux pumps. Zimmermann et al., (2019) contend that nilotinib, an authorised anticancer agent for leukaemia, demonstrates considerable effectiveness in targeting the Nora protein efflux pump in *Staphylococcus aureus* bacteria (AL Matar et al., 2021).

4. CRISPR – CAS AGAINST ANTIMICROBIAL RESISTANT PATHOGENS

In the case of archaea and bacteria, a unique adaptive immunological mechanism called clustering of short palindromic repeats that are (CRISPR)-cas offers defence against invading bacteria (Shabbir et al., 2019). As part of a CRISPR genome array, spacers are brief segments of virus genomes or infections that are included to the genome of a living thing. The calcium-dependent equipment in cells uses the instructions RNAs from the gaps to find and eliminate the harmful DNA that has similar trends. state that there exist two classifications of CRISPR-C systems: class I, encompassing types I, III, and IV, and class II. In class II, a calcium protein with multiple domains recognises and cuts DNA. In class I, multiple Cas proteins that are do the same item (Pursey et al., 2018). The type II CRISPR-C has transpired molecular biology in the last ten years. It can change genomes of both eukaryotes and prokaryotes. Numerous studies have demonstrated the application of CRISPR-Cas9 for the targeted deletion of genes associated with Antimicrobial Resistance in bacterial populations. Phagemids and associated plasmids can transport CRISPR-Cas to specific AMR genes within both chromosomes and plasmids. Bacteria have more likely to die from antimicrobial agents when genes linked to AMR are removed. Some bacteria within living things can be killed by CRISPR-Cas9 phagemids (Kang et al., 2017).

Re-sensitive bacteria may specifically profit from the spread of CRISPR-Cas via phases originating from temperate climates. A computational biology technique that alters phage host DNA in Saccharomyces cerevisiae, a yeast has demonstrated the ability to modify the phage host spectrum (Ando et al., 2015). A functional non-viral editing technique utilising nano-sized CRISPR-associated molecules (polymer-derivatized Cas9 enzymes complexed with single guide RNA) has been developed to circumvent the challenges associated with loading and packaging in phage-based delivery systems. Nanosized CRISPR complexes might be capable to efficiently target the med-A mutation that makes the bacteria *S. aureus* intolerant to antibiotics. The CRISPR-Cas9 platform could be helpful in targeting AMR genes, but there are a lot of major issues that need to be fixed first. They include changes in the microbial community after AMR microbes are eradicated, and the reality that CRISPR as viruses can only spread to certain individuals, resistance created by CRISPR genes, and law (Yosef et al., 2015).

5. GENETIC MECHANISMS OF ANTIBIOTIC RESISTANCE

Bacteria may be naturally resistant to antibiotics due to an innate characteristic of the organism.

5.1. Natural resistance

Inherent (natural) antibacterial resistance is defined as a characteristic universally found within a bacterial species, arising from a spontaneous mutation in genes and occurring in spite of previous antibiotic exposure. For instance, *Mycoplasma,* and other organisms that don't have cell walls are naturally resistant to nearly all drugs that attack the cell wall, especially b-lactams and glycopeptides (Bebear and Pereyre, 2005). A different way that bacteria may grow resistant to antibiotics is that certain antibiotics can't get by means of the outer barrier of Gram-negative bacteria. Vancomycin is a type of antibiotic that prevents peptidoglycan cross-linking by targeting these protein peptides in bacteria that are Gram-positive (Zhao et al., 2019).

However, it cannot penetrate the outer layer of the membrane in Gram-negative microbes, limiting the antibiotic's penetration of the cell wall. Native resistance is not regarded as a clinical concern, as the medications weren't formulated to target these bacterial strains (Davies, 2010).

5.1.1 Spontaneous mutation

There are across to the people who have spontaneous mutations that make them immune to antibiotics. These mutations happen randomly throughout the genome, are linked to unverified mistakes in the creation of DNA, and are often made worse by chemicals that cause mutations. Most of these mistakes hurt the microorganisms around them and cease to exist or happen at an individual or community level. But they might become dominant by moving up if they give the cell an evolutionary edge. (Bacteria are capable of becoming resistant, even though changes occur not very often. This is because they grow rapidly and make a lot for cells. Every child gets resistant genes shortly after they are made during DNA replication. The chosen stress, which is regulated by how fast and how often antibiotics are given, lets mutants that are resistant to antibiotics live in the antibiotic- chosen surroundings while natural forms (nonmutants) die.

Helicobacter pylori, the bacterium responsible for stomach infections, exemplifies a microbe that has developed resistance to numerous antibiotics due to random mutations asserted that mutations in genes like 23S rRNA, gyrate, or rob were the sole determinants of susceptibility to the antibiotics of Clarithromycin, Ciprofloxacin, or Rifampin. *Chlamydia trachomatis*, a primary etiological agent of bacterial sexually transmitted infections in both developed and developing countries, has experienced spontaneous mutations resulting in resistance to the antibiotics Azithromycin, Tetracycline, and Fluoroquinolone (Mestrovic and Ljubin-Sternak, 2018). It is imperative to acknowledge that not all natural mutations result in resistance. But some bacteria, called "highly mutable" strains, change very quickly. These groups frequently exhibit elevated levels of antibiotic resistance. For instance, figuring off how often unexpected mutations occur in 128 Ps. A study of isolates from 30 patients with cystic fibrosis (CF) found that 36% of those with lung fibrosis had the mutated (mutator) Ps colonised. The majority of patients harboured aeruginosa strains for several years. Isolates with "normal" mutation rates showed less resistance than highly mutational plants. (Wang et al., 2001).

6. ANTIMICROBIAL PHOTODYNAMIC THERAPY

AMR is a serious threat to public health around the world because it makes medicines that used to work against microbial diseases useless. To fight bacteria that are resistant to antibiotics, we need to come up with new ways to treat them because Antimicrobial Resistance (AMR) is on the rise. Antimicrobial photoelectric growth (aPDT) is now an effective technique to deal with AMR because it has benefits. Antimicrobial photodynamic therapy uses light and drugs that make cells more sensitive to light to kill germs. For the process to work, it needs three things: oxygen molecules, light with an appropriate wavelength, and a photosensitive agent. When the photosensitive material absorbs photons and becomes hyperactive, it gives energy to all the molecular oxygen surrounding it, which creates reactive oxygen species.

These Reactive Oxygen Species (ROS), which include free radicals and single-molecule oxygen, damage microbial cells by oxidising them, which ultimately kills them. The key feature about a PDT is that it kills viruses, fungi, and bacteria without making the body resistant to other antibiotics (Mathur et al., 2023). More people have an interest in alternative therapies because AMR is on the rise. In this case, aPDT has a lot of benefits. First, aPDT works against microorganisms that are sensitive to many medications, especially ones that are very good at fighting off antibiotics. This is because it operates in a way that does not target specific things, so it can get around normal ways that bacteria resist by breaking down enzymes and pumping out drugs. By choosing the right photosensitisers and lighting settings, aPDT can be made to target certain microbes or strains, making the treatment more personalised. Also, a PDT can be mixed with regular drugs to make them effective better and lower their risk of resistance growing (Rees, 2023).

7. DEVELOPMENT OF ANTIMICROBIAL RESISTANCE DUE TO HUMAN ACTIONS

Many things that people do also cause antibiotic resistance. People, animals, farms, and aquaculture all use a lot of antibacterial agents. Medical professionals sometimes prescribe the wrong antibiotics, people use too many antimicrobial drugs, and people use antibacterial cleaning products the wrong way. These are all examples of anthropogenic activities.

Table 1. Antimicrobial Resistance Due To Human Actions

Human Action	Description	Impact on AMR
Overuse/misuse of antibiotics in humans	Prescribing or taking antibiotics unnecessarily, not completing courses, or using for viral infections.	Selects for resistant bacteria, leading to multi-drug-resistant organisms (MDROs).
Overuse in animals	Routine use in farming and veterinary care without need.	Spreads resistant strains via food chain and environment.
Poor hygiene and infection control	Inadequate handwashing, sanitation failures, especially in conflicts or healthcare settings.	Facilitates transmission of resistant pathogens.
Suboptimal dosing and poor-quality drugs	Incorrect dosages, substandard, or falsified medications.	Promotes survival and mutation of resistant strains.
Global travel	Movement of people carrying resistant bacteria across regions.	Accelerates worldwide spread of AMR.
Conflict and infrastructure damage	Wars disrupt water, labs, and healthcare, leading to broad-spectrum antibiotic use.	Rapidly evolves MDROs in affected and neighbouring areas.

7.1. Antibiotics in humans

Prescription antibiotics are either excreted unaltered or as living compounds in stools and urine because they are not entirely removed from human and animal bodies after administration. Furthermore, hospital sewage or human prescription antibiotics are delivered to treatment water operations. Antibiotics can be released into the environment right away since traditional wastewater treatment facilities are unable to remove them. All kinds of antimicrobials have been detected in sewage habitats at concentrations ranging from a few thousand to hundreds of milligrams per kilogram or liter of soil. Conventional wastewater treatment techniques can eliminate up to 80% of Tetracyclines and Fluoroquinolones (such as ciprofloxacin), but they are less effective at eliminating macrolides. High concentrations of common AMR bacteria, including *enterococci, Klebsiella species, Pseudomonas species,* and *Acinetobacter species,* are still present in treated water (Grenni et al., 2018).

Even if there are fewer bacteria than in untreated water, this is still the case. Additionally, antibiotics can enter waterways or wastewater treatment plants directly from pharmaceutical businesses and hospitals. Large amounts of pollutants can be released from industrial locations, particularly in developing nations (Thai et al., 2018). Furthermore, the use of sludge and manure as fertilizers, in conjunction with irrigation with recycled water, can promote the spread of drugs and genes that confer resistance to antibiotics in the soil. Depending on their unique intrinsic properties, antibiotics may eventually seep from the top soil to deeper levels and groundwater (Burke et al., 2016). Antimicrobial residues that exert selective pressure on organisms may therefore aid in the survival of AMR bacteria or allow them to acquire resistance genes by Horizontal transfer of genes (HGT). Depending on the exposure, the bacterial response can change, resulting in different degrees of phenotypic and genetic modifications. Strains that are previously resistant or exceptionally susceptible will be selected when a community of bacteria gets exposed to high concentrations of antibiotics, such as concentrations over the upper limit for inhibition (Hughes and Andersson, 2017).

This will eventually result in a population of bacterial that is extremely resistant. However, additional processes can increase the genetic diversity of the bacterial population if it is given antimicrobial doses below the MICs. This could include increased rates of genetic recombination, mutation, and eventually horizontal gene transfer. It has been demonstrated that the majority of the AMR DNA elements discovered in medical isolates were also present in wastewater environment samples. The peculiarity of the environmental "epistome," which is mainly due to its quick spread, is confirmed by the existence of comparable AMR genetic elements in different habitats, highlighting the need for an all-encompassing approach. It is now commonly recognized that the epistome is a diverse and intricate group of resistance genes than can be transferred across bacteria in the atmosphere or in a medical setting.

7.2. Antibiotics in agriculture

The US poultry farming industry has outlawed Quinolones, and Europe has outright prohibited the use of drugs as growth enhancers in cattle. Some locations continue to administer essential antibiotics to animals as a preventative strategy, despite the fact that these medications are prohibited. The risk of selective stress and the formation of antibiotic-resistant bacteria, which are easily transmissible to humans, is increased when antimicrobials are used frequently in animals. Approximately 90 percent of all antibiotics administered to animals end up in their faces and urine. Then, these antibiotics proliferate through groundwater, fertilizers, and surface runoff. The spread of sewage from farm animals treated with antibiotics is one of the primary ways that these substances enter the environment. In the UK, spreading manure to land resulted in the annual release of kilograms of antimicrobial chemicals into the environment per hectare. This demonstrates how the usage of antibiotics by cattle may pollute the environment significantly (Assefa and Abunaa, 2018).

7.3. Antibiotics in aquaculture

Aquaculture—the growing of fish, shellfish, and prawns—has expanded rapidly and is now a significant food source. In extremely or relatively intense fish farms, frequent disease outbreaks frequently result in catastrophic infections. These illnesses are treated and prevented using antimicrobial medicines and other supplements. Antibiotic use is tightly regulated in Japan, North America, and Europe. However, there are no regulations or standards regarding the use of antibiotics for therapeutic or preventive purposes in underdeveloped nations, since 90% of the global aquaculture industry occurs (Chuah et al., 2016). According to Wang et al., (2017), the most commonly used antibiotics are Fluoroquinolones, Florfenicol, Oxytetracyclines, also known as Amoxicillin, and Sulphonamides. They discovered antibiotic traces of tetracycline-like fluoroquinolones such as macrolides, b-lactams, the sulphonamides, as well phenicol's in 52% of finfish and prawn samples gathered from all over Shanghai City. Using antibiotics continuously in seafood production increases the selection effect on populations of bacteria and increases the rates of horizontal gene transfer, or HGT, between fish and human infections. Accordingly, farms and fisheries have been dubbed "hotspots for AMR genes" where a great deal of recombination and genome transmission may occur (Watts et al., 2017).

7.4. Prescription of antibiotics

Antimicrobial drug prescription excess and inappropriate use are unquestionably responsible for the escalating problems caused by bacteria that are resistant to antibiotics. According to certain research, from thirty to fifty percent of cases in the hospital setting involved incorrect antibiotic selection, therapeutic indication, or duration of antibiotic therapy. Pneumonia, gastroenteritis, and bacterial meningitis are among the illnesses caused by *S. pneumoniae*. Antibiotics are not necessary to treat about 85% of ear infections caused by bacteria. The fact that nearly all-American children with ear infections might still receive unneeded prescriptions exacerbates antibiotic resistance. Similarly, overuse of Penicillin renders it useless in treating *S. pneumoniae*-induced meningitis (Cheesman et al., 2017). This incorrect prescription's medicinal usefulness is debatable, and patients may suffer grave side effects from taking antibiotics. In the patients who underwent extensive surgery in a public facility and were discharged received an antibiotic by the hospital within a month after their release, according to the Healthcare Safety and Health Council of the Netherlands (De Almeida et al., 2018).

8. CHALLENGES OF ANTIMICROBIAL RESISTANCE

One effective strategy to combat bacterial resistance is to combine non-antibiotic substances with antibiotics such as Amoxicillin and clavulanic acid, which inhibits β-lactamase. This has resulted in an average annual rise in the screening, discovery, and investigation of novel bactericidal and non-antibiotic synergy over the past decade. The goal of this study is to describe antimicrobial synergistic routes and antibacterial potentiators that target existing resistance mechanisms. We also discuss some potential antimicrobial chemicals that can be utilized in combination with antibiotics to overcome medication resistance. These include active ingredients derived from plants, metals and metal oxides, phages and their by-products, and AMPs.

These medications increase the effectiveness of current antibiotics against bacterial resistance, either directly or indirectly, extending their half-life. Globally, antibiotic resistance is on the rise and is linked to higher rates of morbidity and mortality in community or clinical settings. Effective control measures have become more difficult to implement due to the emergence of drug resistance in many contexts and the rise of superbugs. Antibiotic resistance should be prevented and controlled at the local, national, and worldwide levels. Using antimicrobials sparingly, making it more difficult to obtain over-the-counter medications, maintaining clean hands, and taking all reasonable steps to prevent infections from spreading are some of the primary tactics that have been proposed (Ortega et al., 2020).

Adopting antibiotic-resistant solutions is challenging, and there are numerous repercussions. Despite the fact that certain ideas were put out and later implemented, not enough has been taken to address the issue as of yet. Antibiotics are still necessary in all hospitals, and a lack of collaboration between medical, social, and economic endeavours would be disastrous. Simple antibiotic treatment is no longer an option because an increasing number of medications are developing antibiotic resistance. Treatments and prevention strategies must adapt to new therapies and the emergence of bacteria that are resistant to drugs. Continued attention should ideally promote the application of novel research techniques for infection therapy that meet three requirements: the discovery of novel, efficacious treatments, the prevention of resistance, and the preservation of the healthy intestinal microbiota. The best way to accomplish these objectives is to develop innovative combination tactics that incorporate intelligent and local delivery technology.

9. MECHANISMS OF DRUG RESISTANCE

In an identical ecological niche, bacteria and antibiotics coexist, and bacteria build defenses against the negative effects of antibiotic compounds. The four crucial components of bacteria's cells that drugs must target are the cell wall, a membrane that produces proteins, and the generation of nucleic acids. Limiting drug absorption, changing a drug's dosage, dissolving the drug, and boosting active drug efflux are the main mechanisms of resistant bacteria. Bacteria often use mechanisms such drug target change, drug elimination, or drug efflux to develop acquired resistance, whereas uptake limitation and drug elimination, including drug efflux, are the main causes of intrinsic resistance. Because of structural differences, gram-positive and gram-negative bacteria have different levels of drug resistance. Due to their limited ability to use an efflux route to specific drug types and lack of an outer cell membrane containing Lipopolysaccharide (LPS), gram-positive bacteria are less likely to employ the approach of limiting medication absorption (Reynaert,2018). Gram-negative bacteria have been demonstrated to use all four of the primary drug resistance pathways as shown in *Figure 1*.

Figure 1. Mechanisms of Drug Resistance

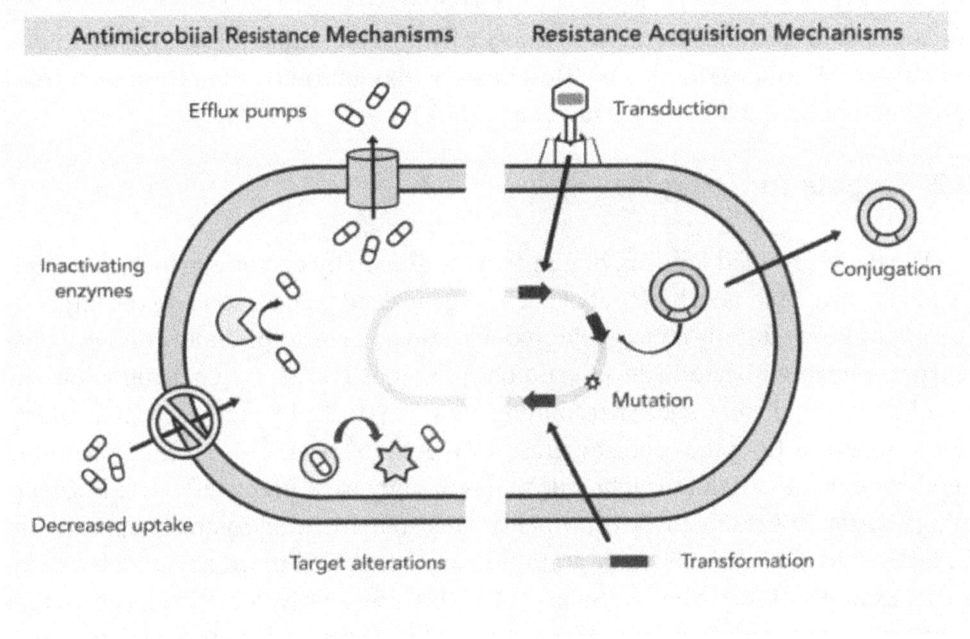

9.1. Limiting Drug Uptake

The main component of the outer membrane of gram-negative bacteria is lipopolysaccharide, a highly acidic lipid that prevents a variety of chemicals, including antibiotics, from penetrating. The inherent resistance of gram-negative bacteria lowers the permeability of certain medications, leading to resistance. Changes in the ability of outer-membrane proteins, especially porin protein, to penetrate can also lead to acquired drug resistance. Porins are the main way that hydrophilic antibiotics including Tetracycline antibiotics, Fluoroquinolones, the antibiotic Chloramphenicol and β-lactams entering the body. According to Choi et al., (2019), the quantity and type of porin proteins affect how these antibiotics penetrate bacterial cells, which in turn affects how vulnerable the bacteria become to these antibiotics. Furthermore, acquired antibiotic resistance may result from modifications that impact porin expression or function. Mutations affecting porin expression led to increased resistance when combined with additional co-occurring mechanisms such as pump efflux and enzymatic antimicrobial degradation (Ghai et al., 2018). By forming biofilms, several bacteria, including the strains of *Enterococcus faecalis, Staphylococcus aureus, Streptococcus viridians, E. coli,* bacteria such as *K. pneumoniae, Proteus mirabilis, or Pseudomonas aeruginosa,* also demonstrate antibiotic resistance. A biofilm is a group of bacteria attached to biotic or abiotic surfaces that are enclosed in their own exopolysaccharide. It has been demonstrated to give bacteria antibiotic resistance and tolerance through a variety of ways, including preventing antibiotic penetration. Furthermore, it may stop bactericidal antibiotic concentrations from growing throughout a colony (Dutt et al., 2022).

9.2. Targets for Drug

The targets needed for drug binding can be altered by bacteria, which can either make the drug bind poorly or not at all. The genes and genes encoding the target of therapy protein naturally undergo this modification. For example, both gram-positive and gram-negative bacteria develop Fluoroquinolone resistance when mutations affect the amino acid tolerance-determining region in the DNA production machinery (topoisomerase II or the topoisomerase IV) (Ashley et al., 2017). Methylation is another target modification technique that is thought to be highly effective in generating resistance. Erm methylases, which are resistant to the antibiotic streptogramin B, lacosamide, or macrolides in gram-positive as well as gram-negative bacteria, are an example of methylation (Saha et al.,.2021). Similarly, it has been shown that methylation of the cfr gene results in resistance in a range of microorganisms, such as *E. coli, Proteus vulgaris,* different types of *Staphylococci, Enterococcus* organisms, and several *Bacillus sp,*. The unique Penicillin-binding protein produced by the macA and mecC genes dramatically lowers Staphylococcus species' affinity for the -lactam antibiotics (Foster, 2017).

9.3. Inactivation of Drug

Antibiotic inactivation by specific bacterial species can lead to drug resistance in a couple of ways: either the antibiotic is really broken down, or a specific chemical compound has been introduced to the antibiotic. Member of the gut bacteria species produce hydrolysing enzymes called βlactamases, which are very efficient at deactivate β-lactam antibiotics. By opening at a precise place, the β-lactamases, formerly known as Penicillinases and cephalosporinases, break down the β-lactam ring structure and prevent the target, also known as Penicillin-binding proteins, from being contained within it. It is thought that the lactamase genes found in many gram-positive bacterial species, such as *S. aureus* and *Enterococcus faecalis,* especially *Enterococcus faecium*, are inherited through horizontal transfer of genes (HGT). Furthermore, the text gene in certain bacteria expresses a molecule that hydrolyzes tetracycline (Blair et al., 2015). The most commonly transferred chemical compounds for drug inactivation are adenyl, phosphoryl, and acetyl groups. Acetylation is the most effective technique against compounds like influenza streptogramins, and chlorine bleach, while phosphate and adenylation methods are known to be mostly used against aminoglycosides.

10. CAUSES OF ANTIMICROBIAL RESISTANCE

The three main causes of antibiotic resistance (AMR) are the misuse and improper use of medicines, the disdain for infection control procedures, and the emergence of bacteria that are resistant to several drugs. The widespread and negligent consumption of antibiotics in both human and animal populations produces selection pressures that promote the evolution of bacteria that can become resistant.

10.1. Over use of Antibiotics

One major issue in the realm of public health is the overuse and insufficient use of antibiotics. Antibiotics can encourage the propagation of AMR strains when they are used improperly or without a genuine necessity. Further risks could result from these resistant strains spreading to additional individuals. The aforementioned circumstances may make it difficult to treat viral infections appropriately, leading to protracted illnesses, long hospital stays, or an increase in medical costs. To stop the emergence and spread of AMR, antibiotics should only be used carefully and only when absolutely required. Following the prescribed dosage and treatment plan is also essential for the finest and most effective therapeutic outcomes. Additionally, getting vaccinated and practicing excellent hygiene can greatly lessen reliance on antimicrobial drugs, which will further lessen the necessity for usage (Maillard et al., 2020).

10.2. Failure of Infection control

A collection of measures employed to stop infectious diseases is referred to as infection control. Because patients in hospitals are more vulnerable to infections because of underlying medical disorders, dedication to infection control standards is crucial. Ignoring appropriate infection control measures can lead to the spread of infections and have serious consequences, such as disease outbreaks and harm to healthcare facilities' reputations. Maintaining high levels of cleanliness, following established norms and recommendations, and keeping surrounds clean and disinfected are all necessary to prevent the failure of disease control systems. This necessitates frequent hand washing, the use of suitable safety precautions, and cautious storage and transportation of contaminated goods. Furthermore, it is crucial to ensure that all medical personnel receive thorough training in techniques for managing infections and are held accountable for their appropriate application (Haque et al., 2020).

10.3. Multiple -Drug-Resistant (MDR) Pathogens

The phrase "infection control" refers to a collection of actions done to prevent infectious diseases. Complete adherence to infection control protocols is essential in hospital environments, where individuals may be more susceptible to infections due to medical histories. Neglecting proper infection control practices can result in the spread for infectious illnesses in addition to having major repercussions, including disease outbreaks and damage to the reputation of healthcare facilities. To keep infection management systems from failing, it is essential to maintain high standards of cleanliness, adhere to accepted standards and guidelines, and keep the environment sanitized. This calls for careful handling and storage of contaminated items, regular hand washing, and the application of appropriate safety measures. Additionally, it is imperative to ensure that all medical staff members receive comprehensive training in infection control techniques and are held responsible for their appropriate application (Haque et al., 2020).

11. MAJOR ANTIBIOTICS DISCOVERIES AND ANTIBIOTIC RESISTANCE

The advanced antibiotic began in 1910, Then Ehrlich and associates discovered salvarsan and neosalvarsan, a manufactured substance, to treat *syphilis* caused by *Treponema pallidum.* Later, salvarsan was gradually replaced by prontosil; this was a sulfur-based prodrug discovered by microbiologist Gerhard Domagk. Selman Waksman, a biochemist and microbial scientist from the United States, is credited with being the first to conduct a systematic investigation of soil bacteria. He examined how these microorganisms could produce substances that are lethal to other microorganisms. He discovered a number of antibiotics in soil-dwelling filamentous actinomycetes. Streptomycin, an antibiotic widely used to treat tuberculosis, was one of these. An antibiotic, according to him, is "a drug made by organisms in order to destroy another microbe." Penicillin was discovered by Scottish physician and microbiologist Sir Alexander Fleming. It originated from the Penicillium rubens mold. The greatest period of the discovery of antibiotics began with this and continued until the middle of the 1950s. The considered to have been the "golden decade" of drug discovery. During that period, the majority of antimicrobial agents still in use today were discovered. Since then, the number of new antibiotic discoveries has gradually declined, and drug-resistant bacteria have developed. Since the beginning of the antibacterial era, bacterial resistance to antibiotics has been recognized (Hutchings et al., 2019). A while before Penicillin was initially used as a medication, first strain of *Staphylococcus* bacteria that was resistant to the antibiotic was discovered.

Methicillin was introduced as a synthetic Penicillin that was indigestible by Penicillinase. Remarkably, a Methicillin-resistant strain of Staphylococcus was discovered in 1960, only a year after the drug's initial release. the glycopeptide Vancomycin was initially utilized as a rescue medication to treat illnesses brought on by Methicillin-resistant Staphylococci. Vancomycin-resistant isolates of resistant Staphylococci appeared, only a few decades later, and only ten years later, vancomycin-resistant status in bacteria called *Enterococcus* was also reported. Due to *S. aureus's* decreased susceptibility to Vancomycin, Methicillin-sensitive *Staphylococcus aureus* and Vancomycin-resistant *Staphylococcus aureus* were discovered, respectively (Uddin et al., 2021). Cephalosporin, also referred to as a beta-lactam antibiotic, and it was used in clinical settings to treat cases of Penicillin resistance. Since then, several varieties of the antibacterial drug have been developed, the most recent of which is now on the market. Initially, it was particularly successful against gram-negative microbes that produce extended beta-lactamases. All of the earlier Penicillin generations—including the fourth generation—have so far developed high levels of resistance. Another significant antibiotic discovered in 1950 was Tetracycline. It was effective for many common diseases, including stomach infections. Tetracycline was claimed to be ineffective against Shigella infections within ten years of its creation. Levofloxacin-resistant Pneumococcus was discovered the same year that levofloxacin, a subsequent-generation fluoroquinolone drug, was included to the list of antibiotics (Zaman et al., 2017).

Cephalosporins fail to cure infections caused by organisms of the bacterial family, carbapenem, a kind of β-lactam, continues to be utilized as a backup medication. Since 2006, reports of carbapenem-resistant enteric bacteria have been made from a number of nations, which corresponds with their rise in frequency during the years (Suay-García et al., 2019). According to the chronology for antibiotic development, pharmaceutical companies only produced novel antibiotics. Following that, there was a significant decline in the rate of discovery. Given that there are far more drug-resistant organisms than antibiotics, critics have sufficient data to claim that we are on the verge of entering a post-antibiotic era. The chronology of the discovery of important antibiotics and the emergence of antibiotic resistance (Iskandar et al., 2022).

12. ETHICAL CHALLENGES IN CRISPR-CAS AND AI-DRIVEN STRATEGIES AGAINST ANTIMICROBIAL RESISTANCE

CRISPR-Cas and AI-driven approaches represent cutting-edge strategies in combating antimicrobial resistance (AMR), yet they introduce profound ethical challenges that demand scrutiny. CRISPR-Cas systems, by precisely targeting resistance genes in pathogenic bacteria, offer a revolutionary alternative to traditional antibiotics, but off-target effects could inadvertently alter non-target microbial genomes, potentially disrupting ecosystems or fostering new resistance mechanisms, as evidenced in early in vivo studies showing variable specificity. Ethical concerns escalate with delivery methods like bacteriophages or nanoparticles, which raise biosafety risks of horizontal gene transfer and unintended environmental release, paralleling broader debates on germline editing's eugenics implications, though bacterial applications intensify fears of bio weaponization without robust international oversight. Meanwhile, AI-driven tools excel in predicting resistance patterns, optimizing antibiotic stewardship, and accelerating drug discovery through machine learning on vast genomic datasets, but they grapple with data privacy breaches under regulations like GDPR, where patient microbiomes could be commodified, and algorithmic biases from underrepresented global populations skew predictions toward wealthier demographics, exacerbating health inequities. The opacity of "black box" AI models further undermines accountability, as clinicians cannot trace erroneous recommendations that might prolong ineffective treatments, while overlapping CRISPR-AI integrations amplify dual-use dilemmas—such as AI-guided CRISPR design for rapid pathogen engineering—necessitating equitable access frameworks, mandatory bias audits, informed consent protocols, and multidisciplinary governance to harmonize innovation with societal trust (Saha et al., 2021).

13. ROLE OF VACCINES IN COMBATING AMR PATHOGENS

Vaccination is an interesting way to stop diseases and/or infections from developing in mammals and humans. It does this by lowering the demand for medicines and stopping the spread and development of resistant microorganisms. The *H. influenzae*, type *B influenza* vaccine and the pneumococci conjugation vaccines are two very clear examples of how well vaccines work to lower AMR. The invention of the hybrid pneumococci conjugate vaccine; there were about 63,000 cases of pneumococcal disease in the US. This caused a big increase in *S. pneumonia's* resistance to Penicillin and other drugs. The introduction of the vaccine not only reduced the prevalence of the disease but also significantly diminished the bacterial colonization of the pathogen, which undoubtedly influenced the spread of AMR isolates (Jansen et al., 2018). Vaccines play a both direct and indirect role in the fight against AMR. Vaccines directly impact resistant diseases by reducing the frequency of transmission and, indirectly, by curtailing the dissemination of isolates that are resistant to non-resistant species. Miceli et al., (2021) say that fewer infections mean fewer antibiotic prescriptions and fewer secondary infections and further infections that would require a lot of antibiotics (Klugman et al., 2018).

The vaccination technique and the establishment of herd immunity are potent strategies against AMR, as they diminish the prevalence of infections that are resistant (Shonen et al., 2017). Recent vaccination campaigns for beef and poultry have resulted in a substantial reduction in antibiotic usage and a concomitant decrease in Antimicrobial Resistance (AMR) within the herd. This trend also confers significant benefits to human health by mitigating the dissemination of AMR characteristics in zoonotic agents. Immunization diminishes the burden of Antimicrobial Resistance and, subsequently, the consumption of antibiotics. Conversely, the excessive use of antibiotics significantly contributes to the development and dissemination of AMR in fish farming, farming, and veterinary medicine. A simple in vivo method for making vaccines against bacteria that don't respond to antibiotics has recently been suggested: making antimicrobial glycoconjugate vaccines. This simple method uses Ply, an oligodactyly transferase, to change the genes of one strain of *E. coli* to make the vaccine that is needed (Holzer et al., 2018).

This enzyme connects a chosen antigenic compound to carrier proteins that have certain N-glycosylation sites. Guided fermentation of certain polysaccharide bacterial antigens can be used to make conjugated vaccines against antimicrobial-resistant pathogens like *Shigella, Flexner, S. aureus, P. aeruginosa, and K. pneumoniae.* This is safe and efficient because there is no need to grow these high-risk pathogens (Riddle et al., 2016). A new way to treat AMR involving antibiotics and vaccines is to use an improbable limited-spectrum vaccination to concentrate on the hardest to kill germs and encourage the use of strains that are more likely to be affected. Antibiotics can then be used to treat these infections (Bochy et al., 2020). Lastly, it is theoretically potential that vaccinations that lower the number of microbes also lower the chances of transferring antibacterial elements for vaccinations against microbes including *S. pneumoniae, S. aureus,* and other members of the *Enterobacter* yeast family, which can then colonize the gastrointestinal tract, skin, throat, and other areas without causing any symptoms Vaccines can help lower the use of antimicrobials (AMU), slow the spreading of AMR bacteria, and stop disease from

AMR infections with bacteria. However, they are not meant to take the place of drugs (Lips itch et al., 2016).

13. CONCLUSION

Antimicrobial Resistance (AMR) is one of the most serious public health issues of our day, endangering a century of advancements in medicine. The extensive usage and abuse of antibiotics in aquaculture, agriculture, and human medicine have led to tremendous selection pressure, which has accelerated the emergence of multidrug-resistant bacteria. The amazing genetic adaptability of bacteria, which use strategies including drug target change, enzymatic inactivation, or efflux pumps to maintain survival, and insufficient infection management exacerbate this issue. The repercussions are dire: longer hospital stays, higher mortality, protracted illnesses, and unmanageable financial strains on healthcare systems around the globe. The academic response to Antimicrobial Resistance (AMR) is developing with encouraging innovation, even if the historical stream of new medicines has diminished. Novel approaches to outwit resistant microorganisms include CRISPR-based modification of genes to disarm resistance, antimicrobial photodynamic treatment, and artificial intelligence for expedited medication discovery. Additionally, by lowering the occurrence of infections and, as a result, the need of therapeutic medicines, the judicious use of vaccines performs a crucial preventative function.

These developments mark a significant change from simply finding new medications to creating more intelligent and focused defences against the resistance mechanisms themselves. But technological fixes by themselves are not enough. A coordinated, complex global plan is required to address the ongoing issues, which include the slow rate of antibiotic discovery, worldwide disparities with regard to medical access, and the ongoing growth of resistance. Strong antimicrobial stewardship initiatives, strict infection prevention guidelines, and improved worldwide surveillance systems are all essential for the sustainable control of AMR. It also necessitates substantial investment in technological advancement as well as legislative changes to control the use of antibiotics in various sectors. In the end, combating AMR is a shared society obligation rather than just a medical and scientific undertaking. Integrating cutting-edge treatments with fundamental public health procedures and encouraging cooperation between medical professionals, researchers, legislators, and the general public are essential to success.

13. REFERENCES

Alanjary, M., Kronmiller, B., Adamek, M., Blin, K., Weber, T., Huson, D., & Medema, M. H. (2017). The Antibiotic-Resistant Target Seeker (ARTS), an exploration engine for antibiotic cluster prioritization and novel drug target discovery. *Nucleic Acids Research, 45*(W1), W42–W48. gkx360DOI: 10.1093/nar/ PMID: 28472505

Ando, H., Lemire, S., Pires, D. P., & Lu, T. K. (2015). Engineering modular viral scaffolds for targeted bacterial population editing. *Cell Systems, 1*(3), 187–196. DOI: 10.1016/j.cels.2015.08.013 PMID: 26973885

Ashley, R. E., Dittmore, A., McPherson, S. A., Turnbough, C. L.Jr, Neuman, K. C., & Osheroff, N. (2017). Activities of gyrase and topoisomerase IV on positively supercoiled DNA. *Nucleic Acids Research, 45*(16), 9611–9624. DOI: 10.1093/nar/gkx649 PMID: 28934496

Assefa, A., & Abunna, F. (2018). Maintenance of fish health in aquaculture: Review of epidemiological approaches for prevention and control of infectious disease of fish. *Veterinary Medicine International, 2018*, 5432497. Advance online publication. DOI: 10.1155/2018/5432497 PMID: 29682272

Ayukekbong, J. A., Ntemgwa, M., & Atabe, A. N. (2017). The threat of Antimicrobial Resistance in developing countries: Causes and control strategies. *Antimicrobial Resistance and Infection Control, 6*, 47. Advance online publication. DOI: 10.1186/s13756-017-0208-x PMID: 28515903

Blair, J. M. A., Webber, M. A., Baylay, A. J., Ogbolu, D. O., & Piddock, L. J. V. (2015). Molecular mechanisms of antibiotic resistance. *Nature Reviews. Microbiology, 13*(1), 42–51. DOI: 10.1038/nrmicro3380 PMID: 25435309

Burke, V., Richter, D., Greskowiak, J., Mehrtens, A., Schulz, L., & Massmann, G. (2016). Occurrence of antibiotics in surface and groundwater of a drinking water catchment area in Germany. *Water Environment Research, 88*(7), 652–665. DOI: 10.2175/106143016X14609975746064 PMID: 27329061

Bush, K. (2024). Commentary on The antibiotic explosion by H. Boyd Woodruff and Richard W. Burg. In Hemodynamics and Immune Defense (pp. 301–306). Elsevier.

Cheesman, M. J., Ilanko, A., Blonk, B., & Cock, I. E. (2017). Developing new antimicrobial therapies: Are synergistic combinations of plant extracts/compounds with conventional antibiotics the solution? *Pharmacognosy Reviews, 11*(22), 57–72. DOI: 10.4103/phrev.phrev_21_17 PMID: 28989242

Choi, U., & Lee, C.-R. (2019). Distinct roles of outer membrane porins in antibiotic resistance and membrane integrity in Escherichia coli. *Frontiers in Microbiology, 10*, 953. DOI: 10.3389/fmicb.2019.00953 PMID: 31114568

Chuah, L.-O., Effarizah, M. E., Goni, A. M., & Rusul, G. (2016). Antibiotic application and emergence of multiple antibiotic resistance (MAR) in global catfish aquaculture. *Current Environmental Health Reports, 3*(2), 118–127. DOI: 10.1007/s40572-016-0091-2 PMID: 27038482

Davies, J., & Davies, D. (2010). Origins and evolution of antibiotic resistance. *Microbiology and Molecular Biology Reviews : MMBR, 74*(3), 417–433. DOI: 10.1128/MMBR.00016-10 PMID: 20805405

De Almeida, M., Gerard, C., Freeman, J. T., Duffy, E., & Roberts, S. A. (2018). Inappropriate prescribing of antibiotics following discharge after major surgery: An area for improvement. *The New Zealand Medical Journal, 131*(1475), 35–43. PMID: 29771900

do Prado, G. V. B., Marchi, A. P., Moreno, L. Z., Rizek, C., Amigo, U., Moreno, A. M., Rossi, F., Guimaraes, T., Levin, A. S., & Costa, S. F. (2016). Virulence and resistance pattern of a novel sequence type of linezolid-resistant Enterococcus faecium identified by whole-genome sequencing. *Journal of Global Antimicrobial Resistance, 6*, 27–31. DOI: 10.1016/j.jgar.2016.02.006 PMID: 27530835

Foster, T. J. (2017). Antibiotic resistance in Staphylococcus aureus. Current status and future prospects. *FEMS Microbiology Reviews, 41*(3), 430–449. DOI: 10.1093/femsre/fux007 PMID: 28419231

Ghai, I., & Ghai, S. (2018). Understanding antibiotic resistance via outer membrane permeability. *Infection and Drug Resistance, 11*, 523–530. DOI: 10.2147/IDR.S156995 PMID: 29695921

Goff, A., Cantillon, D., Muraro Wildner, L., & Waddell, S. J. (2020). Multi-omics technologies applied to tuberculosis drug discovery. *Applied Sciences (Basel, Switzerland), 10*(13), 4629. DOI: 10.3390/app10134629

Grenni, P., Ancona, V., & Caracciolo, A. B. (2018). Ecological effects of antibiotics on natural ecosystems: A review. *Microchemical Journal, 136*, 25–39. DOI: 10.1016/j.microc.2017.02.006

Haque, M., McKimm, J., Sartelli, M., Dhingra, S., Labricciosa, F. M., Islam, S., Jahan, D., Nusrat, T., Chowdhury, T. S., Coccolini, F., Iskandar, K., Catena, F., & Begum, H. A. (2020). Strategies to prevent healthcare-associated infections: A narrative overview. *Risk Management and Healthcare Policy, 13*, 1765–1780. DOI: 10.2147/RMHP.S269315 PMID: 33061710

Hughes, D., & Andersson, D. I. (2017). Environmental and genetic modulation of the phenotypic expression of antibiotic resistance. *FEMS Microbiology Reviews, 41*(3), 374–391. DOI: 10.1093/femsre/fux004 PMID: 28333270

Hutchings, M. I., Truman, A. W., & Wilkinson, B. (2019). Antibiotics: Past, present and future. *Current Opinion in Microbiology, 51*, 72–80. DOI: 10.1016/j.mib.2019.10.008 PMID: 31733401

Iskandar, K., Murugaiyan, J., Hammoudi Halat, D., Hage, S. E., Chibabhai, V., Adukkadukkam, S., Roques, C., Molinier, L., Salameh, P., & Van Dongen, M. (2022). Antibiotic discovery and resistance: The chase and the race. *Antibiotics (Basel, Switzerland), 11*(2), 182. DOI: 10.3390/antibiotics11020182 PMID: 35203785

Jansen, K. U., & Anderson, A. S. (2018). The role of vaccines in fighting Antimicrobial Resistance (AMR). *Human Vaccines & Immunotherapeutics, 14*(9), 2142–2149. DOI: 10.1080/21645515.2018.1476814 PMID: 29787323

Kang, Y. K., Kwon, K., Ryu, J. S., Lee, H. N., Park, C., & Chung, H. J. (2017). Nonviral genome editing based on a polymer-derivatized CRISPR nanocomplex for targeting bacterial pathogens and antibiotic resistance. *Bioconjugate Chemistry, 28*(4), 957–967. DOI: 10.1021/acs.bioconjchem.6b00676 PMID: 28215090

Klugman, K. P., & Black, S. (2018). Impact of existing vaccines in reducing antibiotic resistance: Primary and secondary effects. *Proceedings of the National Academy of Sciences of the United States of America, 115*(51), 12896–12901. DOI: 10.1073/pnas.1721095115 PMID: 30559195

Lakhundi, S., & Zhang, K. (2018). Methicillin-resistant Staphylococcus aureus: Molecular characterization, evolution, and epidemiology. *Clinical Microbiology Reviews, 31*(4), e00020–e18. DOI: 10.1128/CMR.00020-18 PMID: 30209034

Lee, A. S., de Lencastre, H., Garau, J., Kluytmans, J., Malhotra-Kumar, S., Peschel, A., & Harbarth, S. (2018). Methicillin-resistant Staphylococcus aureus. *Nature Reviews. Disease Primers, 4*, 18033. Advance online publication. DOI: 10.1038/nrdp.2018.33 PMID: 29849094

Ma, Y.-X., Wang, C.-Y., Li, Y.-Y., Li, J., Wan, Q.-Q., Chen, J.-H., Tay, F. R., & Niu, L.-N. (2020). Considerations and caveats in combating ESKAPE pathogens against nosocomial infections. *Advancement of Science*, *7*(1), 1901872. DOI: 10.1002/advs.201901872 PMID: 31921562

Maillard, J.-Y., Bloomfield, S. F., Courvalin, P., Essack, S. Y., Gandra, S., Gerba, C. P., Rubino, J. R., & Scott, E. A. (2020). Reducing antibiotic prescribing and addressing the global problem of antibiotic resistance by targeted hygiene in the home and everyday life settings: A position paper. *American Journal of Infection Control*, *48*(9), 1090–1099. DOI: 10.1016/j.ajic.2020.04.011 PMID: 32311380

Mathur, A., Parihar, A. S., Modi, S., & Kalra, A. (2023). Photodynamic therapy for ESKAPE pathogens: An emerging approach to combat Antimicrobial Resistance (AMR). *Microbial Pathogenesis*, *185*, 106307. DOI: 10.1016/j.micpath.2023.106307 PMID: 37604213

Mestrovic, T., & Ljubin-Sternak, S. (2018). Molecular mechanisms of Chlamydia trachomatis resistance to antimicrobial drugs. *Frontiers in Bioscience (Landmark Edition)*, *23*, 656–670. DOI: 10.2741/4611 PMID: 28930567

Ortega, M. A., Guzmán Merino, A., Fraile-Martínez, O., Recio-Ruiz, J., Pekarek, L., Guijarro, L. G., García-Honduvilla, N., Álvarez-Mon, M., Buján, J., & García-Gallego, S. (2020). Dendrimers and dendritic materials: From laboratory to medical practice in infectious diseases. *Pharmaceutics*, *12*(9), 874. DOI: 10.3390/pharmaceutics12090874 PMID: 32937793

Pursey, E., Sünderhauf, D., Gaze, W. H., Westra, E. R., & van Houte, S. (2018). CRISPR-Cas antimicrobials: Challenges and future prospects. *PLoS Pathogens*, *14*(6), e1006990. DOI: 10.1371/journal.ppat.1006990 PMID: 29902258

Rees, T. W., Ho, P. Y., & Hess, J. (2023). Recent advances in metal complexes for antimicrobial photodynamic therapy. *ChemBioChem*, *24*(16), e202200797. DOI: 10.1002/cbic.202200797 PMID: 36917084

Riddle, M. S., Kaminski, R. W., Di Paolo, C., Porter, C. K., Gutierrez, R. L., Clarkson, K. A., Weerts, H. E., Duplessis, C., Castellano, A., Alaimo, C., Paolino, K. M., Gormley, R., & Gambillara Fonck, V. (2016). Safety and immunogenicity of a candidate bioconjugate vaccine against Shigella flexneri 2a administered to healthy adults: A single-blind, randomized phase I study. *Clinical and Vaccine Immunology; CVI*, *23*(12), 908–917. DOI: 10.1128/CVI.00224-16 PMID: 27581434

Román Hurtado, F. (2022). Genome mining of the strain Streptomyces sp. CA-170360: Identification and heterologous expression of secondary metabolite biosynthetic gene clusters [Doctoral dissertation, University of Granada].

Saha, M., & Sarkar, A. (2021). Review on multiple facets of drug resistance: A rising challenge in the 21st century. *Journal of Xenobiotics, 11*(4), 197–214. DOI: 10.3390/jox11040013 PMID: 34940513

Shabbir, M. A. B., Shabbir, M. Z., Wu, Q., Mahmood, S., Sajid, A., Maan, M. K., Ahmed, S., Naveed, U., Hao, H., & Yuan, Z. (2019). CRISPR-cas system: Biological function in microbes and its use to treat antimicrobial resistant pathogens. *Annals of Clinical Microbiology and Antimicrobials, 18*, 21. Advance online publication. DOI: 10.1186/s12941-019-0317-x PMID: 31277669

Shrestha, P., Cooper, B. S., Coast, J., Oppong, R., Do Thi Thuy, N., Phodha, T., Celhay, O., Guerin, P. J., Wertheim, H., & Lubell, Y. (2018). Enumerating the economic cost of Antimicrobial Resistance per antibiotic consumed to inform the evaluation of interventions affecting their use. *Antimicrobial Resistance and Infection Control, 7*, 98. Advance online publication. DOI: 10.1186/s13756-018-0384-3 PMID: 30116525

Singh, S. B., Young, K., & Silver, L. L. (2017). What is an "ideal" antibiotic? Discovery challenges and path forward. *Biochemical Pharmacology, 133*, 63–73. DOI: 10.1016/j.bcp.2017.01.003 PMID: 28087253

Suay-García, B., & Pérez-Gracia, M. T. (2019). Present and future of carbapenem-resistant Enterobacteriaceae (CRE) infections. *Antibiotics (Basel, Switzerland), 8*(3), 122. DOI: 10.3390/antibiotics8030122 PMID: 31430964

Thai, P. K., Ky, L. X., Binh, V. N., Nhung, P. H., Nhan, P. T., Hieu, N. Q., Dang, N. T. T., Tam, N. K. B., & Anh, N. T. K. (2018). Occurrence of antibiotic residues and antibiotic-resistant bacteria in effluents of pharmaceutical manufacturers and other sources around Hanoi, Vietnam. *The Science of the Total Environment, 645*, 393–400. DOI: 10.1016/j.scitotenv.2018.07.126 PMID: 30029118

Uddin, T. M., Chakraborty, A. J., Khusro, A., Zidan, B. R. M., Mitra, S., Emran, T. B., Dhama, K., Ripon, M. K. H., Gajdács, M., Sahibzada, M. U. K., Hossain, M. J., & Koirala, N. (2021). Antibiotic resistance in microbes: History, mechanisms, therapeutic strategies and future prospects. *Journal of Infection and Public Health, 14*(12), 1750–1766. DOI: 10.1016/j.jiph.2021.10.020 PMID: 34756812

Wang, H., Ren, L., Yu, X., Hu, J., Chen, Y., He, G., & Jiang, Q. (2017). Antibiotic residues in meat, milk and aquatic products in Shanghai and human exposure assessment. *Food Control, 80*, 217–225. DOI: 10.1016/j.foodcont.2017.04.034

Yosef, I., Manor, M., Kiro, R., & Qimron, U. (2015). Temperate and lytic bacteriophages programmed to sensitize and kill antibiotic-resistant bacteria. *Proceedings of the National Academy of Sciences of the United States of America, 112*(23), 7267–7272. DOI: 10.1073/pnas.1500107112 PMID: 26060300

Zaman, S. B., Hussain, M. A., Nye, R., Mehta, V., Mamun, K. T., & Hossain, N. (2017). A review on antibiotic resistance: Alarm bells are ringing. *Cureus*, *9*(6), e1403. DOI: 10.7759/cureus.1403 PMID: 28852600

Zhao, F., Liu, J., Shi, W., Huang, F., Liu, L., Zhao, S., & Zhang, J. (2019). Antimicrobial susceptibility and genotyping of Mycoplasma pneumoniae isolates in Beijing, China, from 2014 to 2016. *Antimicrobial Resistance and Infection Control*, *8*, 18. Advance online publication. DOI: 10.1186/s13756-019-0470-1 PMID: 30697421

Zimmermann, S., Klinger-Strobel, M., Bohnert, J. A., Wendler, S., Rödel, J., Pletz, M. W., & Löffler, B. (2019). Clinically approved drugs inhibit the *Staphylococcus aureus* multidrug NorA efflux pump and reduce biofilm formation. *Frontiers in Microbiology*, *10*, 2762. DOI: 10.3389/fmicb.2019.02762 PMID: 31849901

Chapter 13
Revolutionizing Antimicrobial Resistance:
Precision Medicine Strategies in the Fight

Maria Nazir Ahmad
https://orcid.org/0009-0004-6714-6212
Cholistan University of Veterinary and Animal Sciences, Bahawalpur, Pakistan

Syed Sohail Ahmad
https://orcid.org/0009-0001-9652-7565
Rehman College of Allied Health Sciences, Rehman Medical Institute, Peshawar, Pakistan

Abdul Moeez Qureshi
Cholistan University of Veterinary and Animal Sciences, Bahawalpur, Pakistan

ABSTRACT

This chapter examines the transformative impact of precision medicine in combating antimicrobial resistance (AMR), emphasizing the potential of advanced diagnostics, targeted therapies, and personalized treatment strategies. With AMR becoming a significant global health threat, the integration of AI, genomics, synthetic biology, and nanotechnology offers innovative solutions for diagnosing and treating resistant infections. Key technologies such as AI-enhanced diagnostics, phage therapy, and CRISPR-based treatments are poised to revolutionize AMR management by enabling real-time, accurate diagnoses and personalized therapeutic regimens. The chapter also addresses ethical considerations related to the use of genetic data, the development of gene-edited phages, and the challenges of implementing precision medicine in low-resource settings. Additionally, the 2030 roadmap for AMR emphasizes the

DOI: 10.4018/979-8-3373-3825-5.ch013

importance of global collaboration, increased funding for AMR research, and the need for standardized surveillance protocols for AMR. Despite the promising potential of these technologies, significant barriers remain, including cost, regulatory frameworks, and access in underserved regions. The chapter concludes by stressing the need for urgent global action to integrate precision medicine into AMR strategies, offering a sustainable approach to overcoming one of the most pressing public health challenges of the 21st century.

1 INTRODUCTION

Antimicrobial resistance (AMR) is an emergency health-related issue. New statistics on mortality list 10.5 million deaths to AMR every year, exceeding the levels related to HIV/AIDS and malaria (Chambers et al., 2022). Without immediate action, it is estimated that in 2050, AMR will become the single largest cause of death globally, surpassing the effects of malignancy. This poses a significant risk to human life and can destabilize the global economy, potentially leading to a loss exceeding $100 trillion in financial benefits due to diminished productivity and rising healthcare costs. Countries with middle and lower incomes face significant risks; currently, one in five deaths associated with drug-resistant infections occurs in these regions (Alara & Alara, 2024).

Escherichia coli, Klebsiella pneumoniae, and *Pseudomonas aeruginosa* are the primary contributors to this crisis, having developed resistance to a wide range of antibiotics. The European Centre for Disease Prevention and Control (ECDC, 2024) has indicated that 70% of prominent clinical pathogens exhibit resistance to one or more commonly available antibiotics (Tsalidou et al., 2023). This resistance is no longer limited to healthcare settings; it has expanded into community environments, agriculture, and the broader ecosystem. Consequently, healthcare systems worldwide are encountering an increasing challenge, as therapies once considered effective are now perceived as less reliable. This trend is exemplified by the increasing mortality rates associated with AMR, as illustrated in Figure 1, particularly in low- and middle-income countries.

Diet, unbalanced drinking water, and food preservation represent significant areas of concern, as they create an environment beneficial to the development of antimicrobial resistance in fungi, bacteria, and viruses. Nonetheless, these efforts have demonstrated some success in diminishing resistance to a degree. The ongoing overprescription and misuse of antibiotics in low-income areas, where these medications can be obtained without a prescription, remain a significant factor in the crisis. In wealthier regions, the extensive use of antibiotics in agriculture intensifies the pressure on selection processes. Empirical evidence indicates that more than 50 percent of antibiotic prescriptions globally are either unnecessary or inappropriate (Mulchandani et al., 2025). Additionally, the slow pace of new drug development is concerning: currently, there are only 17 antibiotics in late-stage clinical trials, none of which address the majority of the most dangerous resistant pathogens. The slow speed of diagnostics presents a significant challenge, often forcing clinicians to rely on broad-spectrum agents while awaiting culture results, which typically take 72 hours or more. This practice exacerbates the issue of resistance (Singhal et al., 2025). Utilizing genomic data, supported by artificial intelligence and real-time diagnostics, presents a compelling approach to tackling antimicrobial resistance. Precision medicine minimizes the likelihood of resistance development, a common issue with non-selective, broad-spectrum drugs, by creating tailored treatments that align with the characteristics of both the host and the pathogen responsible for the condition. Utilizing genetic information enables clinicians to adopt a more precise, data-driven approach to clinical care, moving away from a generic, one-size-fits-all model (Paulson & Johnson, 2025).

Recent advancements in precision medicine suggest a promising role for it in addressing antimicrobial resistance. The National Health Service (NHS) in the United Kingdom has utilized whole-genome sequencing to enhance the identification of bloodstream pathogens, resulting in a 22% reduction in deaths associated with antimicrobial resistance (AMR) and a 35% decrease in the unnecessary use of broad-spectrum antibiotics (Parcell, 2021). In 2024, AI-enabled diagnostic systems in India decreased the Time needed to predict sepsis patient resistance profiles from 72 hours to just six hours, while simultaneously boosting survival rates by 40%, thereby saving the lives of sepsis patients. Currently, CRISPR-based systems can identify resistance in just one hour, making them essential in critical-care settings. Personalized phage therapy has demonstrated an 85% success rate in treating infections caused by multidrug-resistant P. aeruginosa, a pathogen that is frequently resistant to conventional antibiotics. This collection of case studies highlights the transformative potential of precision medicine in addressing the conventional interventions against antimicrobial resistance. By integrating rapid diagnostics, genomic sequencing, and tailored therapies, precision medicine adopts a forward-thinking, data-centric strategy that improves management outcomes and mitigates the emergence of resistance (Panchpuri et al., 2025). To achieve this goal, it is crucial to implement precision medicine as a primary strategy in addressing the increasing challenge of antimicrobial resistance. The driving forces behind this advancement will be insights gained in diagnostics, synthetic biology, and AI-enabled decision-making, which will empower developers to address resistance and sustain the efficacy of existing antibiotics. A comprehensive response can only be achieved through the collaborative efforts of government, research entities, and policymakers. The enduring viability and maintenance of robust health systems will necessitate the incorporation of precision-medicine principles into both national and international strategies addressing AMR.

2. NEXT-GENERATION PRECISION DIAGNOSTICS FOR AMR

The rising challenge of antimicrobial resistance (AMR) poses a significant threat to the accessibility of healthcare, compelling clinicians to adopt rapid and accurate diagnostic methods to detect potential pathogens and their resistance to treatments. Conventional diagnostic methods, often requiring 48 to 72 hours for results, are associated with significant delays that undermine the promptness of AMR management. On the other hand, recent advancements in innovative diagnostic technologies, including genomic sequencing, CRISPR-based platforms, and microbiome research, have demonstrated improved speed, accuracy, and the potential for personalized intervention strategies. These advancements will mitigate this misuse by empowering clinicians to identify pathogens more quickly, thereby enhancing patient outcomes and enabling health services to more effectively address the escalating challenge of AMR (Lathakumari et al., 2025).

2.1 Genomic and Metagenomic Surveillance

Metagenomic and genomic surveillance is now regarded as essential in the ongoing battle against antimicrobial resistance. The implementation of these technologies enables swift and precise diagnoses through the accurate characterization of pathogen genomes and the profiling of resistance mechanisms. A notable advancement is nanopore sequencing, which enables the real-time identification of resistance genes in clinical samples within approximately four hours, in contrast to conventional methods. Hospitals in the United Kingdom have already implemented systems capable of monitoring outbreaks of multiple drug-resistant pathogens, such as methicillin-resistant Staphylococcus Aureus and carbapenem-resistant Enterobacteriaceae, utilizing nanopore sequencing. This approach facilitates more strategic and prompt responses. Simultaneously, platforms driven by artificial intelligence are being utilized to examine genomic findings and predict resistance patterns with an accuracy of 96.3%, thereby reducing unnecessary antibiotic prescriptions and bolstering efforts in antimicrobial resistance programs (Sukhum et al., 2019).

2.2 CRISPR-Based Diagnostics: Rapid Detection of Resistance

CRISPR-Dx represents a groundbreaking method for tracking antibiotic resistance. The use of the CRISPR enzyme system facilitates these assays, significantly enhancing their speed and specificity in the examination of resistance genes. A recent report demonstrated the capability to screen 20 minutes of NDM-1 carbapenemase, a gene thought to be responsible for resistance to carbapenem (Cell, March 2024). The rapidity of this process is crucial in clinical environments, as swift pathogen identification is essential for guiding evidence-based treatment. The per-test cost of approximately $2 for the CRISPR-based assays makes them accessible, particularly in low and middle-income regions, while traditional methods remain prohibitively expensive. A validation trial using the FDA-approved SHERLOCK platform has demonstrated a sensitivity of 94% in identifying third-generation cephalosporin resistance in Escherichia coli, affirming the diagnostic accuracy of CRISPR-Dx. The application of CRISPR-Dx in sepsis protocols within Mumbai ICU studies demonstrated a 25 percent reduction in mortality, highlighting the clinical relevance of these technologies in enhancing patient outcomes related to causes of death (Hassan et al., 2025). Figure 3 illustrates the capability of CRISPR-Dx technologies to facilitate on-site, real-time identification and detection of AMR markers, thereby offering actionable clinical data to healthcare professionals.

2.3 Microbiome-Based Diagnostics: Personalized Risk Profiles

In recent years, testing methods centered around the microbiome have emerged as a promising approach for predicting and preventing antimicrobial resistance (AMR). A study published in Science Translational Medicine (January 2024) demonstrated that gut microbial signatures in ICU cohorts can predict the occurrence of AMR infections with an impressive precision of 82%, particularly in individuals at higher risk of vancomycin-resistant Enterococcus (VRE) colonization. The findings offer actionable early warning strategies for identifying at-risk populations. The concurrent advancements are currently concentrating on diagnostic methods that employ saliva in pediatric patient populations. In 2024, a study funded by the National Institutes of Health (NIH) reported that salivary tests demonstrate a 90% concordance with traditional blood culture in diagnosing infections in children, offering a non-invasive and rapid method for this purpose. Fecal microbiome transplants (FMT) are currently under investigation as a potential intervention to restore antibiotic-sensitive microbial communities in individuals experiencing recurrent resistant infections. Initial findings suggest that FMT may be a viable therapy for reducing VRE colonization by approximately 70 percent, positioning this approach as a potential adjunct to AMR (Eslami et al., 2025).

The incorporation of experimental diagnostic tools, specifically Genomic surveillance, CRISPR-based platform, and microbiome testing, will drastically modify the way modern antibiotic-resistance control should be approached. The tools provide fast, accurate, and very fine-grained results, thereby helping clinicians optimise their choice of antibiotics, reduce the use of inappropriate antibiotics, and improve their clinical outcomes. Within the context of the increasing incidence of antimicrobial resistance issues, these methodologies provide potential avenues for reducing the burdens of antimicrobial resistance at a regional and global scale, as well as for developing precision-medicine-based applications to address resistant microbial infections (Shukla et al., 2024).

3. BREAKTHROUGH PRECISION THERAPEUTICS FOR AMR: A NEW ERA IN TARGETED TREATMENT STRATEGIES

Modern initiatives in the fight against antimicrobial resistance (AMR) represent a paradigm shift toward precision therapeutics, where the use of interventions is tailored to specific targets. In comparison to broad-spectrum antibiotics, which lack specificity and nonspecifically kill both pathogens and commensals, precision therapeutics target only resistant pathogens, thereby sparing the integrity of the resident microbiome. Such a differential approach diminishes collateral damage and, therefore, negative effects. The new modalities, phage therapy, synthetic biology, and nanotechnology have shown effectiveness in pre-clinical and early-clinical studies and have the potential to assist in future AMR-specific personalized medicine efforts (Olatunji et al., 2024).

3.1 Phage Therapy: Natural precision weapons

The field of phage therapy has experienced a strong revival in recent years, involving the use of bacteriophages to destroy pathogenic bacteria. This new attention is based on the verifiable ability of phages to target specific bacteria and exhibit activity against multidrug-resistant (MDR) infections. Phages also exhibit superior bacterial specificity compared to conventional antibiotics, thereby sparing the native microbial integrity of their hosts. Phage therapy is used to target highly virulent strains that are resistant to conventional antibiotics. The strong evidence was provided in a pooled Phase III clinical trial carried out in May 2024 and reported a 65 percent reduction in ongoing infections of Pseudomonas aeruginosa in cystic fibrosis patients upon receiving personalized phage cocktails, compared to the 28 percent reduction in ongoing infections with standard antibiotic therapy (Sunderland et al., 2017).

Phages demonstrate a significantly higher efficacy in combating biofilm-associated infections, where bacterial communities form protective structures that inhibit the action of antibiotics. Phages eliminate biofilms, thereby facilitating the exposure of resident bacteria to antibiotics and enhancing the effectiveness of antibiotic therapy.

A notable instance of this synergy is found in the study published in Cell Host & Microbe (April 2024), which demonstrated that the combination of phages and antibiotics resulted in bacterial clearance that was 10 times greater than that achieved with antibiotics alone. The findings support the conclusion that the phage-antibiotic strategy markedly improves treatment outcomes (Figure 1).

3.2 Synthetic Biology: Engineering the Next Generation of Antimicrobials

The use of synthetic biology to address the problem of antimicrobial resistance (AMR) has revolutionised modern therapeutic innovation by using methods of genome engineering and computational modelling that can be used to create new agents. CRISPR-encoded antimicrobial components also have been proposed through engineered antimicrobial peptides (AMPs), which are effective in treating antibiotic-resistant infections. These engineered products impart more specific and stronger therapeutic impacts by more unreservedly targeting resistance mechanisms than those of traditional antibiotics (Jaumaux et al., 2020).

Engineered Antimicrobial Peptides (AMPs)

An example of the progress made available by synthetic biology is the advancement of SynAMP-101, a synthetic antimicrobial peptide. Designed to binds to the outer membrane of XDR Acinetobacter baumannii, a pathogen treated by most commercially available antibiotics, SynAMP-101 killed 99 percent of bacteria in murine cell models tested in an article published in February 2024, holding potential in treating antibiotic-resistant infections. In contrast to classic antibiotics that affect specific cellular pathways, SynAMP-101 causes a destruction of the membrane, a mechanism that could be involved in a lower resistant potential (Jaumaux et al., 2020).

CRISPR-Cas Antimicrobials

The upcoming June 2024 publication of a study in Science Advances presents significant progress in the application of CRISPR-Cas systems as antimicrobials. The study demonstrates the application of CRISPR-Cas13a in targeting MRSA, leading to the specific cleavage of bacterial RNA. The system successfully achieved a reduction in bacterial load by 99.99% through the application of lipid nanoparticles as delivery mechanisms. The study emphasizes the crucial adaptability of CRISPR-dependent antimicrobials, allowing practitioners to readily modify the system to address bacterial failures or mutations. CRISPR-based reagents are poised to serve as a viable solution in the ongoing battle against antimicrobial resistance (Bikard & Barrangou, 2017).

Key Advantages of Synthetic Biology

The ease and the precision that synthetic biology offers results in significant benefits relating to AMR control. A rapid redesign synthesis syllabus allows development of therapeutics targeting newly emergent strains resistant phenotypes to be rapidly developed, thus providing the needed time based advantage to keep therapeutic efficacy ahead of evolutionary advantage. In addition, they have constructs with the ability to bind only pathogenic bacteria and therefore leave the commensal microbiota intact. This specificity enables the targeted attack on a small group of vulnerable microorganisms, making synthetic biology an even more attractive approach for the prevention of AMR in the future (Cubillos-Ruiz et al., 2021).

3.3 Nanotechnology: Revolutionizing Drug Delivery and Efficacy

It is universally recognized that nanotechnology can be utilized as a transformational treatment modality to address antimicrobial resistance (AMR), thereby enhancing the delivery, stability, and therapeutic effectiveness of antibiotics. Nano particles have the potential to cross physiological boundaries, e.g., biofilms and the blood-brain barrier, because they have a size range of 1 to 100 nm, thus providing an effective delivery method for therapeutic products to the site of illness. The trait promotes better penetration, reduced side effects, and sustained therapeutic effects, which are beneficial in the treatment of multidrug-resistant and chronic infections (Theivendren et al., 2024). The development of mRNA vaccines is also tuned by nanotechnology and thus offers an immunoprophylaxis to antibiotic treatment. The advantages of using nanotechnology-based treatments to combat antimicrobial resistance, as compared to conventional antibiotics, are outlined below.

Table 1. Nanotechnology's Role in AMR Treatment

Feature	Nanotechnology in AMR Treatment	Traditional Antibiotics	Refernces
Targeting	Direct delivery to infection sites; fewer side effects.	Non-specific spread; more side effects.	(Sultana et al., 2022)
Biofilm Action	Penetrates and disrupts biofilms effectively.	Poor biofilm penetration; reduced efficacy.	(Cai et al., 2021)
Toxicity	Lower systemic toxicity; safer use.	Higher risk of organ and GI toxicity.	(Due, 2023)
Drug Release	Controlled, sustained antibiotic release.	Rapid release; frequent dosing needed.	(Herdiana et al., 2022)
Vaccine Role	Enables mRNA vaccine development for resistant pathogens.	Limited vaccine use against resistance.	(Gebre et al., 2021)
Personalization	Allows infection-specific, tailored therapy.	Standardized dosing; limited customization.	(Chen et al., 2024)
Clinical Stage	Promising trials on nano-antibiotic conjugates.	Established but facing rising resistance.	(Ijaz et al., 2024)
Barrier Penetration	Crosses biofilms and blood-brain barrier.	Limited access to deep or protected sites.	(Hu et al., 2024)

Nanotechnology provides considerable benefits, particularly the ability to combat biofilm-mediated infections, which is a major impediment to conventional antibiotic-based treatments. The ability to pinpoint the site of infections and maintain drug delivery over long durations reduces the need for frequent doses and mitigates the negative consequences.

The Role of Nanotechnology in the Mitigation of Antimicrobial Resistance

It has been proposed that nanotechnology can help address the issue of antimicrobial resistance by providing targeted therapies at the sites of infection, thereby limiting the exposure of microbes to the system and reducing the chances of developing resistance. The nanoparticles have been shown to enter biofilm deposits as well as cross blood-brain barriers and thus can be used to treat infections that are resistant to conventional treatment (Naeem et al., 2023).

4. HOST-TAILORED THERAPEUTIC STRATEGIES

With the growing international interest in antimicrobial resistance (AMR), there is a renewed emphasis on personalized medicine as a form of intervention to develop more specific and targeted treatments. Personalized medicine is based on the idea of tailoring treatment to an individual's genetic makeup, microbiome composition, and other individual-specific factors. New approaches, such as pharmacogenomics and modulation of the microbiome, are on the horizon and have great potential to achieve higher precision, fewer side effects, and lower development of resistance. The core of this system is pharmacogenomics, a field established to understand how genetic variability affects individual responses to different drugs. Currently, medication prescribers can perform pharmacogenomic investigations, thereby improving the decision-making process regarding dose scheduling. The goal will ultimately be to maximize drug efficacy and minimize harmful reactions, which is particularly important to note, as the current dosing paradigm is likely to be incompatible with patients of diverse genetic and metabolic makeup, thereby elevating the risk of antimicrobial resistance (Han et al., 2025).

4.1 Pharmacogenomics: Tailoring Drug Dosing to Individual Profiles

Pharmacogenomics offers a practical approach to combating antimicrobial resistance (AMR) by leveraging a factored study of clinical practice. A good case in point is the targeted use of vancomycin using genotype-based CYP2D6 classification. Despite vancomycin being inevitable in the treatment of methicillin-resistant Staphylococcus aureus (MRSA), its nephrotoxicity, which is accompanied by an increased dosage, is a deadly issue. The results presented in one of the 2024 articles published in Clinical Pharmacology and Therapeutics confirm that CYP2D6 genomic testing significantly reduces kidney damage. Tailoring vancomycin dosage to an individual's CYP2D6 genotype has been shown to reduce nephrotoxicity by up to 40%, thereby increasing both the efficacy and safety of therapy. Pharmacogenomic testing can also play a role in reducing adverse drug reactions (ADRs); an example is prospective testing to detect HLA-B*57:01 status in advance of therapy with HIV medicine abacavir (Dash et al., 2024). This genetic marker can be detected to pre-emptively diagnose individuals at risk of hypersensitivity, allowing for safer treatment regimens to be applied. The figure itself provides an example of the usefulness of pharmacogenomics in overcoming AMR, including CYP2D6-guided vancomycin dosing, which increases its therapeutic effectiveness with decreased related side effects. Much has already been done, but widespread pharmacogenomic testing is hindered by high prices, logistical challenges, and the need to consider site-specific genetic diversity. It is crucial that these factors are addressed to realize the full potential of personalized medicine in the international response to AMR.

4.2 Microbiome Engineering: Restoring Healthy Balance

The human microbiome plays a vital role in maintaining immune system homeostasis and physiological balance. However, there has been a rise in antimicrobial resistance (AMR) that has been linked with the prevalence of antibiotic usage. As a reaction, microbiome-engineering interventions have been considered to restore ecological stability and help address resistant infections. Of these, the fecal microbiota transplantation (FMT) is an idea that is gaining popularity as a potential treatment. This modality involves transferring healthy microbial biota from donors who are pathologically and clinically healthy into the recipient, aiming to restore normal structure and taxonomic diversity (Sivamani et al., 2025). It has been demonstrated that these interventions can be utilized against recurrent Clostridium difficile infections, thereby highlighting their potential as both antibiotic and preventive measures against antibiotic-resistant pathogens. At the same time, precision prebiotics offer a different paradigm that can trigger the fast rise of beneficial microbial lineages, especially in the neonatal stage when xenobiotics are the most vulnerable. Empirical evidence indicates that strategic use of dietary supplementation is sufficient to reduce the risks of AMR by establishing a bacterial ecosystem that can induce an intrinsic defense against pathogenic species. However, several potentially substantial issues remain, including the safety of genome-edited probiotics, particularly in CRISPR-edited strains, and the nature of microbial assemblage variability, which limits the predictive power of clinical outcomes. Based on this, considerations highlight the need for prospective, rigorously designed studies to maximize the safety and therapeutic efficacy of microbial-based interventions (Simon et al., 2025).

5. OVERCOMING BARRIERS AND MOVING FORWARD

Precision medicine is a potentially powerful tool to combat antimicrobial resistance (AMR); however, numerous barriers hinder its widespread adoption. Recent precision tools, of which AI-driven diagnostics, pharmacogenomics, and microbiome engineering are most prominent, provide new opportunities to address AMR. At the same time, the industry faces significant challenges in terms of technology, finance, and regulation. It is of utmost importance that efforts to overcome these obstacles are in place to achieve global health goals in AMR, and that coordinated efforts must be taken. The subsequent discussion identifies the primary obstacles to precision medicine in the context of antimicrobial resistance and outlines a strategic plan beyond 2030 to address these challenges, as well as discusses the initiatives that are likely to characterize management within the context of AMR (Batool et al., 2024).

5.1 Barriers to Implementing Precision Medicine

Precision medicine is now being viewed as a relatively promising approach to tackling antimicrobial resistance (AMR); however, significant financial obstacles, including the high costs of AI-based diagnostic platforms, are still hindering its widespread implementation. Since the application of AI in the healthcare setting of detecting AMR requires a solid infrastructure and advanced data management strategies, both of which significantly increase the annual budget of a facility, it is clear that there is a noticeable addition to the budget of a facility due to AI implementation in healthcare settings. According to a study published in 2024 in JAMA Health Forum, implementing AI-based diagnostics for AMR in a hospital may cost no more than $50,000 per year (Aslam & Aljasir, 2025). Such financial burden is particularly high in low- and middle-income countries, where the introduction of state-of-the-art technology is still limited. Besides, the internal sophistication of AI platforms and the constant necessity to update software increase the expense of operations, thus inhibiting the further spread of these instruments.

The second and related barrier involves the lack of clearly established rules that regulate the emergent AMR therapeutics, like phage therapy. Phage therapy has a significantly high efficacy in treating multidrug-resistant infections, but its clinical application is increasingly limited due to its regulatory status, which restricts its use. The 2024 World Health Organization review reiterated the need to clarify certain standard regulations to promote the clinical use of phage therapy and related medical practices (KEPHALOPOULOS et al., 2024). Without such regulations, large-scale clinical trials would not be feasible, thereby limiting access and slowing the spread of new therapies globally. Further challenges are compounded by the complexity of mixed international regulatory systems: provisions surrounding even the most necessary interventions can become blocked by diverging national demands, further impeding access to populations most at risk.

5.2 Strategic Initiatives for Combating AMR by 2030

There has been significant progress made in precision medicine against antimicrobial resistance (AMR), despite numerous challenges. c The current programmed is systematic in its strategy for Whole Genome Sequencing (WGS) and global surveillance of resistant pathogens, which expedite the diagnosis of cases and enhance accuracy in individual patient care. Moreover, the One Health Approach prioritizes the underlying relationship between human, animal, and environmental health. A surveillance programme was conducted by the United States Department of Agriculture (USDA) and the Environmental Protection Agency (EPA) in 2024 that assessed the use of antimicrobial resistance (AMR) in livestock and also considered the impact of antibiotics in the agricultural industry. By extension, these efforts pose a significant challenge and require long-term, transnational partnerships, as well as improved data sharing and innovation, to manage AMR-related threats effectively (Organization, 2024). Despite these, there are remaining impediments (such as the high costs of implementing precision medicine on a large scale regarding AMR, legal discrepancies, technological drawbacks, and global demographic differences) that cannot be overcome until 2030, making the widespread use of precision medicine regarding AMR unlikely. These barriers and their inherent solutions are represented and described in Table 3. To include precision medicine in AMR management, all these difficulties must be overcome.

Table 3. Challenges in Precision Medicine Implementation

Barrier	Impact on Precision Medicine	Current Solutions and Progress	Key Stakeholders Involved	Regional Impact	Potential Long-Term Solutions	References
High Costs of AI Diagnostics	Limits adoption, especially in low- and middle-income countries (LMICs).	Public-private partnerships and cost-reduction strategies for AI are being explored.	Healthcare providers, tech companies, governments	LMICs, especially rural and underserved areas	Research into cost-effective AI solutions, subsidies, international partnerships to lower costs.	(Rabaan et al., 2022)
Regulatory Gaps in Novel Treatments	Lack of standardized regulations for phage therapy and other novel drugs.	WHO is working on developing global regulatory frameworks for innovative treatments.	WHO, regulatory bodies, pharmaceutical companies	Global, with a focus on developing nations	Global regulatory harmonization, clearer frameworks for fast-tracking approval.	(Dillac et al., 2024)
Technological Barriers	Limited access to WGS and other tools in resource-poor settings.	WHO's Precision AMR 2030 initiative focuses on integrating WGS into global AMR monitoring systems.	WHO, international health organizations	LMICs, conflict zones, and remote regions	Increased infrastructure development, global funding for technology access.	(Batool et al., 2024)
Global Disparities	Exacerbates health inequities and limits access to precision medicine.	Technology transfer programs and global collaborations are expanding access in LMICs.	International organizations, governments, NGOs	LMICs, rural and marginalized populations	Technology transfer, local capacity building, equitable distribution of resources.	(Eke & Cua, 2025)

6. REAL-WORLD APPLICATIONS AND CASE STUDIES

As outcomes, precision medicine has become an everyday concept that has gone beyond a scholarly concept and become an operational plan to combat antimicrobial resistance (AMR). It is currently being deployed in a variety of regions, including modern technologies like artificial intelligence (AI), CRISPR-based gene editing, mRNA vaccination, and precision-medicine-based diagnostics. Such interventions reveal their potential to change how multidrug-resistant pathogens are managed, meaning they have the potential to significantly influence the AMR trend worldwide.

6.1 Case Study 1: AI and CRISPR in Action

A case study released in Texas in 2024 revealed the combined potential of artificial intelligence and CRISPR-based genome editing in addressing a carbapenem-resistant Klebsiella pneumoniae (CR-Kp) outbreak. The epidemic, primarily noted in intensive-care units, was swiftly managed through the implementation of artificial intelligence-driven surveillance and the identification of patients at risk. The elements of natural language processing elucidated the behavior of bacteria, while predictive models of the computations forecasted the pathways of bacterial contamination and interventions. Concurrently, the application of CRISPR genome modification enabled the targeted alteration of factors contributing to antimicrobial resistance. A post-intervention assessment conducted by the CDC (2024) indicates that this hybrid methodology significantly reduced the infection rate and prevented secondary spreading, showcasing the potential of combining AI and CRISPR to address the challenge of antimicrobial resistance (Olatunji et al., 2024).

6.2 Case Study 2: mRNA Vaccines for AMR

The reduction of antibiotic-resistant microorganisms is an emerging focus, driven by the increasing impact of mRNA vaccines as preventive strategies. In 2024, Pfizer made a significant investment in an anticancer mRNA vaccine by initiating a Phase II trial for its mRNA vaccine aimed at Neisseria gonorrhoeae, a sexually transmitted infection that has developed resistance to multiple antibiotics. The trial condition examined a vaccine made of artificially produced bacterial protein antigens that had been developed to stimulate the immune responses before exposure to gonorrhea. Initial findings show a significant immunologic efficacy, a fact that will result in a significant reduction in the number of cases of gonorrhea and consequently reduce the development of gonococcus resistant to antibiotics. This finding highlights a new paradigm of vaccine causal agent development in bacterial pathogen, an area that has been traditionally difficult in comparison to the advancements in the study of viral vaccines (Abusalah et al., 2024).

6.3 Implementing Precision Medicine in Low-Resource Areas

Integration of precision medicine in a resource-constrained setting is a complex issue. Genomic sequencing and AI-based diagnostic paths face challenges in Southeast Asia, Africa, and Latin America, regions with poorly developed health-care infrastructure and limited reporting capacity. The situation is most critical in the African region, where the prevalence of TB and HIV is extremely high and where cost-effective sequential technologies and effective training of the entire health-care workforce are most needed. Ongoing initiatives, such as the Global Health Sequencing Initiative, aim to mitigate these obstacles by providing practitioners with access to tools and training. Southeast Asia has implemented interventions that utilize mHealth applications and telemedicine to support local diagnostic activities. Latin America, on the other hand, is promoting antibiotic stewardship programs and genetic testing, enabling the optimal use of antimicrobial agents. The consistent work done under the directive of the Pan American Health Organization (PAHO) is gradually increasing the reach of precision medicine, even in economically strained settings (Misra et al., 2023).

7. ETHICAL CONSIDERATIONS IN PRECISION MEDICINE FOR AMR

With precision medicine representing a critical paradigm in the modern counterpoint to antimicrobial resistance (AMR), the implementation thereof is not without a range of ethical concerns that must be examined with due diligence. The convergence of genomic information, artificial intelligence, and new methods of treatment, such as genetically modified organisms, will raise new issues related to access to information, personal confidentiality, informed consent, and the ethical implications of modifying living organisms. The primary related challenges are safeguarding patient rights, ensuring procedural fairness, and the potential for unforeseen effects. The issue of urgency, then, is about constructing a balanced regulatory framework that not only protects personal interests but also enables technological advancement (Figure 7).

7.1 Ethical Issues in AI Diagnostics

The recent improvements in antimicrobial resistance (AMR) management in artificial intelligence (AI)- assisted diagnostics propose a multifaceted sphere of ethical challenges. First and foremost clinical data should be safeguarded. Artificial intelligence systems must gather, store, and analyze sensitive data, such as genomic profiles and detailed medical histories. Without strict security measures, these datasets can be hacked, thus exposing patients to privacy breaches, among other things, and unauthorised manipulation. The ethical risk is increased by the fact that sensitive genomic data has the potential to travel without the patients being informed of this (Ito et al., 2025).

Informed permission is a central ethical standard when it comes to the responsive assimilation of AI-based analysis technologies in AMR care. It follows that patients should be provided with detailed explanations of the methods for obtaining, using, storing, and sharing their data, as this field is rapidly evolving. The lack of actual informed consent can unintentionally violate patient privacy, reduce trust in healthcare organizations, and aggravate the adoption of new technologies. It is also necessary to consider the fairness of providing such diagnostic services with the help of AI. Inventions should be shared equally to prevent the worsening of pre-existing inequalities among the population. Conclusively, the diagram below illustrates the key ethical considerations of AI-based diagnostics in the context of AMR, highlighting the importance of sound data governance, patient autonomy, and equity in the AMR agenda (Dhiman & Pandey).

7.2 The Debate Over "Designer Phages"

Altering the phages so that they could be used to edit genes of other organisms for the purpose of the targeted destruction of definite species of bacteria has sparked the question whether such modified phages should be perceived as genetically modified organisms (GMOs). Although phage therapy is largely considered a promising second-generation intervention against multidrug-resistant pathogens, the deployment of CRISPR-mediated editing to phages raises ecological concerns, chief among them the possibility of unintended mutations in non-target microbes and the post-editing proliferation of phage mutants ex vivo. On the one hand, academics call for the introduction of strict regulatory control of gene-edited phages on existing GMO laws, and other commentators describe the constructs to be innovative weapons in the current war against antimicrobial resistance. As a result, the debate has narrowed to the development of a moderate balance between the therapeutic benefit of precise microbial therapies and the risks that are posed by genetically modified microorganisms (Carascal et al., 2022).

7.3 Access to Precision Medicine in Low-Resource Settings

Low- and middle-income countries (LMICs) are characterized by acute resource scarcity that informs the moral need to uphold an ethical obligation to foster equitable access to precision medicine, as discussed in the context of antimicrobial resistance (AMR). As precision-medicine capabilities continue to advance, one predictable consequence is that these new capabilities will likely serve the already wealthy at the expense of LMICs, which will lack access to effective remedies. Thus, the main ethical dilemma encourages, in the first place, meeting the needs of universal access to the implemented innovations and the fairness of treatment decisions even at the level of limited availability of resources (Misra et al., 2023).

8. FUTURE PROSPECTS: EMERGING TECHNOLOGIES AND THEIR IMPACT

The problem of antimicrobial resistance is a long-term issue of public health, acceptance of which will be linked to the implementation of new technologies capable of changing the paradigm of therapeutic practice and diagnostic practice. Modern approaches to the challenge of resistant microorganisms include synthetic biology, phage therapy, nanotechnology, artificial intelligence, and CRISPR-based treatment. Together, such advances will transform pathogen control and detection strategy. Meanwhile the broad-based global health approaches and organized policy-based responses will be paramount in making sure that such inventions are available, fair and can help stop the further resistance growth. The discussion below illustrates the emerging patterns in the diagnosis of antimicrobial resistance, the development of therapeutic research, and the integration of the global health framework, all of which will shape the way forward in the world's response to antimicrobial resistance (Qudrat-Ullah, 2024).

8.1 The Future of AMR Diagnosis

The modern development of diagnostic technologies will redefine the treatment of antimicrobial resistance (AMR). AI-based diagnostic solutions are expected to provide a fast and highly accurate way of detecting pathogens with rates significantly higher than 95% and outperforming conventional culture-based systems. By combining genetic-marker data with discipline-specific current clinical data, such systems can guide antibiotic choice and minimize the inappropriate use of antibiotics, thereby reducing resistance. Simultaneously, there is also an attractive path in nanotechnology: the same diagnostic sensors that deploy nanoparticles can serve as a path to rapid respiratory screening for pathogen-resistant organisms at the point of care. At the same time, studies that aim to block the colonization of medical devices with drug-resistant biofilms, focusing on self-healing materials, seek to mitigate the spread of resistant strains by not only decreasing the rate of hospital-acquired infections but also preventing the emergence of multidrug-resistant strains altogether. The potential synergistic combination of these new diagnostic approaches is a great step forward in the monitoring and detection/treatment of AMR (Tang et al., 2023).

8.2 Advancements in Therapeutic Development

The increasing rates of antimicrobial resistance necessitate the search for new treatment methods, as the effectiveness of traditional antibiotics is declining. Recent evidence suggests that phage therapy holds significant promise in clinical studies, particularly for treating multidrug-resistant infections. The newest designation of several phage-based items by the FDA as Breakthrough Therapies represents the intensifying hold-up of phage-based therapeutic approaches. Similar progress can be cited regarding CRISPR techniques that harness the makeup of bacterial DNA to disable recalcitrant genes of concern in clinics. Parallel, the tools made by synthetic biology are advancing with the creation of specific agents, antimicrobial peptides (AMPs) with effectiveness against different resistant microbes, including Acinetobacter baumannii, and which can perhaps lead to the development of customized treatments based on an individual's genetic makeup (Gunturu, 2025).

8.3 Policy and Global Health Integration

One Health approach and precision medicine, as co-used elements of strategic interventions to reduce antimicrobial resistance (AMR), should be considered in the context of interdependent human, animal, and environmental health. In the Global Action Plan on AMR released by the World Health Organization (WHO), intra-sectoral collaboration is highlighted as a critical need to conduct surveillance and to prevent the spread of resistant pathogens across these areas. The introduction of precision medicine into the One-Health practice will not only streamline clinical and veterinary surveillance and care for antibiotic-resistant organisms but also enhance clinical accuracy. At the same time, it is crucial to strengthen financing processes and establish long-term relationships with the WHO, the G7, and public-private partnerships. These partnerships will not only lead to funding of empirical research, protection of fair access to emerging technologies, but also to address AMR in low and middle-income settings (Gunturu, 2025).

7. CONCLUSION

Precision medicine offers a revolutionary opportunity to protect millions of lives through its integration into the international antimicrobial resistance (AMR) plan. Novel technologies, including artificial intelligence (AI) based diagnostics, whole-genome sequencing, as well as targeted therapeutics, will lead to a paradigm shift of the prevailing approaches of managing AMR, enhancing therapeutic options, and reducing the surreptitious prevalence of resistance. According to the NIH hypotheses (2024), these innovations have the potential to avert 3.2 million deaths each year over the next decade, in the 2030s. Precision medicine holds the promise of improving the efficacy of AMR interventions through enhanced diagnostic accuracy and tailored therapeutic regimens, while also minimizing adverse effects, particularly in the context of multidrug-resistant infections. Nonetheless, the realization of these benefits is contingent upon collective efforts on a global scale. The G7 Declaration (2024) recommends the establishment of an annual investment of 2 billion US dollars in research related to AMR, the implementation of standardized protocols for Whole Genome Sequencing (WGS), enhanced AMR surveillance, and the bolstering of surveillance capacities, especially in low- and middle-income countries (LMICs). To achieve the eventual success of AMR, ongoing investment, robust international collaboration, and extensive monitoring of resistant strains are necessary to shape multinational responses.

REFERENCES

Abusalah, M. A. H., Choudhary, P., Bargui, H., Ahmed, N., Abusalah, M. A. H., & Choudhary, O. P. (2024). A prognostic insight of the mRNA vaccine against antibiotic-resistant bacteria. *Annals of Medicine and Surgery (London), 86*(7), 3801–3805. PMID: 38989193

Alara, J. A., & Alara, O. R. (2024). An overview of the global alarming increase of multiple drug resistant: A major challenge in clinical diagnosis. *Infectious Disorders-Drug TargetsDisorders, 24*(3), 26–42. PMID: 37909431

Aslam, B., & Aljasir, S. F. (2025). Climate Change and AMR: Interconnected Threats and One Health Solutions. *Antibiotics (Basel, Switzerland), 14*(9), 946. PMID: 41009922

Batool, S. P., Fatima, H., & Ul Abadin, M. Z., MD, J. R., Joseph, A., Imran, M., & Hussain, N. (2024). Innovative Therapies In The Fight Against Antimicrobial Resistance Bridging Gaps And Overcoming Barriers. *Frontiers in Health Informatics, 13*(3).

Bikard, D., & Barrangou, R. (2017). Using CRISPR-Cas systems as antimicrobials. *Current Opinion in Microbiology, 37*, 155–160. PMID: 28888103

Cai, X., Tian, J., Zhu, J., Chen, J., Li, L., Yang, C., Chen, J., & Chen, D. (2021). Photodynamic and photothermal co-driven CO-enhanced multi-mode synergistic antibacterial nanoplatform to effectively fight against biofilm infections. *Chemical Engineering Journal, 426*, 131919.

Carascal, M. B., dela Cruz-Papa, D. M., Remenyi, R., Cruz, M. C. B., & Destura, R. V. (2022). Phage revolution against multidrug-resistant clinical pathogens in Southeast Asia. *Frontiers in Microbiology, 13*, 820572. PMID: 35154059

Chambers, H. F., Fowler, V. G.Jr, & Group, A. R. L. (2022). *Confronting antimicrobial resistance together* (Vol. 323). American Physiological Society Rockville.

Chen, J., Liu, Z., Huang, X., Wu, C., Liu, Q., Jiang, G., Pu, Y., Lei, Y., Chen, X., & Wang, X. (2024). When large language models meet personalization: Perspectives of challenges and opportunities. *World Wide Web (Bussum), 27*(4), 42.

Cubillos-Ruiz, A., Guo, T., Sokolovska, A., Miller, P. F., Collins, J. J., Lu, T. K., & Lora, J. M. (2021). Engineering living therapeutics with synthetic biology. *Nature Reviews. Drug Discovery, 20*(12), 941–960. PMID: 34616030

Dash, B., Shireen, M., Kumar, S., Goel, A., Semwal, P., & Rani, R. (2024). A comprehensive review: Pharmacogenomics and personalized medicine customizing drug therapy based on individual genetics profiles. *Chinese. Journal of Applied Physiology (Bethesda, Md.)*, •••, 20240011.

Dhiman, R., & Pandey, R. P. Ethical and Regulatory Considerations for Artificial Intelligence in Managing AMR. In *Artificial Intelligence in Managing Antimicrobial Resistance* (pp. 135–157). CRC Press.

Dillac, L., Christie, W., van Dalen, D., & Adiningrat, R. P. P. (2024). New approaches to combat Antimicrobial Resistance (AMR)? Due, A. (2023). What are side effects? *European Journal for Philosophy of Science*, *13*(1), 16.

Eke, S. M., & Cua, A. (2025). Invisible Engines of Resistance: How Global Inequities Drive Antimicrobial Failure. *Antibiotics (Basel, Switzerland)*, *14*(7), 659. PMID: 40723962

Eslami, M., Naderian, R., Bahar, A., Babaeizad, A., Rezanavaz Gheshlagh, S., Oksenych, V., & Tahmasebi, H. (2025). Microbiota as diagnostic biomarkers: Advancing early cancer detection and personalized therapeutic approaches through microbiome profiling. *Frontiers in Immunology*, *16*, 1559480. PMID: 40406094

Gebre, M. S., Brito, L. A., Tostanoski, L. H., Edwards, D. K., Carfi, A., & Barouch, D. H. (2021). Novel approaches for vaccine development. *Cell*, *184*(6), 1589–1603. PMID: 33740454

Gunturu, S. (2025). Innovative Strategies to Combat Antimicrobial Resistance: Advances in Drug Discovery, Alternative Therapies and Immune Modulation. [AJP]. *Asian Journal of Pharmaceutics*, *19*(2).

Han, E. J., Ahn, J.-S., Chae, Y. J., & Chung, H.-J. (2025). Immunomodulatory Roles of Faecalibacterium prausnitzii and Akkermansia muciniphila in Autoimmune Diseases: Mechanistic Insights and Therapeutic Potential. *Clinical Reviews in Allergy & Immunology*, *68*(1), 77. PMID: 40759811

Hassan, Y. M., Mohamed, A. S., Hassan, Y. M., & El-Sayed, W. M. (2025). Recent developments and future directions in point-of-care next-generation CRISPR-based rapid diagnosis. *Clinical and Experimental Medicine*, *25*(1), 33. PMID: 39789283

Herdiana, Y., Wathoni, N., Shamsuddin, S., & Muchtaridi, M. (2022). Drug release study of the chitosan-based nanoparticles. *Heliyon*, *8*(1). PMID: 35028457

Hu, M., Li, X., You, Z., Cai, R., & Chen, C. (2024). Physiological barriers and strategies of lipid-based nanoparticles for nucleic acid drug delivery. *Advanced Materials*, *36*(22), 2303266. PMID: 37792475

Ijaz, S., Iqbal, J., Abbasi, B. A., Tufail, A., Yaseen, T., Uddin, S., Usman, K., Ullah, R., Bibi, H., & Inam, P. (2024). Current stage of preclinical and clinical development of guggulsterone in cancers: Challenges and promises. *Cell Biology International, 48*(2), 128–142. PMID: 38148708

Ito, H., Wada, T., Ichinose, G., Tanimoto, J., Yoshimura, J., Yamamoto, T., & Morita, S. (2025). Barriers to the widespread adoption of diagnostic artificial intelligence for preventing antimicrobial resistance. *Scientific Reports, 15*(1), 13113. PMID: 40240443

Jaumaux, F., & Gómez de Cadiñanos, P., L., & Gabant, P. (2020). In the age of synthetic biology, will antimicrobial peptides be the next generation of antibiotics? *Antibiotics (Basel, Switzerland), 9*(8), 484. PMID: 32781540

KEPHALOPOULOS, S., COECKE, S., GAWLIK, B. M., QUERCI, M., MARCHINI, A., RUIZ, M. A., CORBISIER, P., PETRILLO, M., RAFFAEL, B., & SPAGNOLO, L. (2024). Antimicrobial resistance: Crowdsourcing JRC Knowledge on AMR, AMR@ JRC Café, 24 October 2023.

Lathakumari, R. H., Vajravelu, L. K., Thulukanam, J., & Narasimhan, A. K. (2025). Next-gen nano biosensor technologies to monitor carbapenem resistance for personalized medicine. *Indian Journal of Microbiology, 65*(1), 277–296. PMID: 40371034

Misra, S., Aguilar-Salinas, C. A., Chikowore, T., Konradsen, F., Ma, R. C., Mbau, L., Mohan, V., Morton, R. W., Nyirenda, M. J., & Tapela, N. (2023). The case for precision medicine in the prevention, diagnosis, and treatment of cardiometabolic diseases in low-income and middle-income countries. *The Lancet. Diabetes & Endocrinology, 11*(11), 836–847. PMID: 37804857

Mulchandani, R., Tiseo, K., Nandi, A., Klein, E., Gandra, S., Laxminarayan, R., & Van Boeckel, T. (2025). Global trends in inappropriate use of antibiotics, 2000–2021: Scoping review and prevalence estimates. *BMJ Public Health, 3*(1). PMID: 40444029

Naeem, M. I., Aziz, S., Akhtar, T., Asghar, M., Tanveer, K., Rehman, A., Zahid, R., Tehseen, U., Arbab, Z., & Ahmad, H. M. (2023). Use of nanotechnology to mitigate antimicrobial resistance.

Olatunji, A. O., Olaboye, J. A., Maha, C. C., Kolawole, T. O., & Abdul, S. (2024). Next-Generation strategies to combat antimicrobial resistance: Integrating genomics, CRISPR, and novel therapeutics for effective treatment. *Engineering Science & Technology Journal, 5*(7), 2284–2303.

Organization, W. H. (2024). *WHO Strategic and Technical Advisory Group for Antimicrobial Resistance (STAG-AMR): report of the fourth meeting 11-13 June 2024*. World Health Organization.

Panchpuri, M., Painuli, R., & Kumar, C. (2025). Artificial intelligence in smart drug delivery systems: A step toward personalized medicine. *RSC Pharmaceutics*.

Parcell, B. J. (2021). *Whole genome sequencing service: investigating healthcare associated infections*. University of St Andrews.

Paulson, D., & Johnson, A. (2025). Integrating Artificial Intelligence with Genomic and Biomarker Data for the Advancement of Personalized Therapeutics in a Human-Centric Framework.

Qudrat-Ullah, H. (2024). Future Prospects and Emerging Technologies. *Sustainable Energy: A Myth or Reality*, 185-202.

Rabaan, A. A., Alhumaid, S., Mutair, A. A., Garout, M., Abulhamayel, Y., Halwani, M. A., Alestad, J. H., Bshabshe, A. A., Sulaiman, T., & AlFonaisan, M. K. (2022). Application of artificial intelligence in combating high antimicrobial resistance rates. *Antibiotics (Basel, Switzerland)*, *11*(6), 784. PMID: 35740190

Shukla, V., Singh, S., Verma, S., Verma, S., Rizvi, A. A., & Abbas, M. (2024). Targeting the microbiome to improve human health with the approach of personalized medicine: Latest aspects and current updates. *Clinical Nutrition ESPEN*, *63*, 813–820. PMID: 39178987

Simon, B. O., Nnaji, N. D., Anumudu, C. K., Aleke, J. C., Ekwueme, C. T., Uhegwu, C. C., Ihenetu, F. C., Obioha, P., Ifedinezi, O. V., & Ezechukwu, P. S. (2025). Microbiome-based interventions for food safety and environmental health. *Applied Sciences (Basel, Switzerland)*, *15*(9), 5219.

Singhal, L., Gupta, P., & Gupta, V. (2025). Diagnostic stewardship in clinical microbiology: An indispensable component of patient care. *Infectious Disorders Drug Targets*, *25*(2), E030724231543. PMID: 38963103

Sivamani, Y., Chakraborty, A., Kounin, A. P., & Elayaperumal, S. (2025). Microbiome Engineering and its Applications. In *Microbiome Engineering* (pp. 13–34). CRC Press.

Sukhum, K. V., Diorio-Toth, L., & Dantas, G. (2019). Genomic and metagenomic approaches for predictive surveillance of emerging pathogens and antibiotic resistance. *Clinical Pharmacology and Therapeutics*, *106*(3), 512–524. PMID: 31172511

Sultana, A., Zare, M., Thomas, V., Kumar, T. S., & Ramakrishna, S. (2022). Nano-based drug delivery systems: Conventional drug delivery routes, recent developments and future prospects. *Medicine in Drug Discovery*, *15*, 100134.

Sunderland, K. S., Yang, M., & Mao, C. (2017). Phage-enabled nanomedicine: From probes to therapeutics in precision medicine. *Angewandte Chemie International Edition*, *56*(8), 1964–1992. PMID: 27491926

Tang, K. W. K., Millar, B. C., & Moore, J. E. (2023). Antimicrobial resistance (AMR). *British Journal of Biomedical Science*, *80*, 11387. PMID: 37448857

Theivendren, P., Kunjiappan, S., Pavadai, P., Ravi, K., Murugavel, A., Dayalan, A., & Santhana Krishna Kumar, A. (2024). Revolutionizing cancer immunotherapy: Emerging nanotechnology-driven drug delivery systems for enhanced therapeutic efficacy. *ACS Measurement Science Au*, *5*(1), 31–55. PMID: 39991031

Tsalidou, M., Stergiopoulou, T., Bostanitis, I., Nikaki, C., Skoumpa, K., Koutsoukou, T., & Papaioannidou, P. (2023). Surveillance of antimicrobial resistance and multidrug resistance prevalence of clinical isolates in a regional hospital in Northern Greece. *Antibiotics (Basel, Switzerland)*, *12*(11), 1595. PMID: 37998797

Chapter 14
Breaking the Resistance Barrier:
Integrating Microbiome Research Into AMR Solutions

Maria Nazir Ahmad
https://orcid.org/0009-0004-6714-6212
Cholistan University of Veterinary and Animal Sciences, Bahawalpur, Pakistan

Syed Sohail Ahmad
https://orcid.org/0009-0001-9652-7565
Rehman College of Allied Health Sciences, Rehman Medical Institute, Pakistan

ABSTRACT

Antimicrobial resistance (AMR) is a growing global health threat, as traditional antibiotics are becoming increasingly ineffective. This chapter explores microbiome-based therapies as innovative solutions to combat AMR. It discusses how engineered probiotics, synthetic antimicrobial peptides (AMPs), and CRISPR gene editing can target resistant pathogens while restoring the balance of the microbiome. The chapter highlights the potential of personalized microbiome medicine to tailor treatments based on individual microbiome profiles, improving effectiveness and reducing resistance. Additionally, it emphasizes the importance of global collaborations in advancing microbiome research and AMR solutions, with efforts from organizations like the WHO. Ultimately, the chapter highlights the transformative potential of microbiome-based interventions in combating AMR, emphasizing the need for ongoing research and international collaboration.

DOI: 10.4018/979-8-3373-3825-5.ch014

1. INTRODUCTION

Antimicrobial resistance (AMR) has rapidly become a global public health concern, posing a significant threat to the progress made in twentieth-century medicine. According to the World Health Organisation (WHO), it is likely that by 2050, AMR may also trigger a total of 10 million deaths annually, becoming the main cause of mortality worldwide, even above cancer (Hussain et al., 2025). *Enterococcus faecium, Staphylococcus aureus, Klebsiella pneumoniae, Acinetobacter baumannii, Pseudomonas aeruginosa, and Enterobacter spp* are primarily responsible for multidrug-resistant infections (Kim et al., 2021). Recent research into the human microbiome has indicated alternative methods of countermeasures that not only address AMR but also suppress its spread. The human microbiome, a combination of microorganisms on and in the body, acts in both directions: it carries and distributes resistance genes, while simultaneously offering therapeutic options to interfere with them. The given discourse presents an overview of the emerging microbiome science that can break through the AMR barrier, focusing on microbial diversity, horizontal gene transfer (HGT), and microbiome-based remedies.

The human microbiome is a diverse, heterogeneous, and interacting assembly of bacteria, fungi, viruses, and archaea, which plays a crucial role in maintaining health and modulating disease. Nevertheless, despite being critical in immune regulation, nutrient assimilation, and vitamin production, it is also involved in maintaining AMR through the horizontal transfer of resistance genes. Take the example of extended-spectrum beta-lactamase (ESBL) and carbapenemases genes, which often transfer to other pathogenic organisms (in the same gut) and in the process initiate multi-drug resistance (Riwu et al., 2020).

Academically, it is currently widely accepted that a healthy, diverse microbiome plays a crucial role in natural resistance to the emergence and spread of antibiotic-resistant pathogens. Within the gastrointestinal tract, the species of commensal bacteria use the mechanisms of competitive inhibition and immunomodulation to limit the colonization of harmful microorganisms. As another example, it has been demonstrated that the metabolism of short-chain fatty acids (SCFAs) by Faecalibacterium prausnitzii is associated with the stability of intestinal epithelia and the reduction of systemic infections (He et al., 2021). Nevertheless, this flora is threatened by antibiotic-related dysbiosis, which eradicates fertile strains while promoting the growth of resistant clones. Events have highlighted a dire need for accuracy in antimicrobial therapies that minimize damage to beneficial biota and provide maximum benefits to pathogenic strains.

It has also been empirically proven that microbial diversity is a key defense against antimicrobial resistance. Existing studies indicate that heterogeneous communities are highly redundant in terms of functionality, in that if one taxonomic group is inhibited by antibiotics, other members of the community can sustain the same functional role and thus evade the development of pathogens. The term colonization resistance illustrates this ability commensal species, such as *Bacteroides* and *Lactobacilli*, block the proliferation of vancomycin-resistant Enterococcus (VRE) through competition to adhere and produce antimicrobial metabolites (Ducarmon et al., 2019).

Microbial diversity is also strongly affected by environmental variables and dietary compositions. Hospitalization and overuse of antibiotics tend to induce the preponderance of antibiotic-resistant bacterial clones, and high fibre diets tend to enrich the populations of beneficial microbial taxa. Recovery of microbiome diversity after the pathophysiological disruption caused by antibiotics, therefore, is a centerpiece of research goals. These measures are probiotic intake, prebiotic and faecal microbiota transplantation (FMT). Both of those strategies aim to restore the equilibrium of destroyed microbial environments and turn the trend towards antimicrobial resistance in a clinical setting (Vliex, 2024).

In modern clinical trials, microbiome-based interventions have proven to be effective in the decrease of antimicrobial resistance (AMR). One notable example includes the Fecal Microbiota Transplantation (FMT), a treatment that made the relapse of Clostridioides difficile in a cohort of patients a relic of the past. FMT has increased microbial diversity and, at the same time, decreased the abundance of multidrug-resistant organisms in the intestinal microbiome. This finding demonstrates that the microbiome restoration process has the potential to prevent repeated carriage of antibiotic-resistant agents and increase the treatment options against AMR (Cusumano et al., 2025).

Phage therapy, which is an alternative to traditional antibiotics, is a further microbiome-based strategy that is in clinical development. They addressed a refractory infection with Pseudomonas aeruginosa, clearing it by treatment with engineered lytic agents (bacteriophages) specific to the resistant strain, thereby demonstrating the bespoke value of using microbiome-derived therapeutics against AMR. Taken together, these findings imply that a microbiome-based intervention can be an effective and specialized approach to AMR (Gordillo Altamirano & Barr, 2019).

The synergetic cooperation of microbiome-centred therapies and next-generation sequencing (NGS) is expected to improve future routes in this area of research. The accuracy of NGSs allows fine-grained interrogation of microbiome makeup, and its use can help clinicians identify resistance determinants, prepare interventions based on patient-level microbial compositions. In addition, the development of synthetic microbiomes (genetically engineered microbial communities meant to out-compete resistant pathogens and restore lost microbial functions), ponders another frontline of the struggle against AMR.

2. MICROBIOME-BASED APPROACHES TO COMBAT AMR

Antimicrobial resistance (AMR) has emerged as a prime health problem of worldwide concern, and traditional management of antibiotic therapy is proving less effective. Because of this, researchers are finding more interest in microbiome as a form of countermeasure. Below the author discusses three such strategies: Fecal Microbiota Transplants (FMT), probiotics and prebiotics, and phage therapy, which are gaining traction in the current movement towards decreasing AMR.

2.1 Fecal Microbiota Transplants (FMT)

FMT is an emerging and swiftly developing therapeutic means of restoring the microbial balance of individuals whose microbial balance has been upset, often by antibiotic usage. The process involves the infusion of feces of a healthy donor into the gastrointestinal tract of the recipient through the lumen. Its main aim is to reseed a heterogeneous population of useful microorganisms, therefore rebalancing the natural microbial ecosystem upon which the health of the gut and resistance to a pathogen onslaught are based.

Restoring the Gut Microbiome as a Therapeutic Strategy Against AMR

Antimicrobial resistance (AMR) is one of the key threats to population health. Antibiotic treatment disrupts the bacterial population randomly, leading to the destabilization of the microbiome and the systematic destruction of both pathogenic and commensal microbes. This disruption decreases microbial diversity, which facilitates the rise of antibiotic-resistant strains. As explained in Figure X, the next microbiomics change enables bacteria resistant to antibiotics to survive and form biofilms that provide invulnerability to similar drug attacks. As a remedy for these harmful effects, the idea of using fecal microbiota transplantation (FMT) as a countermeasure has been suggested, with the intention of reinstating a diverse microbial community and thereby preventing the expansion of resistant pathogens (Cusumano et al., 2025).

Clinical Outcomes: Success in Treating Recurrent Clostridioides difficile Infections

Fecal microbiota transplantation (FMT) has been an innovative intervention against recurrent Clostridioides difficile infection (CDI), which occurs in patients who have received some types of antibacterial therapy. Antibiotics disrupt the delicate balance of the gastrointestinal microbiota, thereby providing *C. difficile* with an opportunity to multiply uncontrollably. Furthermore, a prospective cohort study published in The Lancet (2024) found that FMT was efficacious in curing 91% of patients with recurrent cases of CDI that had been non-responsive to standard regimens, such as long-term treatment with antibiotics (Jarmo et al., 2020).

In addition to the primary effectiveness of treating CDI, FMT offers an important benefit due to its connection with decreased antimicrobial resistance (AMR). Not only did the patients receiving FMT have fewer recurring CDI-inducing episodes, but it also led to a significant decrease in multidrug-resistant organisms (MDR) in the gut microbiota of patients. These results indicate that FMT favors positive microbial microbiota, which overpowers the pathogenic or resistance co-existing bacteria. This way, it can reduce the spread of AMR guns in the long run, providing therapeutic as well as public-health solutions. In fact, a study has listed FMT among the potential interventions to help counter the global threat of AMR (Khanna, 2021). Figure 1 shows the mechanistic foundations of microbiome upheaval caused by antibiotics. Antibiotics kill beneficial but also harmful bacteria, decrease microbial diversity and alter conditions that favor resistant, biofilm-forming microbes and lead to AMR. These ecological imbalances only complicate treatment outcomes and even increase the likelihood of treatment failure.

2.2 Probiotics and Prebiotics: Restoring Gut Health

Biotic probiotics and prebiotics are microbiome-based therapies in antimicrobial resistance (AMR) with therapeutic potential. Probiotics are described as live microorganisms that, when administered in appropriate amounts, provide specific health benefits to the host, especially through the restoration of microbial balance. Prebiotics, on the other hand, are food materials that are not consumed by our body but which play a role in promoting the growth of helpful intestinal microorganisms. Together, both of these modalities have a synergistically stimulating effect, favoring microbial homeostasis and limiting the growth of pathogenic organisms (Al-Habsi et al., 2024).

Probiotics' Role in Reducing the Impact of AMR

Species of Lactobacillus and Bifidobacterium are considered probiotics with the capability of directly addressing antimicrobial resistance (AMR) in a number of ways. It is shown that these organisms have the capacity to keep resistant bacteria at bay through consumption of nutrients and receptor sites, production of antimicrobial products, and strengthening of host protections by making them more sensitive to detect pathogens, and their corresponding destruction. Due to continual administration of antibiotics, it usually affects the homeostasis of the microbes; probiotics help balance this by saving the diversity of microbial organisms and reducing the settlement of greedy pathogens like Enterococcus faecium and Escherichia coli (Aghamohammad & Rohani, 2023).

There is further evidence through recent clinical trials. In a study that was published in Frontiers in microbiology in (2024) showed that participants who were also offered Lactobacillus rhamnosus and Bifidobacterium lactis in combination with antibiotics daily, the frequencies of colonization of antibiotic resistant bacteria were significantly lower, which supports the potential efficiency of probiotics in preventing the spread of AMR (Al-Muslem et al.).

Prebiotics' Contribution to Microbial Balance

Found primarily in foods rich in fiber, prebiotics enhance the growth of beneficial gut microbe that has the capacity to overcome the emergence of antibiotic resistant bacterial form. These beneficial microorganisms prevent the development of the pathogenic infection by maintaining an appropriate microbial habitats. Based on empirical evidence, dietary prebiotics have been shown to increase microbe diversity, which has been associated with reduced antibiotic-resistant bacterial population. It has also been postulated, together with collective evidence, that prebiotics, including inulin and fructooligosaccharides, can enhance the microbial resistance, prevent resistant lineages to dominate once antibiotics are stopped (Basnet et al., 2024).

2.3 Phage Therapy: Targeting Resistant Pathogens

The treatment of antibiotic-resistant infections with bacteriophages (phage therapy) is becoming an increasingly visible way to react to the growing crisis of multidrug-resistant pathogens. Compared to traditional antibiotics, which uncontrollably disrupt entire bacterial populations, bacteriophages will be highly host-specific, thus targeting their killing action to the desired resistant pathogen without causing harm to the commensal and benign microbiome. There are several benefits that such precision can bring to the use of phage therapy as an antimicrobial treatment in the modern age of antimicrobial resistance (Bleriot et al., 2024).

Introduction to Phage Therapy and Its Mechanism

Phage therapy involves the use of bacteriophages that are selected carefully to address resistant species of bacteria to therapy. To enter the cell, the attached phage is able to inject their genetic material into the cytoplasm of the bacterial cell where it eventually lyses it. Since phages are host-specific, this method has the least effects in disturbing the rest of the microbial population and is the most targetted towards clearing the disease-causing bacteria. This makes phage therapy very specific and effective in the treatment of infections involving multidrug-resistant pathogens without causing adverse effects to the stability of the entire microbiome (Strathdee et al., 2023).

Current Studies: Success in Targeting Resistant *P. aeruginosa* and *E. coli*

There is recent clinical confirmation of the therapeutic benefit of phage therapy against recalcitrant Pseudomonas aeruginosa and carbapenem-resistant Escherichia coli. In a 2019 report in Clinical Infectious Diseases, a long-standing non-recurring P. aeruginosa infection that was resistant to many antimicrobials could be cleared and, without adverse effects, removed using a cocktail of genetically designed phages (Clinical Infectious Diseases, 2019). Case series parallelism showed efficacy against carbapenem-resistant E. coli, which could be a treatment option that prevents the rescue in patients who have few and limited treatment options (Science, 2023). Collectively, these findings highlight the potential realization of personalized phage-based therapies against refractory infection hence the potential of personalized antimicrobial modalities that respond to the global problem of antimicrobial resistance (Elfadadny et al., 2024).

3. INNOVATIONS IN DIAGNOSTICS FOR MICROBIOME-BASED AMR SOLUTIONS

With the increasing problem of antimicrobial resistance (AMR), there are growing demands in seeking high-end diagnostics. Traditional methods employed in the identification of pathogens are likely to be time-consuming and difficult to identify other than the already known and defined well-characterized strains. Conversely, novel diagnostic applications such as next-generation sequencing (NGS) and CRISPR diagnostics are changing the way that surveillance is conducted, including full, real-time surveillance. These inventions scan the microbial microbiome and screen at the same time resistance genes linked with AMR. This chapter measures how these strategies can improve AMR detection, surveillance, and the management of AMR therapeutically.

3.1 Next-Generation Sequencing (NGS) for Microbiome Profiling

Next-Generation Sequencing (NGS) has become a revolutionary technology that has rewritten the textbooks not only in terms of microbiome studies but also diagnostic abilities. Since it allows the detailed association of the whole microbial genome, NGS makes it easier to make accurate evaluations of microbial biomass and the existence of antimicrobials resistance (AMR) genes. Unlike the usual culture-based methods that may take several days to weeks, NGS provides quick, marchant results making it very necessary in real-time monitoring of resistance markers. It enables researchers and clinicians to determine resistance genes effectively at the same time and keep track of the total well-being of the microbiome (Wensel et al., 2022).

How NGS is Used to Identify Resistance Genes and Assess Microbiome Health in Real-Time

The NGS analysis continues through the sequencing of the DNA that has been obtained out of clinical specimens such as blood, urine, fecal matter, and others. The result of such sequencing is the full list of microbial species occurring in the specimen, along with detection of AMR genes carried by the species. The leading resistance determinants such as those that play a role in making beta-lactamase and resistance to carbapenems can be identified using specialized bioinformatics algorithms, which match the sequenced information with the databases of the prestigious genes.

The strength of NGS is that the technique can provide an assessment of the health of the microbiome in real time. Such an ability is especially useful to track the way in which the microbiome of a patient changes over the course of antibiotic treatment as such agents may disturb not only the pathogenic factors but also beneficial components. Measurements of microbial diversity based on NGS can shine light on how disturbed the microbial populations are becoming by antibiotic therapy, and whether resistance strains are becoming predominant (Hilt & Ferrieri, 2022).

Technological Breakthroughs: Fast Sequencing Methods to Detect AMR Markers

Recent advances in sequencing modalities have significantly increased profiling accuracy of microbiome and accelerated their rates significantly. Present-day devices, such as Illumina NovaSeq, or Oxford Nanopore Technologies, facilitate high throughput sequencing at the cost of reduced costs of both time and funds. Such developments allow clinicians to question antimicrobial resistance (AMR) labels in a much faster fashion, allowing treatment options to be made with a higher level of temporal precision. Moreover, the real time of next-generation sequencing (NGS) helps identify the emergent resistant strains that are quickly and patient specific therapy (Kaprou et al., 2021).

Figure 2. Illustration of the process used in profiling of microbiome employing NGS. They are processed by DNA extractions, library prep and sequencing, with a subsequent analysis by bioinformatics, detection of AMR markers and reporting of data.

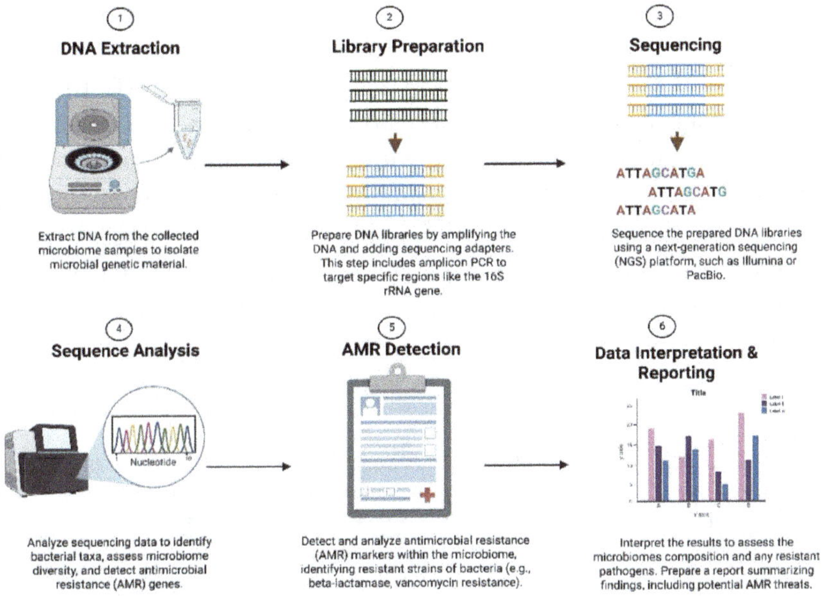

3.2 CRISPR-Based Diagnostics: Targeting AMR Genes

One of the breakthroughs in the field of antimicrobial resistance (AMR) diagnostics is the use of CRISPR technology to produce a speedy and sensitive approach to the detection of resistance genes. In its original form, CRISPR was a platform that was performed gene-editing; however, the technology has been re-contextualized as a diagnostic tool based on its unique molecular specificity in locating a target DNA sequence. Cas-based systems-such as SHERLOCK and DETECTR- are based on engineered CRISPR enzymes to target clinically relevant AMR genes, e.g. NDM-1

(New Delhi metallo-beta lactamase) and KPC (Klebsiella pneumoniae carbapenemase) (Okesanya et al., 2025).

To perform, CRISPR-based assays use guide RNA and bind to a known, fixed region of the DNA measured to the corresponding resistance gene. When identified, the CRISPR-bound enzyme such as Cas12 will be activated and molecularly cut the length of double-stranded DNA producing a signal that can be read. That arrangement offers a fast and exceptionally accurate identification ability, making CRISPR an appealing avenue toward point-of-care prospective diagnostic procedures. The detection ability of the CRISPR systems in real time allows identification of resistant infections early, which is a supreme consideration in any clinical management process (Binnie et al., 2021).

The example of CRISPR diagnostic success is especially effective: i.e., the detection of urinary tract infection (UTI) caused by resistant pathogens. As an example, the DETECTR platform designed with the FDA approval can detect urinary pathogens like E. coli and Klebsiella pneumoniae, which are rather resistant to the so-called common antibiotics like ampicillin and carbapenems. The rapid diagnostic capabilities presented by CRISPR-based diagnostics gives clinicians the ability to make early treatment choices and reduce instances of antibiotic treatment with broad-spectrum antibiotics (Kulkarni et al., 2023).

Table 1. Key CRISPR-Based Diagnostics for AMR Detection

CRISPR Technology Used	Target Pathogen	Resistance Gene Detected	Detection Time	References
SHERLOCK	*Escherichia coli, Klebsiella pneumoniae*	**NDM-1, OXA-48**	20 minutes	(Allander et al., 2022)
DETECTR	*Escherichia coli, Klebsiella pneumoniae*	**KPC, AmpC**	1 hour	(Rodríguez-Guerrero et al., 2022)
CASSI	*Pseudomonas aeruginosa*	**METallo-β-lactamases**	30 minutes	(Ghazaei, 2025)
CRISPR-Cas12	*Staphylococcus aureus*	**MecA (MRSA gene)**	15 minutes	(Li et al., 2022)

The existing antimicrobial resistance (AMR) diagnostics seems to be under the control of a few major CRISPR-based platforms that provide fast results and the ability to identify specific resistance-coding genes of interest. In the process, they empower clinicians with time-sensitive and actionable information needed to support evidence-based therapeutic interventions as explained in table 1.

4. CUTTING-EDGE THERAPEUTIC STRATEGIES USING THE MICROBIOME

The field of microbiome-directed treatments is in an accelerated stage of development, and new methods to treat antimicrobial resistance (AMR) have appeared. These therapies aim to re-establish ecological homeostasis and, in some cases to promote the eradication of resistant pathogens via multifaceted mechanisms by using the intrinsic properties of the microbiome. Examples are found in the field of synthetic-biology and microbiome engineering with enterprises that together hope to prevent and heal infections and allow treatments that are customizable to individual microbial signatures. The discussion below outlines some of the state-of-the-art treatments transforming this landscape of the AMR intercession.

4.1 Synthetic Biology: Creating Microbiome-Targeted Therapies

Synthetic biology is a rapidly developing field of science that deals with the construction of microbes to perform the desired functions. In terms of antimicrobial resistance (AMR), it is an emerging area of research whose application has the potential to revolutionise how we treat resistant bacterial infections through the creation of microbiome-based interventions. By selectively genetically engineering probiotics or producing thoroughly engineered bacterial strains, researchers can engineer interventions that specifically act against harmful micro-organisms at the same time protecting beneficial aspects of the microbiota (Verma et al.).

The Use of Engineered Probiotics and Bacteria to Fight Resistant Infections

Genetically modified organisms that have been designed to provide therapeutic benefits by enhancing the activities of the beneficial organisms or by specifically challenging the pathogens are called engineered probiotics. In this direction, probiotics could be designed to produce antimicrobial peptides (AMPs), proteins consisting of fewer than 100 amino acids that kill or inhibit disease-causing bacteria. Bacteriocins are peptides with natural production through selected Lactobacillus strains that are also integrated to the identification of resistant pathogens like C. difficile and E. coli in the probiotics. Moreover, synthetic probiotics have the capacity to be designed to colonize ecological niches present in the microbiome where otherwise resistant microbes would have excelled hence utilizing competitive exclusion as a biostrategic means of preventing or curbing antibiosis-mediated dysbiosis and eventual overgrowth of intractable organisms (Ma et al., 2022).

Case Studies: Synthetic AMPs (Antimicrobial Peptides) and CRISPR-Cas Antimicrobials

At the same time as some researchers have created a family of synthetic antimicrobial peptides (AMPs) which are active against multidrug-resistant organisms and include Pseudomonas aeruginosa and Staphylococcus aureus. The mechanism of action of such peptides is bactericidal towards the target cell through the destabilization of the cell membrane, which leads to the death of the target cell. There is emerging evidence that synthetic AMPs are effective in treatment of hospital associated infections and therefore hold a viable potential to be used as an alternative to conventional antibiotics. At the same time, CRISPR-based mechanisms have been developed to turn off the particular resistance determinants integrated into chromosomes in bacteria. Antimicrobial intervention using CRISPR is very effective in inhibiting resistance genes like NDM-1 and KPC and this makes it highly precise in targeting resistant pathogens more than the conventional antibiotics (Amen et al., 2025).

4.2 Microbiome Engineering: The Future of Personalized Medicine

The controlled alteration of microbial communities that inhabit the human body to achieve health benefits is what forms microbiome engineering. Techniques like gene-editing approaches- which are symbolized by CRISPR- are used to vary the constitution of microbial populations, which in turn augment resistance to pathogenic attack and assist host immunological operations. Simultaneously, the advent of personalized medicine has offered a structure against which to apply microbiome engineering, whereby clinicians would be able to customize treatment approaches to the unique presentation of the microbiome in an individual patient (Singh & Rastogi, 2024).

Gene Editing Techniques Like CRISPR to Modify Microbiomes for Targeted AMR Resistance

The development of gene-editing technologies--primarily CRISPR and CRISPR/Cas9--allows researchers and practitioners to introduce targeted changes of extremely high substantive precision to the genomes of both human beings and microorganisms. CRISPR/Cas9 particularly allows deletion of resistance or addition of desirable bacteria to enhancing antimicrobial sensitivity of the bacterial population. When used in the microbiome, the strategy can allow the targeted removal of dangerous pathogens even as it is used to promote protective organisms that naturally inhibit the development of antimicrobial resistance (AMR) (Amen et al., 2025).

Personalized Treatments: Custom Microbiome Interventions for Individual Patients

The future development of personalized medicine cannot be separated with the definition of the individual microbiome of each patient. In this regard, evaluating the composition of the microbiome, clinicians can outline the disharmonies and develop the corrections aimed at the restoration of the diversity and the inhibition of resistants. Individualized microbiome-based therapy could include personalized probiotic interventions, diet and lifestyle changes, and antimicrobial intervention that is specific to the resistance profiles found in particular microbial population.

Fecal microbiota transplantation (FMT) is another example of such a treatment modality by which there has been a successful re-establishment of microbial equilibrium in individuals with chronic recurrent infections, like C. difficile. With the development of personalized medicine, there is the prospect of outfitting precision therapeutics through microbiome engineering that anticipates the genetic and microbial-specific aspects of AMR and, thus, allows treatments to be tailored exquisitely with respect to patient specifics (Shukla et al., 2024).

4.3 Microbiome-Based Antibiotic Alternatives

As the worry of the problem of antimicrobial resistance (AMR) has been increasing, more attention is dedicated to alternatives to traditional antibiotics provided by microbiomes. These interventions exploit the inherent antimicrobial potential of the microbial community, such as bacteriocins and antimicrobial peptides and other compounds produced naturally by the beneficial microbial species. In comparison to conventional antibiotics that hamper the resistance crisis cycle, these methods present an optimistic way of controlling the AMR crisis (Ekwueme et al., 2025).

Potential Microbiome-Based Antibiotics and the Role of Bacteriocins in Preventing Resistance

Bacteriocins are a group of antimicrobial peptides produced by certain strains of bacteria, whose toxicity is targeted specifically at either extracellular or intracellular targets in other bacteria, especially pathogens. They may be a solution to the loss of traditional antibiotics because of their species-specific effect allowing them to disrupt the competition of bacteria without interfering with the total microbial population. As an example, some Lactobacillus strains produce bacteriocins that can suppress infection by C. difficile and E. coli thus providing antimicrobial therapeutic potential in resistant infection treatment without using antibiotics (Zhang et al., 2023).

The ongoing research is to design artificial versions of naturally occurring antimicrobial peptides (AMPs) to perform the activity profile of bacteriocins; this way they will limit the antibacterial effect and alleviate resistance. It is envisioned that such synthesized AMPs would have a multitude of uses, such as the drug resistant S. aureus and P. aeruginosa infections. Initial studies show that AMPs may be topically administered, given as oral or used systemically, which offers a new approach to preventing and managing infections without fueling the development of antimicrobial resistance. Table 2 below outlines some of the emerging approaches to microbiome-engineering that have shown promise in terms of fighting antimicrobial resistance, including ways of 'editing genes, microbiome-derived antibiotics, and personalised medicine, alongside their mechanism of action and existing use-cases (Amen et al., 2025).

Table 2. Microbiome Engineering Approaches for AMR Treatment

Approach	Technology Used	Mechanism of Action	Current Applications	Research/Case Studies	References
Gene Editing (CRISPR)	CRISPR/Cas9, CRISPR/Cas12	Editing bacterial genomes to remove resistance genes or insert protective genes	Targeting resistance genes like NDM-1, KPC	CRISPR-Cas12 used to disrupt carbapenemase genes in *Klebsiella pneumoniae* (Nature, 2024)	(Kundar & Gokarn, 2022)
Microbiome-based Antibiotics	Bacteriocins, synthetic AMPs	Using naturally occurring antimicrobial peptides to target specific pathogens	Targeting *C. difficile, E. coli, P. aeruginosa*	Synthetic AMPs developed to treat *Pseudomonas aeruginosa* (Science, 2024)	(Ekwueme et al., 2025)
Personalized Microbiome Therapies	Fecal microbiota transplantation (FMT), personalized probiotics	Restoring microbial balance and suppressing resistant strains based on individual microbiome composition	Treating recurrent infections, restoring microbial diversity	FMT used in treating recurrent *C. difficile* infections	(Ratiner et al., 2024)

5. CHALLENGES IN MICROBIOME-BASED AMR SOLUTIONS

Despite the optimism that microbiome-based therapies will be an efficient solution to the countermeasure of antimicrobial resistance (AMR), the issues are still quite extensive in science, technology and regulatory aspects. The microbiome itself with its innate complex nature and the necessity of critical regulatory control and stringent ethical consideration present an intimidating barrier to large-scale application of microbiome-based interventions. This discussion exhaustively examines these challenges, and provides the possible mitigation strategies.

Technological and Scientific problems

The first challenge related to the creation of microbiome-based treatment of AMR is the nature of the microbiome itself which is a complex system. The human microbiome is a complex multidimensional ecology of trillions of kinds of bacteria, fungi, viruses and archaea with a remarkably complex interaction with the host and the other microbes in the microbiome. Such connections differ significantly across people, which makes the development of general effective treatments highly problematic (Longde et al., 2021).

The concept of interindividual variation is complementary to the complexity issue since it also has a huge influence. Microbiome does not remain constant, but changes based on diet, drugs, exposure to environments, and even genetic make-up. To such a level of variability, it is not possible to establish uniform treatment paradigms. What is effective in treating some individuals clinically is not expected to be efficient in treating another person due to differences in microbiome profile. Probiotics are a case in point: some strains are said to be of benefit, whereas others are said to cause adverse events, especially when they are introduced into a dysbiotic gut. In these circumstances, the selection of the right populations of microbes will still have to be done manually (Alam, 2022).

This simply makes the translational process more difficult due to the relative deficiency of our information on microbial functions and interactions. Even though microbial diversity catalogs have been increasing, the exact contributions of a given microbial taxa and the methods they interact to form the microbial ecosystem are largely unknown. This means that the approaches of treatment that are available now are often implemented in a trial and error system of iteration and not in a systematic system (Liu et al., 2022).

Clinical protocols standardization

Indeed, clear guidelines do not exist around most microbiome-based therapies yet, such as fecal microbiota transplant (FMT), probiotic formulations, and genetically modified bacterial products. Rigid approaches to sample collection, processing, and administration are used in each intervention, which makes replication in different settings very complicated. The FMT specifically can be very variable: screening and storage guidelines, as well as delivery routes, may all make a difference to clinical outcomes. Probiotics also pose such a parallel challenge due to the lack of a clear consensus on what a therapeutic dose entails; in addition, not all strains of probiotics are equally effective, which makes it even challenging to decide on the dose and the overall intervention design (Klumpp-Thomas et al., 2021).

5.2 Regulatory Challenges and Ethical Considerations

The development of preclinical research on microbiome-based therapy into the clinical sphere requires that a number of regulatory barriers are overcome. These obstacles are based on the novelty and complexity of the microbiome as a target of future medicines, which can often not be applied to existing regulatory frameworks.

Regulatory Frameworks for Microbiome Therapies Like FMT, Probiotics, and Genetically Modified Bacteria

Existing regulatory bodies, e.g. the FDA and the EMA, only provide modest directions on microbiome interventions. An example is fecal microbiota transplantation (FMT) which remains experimental in most jurisdictions and as such no ostensibly efficacious indication can be formally approved, such as Clostridioides difficile infection. The issues of donor safety, challenges of standardizing a stool product, and dispute on the ethics of manipulating human biological materials cause regulatory uncertainty about the uses of FMT (Thanush et al., 2023).

Genetically modified bacteria and probiotics have similar regulatory problems. Although probiotics can be seen to be safe, their medicinal properties are not always supported by massive clinical trials, which gives rise to unclear safety assessments, as well as efficacy. Genetically engineered bacteria, which will solve the problem of resistant pathogens to antibiotics, are exposed to further biosafety restrictions. Regulators need to come up with strategies on evaluating the risks involved in the placement of engineered microorganisms into the human microbiome, which can produce unpredictable impacts on the host health or ecosystems (Maor et al., 2025).

Ethical Concerns: Genetic Editing of Human Microbiomes and Balancing Innovation with Safety

There are also a lot of ethical questions that appear when it comes to the genetic editing of a human microbiome. Instead, the introduction of technologies like CRISPR-Cas9 has changed the ability to alter and modify the genomes of microbes and thus allowed to either fix dysbiosis or remove antibiotic-resistance genes in pathogenic microorganisms. Still, what seems even more serious are the potential long-term outcomes, which also comprise ecological destabilizations, horizontal gene transfer, and the emergence of new resistance, which further enhances ethical consideration (Rehman, 2024).

Intervening in the microbiome might also accidentally produce different resistance mechanisms or undermine unavoidable beneficial microorganisms that are of consequence to host health. More to the point, the moral implications of germline editing and the actual necessity of the paperwork needed in the case of such an intervention make it harder to regulate. It will be necessary to carefully regulate the balance, on the one hand, of potential microbiome engineering benefits and, on the other hand, safety and long-term monitoring. The following table 3 can outline the scientific, technological, and regulatory setbacks faced by microbiome-based solutions of antimicrobial resistance (AMR) and potential ways of overcoming them (Singh & Rastogi, 2024).

Table 3. Challenges in Microbiome-Based AMR Solutions

Challenge Type	Description of Challenge	Impact on Microbiome-Based AMR Solutions	Potential Solutions	References
Scientific	Complexity of the microbiome and variability between individuals	Difficulty in creating universal, effective therapies	More research into microbiome function and personalized therapies	(Shukla et al., 2024)
Technological	Lack of standardized protocols for interventions like FMT and probiotics	Variability in treatment outcomes and efficacy across populations	Development of clear guidelines and standardization of protocols	(Servetas et al., 2022)
Regulatory	Lack of regulatory frameworks for novel therapies	Slow approval and inconsistent access to treatments	Establishment of new regulatory pathways for microbiome-based therapies	(Thanush et al., 2023)
Ethical	Ethical concerns around genetic editing and microbiome manipulation	Potential unintended effects on human health and the environment	Comprehensive ethical guidelines and long-term monitoring requirements	(Sharma)

6. FUTURE DIRECTIONS: THE ROAD AHEAD IN MICROBIOME-BASED AMR RESEARCH

As the field of microbiome-based therapies grows up in maturity, new multidisciplinary paradigms are emerging that combine gene editing, immune modulation and personalised microbiome profiling in an effort to combat antimicrobial resistance (AMR). These novel non-antibiotic approaches mainly aim to use the therapeutic potential of the microbiome to the best extent possible, provide precision therapy against drug-resistant pathogens, improve clinical outcomes, and reduce the emergence of future resistance. These methods include, at their center, the development of individualized microbiome engineering, which combines high-tech solutions of combining CRISPR-Cas9 gene editing, engineered probiotics, and immune-system modification in order to give a highly tailored solution to addressing AMR in these individuals.

6.1 Integrating Microbiome Interventions with Conventional AMR Treatments

More recently, microbiome-based treatment approaches are an emerging addition to typical antimicrobials in fighting the rise of antimicrobial resistance (AMR). Instead of replacing antibiotics, such interventions are expected to work in synergy with the known agents to enhance their effectiveness and minimize chances of emergence of resistance. As an example, probiotics and prebiotics may be used simultaneously with antibiotics, which protect the resident microbiome preventing the growth of antibiotic-resistant pathogens. This type of synergetic partnership is likely to lead to better clinical outcomes, reduced adverse reactions and inhibit the development of AMR (Abdulsalam et al., 2024).

6.2 Personalized Microbiome Medicine: The Future of AMR Treatment

An especially high-energy development in this area is the development of personalized microbiome medicine. Questioning the unique microbial flora of each patient, clinicians can work out a personal regimen that responds to the microbiome peculiarities. The chosen antibiotics according to the profile of the microbiome and application of patient-specific probiotics to re-establish homeostasis and develop defensive microbes are examples of therapeutic decisions. The capabilities of microbiome sequencing in this context posit the prediction of treatment response, allow a rational use of antibiotics, and make overall treatment more effective (Shukla et al., 2024).

6.3 Global Research Collaborations and Initiatives

The need to develop international cooperative efforts that utilize combined expertise to explain the links between the microbiome and resistance processes and to catalyze the advancement of microbiome-based autotherapies cannot be overlooked, either. Efforts are being undertaken at the international level including the World Health Organization (WHO) AMR Action Plan to support the development of microbiome surveillance, and the translation of microbial data to clinical practices across the globe. By synchronizing resource and expertise distribution, these projects not only hope to accelerate the identification of new treatment options; they also seek to make AMR approaches to microbiome more standardized (Srivastav et al., 2024).

6.4 Personalized Microbiome Engineering for AMR Treatment

Personalized microbiome engineering is a very interesting direction in the growing area of microbiome-based antimicrobial resistance (AMR)-based therapy. This strategy includes genetic engineering, customised probiotic supplementation and immune system manipulation to deal with AMR on a personalised level. As an example, gene editing-based methods to modify specific bacteria (CRISPR-Cas9) are used in the targeting of AMR-associated genes in resistant bioforms in bacteria, and genetically modified probiotics can provide antimicrobial peptides (AMPs) or bacterium adjuncts to restore microbial homeostasis. Moreover, this ability of boosting the immune system may help in supplementing natural defenses, towards the achievement of better infection control along with reduction of host resistance. All these strategies set up a customized framework of AMR treatment collectively. Microbiome profiling at a patient level will allow clinicians to customize their treatment to maximize its effect in terms of drug action and immune response, providing a comprehensive treatment solution to AMR (Mkilima, 2025).

7. CONCLUSION

Examples have been given how microbiome-focused interventions can be an important paradigm shift in the war on antimicrobial resistance (AMR). Recent research chasing bioengineered probiotics, synthetic antimicrobial peptides (AMPs), CRISPR-based ge ne-editor systems is part of the modern arsenals of efforts to reduce AMR. Together, they can overcome fundamental drivers of resistance, reinstate microbe homeostasis, sabotage antibiotic-tolerant pathogens and reset therapeutic outcomes. As a result of incorporating individual microbiome-level profiling, health-care professionals will be capable of offering treatments based on individual microbial ecologies, reduce reliance on antimicrobials traditionally delivered, and prevent occurrences of secondary resistance.

In spite of such upcoming developments, long-term funding of microbiome-based research is also essential. The complexity of the structure of microbial communities and their dynamic interaction with pathogenic agents also makes the field multidimensional in itself. However, the potential of microbiome-based methods to provide long-term AMR counter measures should be invested in as well. Since AMR is not a localized phenomenon, swarming international efforts, e.g. joint research undertakings, data-sharing platforms, and the development of standard protocols, are crucial to make such therapies equally available to all and to multiply their efficacy.

Finally, microbiome-affecting activities are a highly promising and precise path to dealing with AMR. Combined research and international cooperation via numerous innovations provide prognostic value, allowing the introduction of more effective and individualised AMR therapeutic options and thus, protecting the health of society across the world.

REFERENCES

Abdulsalam, M., Hamisu, A. A., Ahmad, A. M., Wakili, F. B., Annu, F. S., & Garba, M. M. (2024). Microbiome dynamics and strategic management strategies: Exploring synergies between integrative medicine modalities and microbial balance. *Biological Sciences*, *4*(3), 725–735.

Aghamohammad, S., & Rohani, M. (2023). Antibiotic resistance and the alternatives to conventional antibiotics: The role of probiotics and microbiota in combating antimicrobial resistance. *Microbiological Research*, *267*, 127275. PMID: 36493661

Al-Habsi, N., Al-Khalili, M., Haque, S. A., Elias, M., Olqi, N. A., & Al Uraimi, T. (2024). Health benefits of prebiotics, probiotics, synbiotics, and postbiotics. *Nutrients*, *16*(22), 3955. PMID: 39599742

Al-Muslem, L., Al-Qaaneh, A. M., Al-Salem, Z., Rather, I. A., & Rehman, S. The Intricate Relationship between Probiotics and Antimicrobial Resistance. In *Probiotics against Antimicrobial Resistance* (pp. 1–9). CRC Press.

Alam, A. (2022). Educational robotics and computer programming in early childhood education: A conceptual framework for assessing elementary school students' computational thinking for designing powerful educational scenarios. *2022 International Conference on Smart Technologies and Systems for Next Generation Computing (ICSTSN)*

Allander, L., Vickberg, K., Lagerbäck, P., Sandegren, L., & Tängdén, T. (2022). Evaluation of in vitro activity of double-carbapenem combinations against KPC-2-, OXA-48-and NDM-producing Escherichia coli and Klebsiella pneumoniae. [PubMed]. *Antibiotics (Basel, Switzerland)*, *11*(11), 1646.

Amen, R. A., Hassan, Y. M., Essmat, R. A., Ahmed, R. H., Azab, M. M., Shehata, N. R., Elgazzar, M. M., & El-Sayed, W. M. (2025). Harnessing the Microbiome: CRISPR-Based Gene Editing and Antimicrobial Peptides in Combating Antibiotic Resistance and Cancer. *Probiotics and Antimicrobial Proteins*, •••, 1–31. PMID: 40377870

Basnet, J., Eissa, M. A., Yanes Cardozo, L. L., Romero, D. G., & Rezq, S. (2024). Impact of probiotics and prebiotics on gut microbiome and hormonal regulation. *Gastrointestinal Disorders (Basel, Switzerland)*, *6*(4), 801–815. PMID: 39649015

Binnie, A., Fernandes, E., Almeida-Lousada, H., de Mello, R. A., & Castelo-Branco, P. (2021). CRISPR-based strategies in infectious disease diagnosis and therapy. *Infection*, *49*(3), 377–385. PMID: 33393066

Bleriot, I., Pacios, O., Blasco, L., Fernández-García, L., López, M., Ortiz-Cartagena, C., Barrio-Pujante, A., García-Contreras, R., Pirnay, J.-P., & Wood, T. K. (2024). Improving phage therapy by evasion of phage resistance mechanisms. *JAC-Antimicrobial Resistance*, *6*(1), dlae017. PMID: 38343627

Cusumano, G., Flores, G. A., Venanzoni, R., & Angelini, P. (2025). The Impact of Antibiotic Therapy on Intestinal Microbiota: Dysbiosis, Antibiotic Resistance, and Restoration Strategies. *Antibiotics (Basel, Switzerland)*, *14*(4), 371. PMID: 40298495

Ducarmon, Q., Zwittink, R., Hornung, B., Van Schaik, W., Young, V., & Kuijper, E. (2019). Gut microbiota and colonization resistance against bacterial enteric infection. *Microbiology and Molecular Biology Reviews : MMBR*, *83*(3), 00007–00019. DOI: 10.1128/mmbr PMID: 31167904

Ekwueme, C. T., Anyiam, I. V., Ekwueme, D. C., Anumudu, C. K., & Onyeaka, H. (2025). Reconstructing the Antibiotic Pipeline: Natural Alternatives to Antibacterial Agents. *Biomolecules*, *15*(8), 1182. PMID: 40867625

Elfadadny, A., Ragab, R. F., AlHarbi, M., Badshah, F., Ibáñez-Arancibia, E., Farag, A., Hendawy, A. O., De los Ríos-Escalante, P. R., Aboubakr, M., & Zakai, S. A. (2024). Antimicrobial resistance of Pseudomonas aeruginosa: Navigating clinical impacts, current resistance trends, and innovations in breaking therapies. *Frontiers in Microbiology*, *15*, 1374466. PMID: 38646632

Ghazaei, C. (2025). Prevalence of extended-spectrum and metallo β-lactamase production in Pseudomonas aeruginosa isolate. *Reviews and Research in Medical Microbiology*, *36*(1), 9–17.

Gordillo Altamirano, F. L., & Barr, J. J. (2019). Phage therapy in the postantibiotic era. *Clinical Microbiology Reviews*, *32*(2), 00066–00018. DOI: 10.1128/cmr PMID: 30651225

He, X., Zhao, S., & Li, Y. (2021). Faecalibacterium prausnitzii: A next-generation probiotic in gut disease improvement. *The Canadian Journal of Infectious Diseases & Medical Microbiology*, *2021*(1), 6666114.

Hilt, E. E., & Ferrieri, P. (2022). Next generation and other sequencing technologies in diagnostic microbiology and infectious diseases. *Genes*, *13*(9), 1566. PMID: 36140733

Hussain, A., Najeeb, A., & Ali, S. A. (2025). Antimicrobial Resistance: A Modern Plague. In *AI-Driven Breakthroughs in Antimicrobial Resistance* (pp. 27-74). IGI Global Scientific Publishing.

Jarmo, O., Veli-Jukka, A., & Eero, M. (2020). Treatment of Clostridioides (Clostridium) difficile infection. *Annals of Medicine*, *52*(1-2), 12–20. PMID: 31801387

Kaprou, G. D., Bergšpica, I., Alexa, E. A., Alvarez-Ordonez, A., & Prieto, M. (2021). Rapid methods for antimicrobial resistance diagnostics. *Antibiotics (Basel, Switzerland)*, *10*(2), 209. PMID: 33672677

Khanna, S. (2021). My treatment approach to Clostridioides difficile infection. *Mayo Clinic Proceedings*.

Kim, H.-J., Na, S. W., Alodaini, H. A., Al-Dosary, M. A., Nandhakumari, P., & Dyona, L. (2021). Prevalence of multidrug-resistant bacteria associated with polymicrobial infections. [PubMed]. *Journal of Infection and Public Health*, *14*(12), 1864–1869.

Klumpp-Thomas, C., Kalish, H., Drew, M., Hunsberger, S., Snead, K., Fay, M. P., Mehalko, J., Shunmugavel, A., Wall, V., & Frank, P. (2021). Standardization of ELISA protocols for serosurveys of the SARS-CoV-2 pandemic using clinical and at-home blood sampling. *Nature Communications*, *12*(1), 113. PMID: 33397956

Kulkarni, A., Tanga, S., Karmakar, A., Hota, A., & Maji, B. (2023). CRISPR-based precision molecular diagnostics for disease detection and surveillance. *ACS Applied Bio Materials*, *6*(10), 3927–3945. PMID: 37788375

Kundar, R., & Gokarn, K. (2022). CRISPR-Cas system: A tool to eliminate drug-resistant gram-negative bacteria. *Pharmaceuticals*, *15*(12), 1498. PMID: 36558949

Li, Y., Shi, Z., Hu, A., Cui, J., Yang, K., Liu, Y., Deng, G., Zhu, C., & Zhu, L. (2022). Rapid one-tube RPA-CRISPR/Cas12 detection platform for methicillin-resistant Staphylococcus aureus. *Diagnostics (Basel)*, *12*(4), 829. PMID: 35453874

Liu, X., Lu, D., Zhang, A., Liu, Q., & Jiang, G. (2022). Data-driven machine learning in environmental pollution: Gains and problems. *Environmental Science & Technology*, *56*(4), 2124–2133. PMID: 35084840

Longde, S., He, L., Wenyuan, H., Guoxin, L., Rukai, Z., Xu, J., & Siwei, M. (2021). An analysis of major scientific problems and research paths of Gulong shale oil in Daqing Oilfield, NE China. *Petroleum Exploration and Development*, *48*(3), 527–540.

Ma, J., Lyu, Y., Liu, X., Jia, X., Cui, F., Wu, X., Deng, S., & Yue, C. (2022). Engineered probiotics. *Microbial Cell Factories*, *21*(1), 72. PMID: 35477497

Maor, M., Levy Barazany, H., & Kolodkin-Gal, I. (2025). The ladder of regulatory stringency and balance: An application to the US FDA's regulation of bacterial live therapeutics. *Gut Microbes*, *17*(1), 2517377. PMID: 40501442

Mkilima, T. (2025). Engineering artificial microbial consortia for personalized gut microbiome modulation and disease treatment. *Annals of the New York Academy of Sciences*. PMID: 40320966

Okesanya, O. J., Ahmed, M. M., Ogaya, J. B., Amisu, B. O., Ukoaka, B. M., Adigun, O. A., Manirambona, E., Adebusuyi, O., Othman, Z. K., & Oluwakemi, O. G. (2025). Reinvigorating AMR resilience: Leveraging CRISPR–Cas technology potentials to combat the 2024 WHO bacterial priority pathogens for enhanced global health security—a systematic review. *Tropical Medicine and Health*, *53*(1), 43. PMID: 40176174

Ratiner, K., Ciocan, D., Abdeen, S. K., & Elinav, E. (2024). Utilization of the microbiome in personalized medicine. *Nature Reviews. Microbiology*, *22*(5), 291–308. PMID: 38110694

Rehman, S. (2024). Ethical Implications of Genetic Engineering: Balancing Innovation and Responsibility. *Frontiers in Biotechnology and Genetics*, *1*(1), 37–55.

Riwu, K. H. P., Effendi, M. H., & Rantam, F. A. (2020). A Review of Extended Spectrum β-Lactamase (ESBL) Producing Klebsiella pneumoniae and Multidrug Resistant (MDR) on Companion Animals. *Systematic Reviews in Pharmacy*, *11*(7).

Rodríguez-Guerrero, E., Callejas-Rodelas, J. C., Navarro-Marí, J. M., & Gutiérrez-Fernández, J. (2022). Systematic review of plasmid AmpC type resistances in Escherichia coli and Klebsiella pneumoniae and preliminary proposal of a simplified screening method for AmpC. *Microorganisms*, *10*(3), 611. PMID: 35336186

Servetas, S. L., Daschner, P. J., Guyard, C., Thomas, V., Affagard, H., Sergaki, C., Sokol, H., Wargo, J. A., Wu, G. D., & Sabot, P. (2022). Evolution of FMT–From early clinical to standardized treatments. *Biologicals*, *76*, 31–35. PMID: 35086768

Sharma, V. ETHICAL AND SAFETY CONSIDERATIONS: MICROBIAL GENETIC RESEARCH. *MICROBIAL GENETICS*, 85.

Shukla, V., Singh, S., Verma, S., Verma, S., Rizvi, A. A., & Abbas, M. (2024). Targeting the microbiome to improve human health with the approach of personalized medicine: Latest aspects and current updates. *Clinical Nutrition ESPEN*, *63*, 813–820. PMID: 39178987

Singh, V., & Rastogi, M. (2024). Future and Challenges of Microbiome Engineering. In *Microbiome Engineering* (pp. 263–280). CRC Press.

Srivastav, A. K., Das, P., & Srivastava, A. K. (2024). Future trends, innovations, and global collaboration. In *Biotech and IoT: an introduction using cloud-driven labs* (pp. 309–398). Springer.

Strathdee, S. A., Hatfull, G. F., Mutalik, V. K., & Schooley, R. T. (2023). Phage therapy: From biological mechanisms to future directions. *Cell, 186*(1), 17–31. PMID: 36608652

Thanush, D., Basavaraj, H., & Gowrav, M. (2023). Current regulation and initial considerations for successful development and commercialization of microbiome therapies. *Advanced Gut & Microbiome Research, 2023*(1), 6657515.

Verma, A., Vishwakarma, A., Singh, R., & Yadav, P. MICROBIOME-TARGETED THERAPIES: UNLOCKING THE GUT MICROBIOME FOR DISEASE TREATMENT.

Vliex, L. M. M. (2024). The gut microbiome and metabolic health in humans: Individualised impact of antibiotic and prebiotic use.

Wensel, C. R., Pluznick, J. L., Salzberg, S. L., & Sears, C. L. (2022). Next-generation sequencing: Insights to advance clinical investigations of the microbiome. *The Journal of Clinical Investigation, 132*(7). PMID: 35362479

Zhang, D., Zhang, J., Kalimuthu, S., Liu, J., Song, Z.-M., He, B.-b., Cai, P., Zhong, Z., Feng, C., & Neelakantan, P. (2023). A systematically biosynthetic investigation of lactic acid bacteria reveals diverse antagonistic bacteriocins that potentially shape the human microbiome. *Microbiome, 11*(1), 91. PMID: 37101246

Compilation of References

Abdi, G., Jain, M., Barwant, M., Tendulkar, R., Tendulkar, M., Tariq, M., & Amir, A. (2024). Unveiling the dynamic role of bioinformatics in automation for efficient and accurate data processing and interpretation. In *Advances in Bioinformatics* (pp. 279–319). Springer.

Abdulsalam, M., Hamisu, A. A., Ahmad, A. M., Wakili, F. B., Annu, F. S., & Garba, M. M. (2024). Microbiome dynamics and strategic management strategies: Exploring synergies between integrative medicine modalities and microbial balance. *Biological Sciences*, *4*(3), 725–735.

Abedon, S. T., García, P., Mullany, P., & Aminov, R. (2021). Editorial: Phage therapy: Past, present, and future. *Frontiers in Microbiology*, *12*, 658218. DOI: 10.3389/fmicb.2021.658218

Abraham, R., Sahibzada, S., Lee, T., Jordan, D., McMillan, K., Mellor, G., Duffy, L., Lugsomya, K., O'Dea, M., Abraham, S., & Barlow, R. (2026). Antimicrobial resistance, genomic, and public health insights into *Enterococcus* spp. from Australian cattle. *Veterinary Microbiology*, *312*, 110788. PMID: 41308245

Abreu, A. C., McBain, A. J., & Simões, M. (2012). Plants as sources of new antimicrobials and resistance-modifying agents. *Natural Product Reports*, *29*(9), 1007–1021. DOI: 10.1039/C2NP20035J PMID: 22786554

Abusalah, M. A. H., Choudhary, P., Bargui, H., Ahmed, N., Abusalah, M. A. H., & Choudhary, O. P. (2024). A prognostic insight of the mRNA vaccine against antibiotic-resistant bacteria. *Annals of Medicine and Surgery (London)*, *86*(7), 3801–3805. PMID: 38989193

Adedokun, A. I.. (2025). Exploring immunotherapeutic strategies for bacterial and viral diseases. *Exploration of Immunology*, *5*, 1003202.

Aebisher, D.. (2024). Photodynamic therapy in the treatment of cancer—The selection of synthetic photosensitizers. *Pharmaceuticals*, *17*(7), 932.

Afridi, M.. (2022). Combining antibiotics with silver nanoparticles: A potential treatment strategy against antimicrobial resistance. *Main Group Chemistry*, *21*(2), 445–466.

Aghamohammad, S., & Rohani, M. (2023). Antibiotic resistance and the alternatives to conventional antibiotics: The role of probiotics and microbiota in combating antimicrobial resistance. *Microbiological Research*, *267*, 127275. PMID: 36493661

Agyeman, W. Y., Bisht, A., Gopinath, A., Cheema, A. H., Chaludiya, K., Khalid, M., Nwosu, M., Konka, S., & Khan, S. (2022). A systematic review of antibiotic resistance trends and treatment options for hospital-acquired multidrug-resistant infections. *Cureus*, *14*(10). PMID: 36381838

Ahlstrom, C. A., Bonnedahl, J., Woksepp, H., Hernandez, J., Olsen, B., & Ramey, A. M. (2018). Acquisition and dissemination of cephalosporin-resistant E. coli in migratory birds sampled at an Alaska landfill as inferred through genomic analysis. *Scientific Reports*, *8*(1), 7361. DOI: 10.1038/s41598-018-25474-w PMID: 29743625

Ahmad, N., Ahuja, S. D., Akkerman, O. W., Alffenaar, J.-W. C., Anderson, L. F., Baghaei, P., Bang, D., Barry, P. M., Bastos, M. L., Behera, D., Benedetti, A., Bisson, G. P., Boeree, M. J., Bonnet, M., Brode, S. K., Brust, J. C. M., Cai, Y., Caumes, E., Cegielski, J. P., & Centis, R. (2018). Treatment correlates of successful outcomes in pulmonary multidrug-resistant tuberculosis: An individual patient data meta-analysis. *Lancet*, *392*(10150), 821–834. https://doi.org/10.1016/s0140-6736(18)31644-1

Ahmed, M. M.. (2024). CRISPR-Cas systems in the fight against antimicrobial resistance: Current status, potentials, and future directions. *Infection and Drug Resistance*, •••, 5229–5245.

Ahmed, O. B. (2022). Detection of Antibiotic Resistance Genes in Pseudomonas aeruginosa by Whole Genome Sequencing. *Infection and Drug Resistance*, •••, 6703–6709. DOI: 10.2147/idr.s389959 PMID: 36425153

Ahmed, S. K. (2024). Artificial intelligence in nursing: Current trends, possibilities and pitfalls. *Journal of Medicine, Surgery, and Public Health*, *3*, 100072.

Akegbe, H., Onyeaka, H., Mazi, I. M., Olowolafe, O. A., Omotosho, A. D., Oladunjoye, I. O., Tajudeen, Y. A., & Ofeh, A. S. (2023). The need for Africa to develop capacity for vaccinology as a means of curbing antimicrobial resistance. *Vaccine: X*, *14*, 100320. PMID: 37293248

Akova, M. (2016). Epidemiology of antimicrobial resistance in bloodstream infections. *Virulence*, *7*(3), 252–266. PMID: 26984779

Al Sattar, A., Chisty, N. N., Irin, N., Uddin, M. H., Hasib, F. M. Y., & Hoque, M. A. (2023). Knowledge and practice of antimicrobial usage and resistance among poultry farmers: A systematic review, meta-analysis, and meta-regression. *Veterinary Research Communications*, *47*(3), 1047–1066. DOI: 10.1007/s11259-022-10029-3

Alam, A. (2022). Educational robotics and computer programming in early childhood education: A conceptual framework for assessing elementary school students' computational thinking for designing powerful educational scenarios. *2022 International Conference on Smart Technologies and Systems for Next Generation Computing (ICSTSN)*

Alam, M. M., Islam, N., Hossain Hawlader, M. D., Ahmed, S., Wahab, A., Islam, M., Uddin, K. R., & Hossain, A. (2021). Prevalence of multidrug resistance bacterial isolates from infected wound patients in Dhaka, Bangladesh: A cross-sectional study. *International Journal of Surgery Open*, *28*, 56–62. DOI: 10.1016/j.ijso.2020.12.002

Alanjary, M., Kronmiller, B., Adamek, M., Blin, K., Weber, T., Huson, D., & Medema, M. H. (2017). The Antibiotic-Resistant Target Seeker (ARTS), an exploration engine for antibiotic cluster prioritization and novel drug target discovery. *Nucleic Acids Research*, *45*(W1), W42–W48. gkx360DOI: 10.1093/nar/ PMID: 28472505

Alara, J. A., & Alara, O. R. (2024). An overview of the global alarming increase of multiple drug resistant: A major challenge in clinical diagnosis. *Infectious Disorders-Drug TargetsDisorders*, *24*(3), 26–42. PMID: 37909431

Al-Habsi, N., Al-Khalili, M., Haque, S. A., Elias, M., Olqi, N. A., & Al Uraimi, T. (2024). Health benefits of prebiotics, probiotics, synbiotics, and postbiotics. *Nutrients*, *16*(22), 3955. PMID: 39599742

Al-Khalaifah, H.. (2025). A One-Health Perspective of Antimicrobial Resistance (AMR): Human, Animals and Environmental Health. *Life (Chicago, Ill.)*, *15*(10), 1598.

Allander, L., Vickberg, K., Lagerbäck, P., Sandegren, L., & Tängdén, T. (2022). Evaluation of in vitro activity of double-carbapenem combinations against KPC-2-, OXA-48-and NDM-producing Escherichia coli and Klebsiella pneumoniae. [PubMed]. *Antibiotics (Basel, Switzerland)*, *11*(11), 1646.

Allegranzi, B., Bagheri Nejad, S., Combescure, C., Graafmans, W., Attar, H., Donaldson, L., & Pittet, D. (2011). Burden of endemic health-care-associated infection in developing countries: Systematic review and meta-analysis. *Lancet*, *377*(9761), 228–241. PMID: 21146207

Allen, H. K., Traxler, M. F., & Barker, M. (2021). Mechanisms and ecological impacts of antibiotic resistance evolution. *Nature Reviews. Microbiology, 19*(7), 416–429. DOI: 10.1038/s41579-021-00530-6

Al-Muslem, L., Al-Qaaneh, A. M., Al-Salem, Z., Rather, I. A., & Rehman, S. The Intricate Relationship between Probiotics and Antimicrobial Resistance. In *Probiotics against Antimicrobial Resistance* (pp. 1–9). CRC Press.

AL-Tameemi, Z. A., et al. (2023). Systematic study of aminoglycoside group antibiotics drug resistance. *WORLD (Oakland, Calif.), 2*(6).

Ambreetha, S., & Singh, V. (2023). Genetic and environmental determinants of surface adaptations in Pseudomonas aeruginosa. *Microbiology (United Kingdom), 169*(6). Advance online publication. DOI: 10.1099/MIC.0.001335 PMID: 37276014

Amen, R. A., Hassan, Y. M., Essmat, R. A., Ahmed, R. H., Azab, M. M., Shehata, N. R., Elgazzar, M. M., & El-Sayed, W. M. (2025). Harnessing the Microbiome: CRISPR-Based Gene Editing and Antimicrobial Peptides in Combating Antibiotic Resistance and Cancer. *Probiotics and Antimicrobial Proteins*, •••, 1–31. PMID: 40377870

Ammoura, J. E. O., Saad, N., Elamin, A. B., & Chambuso, R. (2025). Antimicrobial Resistance and Microbiological Gap Analysis for Central Nervous System Infections Bacterial Pathogens in Nigeria. medRxiv, 2025.2008. 2012.25333494.

Andam, C. P. (2019). Clonal yet Different: Understanding the Causes of Genomic Heterogeneity in Microbial Species and Impacts on Public Health. *mSystems, 4*(3). Advance online publication. DOI: 10.1128/msystems.00097-19 PMID: 31219786

Anderson, J. K., Huang, J. Y., Wreden, C., Sweeney, E. G., Goers, J., Remington, S. J., & Guillemin, K. (2015). Chemorepulsion from the quorum signal autoinducer-2 promotes *Helicobacter pylori* biofilm dispersal. *Molecular Biology, 6*(4), e00379–e15. DOI: 10.1128/mBio.00379-15 PMID: 26152582

Ando, H., Lemire, S., Pires, D. P., & Lu, T. K. (2015). Engineering modular viral scaffolds for targeted bacterial population editing. *Cell Systems, 1*(3), 187–196. DOI: 10.1016/j.cels.2015.08.013 PMID: 26973885

Antimicrobial Resistance Collaborators. (2022). Global Burden of Bacterial Antimicrobial Resistance in 2019: A Systematic Analysis. *Lancet, 399*(10325), 629–655. https://doi.org/10.1016/S0140-6736(21)02724-0

Antonelli, A.. (2024). Healthcare-associated infections and antimicrobial use in acute care hospitals: A point prevalence survey in Lombardy, Italy, in 2022. *BMC Infectious Diseases, 24*(1), 632.

Ardila, C. M., González-Arroyave, D., & Tobón, S. (2025). Machine learning for predicting antimicrobial resistance in critical and high-priority pathogens: A systematic review considering antimicrobial susceptibility tests in real-world healthcare settings. *PLoS One*, *20*(2), e0319460. PMID: 39999193

Arias-Andres, M.. (2018). Microplastic pollution increases gene exchange in aquatic ecosystems. *Environmental Pollution*, *237*, 253–261.

Arip, M.. (2022). Review on plant-based management in combating antimicrobial resistance: A mechanistic perspective. *Frontiers in Pharmacology*, *13*, 879495.

Arnold, K. E., Laing, G., McMahon, B. J., Fanning, S., Stekel, D. J., Pahl, O., Coyne, L., Latham, S. M., & McIntyre, K. M. (2024). The need for One Health systems-thinking approaches to understand multiscale dissemination of antimicrobial resistance. *The Lancet. Planetary Health*, *8*(2), e124–e133. PMID: 38331529

Arthur, M., Molinas, C., & Courvalin, P. (1996). The vanS and vanR genes of *Tn1546* are required for glycopeptide resistance in *Enterococcus faecium* BM4147. *Journal of Bacteriology*, *175*(1), 117–127. DOI: 10.1128/jb.175.1.117-127.1993

Asamenew, T., Worku, S., Motbainor, H., Mekonnen, D., & Deribe, A. (2023). Antimicrobial Resistance Profile of Pseudomonas aeruginosa from Different Clinical Samples in Debre Tabor Comprehensive Specialized Hospital, Northwest Ethiopia. *Ethiopian Journal of Health Sciences*, *33*(3), 423–432. DOI: 10.4314/EJHS.V33I3.5 PMID: 37576170

Asantewaa, A. A., Odoom, A., Owusu-Okyere, G., & Donkor, E. S. (2024). Cholera Outbreaks in Low-and Middle-Income Countries in the Last Decade: A systematic review and meta-analysis. *Microorganisms*, *12*(12), 2504. PMID: 39770707

Ashbolt, N. J., Amézquita, A., Backhaus, T., Borriello, P., Brandt, K. K., Collignon, P., Coors, A., Finley, R., Gaze, W. H., Heberer, T., Lawrence, J. R., Larsson, D. G. J., McEwen, S. A., Ryan, J. J., Schönfeld, J., Silley, P., Snape, J. R., Van den Eede, C., & Topp, E. (2013). Human health risk assessment (HHRA) for environmental development and transfer of antibiotic resistance. *Environmental Health Perspectives*, *121*(9), 993–1001. DOI: 10.1289/ehp.1206316 PMID: 23838256

Ashley, R. E., Dittmore, A., McPherson, S. A., Turnbough, C. L.Jr, Neuman, K. C., & Osheroff, N. (2017). Activities of gyrase and topoisomerase IV on positively supercoiled DNA. *Nucleic Acids Research*, *45*(16), 9611–9624. DOI: 10.1093/nar/gkx649 PMID: 28934496

Aslam, B., & Aljasir, S. F. (2025). Climate Change and AMR: Interconnected Threats and One Health Solutions. *Antibiotics (Basel, Switzerland)*, *14*(9), 946. PMID: 41009922

Assefa, A., & Abunna, F. (2018). Maintenance of fish health in aquaculture: Review of epidemiological approaches for prevention and control of infectious disease of fish. *Veterinary Medicine International*, *2018*, 5432497. Advance online publication. DOI: 10.1155/2018/5432497 PMID: 29682272

Attri, I., Vanita, B., Rajput, R., Awasthi, L. K., Thakur, A., Tripathi, D., Pathak, V., Shukla, P., & Gupta, D. (•••). SAAM-VetNet: An attention-based multi-task framework for animal disease detection and severity grading. *Annals of Medicine and Surgery (London)*, *10*, 1097.

Awanye, A. M., Ibezim, C. N., Stanley, C. N., Onah, H., Okonko, I. O., & Egbe, N. E. (2022). Multidrug-Resistant and Extremely Drug-Resistant Pseudomonas aeruginosa in Clinical Samples From a Tertiary Healthcare Facility in Nigeria. *Turkish Journal of Pharmaceutical Sciences*, *19*(4), 447–454. DOI: 10.4274/TJPS.GALENOS.2021.66066 PMID: 36047595

Ayukekbong, J. A., Ntemgwa, M., & Atabe, A. N. (2017). The threat of antimicrobial resistance in developing countries: causes and control strategies. *Antimicrobial Resistance & Infection Control 2017 6:1*, *6*(1), 47-. https://doi.org/DOI: 10.1186/S13756-017-0208-X

Ayukekbong, J. A., Ntemgwa, M., & Atabe, A. N. (2017). The threat of Antimicrobial Resistance in developing countries: Causes and control strategies. *Antimicrobial Resistance and Infection Control*, *6*, 47. Advance online publication. DOI: 10.1186/s13756-017-0208-x PMID: 28515903

Azimzadeh, M., Greco, G., Farmani, A., Nourian, A., Pourhajibagher, M., Taherkhani, A., Alikhani, M. Y., & Bahador, A. (2025). Biofilm inhibition of multidrug-resistant Pseudomonas aeruginosa using green-synthesized silver nanoparticles and colistin. *Scientific Reports*, *15*(1), 1–15. DOI: 10.1038/S41598-025-00005-6 PMID: 40301384

Azzaya, D., Gantuya, B., Oyuntsetseg, K., Davaadorj, D., Matsumoto, T., Akada, J., & Yamaoka, Y. (2020). High antibiotic resistance of *Helicobacter pylori* and its associated novel gene mutations among the Mongolian population. *Microorganisms*, *8*(7), 1062. DOI: 10.3390/microorganisms8071062 PMID: 32708761

Baker-Austin, C., Wright, M. S., Stepanauskas, R., & McArthur, J. V. (2006). Co-selection of antibiotic and metal resistance. *Trends in Microbiology*, *14*(4), 176–182. DOI: 10.1016/j.tim.2006.02.006

Baker, S., Thomson, N., Weill, F.-X., & Holt, K. E. (2018). Genomic insights into the emergence and spread of antimicrobial-resistant bacterial pathogens. *Science, 360*(6390), 733–738. https://doi.org/10.1126/science.aar3777

Balaban, N. Q., Helaine, S., Lewis, K., Ackermann, M., Aldridge, B., Andersson, D. I., & Levin, B. R. (2019). Definitions and guidelines for research on antibiotic persistence. *Nature Reviews. Microbiology, 17*(7), 441–448. DOI: 10.1038/s41579-019-0196-3

Banerjee, R., Teng, C. B., Cunningham, S. A., Ihde, S. M., Steckelberg, J. M., Moriarty, J. P., Shah, N. D., Mandrekar, J. N., & Patel, R. (2015). Randomized trial of rapid multiplex polymerase chain reaction–based blood culture identification and susceptibility testing. *Clinical Infectious Diseases, 61*(7), 1071–1080. DOI: 10.1093/cid/civ447 PMID: 26197846

Baquero, F., Martinez, J. L. F., Lanza, V., Rodríguez-Beltrán, J., Galán, J. C., San Millán, A., Cantón, R., & Coque, T. M. (2021). Evolutionary pathways and trajectories in antibiotic resistance. *Clinical Microbiology Reviews, 34*(4), e00050–e00019. PMID: 34190572

Barlam, T. F., Cosgrove, S. E., Abbo, L. M., MacDougall, C., Schuetz, A. N., Septimus, E. J., Srinivasan, A., Dellit, T. H., Falck-Ytter, Y. T., Fishman, N. O., Hamilton, C. W., Jenkins, T. C., Lipsett, P. A., Malani, P. N., May, L. S., Moran, G. J., Neuhauser, M. M., Newland, J. G., Ohl, C. A., & Trivedi, K. K. (2016). Implementing an antibiotic stewardship program: Guidelines by the Infectious Diseases Society of America and the Society for Healthcare Epidemiology of America. *Clinical Infectious Diseases, 62*(10), e51–e77. DOI: 10.1093/cid/ciw118 PMID: 27080992

Basnet, J., Eissa, M. A., Yanes Cardozo, L. L., Romero, D. G., & Rezq, S. (2024). Impact of probiotics and prebiotics on gut microbiome and hormonal regulation. *Gastrointestinal Disorders (Basel, Switzerland), 6*(4), 801–815. PMID: 39649015

Bassetti, M., Vena, A., Croxatto, A., Righi, E., & Guery, B. (2018). How to manage Pseudomonas aeruginosa infections. *Drugs in Context, 7*, 212527. DOI: 10.7573/DIC.212527 PMID: 29872449

Batool, S. P., Fatima, H., & Ul Abadin, M. Z., MD, J. R., Joseph, A., Imran, M., & Hussain, N. (2024). Innovative Therapies In The Fight Against Antimicrobial Resistance Bridging Gaps And Overcoming Barriers. *Frontiers in Health Informatics, 13*(3).

Baum, J. H., Dörre, A., Reichert, F., Noll, I., Feig, M., Eckmanns, T., Sandfort, M., & Haller, S. (2025). Changes in incidence and epidemiology of antimicrobial resistant pathogens before and during the COVID-19 pandemic in Germany, 2015–2022. *BMC Microbiology*, *25*(1), 51. PMID: 39875841

Baur, D., Gladstone, B. P., Burkert, F., Carrara, E., Foschi, F., Döbele, S., & Tacconelli, E. (2019). Effect of antibiotic stewardship on the incidence of infection and colonisation with antibiotic-resistant bacteria and Clostridium difficile infection: A systematic review and meta-analysis. *The Lancet. Infectious Diseases*, *19*(9), 998–1008. DOI: 10.1016/S1473-3099(19)30038-3

Bearman, G., Rosato, A. E., Elam, K., Stevens, M. P., & Wenzel, R. P. (2023). Genomic epidemiology of methicillin-resistant Staphylococcus aureus transmission. *Infection Control and Hospital Epidemiology*, *44*(6), 889–897. DOI: 10.1017/ice.2022.297

Bédard, E., Laferrière, C., Déziel, E., & Prévost, M. (2018). Impact of stagnation and sampling volume on water microbial quality monitoring in large buildings. *PLoS One*, *13*(6), e0199429. https://doi.org/10.1371/journal.pone.0199429

Belay, W. Y.. (2024). Mechanism of antibacterial resistance, strategies and next-generation antimicrobials to contain antimicrobial resistance: A review. *Frontiers in Pharmacology*, *15*, 1444781.

Bello-López, J. M.. (2019). Horizontal gene transfer and its association with antibiotic resistance in the genus Aeromonas spp. *Microorganisms*, *7*(9), 363.

Berendonk, T. U., Manaia, C. M., Merlin, C., Fatta-Kassinos, D., Cytryn, E., Walsh, F., Bürgmann, H., Sørum, H., Norström, M., Pons, M.-N., Kreuzinger, N., Huovinen, P., Stefani, S., Schwartz, T., Kisand, V., Baquero, F., & Martinez, J. L. (2015). Tackling antibiotic resistance: The environmental framework. *Nature Reviews. Microbiology*, *13*(5), 310–317. DOI: 10.1038/nrmicro3439 PMID: 25817583

Besser, J. M. (2018). Salmonella epidemiology: A whirlwind of change. *Food Microbiology*, *71*, 55–59.

Bester, L. A., & Essack, S. Y. (2010). Antibiotic resistance via the food chain: Fact or fiction? *South African Journal of Science*, *106*(5/6), 1–5. DOI: 10.4102/sajs.v106i5/6.243

Bettiol, E.. (2014). Improved treatment of multidrug-resistant bacterial infections: Utility of clinical studies. *Future Microbiology*, *9*(6), 757–771.

Bianconi, I., Aschbacher, R., & Pagani, E. (2023). Current uses and future perspectives of genomic technologies in clinical microbiology. *Antibiotics (Basel, Switzerland)*, *12*(11), 1580. PMID: 37998782

Bielskė, K.. (2025). Broadly reactive monoclonal antibodies against beta-lactamases for immunodetection of bacterial resistance to antibiotics. *Scientific Reports*, *15*(1), 19094.

Bikard, D., & Barrangou, R. (2017). Using CRISPR-Cas systems as antimicrobials. *Current Opinion in Microbiology*, *37*, 155–160. PMID: 28888103

Bikard, D., & Barrangou, R. (2020). Using CRISPR–Cas systems as antimicrobials. *Nature Biotechnology*, *38*(2), 143–155.

Bikard, D., Euler, C. W., Jiang, W., Nussenzweig, P. M., Goldberg, G. W., Duportet, X., & Fischetti, V. A. (2020). Exploiting CRISPR-Cas nucleases to combat antimicrobial resistance. *Nature Reviews. Microbiology*, *18*(10), 611–622. DOI: 10.1038/s41579-020-0386-z

Billings, N., Birjiniuk, A., Samad, T. S., Doyle, P. S., & Ribbeck, K. (2015). Material properties of biofilms A review of methods for understanding permeability and mechanics. *Reports on Progress in Physics*, *78*(3), 036601. DOI: 10.1088/0034-4885/78/3/036601 PMID: 25719969

Binnie, A., Fernandes, E., Almeida-Lousada, H., de Mello, R. A., & Castelo-Branco, P. (2021). CRISPR-based strategies in infectious disease diagnosis and therapy. *Infection*, *49*(3), 377–385. PMID: 33393066

Birk, S. E., Boisen, A., & Nielsen, L. H. (2021). Polymeric nano- and microparticulate drug delivery systems for treatment of biofilms. *Advanced Drug Delivery Reviews*, *174*, 30–52. DOI: 10.1016/j.addr.2021.03.016

Biswas, S., Brunel, J.-M., Dubus, J.-C., Reynaud-Gaubert, M., & Rolain, J.-M. (2012). Colistin: An update on the antibiotic of the 21st century. *Expert Review of Anti-Infective Therapy*, *10*(8), 917–934. PMID: 23030331

Blair, J. M., Webber, M. A., Baylay, A. J., Ogbolu, D. O., & Piddock, L. J. (2015). Molecular mechanisms of antibiotic resistance. *Nature Reviews. Microbiology*, *13*(1), 42–51. DOI: 10.1038/nrmicro3380

Bleriot, I., Pacios, O., Blasco, L., Fernández-García, L., López, M., Ortiz-Cartagena, C., Barrio-Pujante, A., García-Contreras, R., Pirnay, J.-P., & Wood, T. K. (2024). Improving phage therapy by evasion of phage resistance mechanisms. *JAC-Antimicrobial Resistance*, *6*(1), dlae017. PMID: 38343627

Bonomo, R. A., Burd, E. M., Conly, J., Limbago, B. M., Poirel, L., Segre, J. A., & Westblade, L. F. (2018). Carbapenemase-producing organisms. *Clinical Infectious Diseases*, *66*(8), 1290–1297. DOI: 10.1093/cid/cix893 PMID: 29165604

Borgatta, B., Gattarello, S., Mazo, C. A., Imbiscuso, A. T., Larrosa, M. N., Lujàn, M., & Rello, J. (2017). The clinical significance of pneumonia in patients with respiratory specimens harbouring multidrug-resistant Pseudomonas aeruginosa: A 5-year retrospective study following 5667 patients in four general ICUs. *European Journal of Clinical Microbiology & Infectious Diseases*, *36*(11), 2155–2163. DOI: 10.1007/S10096-017-3039-Z/TABLES/4 PMID: 28624864

Borromeo, A. S., Manaloto, A. M., & Antonio, R. P. (2025). Southeast–Asian landscape of antimicrobial resistance research (2014–2024): A bibliometric analysis. *Journal of Global Antimicrobial Resistance*, *45*, 125–133. PMID: 40983143

Bouza, E., Guinea, J., & Guembe, M. (2014). The role of antifungals against *Candida* biofilm in catheter-related candidemia. *Antibiotics (Basel, Switzerland)*, *4*(1), 1–17. DOI: 10.3390/antibiotics4010001 PMID: 27025612

Branda, F., & Scarpa, F. (2024). Implications of artificial intelligence in addressing antimicrobial resistance: Innovations, global challenges, and healthcare's future. *Antibiotics (Basel, Switzerland)*, *13*(6), 502. PMID: 38927169

Breijyeh, Z.. (2020). Resistance of gram-negative bacteria to current antibacterial agents and approaches to resolve it. *Molecules (Basel, Switzerland)*, *25*(6), 1340.

Brives, C., & Pourraz, J. (2020). Phage therapy as a potential solution in the fight against AMR: Obstacles and possible futures. *Palgrave Communications*, *6*(1), 1–11.

Browne, K.. (2020). A new era of antibiotics: The clinical potential of antimicrobial peptides. *International Journal of Molecular Sciences*, *21*(19), 7047.

Bruenke, J., Roschke, I., Agarwal, S., Riemann, T., & Greiner, A. (2016). Quantitative comparison of the antimicrobial efficiency of leaching versus nonleaching polymer materials. *Macromolecular Bioscience*, *16*(5), 647–654. DOI: 10.1002/mabi.201500370 PMID: 26806336

Burke, V., Richter, D., Greskowiak, J., Mehrtens, A., Schulz, L., & Massmann, G. (2016). Occurrence of antibiotics in surface and groundwater of a drinking water catchment area in Germany. *Water Environment Research*, *88*(7), 652–665. DOI: 10.2175/106143016X14609975746064 PMID: 27329061

Bush, K. (2024). Commentary on The antibiotic explosion by H. Boyd Woodruff and Richard W. Burg. In Hemodynamics and Immune Defense (pp. 301–306). Elsevier.

Bush, K., & Bradford, P. A. (2016). β-Lactams and β-lactamase inhibitors: An overview. *Cold Spring Harbor Perspectives in Medicine*, *6*(8), a025247. DOI: 10.1101/cshperspect.a025247

Bwanali, A. N.. (2025). Trends and patterns of antimicrobial resistance among common pathogens isolated from adult bloodstream and urinary tract infections in public health facilities in Malawi, 2020–2024. *BMC Infectious Diseases*, *25*(1), 946.

Cai, X., Tian, J., Zhu, J., Chen, J., Li, L., Yang, C., Chen, J., & Chen, D. (2021). Photodynamic and photothermal co-driven CO-enhanced multi-mode synergistic antibacterial nanoplatform to effectively fight against biofilm infections. *Chemical Engineering Journal*, *426*, 131919.

Carascal, M. B., dela Cruz-Papa, D. M., Remenyi, R., Cruz, M. C. B., & Destura, R. V. (2022). Phage revolution against multidrug-resistant clinical pathogens in Southeast Asia. *Frontiers in Microbiology*, *13*, 820572. PMID: 35154059

Carattoli, A. (2013). Plasmids and the spread of resistance. *International Journal of Medical Microbiology*, *303*(6-7), 298–304. DOI: 10.1016/j.ijmm.2013.02.001

Carlet, J.. (2014). Antibiotic resistance: A geopolitical issue. *Clinical Microbiology and Infection*, *20*(10), 949–953.

Carlson, E. E.. (2025). Decoding the Penicillin-Binding Proteins with Activity-Based Probes. *Accounts of Chemical Research*, *58*(11), 1754–1763.

Castanheira, M.. (2021). Extended-spectrum β-lactamases: An update on their characteristics, epidemiology and detection. *JAC-Antimicrobial Resistance*, *3*(3), dlab092.

Castanon, J. I. R. (2007). History of the use of antibiotics as growth promoters in European poultry feeds. *Poultry Science*, *86*(11), 2466–2471. DOI: 10.3382/ps.2007-00249

CDC. (2022). *Antibiotic resistance threats in the United States, 2022*. Centers for Disease Control and Prevention.

CDC. (2023). *Healthcare-associated infections progress report*. Centers for Disease Control and Prevention.

CDC. (2024). *Antimicrobial resistance threats in the United States*. Centers for Disease Control and Prevention.

Chakraborty, A., Diwan, A., & Tatake, J. (2023). Prospect of nanomaterials as antimicrobial and antiviral regimen. *AIMS Microbiology*, *9*(3), 444–466. PMID: 37649798

Chakraborty, P.. (2021). Biofilm formation in the lung contributes to virulence and drug tolerance of Mycobacterium tuberculosis. *Nature Communications*, *12*(1), 1606.

Chambers, H. F., Fowler, V. G.Jr, & Group, A. R. L. (2022). *Confronting antimicrobial resistance together* (Vol. 323). American Physiological Society Rockville.

Chandal, N.. (2025). In Vitro and In Vivo Investigations into the Potential of Quinazoline and Quinoline Derivatives as NorA Efflux Pump Inhibitors Against Resistant Staphylococcus aureus Strains. *Antibiotics (Basel, Switzerland)*, *14*(4), 339.

Chang, S.-K., Lo, D.-Y., Wei, H.-W., & Kuo, H.-C. (2015). Antimicrobial resistance of Escherichia coli isolates from canine urinary tract infections. *The Journal of Veterinary Medical Science*, *77*(1), 59–65. DOI: 10.1292/jvms.14-0009 PMID: 25720807

Chan, K.-G.. (2015). Inhibiting N-acyl-homoserine lactone synthesis and quenching Pseudomonas quinolone quorum sensing to attenuate virulence. *Frontiers in Microbiology*, *6*, 1173.

Chao, Y., Marks, L. R., Pettigrew, M. M., & Hakansson, A. P. (2014). *Streptococcus pneumoniae* biofilm formation and dispersion during colonization and disease. *Frontiers in Cellular and Infection Microbiology*, *4*, 194. DOI: 10.3389/fcimb.2014.00194 PMID: 25629011

Chaw, P. S., Hopner, J., & Mikolajczyk, R. (2018). The knowledge, attitude and practice of health practitioners towards antibiotic prescribing and resistance in developing countries—A systematic review. *Journal of Clinical Pharmacy and Therapeutics*, *43*(5), 606–613. DOI: 10.1111/jcpt.12730 PMID: 29959783

Cheesman, M. J., Ilanko, A., Blonk, B., & Cock, I. E. (2017). Developing new antimicrobial therapies: Are synergistic combinations of plant extracts/compounds with conventional antibiotics the solution? *Pharmacognosy Reviews*, *11*(22), 57–72. DOI: 10.4103/phrev.phrev_21_17 PMID: 28989242

Chegini, Z., Khoshbayan, A., Taati Moghadam, M., Farahani, I., Jazireian, P., & Shariati, A. (2020). Bacteriophage therapy against Pseudomonas aeruginosa biofilms: a review. *Annals of Clinical Microbiology and Antimicrobials 2020 19:1*, *19*(1), 1–17. https://doi.org/DOI: 10.1186/S12941-020-00389-5

Chen, J., Liu, Z., Huang, X., Wu, C., Liu, Q., Jiang, G., Pu, Y., Lei, Y., Chen, X., & Wang, X. (2024). When large language models meet personalization: Perspectives of challenges and opportunities. *World Wide Web (Bussum)*, *27*(4), 42.

Chen, L., Qu, X., Su, J., Yao, H., Yuan, Q., Wang, Y., Li, N., Wu, G., Liu, X., Hu, J., & Zhang, J. (2023). The dilemma of antibiotic susceptibility and clinical decision-making in a multi-drug-resistant Pseudomonas aeruginosa bloodstream infection. *Frontiers in Pharmacology*, *14*, 1183332. DOI: 10.3389/FPHAR.2023.1183332 PMID: 37324460

Cheraghi, M., Amiri, M., Andarzgoo, S., Zarei, F., Seghatoleslami, Z. S., Centis, R., Migliori, G. B., Visca, D., & Pontali, E. (2025). Bedaquiline and linezolid regimens for multidrug-resistant tuberculosis: A systematic review and meta-analysis. *Jornal Brasileiro de Pneumologia : Publicaçao Oficial da Sociedade Brasileira de Pneumologia e Tisilogia, 51*(1), e20240391. DOI: 10.36416/1806-3756/e20240391

Chigozie, V. U., Aniokete, C. U., Ogbonna, P. I., & Iroha, R. I. (2025). Transforming antimicrobial resistance mitigation: The genomic revolution in one health and public health. *Discover Applied Sciences, 7*(10), 1187.

Chin, C. D., Linder, V., & Sia, S. K. (2017). Commercialization of microfluidic point-of-care diagnostic devices. *Lab on a Chip, 12*(12), 2118–2134. DOI: 10.1039/C2LC21204H

Chindelevitch, L., Jauneikaite, E., Wheeler, N. E., Allel, K., Ansiri-Asafoakaa, B. Y., Awuah, W. A., Bauer, D. C., Beisken, S., Fan, K., & Grant, G. (2022). Applying data technologies to combat AMR: current status, challenges, and opportunities on the way forward. *arXiv preprint arXiv:2208.04683.*

Choi, U., & Lee, C.-R. (2019). Distinct roles of outer membrane porins in antibiotic resistance and membrane integrity in Escherichia coli. *Frontiers in Microbiology, 10*, 953. DOI: 10.3389/fmicb.2019.00953 PMID: 31114568

Chokshi, A., Sifri, Z., Cennimo, D., & Horng, H. (2019). Global contributors to antibiotic resistance. *Journal of Global Infectious Diseases, 11*(1), 36–42. DOI: 10.4103/jgid.jgid_110_18

Chowdhary, A., Sharma, C., & Meis, J. F. (2017). Candida auris: A rapidly emerging cause of hospital-acquired multidrug-resistant fungal infections globally. *PLoS Pathogens, 13*(5), e1006290. https://doi.org/10.1371/journal.ppat.1006290

Chuah, L.-O., Effarizah, M. E., Goni, A. M., & Rusul, G. (2016). Antibiotic application and emergence of multiple antibiotic resistance (MAR) in global catfish aquaculture. *Current Environmental Health Reports, 3*(2), 118–127. DOI: 10.1007/s40572-016-0091-2 PMID: 27038482

Churchyard, G. J., Swindells, S., Gupta, A., Shah, N. S., Hughes, M., Kim, S., Fox, G. J., Harrington, M., Chaisson, R. E., & Hesseling, A. C. (2025). Preventing multidrug-resistant tuberculosis: The dawn of a new era. *Clinical Infectious Diseases, 81*(6), 1135–1140. https://doi.org/10.1093/cid/ciaf426

Cieplik, F.. (2013). Photodynamic biofilm inactivation by SAPYR—An exclusive singlet oxygen photosensitizer. *Free Radical Biology & Medicine, 65*, 477–487.

Citorik, R. J., Mimee, M., & Lu, T. K. (2019). CRISPR-based antimicrobials. *Nature Reviews. Microbiology, 17*(3), 153–164. DOI: 10.1038/s41579-018-0135-3

Clancy, C., & Nguyen, M. (2020). Coronavirus disease 2019, superinfections, and antimicrobial development: What can we expect? *Clinical Infectious Diseases, 71*(10), 2736–2743. PMID: 32361747

Claycamp, H. G. (2015). Risk assessment of antimicrobial resistance. In Chen, C.-Y., Yan, X., & Jackson, C. R. (Eds.), *Antimicrobial Resistance and Food Safety* (pp. 283–302). Academic Press., DOI: 10.1016/B978-0-12-801214-7.00014-3

Clemens, J., et al. "Cholera Lancet, 390 (2017)." View PDF View article View in Scopus: 1539-1549.

CLSI. (2023). *Analysis and presentation of cumulative antimicrobial susceptibility test data* (5th ed.). Clinical and Laboratory Standards Institute.

CLSI. (2024). *Performance standards for antimicrobial susceptibility testing* (34th ed.). Clinical and Laboratory Standards Institute.

Cochran, W. L., McFeters, G. A., & Stewart, P. S. (2000). Reduced susceptibility of thin *Pseudomonas aeruginosa* biofilms to hydrogen peroxide and monochloramine. *Journal of Applied Microbiology, 88*(1), 22–30. DOI: 10.1046/j.1365-2672.2000.00871.x PMID: 10735239

Codda, G. (2024). Next Generation Sequencing-based detection and characterization of microbial pathogens causing invasive infections and outbreaks in ICU: Towards improved management of the high-risk patient.

Codjoe, F. S., & Donkor, E. S. (2017). Carbapenem resistance: A review. *Medical Science, 6*(1), 1.

Coque, T. M., Cantón, R., Pérez-Cobas, A. E., Fernández-de-Bobadilla, M. D., & Baquero, F. (2023). Antimicrobial resistance in the global health network: Known unknowns and challenges for efficient responses in the 21st century. *Microorganisms, 11*(4), 1050. PMID: 37110473

Courbet, A., et al. (2015). "Detection of pathological biomarkers in human clinical samples via amplifying genetic switches and logic gates." Science translational medicine 7(289): 289ra283-289ra283.

Cubillos-Ruiz, A., Guo, T., Sokolovska, A., Miller, P. F., Collins, J. J., Lu, T. K., & Lora, J. M. (2021). Engineering living therapeutics with synthetic biology. *Nature Reviews. Drug Discovery, 20*(12), 941–960. PMID: 34616030

Cusumano, G., Flores, G. A., Venanzoni, R., & Angelini, P. (2025). The Impact of Antibiotic Therapy on Intestinal Microbiota: Dysbiosis, Antibiotic Resistance, and Restoration Strategies. *Antibiotics (Basel, Switzerland)*, *14*(4), 371. PMID: 40298495

D'Aquila, P., De Rose, E., Sena, G., Scorza, A., Cretella, B., Passarino, G., & Bellizzi, D. (2024). Quorum quenching approaches against bacterial-biofilm-induced antibiotic resistance. *Antibiotics (Basel, Switzerland)*, *13*(7), 619. DOI: 10.3390/antibiotics13070619 PMID: 39061301

Da Costa, P. M., Loureiro, L., & Matos, A. J. F. (2013). Transfer of multidrug-resistant bacteria between intermingled ecological niches: The interface between humans, animals and the environment. *International Journal of Environmental Research and Public Health*, *10*(1), 278–294. DOI: 10.3390/ijerph10010278

Dabhi, M.. (2024). Penicillin-binding proteins: The master builders and breakers of bacterial cell walls and its interaction with β-lactam antibiotics. *Journal of Proteins and Proteomics*, *15*(2), 215–232.

Dadgostar, P. (2019). Antimicrobial resistance: Implications and costs. *Infection and Drug Resistance*, *12*, 3903–3910. DOI: 10.2147/IDR.S234610 PMID: 31908502

Dan, B., Dai, H., Zhou, D., Tong, H., & Zhu, M. (2023). Relationship between drug resistance characteristics and biofilm formation in *Klebsiella pneumoniae* strains. *Infection and Drug Resistance*, *16*, 985–998. DOI: 10.2147/IDR.S395098 PMID: 36824066

Darby, E. M.. (2023). Molecular mechanisms of antibiotic resistance revisited. *Nature Reviews. Microbiology*, *21*(5), 280–295.

Dash, B., Shireen, M., Kumar, S., Goel, A., Semwal, P., & Rani, R. (2024). A comprehensive review: Pharmacogenomics and personalized medicine customizing drug therapy based on individual genetics profiles. *Chinese. Journal of Applied Physiology (Bethesda, Md.)*, ●●●, 20240011.

Das, P. K., & Samal, S. (2018). Microbial biofilms: Pathogenicity and treatment strategies. *PharmaTutor*, *6*(1), 16–22.

Davenport, E. K., Call, D. R., & Beyenal, H. (2014). Differential protection from tobramycin by extracellular polymeric substances from *Acinetobacter baumannii* and *Staphylococcus aureus* biofilms. *Antimicrobial Agents and Chemotherapy*, *58*(8), 4755–4761. DOI: 10.1128/AAC.03071-14 PMID: 24913166

David, S., Caballero, J. D., Couto, N., Abudahab, K., Alikhan, N.-F., Yeats, C., Underwood, A., Molloy, A., Connor, D., Shane, H. M., Ashton, P. M., Grundmann, H., Holden, M. T. G., Feil, E. J., Sia, S. B., Donado-Godoy, P., Lingegowda, R. K., Okeke, I. N., Argimón, S., & Aanensen, D. M. (2025). Monitoring antimicrobial resistance trends from global genomics data: Amr.watch. *PLOS Global Public Health*, *5*(11), e0005256. https://doi.org/10.1371/journal.pgph.0005256

Davies, D. (2003). Understanding biofilm resistance to antibacterial agents. *Nature Reviews. Drug Discovery*, *2*(2), 114–122. DOI: 10.1038/nrd1008 PMID: 12563302

Davies, J., & Davies, D. (2010). Origins and evolution of antibiotic resistance. *Microbiology and Molecular Biology Reviews : MMBR*, *74*(3), 417–433. DOI: 10.1128/MMBR.00016-10 PMID: 20805405

De Almeida, M., Gerard, C., Freeman, J. T., Duffy, E., & Roberts, S. A. (2018). Inappropriate prescribing of antibiotics following discharge after major surgery: An area for improvement. *The New Zealand Medical Journal*, *131*(1475), 35–43. PMID: 29771900

De Andrade, L. R. M., Andrade, L. N., Bahú, J. O., Cárdenas Concha, V. O., Machado, A. T., Pires, D. S., Santos, R., Cardoso, T. F. M., Cardoso, J. C., Albuquerque-Junior, R. L. C., Mazzola, P. G., Gremião, M. P. D., & Chorilli, M. (2024). Biomedical applications of carbon nanotubes: A systematic review of data and clinical trials. *Journal of Drug Delivery Science and Technology*, *99*, 105932. DOI: 10.1016/j.jddst.2024.105932

de Carvalho Leonel, L.. (2019). Photodynamic Antimicrobial Chemotherapy (PACT) using methylene blue inhibits the viability of the biofilm produced by Candida albicans. *Photodiagnosis and Photodynamic Therapy*, *26*, 316–323.

De Gaetano, G. V.. (2023). Antimicrobial resistance: Two-component regulatory systems and multidrug efflux pumps. *Antibiotics (Basel, Switzerland)*, *12*(6), 965.

De Souza, G. H., Rossato, L., de Oliveira, A. R., & Simionatto, S. (2023). Antimicrobial peptides against polymyxin-resistant Klebsiella pneumoniae: A patent review. *World Journal of Microbiology & Biotechnology*, *39*(3), 1–10. PMID: 36720739

Dehari, D.. (2023). A bacteriophage microgel effectively treats the multidrug-resistant Acinetobacter baumannii bacterial infections in burn wounds. *Pharmaceuticals*, *16*(7), 942.

Desai, S., Patel, V., Nagare, S. D., Patil, R., & More, M. J. (2025). Microbial genomics and infectious disease forecasting. In *Host Adaptation, Virulence, and Evolution* (pp. 193-223). Academic Press.

Dettori, S., Portunato, F., Vena, A., Giacobbe, D. R., & Bassetti, M. (2023). Severe infections caused by difficult-to-treat Gram-negative bacteria. In *Current Opinion in Critical Care* (Vol. 29, Issue 5, pp. 438–445). Lippincott Williams and Wilkins. https://doi.org/DOI: 10.1097/MCC.0000000000001074

Devi, M., Manokaran, D., Sehgal, R. K., Shariff, S. A., & Vettriselvan, R. (2025). Precision Medicine, Personalized Treatment, and Network-Driven Innovations: Transforming Healthcare With AI. In *AI for Large Scale Communication Networks* (pp. 303-322). IGI Global.

Dhiman, R., & Pandey, R. P. Ethical and Regulatory Considerations for Artificial Intelligence in Managing AMR. In *Artificial Intelligence in Managing Antimicrobial Resistance* (pp. 135–157). CRC Press.

Didelot, X., Bowden, R., Wilson, D. J., Peto, T. E., & Crook, D. W. (2019). Transforming clinical microbiology with bacterial genome sequencing. *Nature Reviews. Genetics*, *20*(10), 601–612. DOI: 10.1038/s41576-019-0153-6

Didelot, X., Fraser, C., Gardy, J., & Colijn, C. (2021). Genomic epidemiology analysis of bacterial pathogens. *Nature Reviews. Genetics*, *22*(9), 593–610. DOI: 10.1038/s41576-021-00345-3

Dillac, L., Christie, W., van Dalen, D., & Adiningrat, R. P. P. (2024). New approaches to combat Antimicrobial Resistance (AMR)? Due, A. (2023). What are side effects? *European Journal for Philosophy of Science*, *13*(1), 16.

Dimitriu, T. (2022). Evolution of horizontal transmission in antimicrobial resistance plasmids. *Microbiology*, *168*(7), 001214. PMID: 35849537

Dissanayake, U., Ukhanova, M., Moye, Z. D., Sulakvelidze, A., & Mai, V. (2019). Bacteriophages reduce pathogenic Escherichia coli counts in mice without distorting gut microbiota. *Frontiers in Microbiology*, *10*, 1984. PMID: 31551950

Djordjevic, S. P., Jarocki, V. M., Seemann, T., Cummins, M. L., Watt, A. E., Drigo, B., Wyrsch, E. R., Reid, C. J., Donner, E., & Howden, B. P. (2024). Genomic surveillance for antimicrobial resistance—A One Health perspective. *Nature Reviews. Genetics*, *25*(2), 142–157. PMID: 37749210

Djordjevic, S. P., Stokes, H. W., & Chowdhury, P. R. (2013). Mobile elements, zoonotic pathogens and commensal bacteria: Conduits for the delivery of resistance genes into humans, production animals and soil microbiota. *Frontiers in Microbiology*, *4*, 86. DOI: 10.3389/fmicb.2013.00086 do Prado, G. V. B., Marchi, A. P., Moreno, L. Z., Rizek, C., Amigo, U., Moreno, A. M., Rossi, F., Guimaraes, T., Levin, A. S., & Costa, S. F. (2016). Virulence and resistance pattern of a novel sequence type of linezolid-resistant Enterococcus faecium identified by whole-genome sequencing. *Journal of Global Antimicrobial Resistance*, *6*, 27–31. DOI: 10.1016/j.jgar.2016.02.006 PMID: 27530835

Dolejska, M., & Literak, I. (2019). Wildlife is overlooked in the epidemiology of medically important antibiotic-resistant bacteria. *Antimicrobial Agents and Chemotherapy*, *63*(8), e01167–e19. DOI: 10.1128/AAC.01167-19 PMID: 31209001

Dong, H., Xiang, Y., & Fang, W. (2021). Phage-delivered CRISPR-Cas systems for precision antimicrobial applications. *Trends in Biotechnology*, *39*(10), 1049–1062. DOI: 10.1016/j.tibtech.2021.03.008

Doran, P. M. (2024). Foreign protein degradation and instability in plants and plant tissue cultures. *Trends in Biotechnology*, *24*(9), 426–432. PMID: 16843560

Du Plessis, G. M. (2017). *Microbial geopolitics: Living with danger and the future of security* [Doctoral dissertation, University of Pretoria].

Ducarmon, Q., Zwittink, R., Hornung, B., Van Schaik, W., Young, V., & Kuijper, E. (2019). Gut microbiota and colonization resistance against bacterial enteric infection. *Microbiology and Molecular Biology Reviews : MMBR*, *83*(3), 00007–00019. DOI: 10.1128/mmbr PMID: 31167904

Du, D., Wang-Kan, X., Neuberger, A., van Veen, H. W., Pos, K. M., Piddock, L. J., & Luisi, B. F. (2018). Multidrug efflux pumps: Structure, function and regulation. *Nature Reviews. Microbiology*, *16*(9), 523–539.

Đukanović, S.. (2022). Elucidating the antibiofilm activity of Frangula emodin against Staphylococcus aureus biofilms. *Journal of Applied Microbiology*, *132*(3), 1840–1855.

Dutt, Y., Dhiman, R., Singh, T., Vibhuti, A., Gupta, A., Pandey, R. P., Raj, V. S., Chang, C.-M., & Priyadarshini, A. (2022). The association between biofilm formation and antimicrobial resistance with possible ingenious bio-remedial approaches. *Antibiotics (Basel, Switzerland)*, *11*(7), 930. DOI: 10.3390/antibiotics11070930 PMID: 35884186

Dyary, H.. (2023). History, current situation, and future perspectives on antibiotics and antibiotic Resistance. *International Journal of Agriculture and Biosciences*, *2*, 109–118.

Eccleston-Turner, M., & Upton, H. (2021). International collaboration to ensure equitable access to vaccines for COVID-19: The ACT-Accelerator and the COVAX facility. *The Milbank Quarterly*, *99*(2), 426–449. PMID: 33650737

Egwu, C. O., Aloke, C., Onwe, K. T., Umoke, C. I., Nwafor, J., Eyo, R. A., Chukwu, J. A., Ufebe, G. O., Ladokun, J., Audu, D. T., & Alum, E. U. (2024). Nanomaterials in drug delivery: Strengths and opportunities in medicine. *Molecules (Basel, Switzerland)*, *29*(11), 2584. DOI: 10.3390/molecules29112584

Eke, S. M., & Cua, A. (2025). Invisible Engines of Resistance: How Global Inequities Drive Antimicrobial Failure. *Antibiotics (Basel, Switzerland)*, *14*(7), 659. PMID: 40723962

Ekwueme, C. T., Anyiam, I. V., Ekwueme, D. C., Anumudu, C. K., & Onyeaka, H. (2025). Reconstructing the Antibiotic Pipeline: Natural Alternatives to Antibacterial Agents. *Biomolecules*, *15*(8), 1182. PMID: 40867625

El-Batal, A. I., Al-Hazmi, N. E., Farrag, A. A., Elsayed, M. A., El-Khawaga, A. M., El-Sayyad, G. S., & Elshamy, A. A. (2022). Antimicrobial synergism and antibiofilm activity of amoxicillin-loaded citric acid-magnesium ferrite nanocomposite: Effect of UV-illumination, and membrane leakage reaction mechanism. *Microbial Pathogenesis*, *164*, 105–440. DOI: 10.1016/j.micpath.2022.105440

Elbehiry, A., & Abalkhail, A. (2025). Metagenomic next-generation sequencing in infectious diseases: Clinical applications, translational challenges, and future directions. *Diagnostics (Basel)*, *15*(16), 1991. PMID: 40870843

Elfadadny, A., Ragab, R. F., AlHarbi, M., Badshah, F., Ibáñez-Arancibia, E., Farag, A., Hendawy, A. O., De los Ríos-Escalante, P. R., Aboubakr, M., Zakai, S. A., & Nageeb, W. M. (2024). Antimicrobial resistance of Pseudomonas aeruginosa: Navigating clinical impacts, current resistance trends, and innovations in breaking therapies. *Frontiers in Microbiology*, *15*, 1374466. DOI: 10.3389/FMICB.2024.1374466/XML/NLM PMID: 38646632

Elguoshy, A., & Hashem, A. M. (2024). Introduction to genomic-based clinical applications. In *Microbial Genomics: Clinical, Pharmaceutical, and Industrial Applications* (pp. 97-115). Academic Press.

Ellington, M. J., Ekelund, O., & Aarestrup, F. M.. (2017). The role of whole genome sequencing in antimicrobial susceptibility testing of bacteria: Report from EUCAST Subcommittee. *Clinical Microbiology and Infection*, *23*(1), 2–22. DOI: 10.1016/j.cmi.2016.11.012

Elmassry, M. M., Colmer-Hamood, J. A., Kopel, J., San Francisco, M. J., & Hamood, A. N. (2023). Anti-Pseudomonas aeruginosa Vaccines and Therapies: An Assessment of Clinical Trials. *Microorganisms 2023, Vol. 11, Page 916, 11*(4), 916. https://doi.org/DOI: 10.3390/MICROORGANISMS11040916

Elmongui, E.. (2025). Evaluating anti-MRSA antibiotic stewardship with a focus on trends in consumption and resistance in a tertiary hospital in Alexandria, Egypt from 2019 to 2023. *Archives of Public Health = Archives Belges de Santé Publique, 83*(1), 133.

El-Sapagh, S., El-Shenody, R., Pereira, L., & Elshobary, M. (2023). Unveiling the potential of algal extracts as promising antibacterial and antibiofilm agents against multidrug-resistant *Pseudomonas aeruginosa*: In vitro and in silico studies including molecular docking. *Plants, 12*(19), 3324. DOI: 10.3390/plants12193324 PMID: 37765485

Elshobary, M. E., Badawy, N. K., Ashraf, Y., Zatioun, A. A., Masriya, H. H., Ammar, M. M., Mohamed, N. A., Mourad, S., & Assy, A. M. (2025). Combating Antibiotic Resistance: Mechanisms, Multidrug-Resistant Pathogens, and Novel Therapeutic Approaches: An Updated Review. *Pharmaceuticals 2025, Vol. 18, Page 402, 18*(3), 402. https://doi.org/DOI: 10.3390/PH18030402

Elshobary, M. E.. (2025). Combating antibiotic resistance: Mechanisms, multidrug-resistant pathogens, and novel therapeutic approaches: An updated review. *Pharmaceuticals, 18*(3), 402.

Elumalai, K., Srinivasan, S., & Shanmugam, A. (2024). Review of the efficacy of nanoparticle-based drug delivery systems for cancer treatment. *Biomedical Technology, 5*, 109–122.

Erkihun, M., Asmare, Z., Endalamew, K., Getie, B., Kiros, T., & Berhan, A. (2024). Medical scope of biofilm and quorum sensing during biofilm formation: Systematic review. *Bacteria, 3*(2), 118–135. DOI: 10.3390/bacteria3020009

Eslami, M., Naderian, R., Bahar, A., Babaeizad, A., Rezanavaz Gheshlagh, S., Oksenych, V., & Tahmasebi, H. (2025). Microbiota as diagnostic biomarkers: Advancing early cancer detection and personalized therapeutic approaches through microbiome profiling. *Frontiers in Immunology, 16*, 1559480. PMID: 40406094

Esposito, S., Amirthalingam, G., Bassetti, M., Blasi, F., De Rosa, F. G., Halasa, N. B., Huttner, A., Martin-Loeches, I., Pollard, A. J., Rello, J., Schultsz, C., Tumbarello, M., & Kantele, A. (2023). Monoclonal antibodies for prophylaxis and therapy of respiratory syncytial virus, SARS-CoV-2, human immunodeficiency virus, rabies and bacterial infections. *Frontiers in Immunology, 14*, 1172054. PMID: 37256125

Esposito, S., Purrello, S. M., Bonnet, E., Novelli, A., Tripodi, F., Pascale, R., Unal, S., & Milkovich, G. (2013). Central venous catheter-related biofilm infections: An up-to-date focus on meticillin-resistant *Staphylococcus aureus. Journal of Global Antimicrobial Resistance, 1*(2), 71–78. DOI: 10.1016/j.jgar.2013.04.003 PMID: 27873581

European Centre for Disease Prevention and Control. (2025). *Antimicrobial resistance in the EU/EEA (EARS-Net) — Annual Epidemiological Report for 2024*. ECDC.

European Medicines Agency. (2015). *Reflection paper on the risk of antimicrobial resistance transfer from companion animals* (EMA/CVMP/CHMP/682198/2014). https://www.ema.europa.eu/en/documents/scientific-guideline/reflection-paper-risk-antimicrobial-resistance-transfer-companion-animals_en.pdf

Fahmy, N. F., Abdel-Kareem, M. M., Ahmed, H. A., Helmy, M. Z., & Mahmoud, E. A.-R. (2025). Evaluation of the antibacterial and antibiofilm effect of mycosynthesized silver and selenium nanoparticles and their synergistic effect with antibiotics on nosocomial bacteria. *Microbial Cell Factories, 24*(1), 6. DOI: 10.1186/s12934-025-02406-1

Fang, K.. (2018). Probiotic Escherichia coli inhibits biofilm formation of pathogenic E. coli via extracellular activity of DegP. *Scientific Reports, 8*(1), 4939.

Farzi, N., Oloomi, M., Bahramali, G., Siadat, S. D., & Bouzari, S. (2023). Antibacterial properties and efficacy of LL-37 fragment GF-17D3 and scolopendin A2 peptides against resistant clinical strains of *Staphylococcus aureus, Pseudomonas aeruginosa*, and *Acinetobacter baumannii* in vitro and in vivo model studies. *Probiotics and Antimicrobial Proteins, 15*(5), 1–19. DOI: 10.1007/s12602-023-10053-x PMID: 37148452

Fauzia, K. A., Miftahussurur, M., Syam, A. F., Waskito, L. A., Doohan, D., Rezkitha, Y. A. A., Matsumoto, T., Tuan, V. P., Akada, J., Yonezawa, H., & Yamaoka, Y. (2020). Biofilm formation and antibiotic resistance phenotype of *Helicobacter pylori* clinical isolates. *Toxins, 12*(8), 473. DOI: 10.3390/toxins12080473 PMID: 32722296

Fernández-Barat, L., Ferrer, M., De Rosa, F., Gabarrús, A., Esperatti, M., Terraneo, S., Rinaudo, M., Li Bassi, G., & Torres, A. (2017). Intensive care unit-acquired pneumonia due to Pseudomonas aeruginosa with and without multidrug resistance. *The Journal of Infection, 74*(2), 142–152. DOI: 10.1016/j.jinf.2016.11.008 PMID: 27865895

Fernández-Billón, M., Llambías-Cabot, A. E., Jordana-Lluch, E., Oliver, A., & Macià, M. D. (2023). Mechanisms of antibiotic resistance in Pseudomonas aeruginosa biofilms. *Biofilm*, *5*, 100129. DOI: 10.1016/J.BIOFLM.2023.100129 PMID: 37205903

Fernández, L., Gooderham, W. J., & Hancock, R. E. W. (2010). Adaptive resistance to the "last hope" antibiotics colistin and polymyxin B in Pseudomonas aeruginosa is mediated by activation of the arn operon. *Antimicrobial Agents and Chemotherapy*, *54*(8), 3372–3377. DOI: 10.1128/AAC.00216-10

Ferri, M., Ranucci, E., Romagnoli, P., & Giaccone, V. (2017). Antimicrobial resistance: A global emerging threat to public health systems. *Critical Reviews in Food Science and Nutrition*, *57*(13), 2857–2876. PMID: 26464037

Fisher, M. C., Burnett, F., Chandler, C., Gow, N. A. R., Gurr, S., Hart, A., Holmes, A., May, R. C., Quinn, J., Soliman, T., Talbot, N. J., White, P. L., Bromley, M., & Armstrong-James, D. (2024). A One Health roadmap towards understanding and mitigating emerging fungal antimicrobial resistance: fAMR. npj Antimicrobials and Resistance, 2(36), Article 36. https://doi.org/10.1038/s44259-024-00055-2

Fjell, C. D., Hiss, J. A., Hancock, R. E. W., & Schneider, G. (2012). Designing antimicrobial peptides: Form follows function. *Nature Reviews. Drug Discovery*, *11*(1), 37–51. DOI: 10.1038/nrd3591

Fleming, D., & Rumbaugh, K. (2018). The consequences of biofilm dispersal on the host. *Scientific Reports*, *8*(1), 10738.

Flemming, H. C., & Wuertz, S. (2019). Bacteria and archaea on Earth and their abundance in biofilms. *Nature Reviews. Microbiology*, *17*(4), 247–260.

Flores-Vega, V. R., Partida-Sanchez, S., Ares, M. A., Ortiz-Navarrete, V., & Rosales-Reyes, R. (2025). High-risk Pseudomonas aeruginosa clones harboring β-lactamases: 2024 update. *Heliyon*, *11*(1), e41540. DOI: 10.1016/J.HELIYON.2024.E41540 PMID: 39850428

Food and Agriculture Organization of the United Nations & World Health Organization. (2002). *Guidelines for the evaluation of probiotics in food*. FAO/WHO. ftp://ftp.fao.org/es/esn/food/wgreport2.pdf

Foster, T. J. (2017). Antibiotic resistance in Staphylococcus aureus. Current status and future prospects. *FEMS Microbiology Reviews*, *41*(3), 430–449. DOI: 10.1093/femsre/fux007 PMID: 28419231

Foudraine, D. E.. (2021). Exploring antimicrobial resistance to beta-lactams, aminoglycosides and fluoroquinolones in E. coli and K. pneumoniae using proteogenomics. *Scientific Reports*, *11*(1), 12472.

Founou, L. L., Founou, R. C., & Essack, S. Y. (2016). Antibiotic resistance in the food chain: A developing country-perspective. *Frontiers in Microbiology*, *7*, 18–81. DOI: 10.3389/fmicb.2016.01881

Fridkin, S. K. (2001). Vancomycin-intermediate and -resistant Staphylococcus aureus: What the infectious disease specialist needs to know. *Clinical Infectious Diseases*, *32*(1), 108–115. PMID: 11118389

Fux, C. A., Costerton, J. W., Stewart, P. S., & Stoodley, P. (2005). Survival strategies of infectious biofilms. *Trends in Microbiology*, *13*(1), 34–40. DOI: 10.1016/j.tim.2004.11.010 PMID: 15639630

Gach, M. W.. (2024). Antimicrobial resistance among common bacterial pathogens in Indonesia: A systematic review. *The Lancet Regional Health. Southeast Asia*, •••, 26.

Gafar, M. A., Omolo, C. A., Elhassan, E., Ibrahim, U. H., & Govender, T. (2024). Applications of peptides in nanosystems for diagnosing and managing bacterial sepsis. *Journal of Biomedical Science*, *31*(1), 40. DOI: 10.1186/s12929-024-00978-7

Ganesan, N., Mishra, B., Felix, L., & Mylonakis, E. (2023). Antimicrobial peptides and small molecules targeting the cell membrane of Staphylococcus aureus. *Microbiology and Molecular Biology Reviews : MMBR*, *87*(2), e0003722. PMID: 37129495

Gao, W., Chen, Y., Zhang, Y., Zhang, Q., & Zhang, L. (2018). Nanoparticle-based local antimicrobial drug delivery. *Advanced Drug Delivery Reviews*, *127*, 46–57. DOI: 10.1016/j.addr.2017.12.008

Garcillán-Barcia, M. P., Pluta, R., Lorenzo-Díaz, F., Bravo, A., & Espinosa, M. (2022). The facts and family secrets of plasmids that replicate via the rolling-circle mechanism. *Microbiology and Molecular Biology Reviews : MMBR*, *86*(1), e00222–e00220. PMID: 34878299

Gebre, M. S., Brito, L. A., Tostanoski, L. H., Edwards, D. K., Carfi, A., & Barouch, D. H. (2021). Novel approaches for vaccine development. *Cell*, *184*(6), 1589–1603. PMID: 33740454

Gerits, E., Spincemaille, P., De Cremer, K., De Brucker, K., Beullens, S., Thevissen, K., Cammue, B. P. A., Vandamme, K., Fauvart, M., Verstraeten, N., & Michiels, J. (2017). Repurposing AM404 for the treatment of oral infections by *Porphyromonas gingivalis*. *Clinical and Experimental Dental Research*, *3*(2), 69–76. DOI: 10.1002/cre2.61 PMID: 29744181

Ghai, I., & Ghai, S. (2018). Understanding antibiotic resistance via outer membrane permeability. *Infection and Drug Resistance, 11*, 523–530. DOI: 10.2147/IDR.S156995 PMID: 29695921

Ghazaei, C. (2025). Prevalence of extended-spectrum and metallo β-lactamase production in Pseudomonas aeruginosa isolate. *Reviews and Research in Medical Microbiology, 36*(1), 9–17.

Gillieatt, B. F., & Coleman, N. V. (2024). Unravelling the mechanisms of antibiotic and heavy metal resistance co-selection in environmental bacteria. *FEMS Microbiology Reviews, 48*(2), fuae017. Advance online publication. DOI: 10.1093/femsre/fuae017 PMID: 38897736

Gillings, M. R. (2014). Integrons: Past, present, and future. *Microbiology and Molecular Biology Reviews : MMBR, 78*(2), 257–277. DOI: 10.1128/MMBR.00056-13

Godoy-Gallardo, M.. (2021). Antibacterial approaches in tissue engineering using metal ions and nanoparticles: From mechanisms to applications. *Bioactive Materials, 6*(12), 4470–4490.

Goff, A., Cantillon, D., Muraro Wildner, L., & Waddell, S. J. (2020). Multi-omics technologies applied to tuberculosis drug discovery. *Applied Sciences (Basel, Switzerland), 10*(13), 4629. DOI: 10.3390/app10134629

Goleanu, C. D.. (2025). Trends in antibiotic resistance of Escherichia coli strains isolated from clinical samples (2019–2023): A hospital-based retrospective analysis. *Pathogens (Basel, Switzerland), 14*(9), 927.

Gomes, D., Santos, R., Soares, R. S., Reis, S., Carvalho, S., Rego, P., Peleteiro, M. C., Tavares, L., & Oliveira, M. (2020). Pexiganan in combination with nisin to control polymicrobial diabetic foot infections. *Antibiotics (Basel, Switzerland), 9*(3), 128. PMID: 32244862

Goniewicz, K.. (2025). Transforming global public health: Climate collaboration, political challenges, and systemic change. *Journal of Infection and Public Health, 18*(1), 102615.

Gordillo Altamirano, F. L., & Barr, J. J. (2019). Phage therapy in the postantibiotic era. *Clinical Microbiology Reviews, 32*(2), e00066–e18. DOI: 10.1128/CMR.00066-18

Götz, F. (2002). *Staphylococcus* and biofilms. *Molecular Microbiology, 43*(6), 1367–1378. DOI: 10.1046/j.1365-2958.2002.02827.x PMID: 11952892

Grande, R., Campli, E. D., Bartolomeo, S. D., Verginelli, F., Giulio, M. D., Baffoni, M., Bessa, L. J., & Cellini, L. (2012). *Helicobacter pylori* biofilm: A protective environment for bacterial recombination. *Journal of Applied Microbiology, 113*(3), 669–676. DOI: 10.1111/j.1365-2672.2012.05366.x PMID: 22639839

Grande, R., Nistico, L., Sambanthamoorthy, K., Longwell, M., Iannitelli, A., Cellini, L., Di Stefano, A., Hall Stoodley, L., & Stoodley, P. (2014). Temporal expression of *agrB, cidA*, and *alsS* in the early development of *Staphylococcus aureus* UAMS-1 biofilm formation and the structural role of extracellular DNA and carbohydrates. *Pathogens and Disease, 70*(3), 414–422. DOI: 10.1111/j.1365-2672.2012.05350.x PMID: 24535842

Grass, G., Rensing, C., & Solioz, M. (2011). Metallic copper as an antimicrobial surface. *Applied and Environmental Microbiology, 77*(5), 1541–1547. DOI: 10.1128/AEM.02766-10 PMID: 21193661

Grenni, P., Ancona, V., & Caracciolo, A. B. (2018). Ecological effects of antibiotics on natural ecosystems: A review. *Microchemical Journal, 136*, 25–39. DOI: 10.1016/j.microc.2017.02.006

Guerra, M. E. S., Destro, G., Vieira, B., Lima, A. S., Ferraz, L. F. C., Hakansson, A. P., Darrieux, M., & Converso, T. R. (2022). Klebsiella pneumoniae biofilms and their role in disease pathogenesis. *Frontiers in Cellular and Infection Microbiology, 12*, 877995. PMID: 35646720

Gu, H., Hou, S., Yongyat, C., De Tore, S., & Ren, D. (2013). Patterned biofilm formation reveals a mechanism for structural heterogeneity in bacterial biofilms. *Langmuir, 29*(35), 11145–11153. DOI: 10.1021/la402608z PMID: 23919925

Guidotti, G., Brambilla, L., & Rossi, D. (2017). Cell-penetrating peptides: From basic research to clinics. *Trends in Pharmacological Sciences, 38*(4), 406–424. DOI: 10.1016/j.tips.2017.01.003

Guiyoule, A., Gerbaud, G., Buchrieser, C., Galimand, M., Rahalison, L., Chanteau, S. P., & Carniel, E. (2001). Transferable plasmid-mediated resistance to streptomycin in a clinical isolate of Yersinia pestis. *Emerging Infectious Diseases, 7*(1), 43–48. DOI: 10.3201/eid0701.010106 PMID: 11266293

Gunther, T., Kramer-Schadt, S., Fuhrmann, M., & Belik, V. (2022). Environmental factors associated with the prevalence of ESBL/AmpC-producing *Escherichia coli* in wild boar (*Susscrofa*). *Frontiers in Veterinary Science, 9*, 980554. DOI: 10.3389/fvets.2022.980554 PMID: 36311652

Gunturu, S. (2025). Innovative Strategies to Combat Antimicrobial Resistance: Advances in Drug Discovery, Alternative Therapies and Immune Modulation. [AJP]. *Asian Journal of Pharmaceutics*, *19*(2).

Guo, Y., Ding, L., Han, R., Yin, D., Wu, S., Yang, Y., Wang, F., Zhu, D., & Hu, F. (2025). Antimicrobial resistance profile of clinical isolates from hospitals across China: CHINET 2024 surveillance report. *One Health Advances 2025 3:1, 3*(1), 23-. https://doi.org/DOI: 10.1186/S44280-025-00092-0

Guo, J., Li, J., Chen, H., Bond, P. L., & Yuan, Z. (2017). Metagenomic analysis reveals wastewater treatment plants as hotspots of antibiotic resistance genes and mobile genetic elements. *Water Research*, *123*, 468–478. DOI: 10.1016/j.watres.2017.07.002 PMID: 28689130

Guo, Y. (2021). Removal Ability of Antibiotic Resistant Bacteria (Arb) and Antibiotic Resistance Genes (Args) by Membrane Filtration Process. *IOP Conference Series. Earth and Environmental Science*, *801*(1), 12004. DOI: 10.1088/1755-1315/801/1/012004

Guo, Z., Yuan, M., & Chai, J. (2024). Advantages and limitations of lytic phages compared with chemical antibiotics to combat bacterial infections. *Heliyon*, *10*(7), e34849. PMID: 39148970

Gupta, Y. D., & Bhandary, S. (2024). Artificial intelligence for understanding mechanisms of antimicrobial resistance and antimicrobial discovery: a new age model for translational research. *Artificial Intelligence and Machine Learning in Drug Design and Development*, 117-156.

Gupta, P., & Mandal, B. B. (2021). Silk biomaterials for vascular tissue engineering applications. *Acta Biomaterialia*, *134*, 79–106. DOI: 10.1016/j.actbio.2021.08.024

Gupta, P., Sarkar, S., Das, B., Bhattacharjee, S., & Tribedi, P. (2016). Biofilm, pathogenesis and prevention A journey to break the wall: A review. *Archives of Microbiology*, *198*(1), 1–15. DOI: 10.1007/s00203-015-1148-6 PMID: 26377585

Gupta, R. K.. (2015). RNAIII of the Staphylococcus aureus agr system activates global regulator MgrA by stabilizing mRNA. *Proceedings of the National Academy of Sciences of the United States of America*, *112*(45), 14036–14041.

Guzman, J., & Vilcinskas, A. (2020). Bacteria associated with cockroaches: Health risk or biotechnological opportunity? *Applied Microbiology and Biotechnology*, *104*(24), 10369–10387. DOI: 10.1007/s00253-020-10973-6 PMID: 33128616

Hall, C. W., & Mah, T.-F. (2017). Molecular mechanisms of biofilm-based antibiotic resistance and tolerance in pathogenic bacteria. *FEMS Microbiology Reviews*, *41*(3), 276–301. DOI: 10.1093/femsre/fux010

Han, B.. (2022). The source, fate and prospect of antibiotic resistance genes in soil: A review. *Frontiers in Microbiology*, *13*, 976657.

Han, E. J., Ahn, J.-S., Chae, Y. J., & Chung, H.-J. (2025). Immunomodulatory Roles of Faecalibacterium prausnitzii and Akkermansia muciniphila in Autoimmune Diseases: Mechanistic Insights and Therapeutic Potential. *Clinical Reviews in Allergy & Immunology*, *68*(1), 77. PMID: 40759811

Haniffa, R.. (2018). Improving ICU services in resource-limited settings: Perceptions of ICU workers from low-middle-, and high-income countries. *Journal of Critical Care*, *44*, 352–356.

Haque, M., McKimm, J., Sartelli, M., Dhingra, S., Labricciosa, F. M., Islam, S., Jahan, D., Nusrat, T., Chowdhury, T. S., Coccolini, F., Iskandar, K., Catena, F., & Begum, H. A. (2020). Strategies to prevent healthcare-associated infections: A narrative overview. *Risk Management and Healthcare Policy*, *13*, 1765–1780. DOI: 10.2147/RMHP.S269315 PMID: 33061710

Harun, M. G. D., Sumon, S. A., Hasan, I., Akther, F. M., Islam, M. S., & Anwar, M. M. U. (2024). Barriers, facilitators, perceptions and impact of interventions in implementing antimicrobial stewardship programs in hospitals of low-middle and middle countries: a scoping review. *Antimicrobial Resistance & Infection Control 2024 13:1*, *13*(1), 8-. https://doi.org/DOI: 10.1186/S13756-024-01369-6

Hasan, G. M., Mohammad, T., Shamsi, A., Sohal, S. S., & Hassan, M. I. (2025). Applications of Genome Sequencing in Infectious Diseases: From Pathogen Identification to Precision Medicine. *Pharmaceuticals*, *18*(11), 1687. PMID: 41304932

Hasan, M., & Ahn, J. (2022). Evolutionary dynamics between phages and bacteria as a possible approach for designing effective phage therapies against antibiotic-resistant bacteria. *Antibiotics (Basel, Switzerland)*, *11*(7), 915.

Hashemi Shahraki, A., & Mirsaeidi, M. (2021). Phage therapy for Mycobacterium abscessus and strategies to improve outcomes. *Microorganisms*, *9*(3), 596.

Hassan, S. A., Isak, M. J., Osman, A. M., Hassan, Y. M., Ahmed, A. M., Mire, S. A., Jimale, K. A., Omar, A. I., & Ahmed, N. R. (2025). Effectiveness of an e-Bug–based antimicrobial resistance education intervention: A prospective quasi-experimental study among Grade 12 students in Mogadishu, Somalia. *IJID Regions*, *17*, 100771. PMID: 41143070

Hassan, Y. M., Mohamed, A. S., Hassan, Y. M., & El-Sayed, W. M. (2025). Recent developments and future directions in point-of-care next-generation CRISPR-based rapid diagnosis. *Clinical and Experimental Medicine*, *25*(1), 33. PMID: 39789283

Hatfull, G. F., Dedrick, R. M., & Schooley, R. T. (2022). Phage therapy for antibiotic-resistant bacterial infections. *Annual Review of Medicine*, *73*, 197–211. PMID: 34428079

Hayet, S.. (2023). Titanium complexes affect Bacillus subtilis biofilm formation. *RSC Medicinal Chemistry*, *14*(5), 983–991.

Heilbronner, S.. (2021). The microbiome-shaping roles of bacteriocins. *Nature Reviews. Microbiology*, *19*(11), 726–739.

Henderson, R. K.. (2019). Coupling efficiency of secondary active transporters. *Current Opinion in Biotechnology*, *58*, 62–71.

Hendriksen, R. S., Munk, P., Njage, P., van Bunnik, B., McNally, L., Lukjancenko, O., & Aarestrup, F. M. (2019). Global monitoring of antimicrobial resistance based on metagenomics analyses of urban sewage. *Nature Communications*, *10*(1), 1124.

Herdiana, Y., Wathoni, N., Shamsuddin, S., & Muchtaridi, M. (2022). Drug release study of the chitosan-based nanoparticles. *Heliyon*, *8*(1). PMID: 35028457

He, X., Zhao, S., & Li, Y. (2021). Faecalibacterium prausnitzii: A next-generation probiotic in gut disease improvement. *The Canadian Journal of Infectious Diseases & Medical Microbiology*, *2021*(1), 6666114.

Hickson, S. M., et al. (2025). "Emerging antimicrobial therapies for Gram-negative infections in human clinical use." npj Antimicrobials and Resistance 3(1): 16.

Hilt, E. E., & Ferrieri, P. (2022). Next generation and other sequencing technologies in diagnostic microbiology and infectious diseases. *Genes*, *13*(9), 1566. PMID: 36140733

Hlanze, H. (2024). *The evolution of drug resistance in the different lineages of the Mycobacterium tuberculosis complex*. University of Pretoria.

Hoffmann, A., Grubwieser, P., Bumann, D., Haschka, D., & Weiss, G. (2025). Tackling microbial iron homeostasis: Novel antimicrobial strategies. *Trends in Pharmacological Sciences*, *46*(10), 1004–1017. PMID: 40914687

Hokken, M. W. J., Zwaan, B. J., Melchers, W. J. G., & Verweij, P. E. (2019). Facilitators of adaptation and antifungal resistance mechanisms in clinically relevant fungi. *Fungal Genetics and Biology*, *132*, 103254. DOI: 10.1016/j.fgb.2019.103254 PMID: 31326470

Holmes, A. H., Moore, L. S., Sundsfjord, A., Steinbakk, M., Regmi, S., Karkey, A., & Piddock, L. J. (2019). Understanding the mechanisms and drivers of antimicrobial resistance. *Lancet*, *387*(10014), 176–187.

Hong, T. C., El-Omar, E. M., Kuo, Y. T., Wu, J. Y., Chen, M. J., Chen, C. C., Fang, Y. J., Leow, A. H. R., Lu, H., Lin, J. T., & Wu, M. S. (2024). Primary antibiotic resistance of *Helicobacter pylori* in the Asia-Pacific region between 1990 and 2022: An updated systematic review and meta-analysis. *The Lancet. Gastroenterology & Hepatology*, *9*(1), 56–67. DOI: 10.1016/S2468-1253(23)00306-9 PMID: 37972625

Hosny, S., Elshobary, M. E., & El-Sheekh, M. M. (2025). Unleashing the power of microalgae: A pioneering path to sustainability and achieving the sustainable development goals. *Environmental Science and Pollution Research International*, *32*, 1–31. DOI: 10.1007/s11356-025-36181-1 PMID: 39920498

Howell, M., ... (2022). Exploring synergy and its role in antimicrobial peptide biology. Methods in Enzymology, Elsevier. 663: 99-130.

Huang, S. S., Septimus, E., Kleinman, K., Moody, J., Hickok, J., Avery, T. R., Lankiewicz, J., Gombosev, A., Terpstra, L., Hartford, F., Hayden, M. K., Jernigan, J. A., Weinstein, R. A., & Fraser, V. J. (2013). Targeted versus universal decolonization to prevent ICU infection. *The New England Journal of Medicine*, *368*(24), 2255–2265. https://doi.org/10.1056/NEJMoa1207290

Huang, T.. (2016). Low-concentration ciprofloxacin selects plasmid-mediated quinolone resistance encoding genes and affects bacterial taxa in soil containing manure. *Frontiers in Microbiology*, *7*, 1730.

HUDA, M., et al. (2025). "Prevalence of ACRA, ACRB, and TOLC efflux pump genes among multiple-drug resistant escherichia coli strains in isolates obtained from patients with diabetes mellitus." Laboratory diagnostics. Eastern Europe Учредители: УП" Профессиональные издания", ООО «Вилин–Профессиональные издания» 14(1): 63-74.

Hudson, J. A., Frewer, L. J., Jones, G., Brereton, P. A., Whittingham, M. J., & Stewart, G. (2017). The agri-food chain and antimicrobial resistance: A review. *Trends in Food Science & Technology*, *69*, 131–147. DOI: 10.1016/j.tifs.2017.09.007

Hughes, D., & Andersson, D. I. (2017). Environmental and genetic modulation of the phenotypic expression of antibiotic resistance. *FEMS Microbiology Reviews*, *41*(3), 374–391. DOI: 10.1093/femsre/fux004 PMID: 28333270

Hu, M., Li, X., You, Z., Cai, R., & Chen, C. (2024). Physiological barriers and strategies of lipid-based nanoparticles for nucleic acid drug delivery. *Advanced Materials*, *36*(22), 2303266. PMID: 37792475

Hussain, A., Najeeb, A., & Ali, S. A. (2025). Antimicrobial Resistance: A Modern Plague. In *AI-Driven Breakthroughs in Antimicrobial Resistance* (pp. 27-74). IGI Global Scientific Publishing.

Hussein, S., Qurbani, K., & Ahmed, S. K. (2023). Potential increase in Crimean–Congo hemorrhagic fever incidence in Iraq post Eid-al-Adha, 2023. *New Microbes and New Infections*, *54*, 101175. PMID: 37727502

Hutchings, M. I.. (2019). Antibiotics: Past, present and future. *Current Opinion in Microbiology*, *51*, 72–80.

Hwang, S. M., Cho, H. W., Kim, T. Y., Park, J. S., Jung, J., Song, K.-H., Lee, H., Kim, E. S., Kim, H. B., & Park, K. U. (2021). Whole-genome sequencing for investigating a health care-associated outbreak of carbapenem-resistant Acinetobacter baumannii. *Diagnostics (Basel)*, *11*(2), 201. PMID: 33573077

Idigo, A. J., Wells, J. M., Brown, M. L., Wiener, H. W., Griffin, R. L., Cutter, G., Shrestha, S., & Lee, R. A. (2022). Clinical risk factors for admission with Pseudomonas and multidrug-resistant Pseudomonas community-acquired pneumonia. *Antimicrobial Resistance and Infection Control*, *11*(1), 1–10. DOI: 10.1186/S13756-022-01137-4/TABLES/4 PMID: 35836272

Ijaz, S., Iqbal, J., Abbasi, B. A., Tufail, A., Yaseen, T., Uddin, S., Usman, K., Ullah, R., Bibi, H., & Inam, P. (2024). Current stage of preclinical and clinical development of guggulsterone in cancers: Challenges and promises. *Cell Biology International*, *48*(2), 128–142. PMID: 38148708

Iskandar, K., Murugaiyan, J., Hammoudi Halat, D., Hage, S. E., Chibabhai, V., Adukkadukkam, S., Roques, C., Molinier, L., Salameh, P., & Van Dongen, M. (2022). Antibiotic discovery and resistance: The chase and the race. *Antibiotics (Basel, Switzerland)*, *11*(2), 182. DOI: 10.3390/antibiotics11020182 PMID: 35203785

Islam, M. R., Summers, A. O., & Arpinar, I. B. (2025). Knowledge Graph-Based Framework for Detecting Horizontal Gene Transfer Events Driving Antimicrobial Resistance. bioRxiv, 2025.2006. 2009.658534.

Isuranga, M., & Danthanarayana, D. N. (2025). Antimicrobial Potential of Phytochemicals from Coccinia grandis Leaves: A Molecular Docking Study Against Penicillin-Binding Protein 5 of Escherichia coli and DNA Topoisomerase IV Subunit B (ParE 24kDa) of Staphylococcus aureus and Escherichia coli. *Biology, Medicine, & Natural Product Chemistry*, *14*(1), 541–552.

Ito, H., Wada, T., Ichinose, G., Tanimoto, J., Yoshimura, J., Yamamoto, T., & Morita, S. (2025). Barriers to the widespread adoption of diagnostic artificial intelligence for preventing antimicrobial resistance. *Scientific Reports*, *15*(1), 13113. PMID: 40240443

Jain, M., Stitt, G., Son, L., & Enioutina, E. Y. (2023). Probiotics and their bioproducts: A promising approach for targeting methicillin-resistant Staphylococcus aureus and vancomycin-resistant Enterococcus. *Microorganisms*, *11*(10), 2393. PMID: 37894051

James, C., James, S. J., Onarinde, B. A., Dixon, R. A., & Williams, N. (2017). A critical review of AMR risks arising as a consequence of using biocides and certain metals in food animal production. *Antibiotics (Basel, Switzerland)*, *12*(10), 1569. DOI: 10.3390/antibiotics12101569 PMID: 37998771

Jangra, V., Sharma, N., & Chhillar, A. K. (2022). Therapeutic approaches for combating Pseudomonas aeruginosa infections. *Microbes and Infection*, *24*(4), 104950. DOI: 10.1016/J.MICINF.2022.104950 PMID: 35139390

Jansen, K. U., & Anderson, A. S. (2018). The role of vaccines in fighting Antimicrobial Resistance (AMR). *Human Vaccines & Immunotherapeutics*, *14*(9), 2142–2149. DOI: 10.1080/21645515.2018.1476814 PMID: 29787323

Jarmo, O., Veli-Jukka, A., & Eero, M. (2020). Treatment of Clostridioides (Clostridium) difficile infection. *Annals of Medicine*, *52*(1-2), 12–20. PMID: 31801387

Jaumaux, F., & Gómez de Cadiñanos, P., L., & Gabant, P. (2020). In the age of synthetic biology, will antimicrobial peptides be the next generation of antibiotics? *Antibiotics (Basel, Switzerland)*, *9*(8), 484. PMID: 32781540

Javed, W. (2020). *Study of the conformational states of a bacterial multidrug ABC transporter BmrA*. Université Grenoble Alpes. [2020-....]

Jayaraman, P.. (2017). Repurposing a two-component system-based biosensor for the killing of Vibrio cholerae. *ACS Synthetic Biology*, *6*(7), 1403–1415.

Jiang, W. (2025). Addressing Antimicrobial Resistance: Evidence-Based Strategies And Innovations. *Transactions on Materials. Biotechnology and Life Sciences*, *8*, 357–364.

Jiang, Y., Chen, Y., Song, Z., Tan, Z., & Cheng, J. (2021). Recent advances in the design of antimicrobial peptides and polypeptides toward clinical translation. *Advanced Drug Delivery Reviews, 170*, 261–280. DOI: 10.1016/j.addr.2020.12.003

Joerger, R. D. (2003). Alternatives to antibiotics: Bacteriocins, antimicrobial peptides and bacteriophages. *Poultry Science, 82*(4), 640–647. DOI: 10.1093/ps/82.4.640

Johnston, C.. (2014). Bacterial transformation: Distribution, shared mechanisms and divergent control. *Nature Reviews. Microbiology, 12*(3), 181–196.

Jones, A. D. (2024). Microbial risk assessment. *Human and Ecological Risk Assessment: Theory and Practice, 2*, 779–832.

Joo, H.-S., & Otto, M. (2012). Molecular basis of in vivo biofilm formation by bacterial pathogens. *Chemistry & Biology, 19*(12), 1503–1513. DOI: 10.1016/j.chembiol.2012.10.022 PMID: 23261595

Jorgensen, J. H., & Ferraro, M. J. (2009). Antimicrobial susceptibility testing: A review of general principles and contemporary practices. *Clinical Infectious Diseases, 49*(11), 1749–1755. DOI: 10.1086/647952

Joshi, M. P., Hafner, T., Twesigye, G., Ndiaye, A., Kiggundu, R., Mekonnen, N., Kusu, N., Berthé, S., Lusaya, E. P., & Acho, A. (2021). Strengthening multisectoral coordination on antimicrobial resistance: A landscape analysis of efforts in 11 countries. *Journal of Pharmaceutical Policy and Practice, 14*(1), 27. PMID: 33648589

Jurado-Martín, I., Sainz-Mejías, M., & McClean, S. (2021). Pseudomonas aeruginosa: An Audacious Pathogen with an Adaptable Arsenal of Virulence Factors. *International Journal of Molecular Sciences 2021, Vol. 22, Page 3128, 22*(6), 3128. https://doi.org/DOI: 10.3390/IJMS22063128

Kakkar, A. K., Shafiq, N., Singh, G., Ray, P., Gautam, V., Agarwal, R., Muralidharan, J., & Arora, P. (2020). Antimicrobial Stewardship Programs in Resource Constrained Environments: Understanding and Addressing the Need of the Systems. *Frontiers in Public Health, 8*, 502288. DOI: 10.3389/FPUBH.2020.00140/BIBTEX PMID: 32411647

Kakkar, A. K., Shafiq, N., Singh, R., Ray, P., Gautam, V., Agarwal, R., Muralidharan, J., & Arora, P. (2020). Antimicrobial stewardship programs in resource-constrained environments: Understanding and addressing the need of the systems. *Frontiers in Public Health, 8*, 140. https://doi.org/10.3389/fpubh.2020.00140

Kakoullis, L., Papachristodoulou, E., Chra, P., & Panos, G. (2021). Mechanisms of antibiotic resistance in important Gram-positive and Gram-negative pathogens and novel antibiotic solutions. *Antibiotics (Basel, Switzerland), 10*(4), 415. DOI: 10.3390/antibiotics10040415 PMID: 33920199

Kaluba, C. K., Samutela, M. T., Kapesa, C., Muma, J. B., Hang'ombe, B. M., Hachaambwa, L., Mukomena, P., & Yamba, K. (2021). Carbapenem resistance in Pseudomonas aeruginosa and Acinetobacter species at a large tertiary referral hospital in Lusaka, Zambia. *Scientific African, 13*, e00908. DOI: 10.1016/J.SCIAF.2021.E00908

Kang, Y. K., Kwon, K., Ryu, J. S., Lee, H. N., Park, C., & Chung, H. J. (2017). Nonviral genome editing based on a polymer-derivatized CRISPR nanocomplex for targeting bacterial pathogens and antibiotic resistance. *Bioconjugate Chemistry, 28*(4), 957–967. DOI: 10.1021/acs.bioconjchem.6b00676 PMID: 28215090

Kaprou, G. D., Bergšpica, I., Alexa, E. A., Alvarez-Ordonez, A., & Prieto, M. (2021). Rapid methods for antimicrobial resistance diagnostics. *Antibiotics (Basel, Switzerland), 10*(2), 209. PMID: 33672677

Kariuki, S., Keddy, K. H., Antonio, M., & Okeke, I. N. (2018). Antimicrobial resistance surveillance in Africa: Successes, gaps and a roadmap for the future. *African Journal of Laboratory Medicine, 7*(2), a924. https://doi.org/10.4102/ajlm.v7i2.924

Karruli, A., Catalini, C., D'Amore, C., Foglia, F., Mari, F., Harxhi, A., Galdiero, M., & Durante-Mangoni, E. (2023). Evidence-Based Treatment of Pseudomonas aeruginosa Infections: A Critical Reappraisal. *Antibiotics 2023, Vol. 12, Page 399, 12*(2), 399. https://doi.org/DOI: 10.3390/ANTIBIOTICS12020399

Kästner, M., Miltner, A., Thiele-Bruhn, S., & Liang, C. (2021). Microbial Necromass in Soils—Linking Microbes to Soil Processes and Carbon Turnover. *Frontiers in Environmental Science*. Advance online publication. DOI: 10.3389/fenvs.2021.756378

Katsarou, A.. (2025). β-lactam/β-lactamase inhibitor combination antibiotics Under development. *Pathogens (Basel, Switzerland), 14*(2), 168.

Kaur, H., ... (2023). Antimicrobial nanoparticles: Synthesis, mechanism of actions. Antimicrobial activity of nanoparticles, Elsevier: 155-202.

Keenan, K., Kiffer, C. R. V., Carmo, É. V. S., Corrêa, J. S., Abreu, A. L. d., Massuda, A., Gales, A. C., & Colombo, A. L. (2025). Antimicrobial resistance burden estimates from the bottom-up: Research priorities for estimating the impact of antimicrobial resistance in Brazil. *IJID Regions, 14*, 100558. PMID: 39911748

Kelbrick, M.. (2023). Cultivating antimicrobial resistance: How intensive agriculture ploughs the way for antibiotic resistance. *Microbiology, 169*(8), 001384.

KEPHALOPOULOS, S., COECKE, S., GAWLIK, B. M., QUERCI, M., MARCHINI, A., RUIZ, M. A., CORBISIER, P., PETRILLO, M., RAFFAEL, B., & SPAGNOLO, L. (2024). Antimicrobial resistance: Crowdsourcing JRC Knowledge on AMR, AMR@ JRC Café, 24 October 2023.

Khameneh, B.. (2021). Phytochemicals: A promising weapon in the arsenal against antibiotic-resistant bacteria. *Antibiotics (Basel, Switzerland), 10*(9), 1044.

Khangai, A., Saruuljavkhlan, B., Azzaya, D., Gantuya, B., Oyuntsetseg, K., Akada, J., Matsumoto, T., & Yamaoka, Y. (2023). Exploring alternative treatment choices for multidrug-resistant clinical strains of *Helicobacter pylori* in Mongolia. *Microorganisms, 11*(12), 2852. DOI: 10.3390/microorganisms11122852 PMID: 38137996

Khan, I.. (2019). Nanoparticles: Properties, applications and toxicities. *Arabian Journal of Chemistry, 12*(7), 908–931.

Khanna, S. (2021). My treatment approach to Clostridioides difficile infection. *Mayo Clinic Proceedings.*

Khan, W., Bernier, S. P., Kuchma, S. L., Hammond, J. H., Hasan, F., & O'Toole, G. A. (2010). Aminoglycoside resistance of *Pseudomonas aeruginosa* biofilms modulated by extracellular polysaccharide. *International Microbiology, 13*(4), 207–212. DOI: 10.2436/20.1501.01.123 PMID: 21404215

Khazaal, S. S., Al-Saryi, N., & Ibrahim, S. A. (2020). Immunomodulation by *Acinetobacter baumannii* of endotracheal tube biofilm in ventilator-associated pneumonia. *Meta Gene, 24*, 100672. DOI: 10.1016/j.mgene.2020.100672

Kiggundu, R., Waswa, J. P., Konduri, N., Kasujja, H., Murungi, M., Vudriko, P., Akello, H., Lugada, E., Muiva, C., Were, E., Tjipura, D., Kajumbula, H., Kikule, K., Nfor, E., & Joshi, M. P. (2019). [Title of 2019 article needed for citation].

Kiggundu, R., Waswa, J. P., Konduri, N., Kasujja, H., Murungi, M., Vudriko, P., Akello, H., Lugada, E., Muiva, C., Were, E., Tjipura, D., Kajumbula, H., Kikule, K., Nfor, E., & Joshi, M. P. (2024). A One Health approach to fight antimicrobial resistance in Uganda: Implementation experience, results, and lessons learned. *Biosafety and Health.* PMID: 40078942

Killough, M., Rodgers, A. M., & Ingram, R. J. (2022). Pseudomonas aeruginosa: Recent Advances in Vaccine Development. *Vaccines 2022, Vol. 10, Page 1100, 10*(7), 1100. https://doi.org/DOI: 10.3390/VACCINES10071100

Kim, D.. (2023). Structural insights for β-lactam antibiotics. *Biomolecules & Therapeutics*, *31*(2), 141.

Kim, H.-J., Na, S. W., Alodaini, H. A., Al-Dosary, M. A., Nandhakumari, P., & Dyona, L. (2021). Prevalence of multidrug-resistant bacteria associated with polymicrobial infections. [PubMed]. *Journal of Infection and Public Health*, *14*(12), 1864–1869.

Kim, J. I., Maguire, F., Tsang, K. K., Gouliouris, T., Peacock, S. J., McAllister, T. A., McArthur, A. G., & Beiko, R. G. (2022). Machine learning for antimicrobial resistance prediction: Current practice, limitations, and clinical perspective. *Clinical Microbiology Reviews*, *35*(3), e00179–e00121. PMID: 35612324

Kim, J.. (2021). Structural insights into transporter-mediated drug resistance in infectious diseases. *Journal of Molecular Biology*, *433*(16), 167005.

Kincses, A.. (2025). Repurposed Drugs and Efflux Pump Inhibitors Against Gram-Negative Urinary Tract Pathogenic Bacteria. *Antibiotics (Basel, Switzerland)*, *14*(10), 988.

Kirby, J. E., Brennan-Krohn, T., & Smith, K. P. (2019). Bringing Antimicrobial Susceptibility Testing for New Drugs into the Clinical Laboratory: Removing Obstacles in Our Fight against Multidrug-Resistant Pathogens. *Journal of Clinical Microbiology*, *57*(12). Advance online publication. https://doi.org/10.1128/jcm.01270-19

Klein, E. Y., Impalli, I., Poleon, S., Denoel, P., Cipriano, M., Van Boeckel, T. P., Pecetta, S., Bloom, D. E., & Nandi, A. (2024). Global trends in antibiotic consumption during 2016–2023 and future projections through 2030. *Proceedings of the National Academy of Sciences of the United States of America*, *121*(49). Advance online publication. https://doi.org/10.1073/pnas.2411919121

Klobucar, K., & Brown, E. D. (2022). New potentiators of ineffective antibiotics: Targeting the Gram-negative outer membrane to overcome intrinsic resistance. *Current Opinion in Chemical Biology*, *66*, 102099.

Klugman, K. P., & Black, S. (2018). Impact of existing vaccines in reducing antibiotic resistance: Primary and secondary effects. *Proceedings of the National Academy of Sciences of the United States of America*, *115*(51), 12896–12901. DOI: 10.1073/pnas.1721095115 PMID: 30559195

Klumpp-Thomas, C., Kalish, H., Drew, M., Hunsberger, S., Snead, K., Fay, M. P., Mehalko, J., Shunmugavel, A., Wall, V., & Frank, P. (2021). Standardization of ELISA protocols for serosurveys of the SARS-CoV-2 pandemic using clinical and at-home blood sampling. *Nature Communications*, *12*(1), 113. PMID: 33397956

Kmet, V., Cuvalová, A., & Stanko, M. (2018). Small mammals as sentinels of antimicrobial-resistant staphylococci. *Folia Microbiologica, 63*(5), 665–668. DOI: 10.1007/s12223-018-0602-7 PMID: 29524153

Knapp, C. W.. (2011). Antibiotic resistance gene abundances correlate with metal and geochemical conditions in archived Scottish soils. *PLoS One*, *6*(11), e27300.

Knight, D. R. (2018). Comparative phylogenomics and antimicrobial resistance in livestock-associated lineages of Clostridium difficile.

Kofteridis, D. P., Andrianaki, A. M., Maraki, S., Mathioudaki, A., Plataki, M., Alexopoulou, C., Ioannou, P., Samonis, G., & Valachis, A. (2020). Treatment pattern, prognostic factors, and outcome in patients with infection due to pan-drug-resistant gram-negative bacteria. *European Journal of Clinical Microbiology & Infectious Diseases*, *39*(5), 965–970. PMID: 31933017

Kolanjinathan, K., Rajasekar, M., Harinathan, B., Saranraj, P., & Manigandan, M. (2024). Assessment of the antimicrobial and mosquito larvicidal efficacy of medicinal herb *Elytraria acaulis. International Journal of Entomological Research*, *9*(11), 225–228.

Kolawole, T. O., Mustapha, A. Y., Mbata, A. O., Tomoh, B. O., Forkuo, A. Y., & Kelvin-Agwu, M. (2023). *Innovative strategies for reducing antimicrobial resistance: A review of global policy and practice*. Journal Name Missing.

Kollef, M. H., Shorr, A. F., Bassetti, M., Timsit, J.-F., Micek, S. T., Michelson, A. P., & Garnacho-Montero, J. (2021). Timing of antibiotic therapy in the ICU. *Critical Care*, *25*(1), 360. PMID: 34654462

Konwar, A. N.. (2022). Emerging non-traditional approaches to combat antibiotic resistance. *Current Microbiology*, *79*(11), 330.

Köser, C. U., Ellington, M. J., & Peacock, S. J. (2014). Whole-genome sequencing to control antimicrobial resistance. *Trends in Genetics*, *30*(9), 401–407. https://doi.org/10.1016/j.tig.2014.07.003

Kothari, A., Jain, N., Kumar, S. K., Kumar, A., Kaushal, K., Kaur, S., Pandey, A., Gaurav, A., & Omar, B. J. (2022). Potential Synergistic Antibiotic Combinations against Fluoroquinolone-Resistant Pseudomonas aeruginosa. *Pharmaceuticals*, *15*(2), 243. DOI: 10.3390/PH15020243/S1 PMID: 35215357

Kraemer, S. A., Ramachandran, A., & Perron, G. G. (2019). Antibiotic pollution in the environment: From microbial ecology to public policy. *Microorganisms*, *7*(6), 180.

Krause, K. M.. (2016). Aminoglycosides: An overview. *Cold Spring Harbor Perspectives in Medicine, 6*(6), a027029.

Krul, D.. (2025). Spread of antimicrobial-resistant clones of the ESKAPEE group: From the clinical setting to hospital effluent. *The Science of the Total Environment, 973*, 179124.

Krysiak, K., Konkol, D., & Korczyński, M. (2021). Overview of the use of probiotics in poultry production. *Animals (Basel), 11*(6), 1620. DOI: 10.3390/ani11061620

Kulkarni, A., Tanga, S., Karmakar, A., Hota, A., & Maji, B. (2023). CRISPR-based precision molecular diagnostics for disease detection and surveillance. *ACS Applied Bio Materials, 6*(10), 3927–3945. PMID: 37788375

Kumar, B., Sharma, D., Sharma, P., Katoch, V. M., Venkatesan, K., & Bisht, D. (2013). Proteomic analysis of *Mycobacterium tuberculosis* isolates resistant to kanamycin and amikacin. *Journal of Proteomics, 94*, 68–77. DOI: 10.1016/j.jprot.2013.08.025 PMID: 24036035

Kumari, L. S., Siriwardhana, D. M., Liyanapathirana, V., Jinadasa, R., & Wijesinghe, P. (2025). Rapid whole genome sequencing for AMR surveillance in low-and middle-income countries: Oxford Nanopore Technology reveals multidrug-resistant Enterobacter cloacae complex from dairy farms in Sri Lanka. *BMC Veterinary Research, 21*(1), 351. PMID: 40382559

Kundar, R., & Gokarn, K. (2022). CRISPR-Cas system: A tool to eliminate drug-resistant gram-negative bacteria. *Pharmaceuticals, 15*(12), 1498. PMID: 36558949

Kwong, J. C., Mccallum, N., Sintchenko, V., & Howden, B. P. (2015). Whole genome sequencing in clinical and public health microbiology. *Pathology, 47*(3), 199–210. https://doi.org/10.1097/pat.0000000000000235

Lade, H., & Kim, J.-S. (2023). Molecular determinants of β-lactam resistance in methicillin-resistant Staphylococcus aureus (MRSA): An updated review. *Antibiotics (Basel, Switzerland), 12*(9), 1362. DOI: 10.3390/antibiotics12091362

Lak Hondori, M.. (2025). Frequency of Beta-lactamase Genes (blaSHV, blaTEM, blaCTX-M-15, blaKPC, blaOXA-48) in Multidrug-resistant Klebsiella pneumoniae. *International Journal of Molecular and Clinical Microbiology, 15*(1), 2180–2189.

Lakhundi, S., & Zhang, K. (2018). Methicillin-resistant Staphylococcus aureus: Molecular characterization, evolution, and epidemiology. *Clinical Microbiology Reviews, 31*(4), e00020–e18. DOI: 10.1128/CMR.00020-18 PMID: 30209034

Lanckohr, C., & Bracht, H. (2022). Antimicrobial stewardship. *Current Opinion in Critical Care*, *28*(5), 551–556. DOI: 10.1097/MCC.0000000000000967 PMID: 35942707

Langford, B. J., Leung, V., Lo, J., Akl, E. A., Nieuwlaat, R., Schwartz, K. L., & Daneman, N. (2023). Antibiotic prescribing guideline recommendations in COVID-19: A systematic survey. *EClinicalMedicine*, *65*, 102257. https://doi.org/10.1016/j.eclinm.2023.102257

Larsson, D. J., & Flach, C.-F. (2022). Antibiotic resistance in the environment. *Nature Reviews. Microbiology*, *20*(5), 257–269.

Lata, M., Sharma, D., Deo, N., Tiwari, P. K., Bisht, D., & Venkatesan, K. (2015). Proteomic analysis of ofloxacin-mono resistant *Mycobacterium tuberculosis* isolates. *Journal of Proteomics, 127*(Pt A), 114–121. https://doi.org/DOI: 10.1016/j.jprot.2015.07.031

Lathakumari, R. H., Vajravelu, L. K., Thulukanam, J., & Narasimhan, A. K. (2025). Next-gen nano biosensor technologies to monitor carbapenem resistance for personalized medicine. *Indian Journal of Microbiology*, *65*(1), 277–296. PMID: 40371034

Laxminarayan, R., Van Boeckel, T., Frost, I., Kariuki, S., Khan, E. A., Limmathurotsakul, D., Larsson, D. G. J., Levy-Hara, G., Mendelson, M., Outterson, K., Peacock, S. J., & Srikantiah, P. (2020). The Lancet Infectious Diseases Commission on antimicrobial resistance: 6 years later. *The Lancet. Infectious Diseases*, *20*(4), e51–e60. DOI: 10.1016/S1473-3099(20)30003-7 PMID: 32059790

Lebeaux, D., Chauhan, A., Rendueles, O., & Beloin, C. (2013). From in vitro to in vivo models of bacterial biofilm-related infections. *Pathogens (Basel, Switzerland)*, *2*(2), 288–356. DOI: 10.3390/pathogens2020288 PMID: 25437038

Lee, A. S., de Lencastre, H., Garau, J., Kluytmans, J., Malhotra-Kumar, S., Peschel, A., & Harbarth, S. (2018). Methicillin-resistant Staphylococcus aureus. *Nature Reviews. Disease Primers*, *4*, 18033. Advance online publication. DOI: 10.1038/nrdp.2018.33 PMID: 29849094

Lee, Y., Lim, W. I., Bloom, C. I., Moore, S., Chung, E., & Marzella, N. (2017). Bezlotoxumab (Zinplava) for Clostridium difficile infection: The first monoclonal antibody approved to prevent the recurrence of a bacterial infection. *P&T : a Peer-Reviewed Journal for Formulary Management*, *42*(12), 735–738. PMID: 29234211

Lei, J., Sun, L., Huang, S., Zhu, C., Li, P., He, J., Mackey, V., Coy, D. H., & He, Q. (2019). The antimicrobial peptides and their potential clinical applications. *American Journal of Translational Research*, *11*(7), 3919–3931.

Leptihn, S., & Loh, B. (2022). Complexity, challenges and costs of implementing phage therapy. *Future Microbiology*, *17*(8), 643–646. PMID: 35400196

Letizia, M., Diggle, S. P., & Whiteley, M. (2025). Pseudomonas aeruginosa: ecology, evolution, pathogenesis and antimicrobial susceptibility. *Nature Reviews Microbiology 2025 23:11, 23*(11), 701–717. https://doi.org/DOI: 10.1038/s41579-025-01193-8

Lewis, K. (2008). Multidrug tolerance of biofilms and persister cells. *Current Topics in Microbiology and Immunology*, *322*, 107–131. DOI: 10.1007/978-3-540-75418-3_6 PMID: 18453274

Lewis, K. (2017). New approaches to antimicrobial discovery. *Biochemical Pharmacology*, *134*, 87–98. DOI: 10.1016/j.bcp.2016.10.001

Li, S., Carss, K. J., Halldorsson, B. V., Cortes, A., & Consortium, U. B. W.-G. S. (2023). Whole-genome sequencing of half-a-million UK Biobank participants. *medRxiv*, 2023.2012. 2006.23299426.

Liao, S. (2023). *A Study on the Application of Generative Artificial Intelligence Technology in Image Design*. https://doi.org/DOI: 10.2991/978-94-6463-266-8_36

Liesenfeld, O., Lehman, L., Hunfeld, K. P., & Kost, G. (2014). Molecular diagnosis of sepsis: New aspects and recent developments. *European Journal of Microbiology & Immunology*, *4*(1), 1–25. DOI: 10.1556/EuJMI.4.2014.1.1

Li, J.. (2018). Global survey of antibiotic resistance genes in air. *Environmental Science & Technology*, *52*(19), 10975–10984.

Li, J., Koh, J. J., Liu, S., Lakshminarayanan, R., Verma, C. S., & Beuerman, R. W. (2021). Membrane-active antimicrobial peptides: Translating mechanistic insights to design. *Frontiers in Neuroscience*, *15*, 633625. DOI: 10.3389/fnins.2021.633625

Li, L., Mendis, N., Trigui, H., Oliver, J. D., & Faucher, S. P. (2014). The importance of the viable but non-culturable state in human bacterial pathogens. *Frontiers in Microbiology*, *5*, 258. DOI: 10.3389/fmicb.2014.00258 PMID: 24917854

Li, M.-c., Lu, J., Lu, Y., Xiao, T.-y., Liu, H.-c., Lin, S.-q., Xu, D., Li, G.-l., Zhao, X.-q., & Liu, Z.-g. (2021). rpoB mutations and effects on rifampin resistance in Mycobacterium tuberculosis. *Infection and Drug Resistance*, **•••**, 4119–4128. PMID: 34675557

Lin, D. M., Koskella, B., & Lin, H. C. (2022). Phage therapy: An alternative to antibiotics in the age of multidrug resistance. *World Journal of Gastrointestinal Pharmacology and Therapeutics*, *13*(3), 77–91. DOI: 10.4292/wjgpt.v13.i3.77

Ling-Hu, T., Rios-Guzman, E., Lorenzo-Redondo, R., Ozer, E. A., & Hultquist, J. F. (2022). Challenges and opportunities for global genomic surveillance strategies in the COVID-19 era. *Viruses*, *14*(11), 2532. PMID: 36423141

Li, Q. Y., Liu, B., & Liu, L. (2021). Successfully controlling the incidence of multidrug-resistant Pseudomonas aeruginosa through antibiotic stewardship and infection control programmes at a Chinese university hospital. *Journal of Clinical Pharmacy and Therapeutics*, *46*(5), 1357–1366. DOI: 10.1111/JCPT.13446;SUBPAGE:STRING:FULL PMID: 34096086

Littmann, J., & Viens, A. M. (2015). The ethical significance of antimicrobial resistance. *Public Health Ethics*, *8*(3), 209–224. PMID: 26566395

Liu, C. S. C., & Pandey, R. (2024). Integrative genomics would strengthen AMR understanding through ONE health approach. *Heliyon*, *10*(14). PMID: 39816336

Liu, J.. (2019). Mutations in efflux pump Rv1258c (Tap) cause resistance to pyrazinamide, isoniazid, and streptomycin in M. tuberculosis. *Frontiers in Microbiology*, *10*, 216.

Liu, Q., Yin, L., Zhang, X., Zhu, G., Liu, H., Bai, F., Cheng, Z., Wu, W., & Jin, Y. (2022). Reversion of ceftazidime resistance in *Pseudomonas aeruginosa* under clinical setting. *Microorganisms*, *10*(12), 2395. DOI: 10.3390/microorganisms10122395 PMID: 36557649

Liu, X., Liu, S., Mai, B., Su, X., Guo, X., Chang, Y., Dong, W., Wang, W., & Feng, X. (2022). Synergistic gentamicin-photodynamic therapy against resistant bacteria in burn wound infections. *Photodiagnosis and Photodynamic Therapy*, *39*, 103034. PMID: 35882288

Liu, X., Lu, D., Zhang, A., Liu, Q., & Jiang, G. (2022). Data-driven machine learning in environmental pollution: Gains and problems. *Environmental Science & Technology*, *56*(4), 2124–2133. PMID: 35084840

Liu, Y.. (2015). Antibacterial photodynamic therapy: Overview of a promising approach to fight antibiotic-resistant bacterial infections. *Journal of Clinical and Translational Research*, *1*(3), 140.

Liu, Y., Tong, Z., Liu, S., Chen, Y., & Li, J. (2024). Artificial intelligence for antimicrobial resistance prediction. *Briefings in Bioinformatics*, *25*(1), bbad497. Advance online publication. DOI: 10.1093/bib/bbad497

Liu, Y.-Y., Wang, Y., & Walsh, T. R.. (2016). Emergence of plasmid-mediated colistin resistance mechanism MCR-1 in animals and human beings in China: A microbiological and molecular biological study. *The Lancet. Infectious Diseases, 16*(2), 161–168. DOI: 10.1016/S1473-3099(15)00424-7

Li, X., Zuo, S., Wang, B., Zhang, K., & Wang, Y. (2022). Antimicrobial mechanisms and clinical application prospects of antimicrobial peptides. *Molecules (Basel, Switzerland), 27*(9), 2675. DOI: 10.3390/molecules27092675

Li, Y., Roberts, J. A., Walker, M. M., Aslan, A. T., Harris, P. N. A., & Sime, F. B. (2024). The global epidemiology of ventilator-associated pneumonia caused by multi-drug resistant Pseudomonas aeruginosa: A systematic review and meta-analysis. *International Journal of Infectious Diseases, 139*, 78–85. DOI: 10.1016/J.IJID.2023.11.023 PMID: 38013153

Li, Y., Shi, Z., Hu, A., Cui, J., Yang, K., Liu, Y., Deng, G., Zhu, C., & Zhu, L. (2022). Rapid one-tube RPA-CRISPR/Cas12 detection platform for methicillin-resistant Staphylococcus aureus. *Diagnostics (Basel), 12*(4), 829. PMID: 35453874

Llor, C., & Bjerrum, L. (2014). Antimicrobial resistance: Risk associated with antibiotic overuse and initiatives to reduce the problem. *Therapeutic Advances in Drug Safety, 5*(6), 229–241. PMID: 25436105

Lockhart, S. R., Etienne, K. A., Vallabhaneni, S., Farooqi, J., Chowdhary, A., Govender, N. P., Colombo, A. L., Calvo, B., Cuomo, C. A., Desjardins, C. A., Berkow, E. L., Castanheira, M., Magobo, R. E., Jabeen, K., Asghar, R. J., Meis, J. F., Jackson, B., Chiller, T., & Litvintseva, A. P. (2016). Simultaneous Emergence of Multidrug-Resistant *Candida auris* on 3 Continents Confirmed by Whole-Genome Sequencing and Epidemiological Analyses. *Clinical Infectious Diseases, 64*(2), 134–140. https://doi.org/10.1093/cid/ciw691

Logan, L. K., & Weinstein, R. A. (2017). The epidemiology of carbapenem-resistant Enterobacteriaceae: The impact and evolution of a global menace. *The Journal of Infectious Diseases, 215*(Suppl. 1), S28–S36. https://doi.org/10.1093/infdis/jiw282

Longde, S., He, L., Wenyuan, H., Guoxin, L., Rukai, Z., Xu, J., & Siwei, M. (2021). An analysis of major scientific problems and research paths of Gulong shale oil in Daqing Oilfield, NE China. *Petroleum Exploration and Development, 48*(3), 527–540.

Luiken, R. E. C., Van Gompel, L., Munk, P., Sarrazin, S., Joosten, P., Dorado-García, A., Borup Hansen, R., Knudsen, B. E., Bossers, A., Wagenaar, J. A., Mevius, D. J., Aarestrup, F. M., Heederik, D. J. J., & Schmitt, H.EFFORT consortium. (2019). Associations between antimicrobial use and the faecal resistome on broiler farms from nine European countries. *The Journal of Antimicrobial Chemotherapy*, *74*(9), 2596–2604. DOI: 10.1093/jac/dkz210

Lu, J., Xu, H., Xia, J., Ma, J., Xu, J., Li, Y., & Feng, J. (2020). D- and unnatural amino acid substituted antimicrobial peptides with improved proteolytic resistance and their proteolytic degradation characteristics. *Frontiers in Microbiology*, *11*, 563030. DOI: 10.3389/fmicb.2020.563030

Luong, T.. (2020). Phage therapy in the resistance era: Where do we stand and where are we going? *Clinical Therapeutics*, *42*(9), 1659–1680.

Lynch, J. P., & Zhanel, G. G. (2022). Pseudomonas aeruginosa Pneumonia: Evolution of Antimicrobial Resistance and Implications for Therapy. *Seminars in Respiratory and Critical Care Medicine*, *43*(2), 191–218. DOI: 10.1055/S-0041-1740109/ID/JR220203-19/BIB PMID: 35062038

Ma, D., Cai, F., & Zhang, T. (2025). Advances in the detection of Drug-Resistant bacteria: Current trends and innovations. *European Journal of Clinical Microbiology & Infectious Diseases*, •••, 1–17. PMID: 40974457

Magill, S. S., Edwards, J. R., & Bamberg, W.. (2014). Multistate point-prevalence survey of health care-associated infections. *The New England Journal of Medicine*, *370*(13), 1198–1208. DOI: 10.1056/NEJMoa1306801

Magiorakos, A. P., Srinivasan, A., Carey, R. B., Carmeli, Y., Falagas, M. E., Giske, C. G., & Monnet, D. L. (2012). Multidrug-resistant, extensively drug-resistant, and pandrug-resistant bacteria: An international expert proposal for interim standard definitions for acquired resistance. *Clinical Microbiology and Infection*, *18*(3), 268–281. DOI: 10.1111/j.1469-0691.2011.03570.x

Magiorakos, A.-P.. (2012). Multidrug-resistant, extensively drug-resistant and pandrug-resistant bacteria: An international expert proposal for interim standard definitions for acquired resistance. *Clinical Microbiology and Infection*, *18*(3), 268–281.

Magnet, S., Courvalin, P., & Lambert, T. (2001). Resistance-nodulation-cell division-type efflux pump involved in aminoglycoside resistance in *Acinetobacter baumannii* strain BM4454. *Antimicrobial Agents and Chemotherapy*, *45*(12), 3375–3380. DOI: 10.1128/AAC.45.12.3375-3380.2001 PMID: 11709311

Mahlapuu, M., Björn, C., & Ekblom, J. (2020). Antimicrobial peptides as therapeutic agents: Opportunities and challenges. *Critical Reviews in Biotechnology, 40*(7), 978–992. DOI: 10.1080/07388551.2020.1796576

Mah, T.-F., & O'Toole, G. A. (2001). Mechanisms of biofilm resistance to antimicrobial agents. *Trends in Microbiology, 9*(1), 34–39. DOI: 10.1016/S0966-842X(00)01913-2 PMID: 11166241

Mahto, K. U., Kumari, S., & Das, S. (2022). Unraveling the complex regulatory networks in biofilm formation in bacteria and relevance of biofilms in environmental remediation. *Critical Reviews in Biochemistry and Molecular Biology, 57*(3), 305–332. DOI: 10.1080/10409238.2021.2015747 PMID: 34937434

Maillard, J.-Y., Bloomfield, S. F., Courvalin, P., Essack, S. Y., Gandra, S., Gerba, C. P., Rubino, J. R., & Scott, E. A. (2020). Reducing antibiotic prescribing and addressing the global problem of antibiotic resistance by targeted hygiene in the home and everyday life settings: A position paper. *American Journal of Infection Control, 48*(9), 1090–1099. DOI: 10.1016/j.ajic.2020.04.011 PMID: 32311380

Ma, J., Lyu, Y., Liu, X., Jia, X., Cui, F., Wu, X., Deng, S., & Yue, C. (2022). Engineered probiotics. *Microbial Cell Factories, 21*(1), 72. PMID: 35477497

Maldonado, K. V. M.. (2025). Widespread Distribution of Carbapenem-Resistant Klebsiella spp. in Clinical and Environmental Settings. *Antibiotics (Basel, Switzerland), 14*(11), 1140.

Mancuso, G.. (2021). Bacterial antibiotic resistance: The most critical pathogens. *Pathogens (Basel, Switzerland), 10*(10), 1310.

Manigandan, M. (2014). Mass cultivation and determination of biochemical composition of Spirulina platensis in three different medium. *International Journal of Pharmacy and Biological Sciences, 5*(3), 847–854.

Maor, M., Levy Barazany, H., & Kolodkin-Gal, I. (2025). The ladder of regulatory stringency and balance: An application to the US FDA's regulation of bacterial live therapeutics. *Gut Microbes, 17*(1), 2517377. PMID: 40501442

Marshall, B. M., & Levy, S. B. (2011). Food animals and antimicrobials: Impacts on human health. *Clinical Microbiology Reviews, 24*(4), 718–733. PMID: 21976606

Martin, J.. (2017). Covert dissemination of carbapenemase-producing Klebsiella pneumoniae (KPC) in a successfully controlled outbreak: Long-and short-read whole-genome sequencing demonstrate multiple genetic modes of transmission. *The Journal of Antimicrobial Chemotherapy, 72*(11), 3025–3034.

Masclaux, F. G.. (2013). Concentration of airborne Staphylococcus aureus (MRSA and MSSA), total bacteria, and endotoxins in pig farms. *The Annals of Occupational Hygiene*, *57*(5), 550–557.

Maslikowska, J.. (2016). Impact of infection with extended-spectrum β-lactamase-producing Escherichia coli or Klebsiella species on outcome and hospitalization costs. *The Journal of Hospital Infection*, *92*(1), 33–41.

Mathur, A., Parihar, A. S., Modi, S., & Kalra, A. (2023). Photodynamic therapy for ESKAPE pathogens: An emerging approach to combat Antimicrobial Resistance (AMR). *Microbial Pathogenesis*, *185*, 106307. DOI: 10.1016/j.micpath.2023.106307 PMID: 37604213

Mathur, S., & Singh, R. (2005). Antibiotic resistance in food lactic acid bacteria—A review. *International Journal of Food Microbiology*, *105*(3), 281–295. DOI: 10.1016/j.ijfoodmicro.2005.03.025 PMID: 16289406

Matuszewska, M., Maciąg, T., Rajewska, M., Wierzbicka, A., & Jafra, S. (2021). The carbon source-dependent pattern of antimicrobial activity and gene expression in Pseudomonas donghuensis P482. *Scientific Reports 2021 11:1, 11*(1), 1–17. https://doi.org/DOI: 10.1038/s41598-021-90488-w

Maurice, N. M., Bedi, B., & Sadikot, R. T. (2018). Pseudomonas aeruginosa biofilms: Host response and clinical implications in lung infections. *American Journal of Respiratory Cell and Molecular Biology*, *58*(4), 428–439. DOI: 10.1165/RCMB.2017-0321TR/SUPPL_FILE/DISCLOSURES.PDF$AUTHORDISCLOSURES PMID: 29372812

Ma, Y.-X., Wang, C.-Y., Li, Y.-Y., Li, J., Wan, Q.-Q., Chen, J.-H., Tay, F. R., & Niu, L.-N. (2020). Considerations and caveats in combating ESKAPE pathogens against nosocomial infections. *Advancement of Science*, *7*(1), 1901872. DOI: 10.1002/advs.201901872 PMID: 31921562

Mazur, N. I., Terstappen, J., Baral, R., Bardají, A., Beutels, P., Buchholz, U. J., Cohen, C., Crowe, J. E., Cutland, C. L., Eckert, L., Feikin, D., Fitzpatrick, T., Graham, B. S., Heikkinen, T., Higgins, D., Hirve, S., Klugman, K. P., Kragten-Tabatabaie, L., Lemey, P., & Bont, L. J. (2023). Respiratory syncytial virus prevention within reach: The vaccine and monoclonal antibody landscape. *The Lancet. Infectious Diseases*, *23*(1), e2–e21. PMID: 35952703

McCallum, N., Berger-Bächi, B., & Senn, M. M. (2010). Regulation of antibiotic resistance in Staphylococcus aureus. *International Journal of Medical Microbiology*, *300*(2–3), 118–129. DOI: 10.1016/J.IJMM.2009.08.015 PMID: 19800843

McCulloch, T. R., Wells, T. J., & Souza-Fonseca-Guimaraes, F. (2022). Towards efficient immunotherapy for bacterial infection. *Trends in Microbiology*, *30*(2), 158–169. PMID: 34253452

Mendelsohn, E., Ross, N., Zambrana-Torrelio, C., Van Boeckel, T. P., Laxminarayan, R., & Daszak, P. (2023). Global patterns and correlates in the emergence of antimicrobial resistance in humans. Proceedings of the Royal Society B: Biological Sciences, 290(2007), 20231085. https://doi.org/10.1098/rspb.2023.1085

Mendes Pedro, D., Paulo, S. E., Santos, C. M., Fonseca, A. B., Melo Cristino, J., Pereira, Á. A., & Caneiras, C. (2024). Extensively drug-resistant Pseudomonas aeruginosa: Clinical features and treatment with ceftazidime/avibactam and ceftolozane/tazobactam in a tertiary care university hospital center in Portugal – A cross-sectional and retrospective observational study. *Frontiers in Microbiology*, *15*, 1347521. DOI: 10.3389/FMICB.2024.1347521/BIBTEX PMID: 38414772

Merakou, C., Schaefers, M. M., & Priebe, G. P. (2018). Progress toward the elusive pseudomonas aeruginosa vaccine. *Surgical Infections*, *19*(8), 757–768. DOI: 10.1089/SUR.2018.233;WGROUP:STRING:PUBLICATION PMID: 30388058

Meşe, E. A., Carrara, E., Tartari, E., Mutters, N. T., Tsioutis, C., Birgand, G., & Tacconelli, E. (2025). Prioritizing isolation precautions: A patient-centered approach to infection prevention and control. *Antimicrobial Stewardship & Healthcare Epidemiology : ASHE*, *5*(1), e123. DOI: 10.1017/ASH.2025.173 PMID: 40528936

Mestrovic, T., & Ljubin-Sternak, S. (2018). Molecular mechanisms of Chlamydia trachomatis resistance to antimicrobial drugs. *Frontiers in Bioscience (Landmark Edition)*, *23*, 656–670. DOI: 10.2741/4611 PMID: 28930567

Migliaccio, A.. (2022). Inhibition of AdeB, AceI, and AmvA efflux pumps restores chlorhexidine and benzalkonium susceptibility in Acinetobacter baumannii ATCC 19606. *Frontiers in Microbiology*, *12*, 790263.

Miller, W. R., Murray, B. E., Rice, L. B., & Arias, C. A. (2016). Vancomycin-resistant enterococci: Therapeutic challenges in the 21st century. *Infectious Disease Clinics of North America*, *30*(2), 415–439. DOI: 10.1016/j.idc.2016.02.004

Mishra, A.. (2024). Medical device-associated infections caused by biofilm-forming microbial pathogens and controlling strategies. *Antibiotics (Basel, Switzerland)*, *13*(7), 623.

Misra, S., Aguilar-Salinas, C. A., Chikowore, T., Konradsen, F., Ma, R. C., Mbau, L., Mohan, V., Morton, R. W., Nyirenda, M. J., & Tapela, N. (2023). The case for precision medicine in the prevention, diagnosis, and treatment of cardiometabolic diseases in low-income and middle-income countries. *The Lancet. Diabetes & Endocrinology*, *11*(11), 836–847. PMID: 37804857

Mitra, S., Sultana, S. A., Prova, S. R., Uddin, T. M., Islam, F., Das, R., Nainu, F., Sartini, S., Chidambaram, K., & Alhumaydhi, F. A. (2022). Investigating forthcoming strategies to tackle deadly superbugs: Current status and future vision. *Expert Review of Anti-Infective Therapy*, *20*(10), 1309–1332. PMID: 36069241

Mitton, D., & Ackroyd, R. (2008). A brief overview of photodynamic therapy in Europe. *Photodiagnosis and Photodynamic Therapy*, *5*(2), 103–111. PMID: 19356640

Mittra, J.. (2021). Regulatory and market influences on innovation pathways for the development of new antimicrobial drugs. *Technology Analysis and Strategic Management*, *33*(3), 283–295.

Miyauchi, H.. (2017). Structural basis for xenobiotic extrusion by eukaryotic MATE transporter. *Nature Communications*, *8*(1), 1633.

Mkilima, T. (2025). Engineering artificial microbial consortia for personalized gut microbiome modulation and disease treatment. *Annals of the New York Academy of Sciences*. PMID: 40320966

Mnyambwa, N. P. (2019). *Characterization of mutations in drug resistant tuberculosis and diagnostic challenges in referral health facilities*. NM-AIST.

Modgil, V., Sahay, S., Taneja, N., Mukherjee, A., Joshi, N., Mitra, A., Soman, B., Singh, R., Sinha, O., & Surial, R. (2025). Enhancing access to antimicrobial resistance diagnostics for the marginalised: Challenges and opportunities of point-of-care technologies. *Journal of Global Antimicrobial Resistance*, *44*, 281–286. PMID: 40645328

Mohammed, A. M., Oleiwi, J. K., Osman, A. F., Adam, T., Betar, B. O., Gopinath, S. C., & Ihmedee, F. H. (2025). Enhancing antimicrobial resistance strategies: Leveraging artificial intelligence for improved outcomes. *South African Journal of Chemical Engineering*, *51*(1), 272–286.

Mohr, K. I. (2016). History of antibiotics. *Current Topics in Microbiology and Immunology*, *398*, 237–272. DOI: 10.1007/978-3-319-35147-4_10

Moossavi, S. (2014). The necessity for an Iranian gut microbiome initiative. *Middle East Journal of Digestive Diseases*, *6*(2), 109–110. PMID: 24872871

Morales, E., Cots, F., Sala, M., Comas, M., Belvis, F., Riu, M., Salvadá, M., Grau, S., Horcajada, J. P., Montero, M. M., & Castells, X. (2012). Hospital costs of nosocomial multi-drug resistant Pseudomonas aeruginosa acquisition. *BMC Health Services Research 2012 12:1, 12*(1), 122-. https://doi.org/DOI: 10.1186/1472-6963-12-122

Moran, R. A., Anantham, S., Holt, K. E., & Hall, R. M. (2016). Prediction of antibiotic resistance from antibiotic resistance genes detected in antibiotic-resistant commensal *Escherichia coli* using PCR or WGS. *The Journal of Antimicrobial Chemotherapy*, •••, dkw511. Advance online publication. https://doi.org/10.1093/jac/dkw511

Mora-Ochomogo, M., & Lohans, C. T. (2021). β-Lactam antibiotic targets and resistance mechanisms: From covalent inhibitors to substrates. *RSC Medicinal Chemistry*, *12*(10), 1623–1639.

Morgan, D. J., Malani, P., & Diekema, D. J. (2017). Diagnostic stewardship—Leveraging the laboratory to improve antimicrobial use. *Journal of the American Medical Association*, *318*(7), 607–608. DOI: 10.1001/jama.2017.8531 PMID: 28759678

Morin, C. D., Déziel, E., Gauthier, J., Levesque, R. C., & Lau, G. W. (2021). An Organ System-Based Synopsis of Pseudomonas aeruginosa Virulence. *Virulence*, *12*(1), 1469–1507. DOI: 10.1080/21505594.2021.1926408 PMID: 34180343

Morio, F., Jensen, R. H., Le Pape, P., & Arendrup, M. C. (2017). Molecular basis of antifungal drug resistance in yeasts. *International Journal of Antimicrobial Agents*, *50*(5), 599–606. DOI: 10.1016/j.ijantimicag.2017.05.012 PMID: 28669835

Morton, E. R., Lynch, J., Froment, A., Lafosse, S., Heyer, E., Przeworski, M., Segurel, L., & Quintana-Murci, L. (2015). Variation in rural African gut microbiota is strongly correlated with colonization by entamoeba and subsistence. *PLOS Genetics*, *11*(11), e1005658. DOI: 10.1371/journal.pgen.1005658 PMID: 26619199

Motbainor, H., Bereded, F., & Mulu, W. (2020). Multi-drug resistance of blood stream, urinary tract and surgical site nosocomial infections of Acinetobacter baumannii and Pseudomonas aeruginosa among patients hospitalized at Felegehiwot referral hospital, Northwest Ethiopia: A cross-sectional study. *BMC Infectious Diseases*, *20*(1), 1–11. DOI: 10.1186/S12879-020-4811-8/TABLES/5 PMID: 32000693

Mukherjee, A. S., & Sahay, S. (2023). Systems thinking based approaches to engage with health inequities shaping Antimicrobial Resistance in low and lower-middle-income countries. *Journal of Infection and Public Health*, *16*, 129–133. PMID: 37977980

Mulani, M. S., Kamble, E. E., Kumkar, S. N., Tawre, M. S., & Pardesi, K. R. (2019). Emerging strategies to combat ESKAPE pathogens in the era of antimicrobial resistance: A review. *Frontiers in Microbiology, 10*, 539. DOI: 10.3389/fmicb.2019.00539 PMID: 30988669

Mulchandani, R., Tiseo, K., Nandi, A., Klein, E., Gandra, S., Laxminarayan, R., & Van Boeckel, T. (2025). Global trends in inappropriate use of antibiotics, 2000–2021: Scoping review and prevalence estimates. *BMJ Public Health, 3*(1). PMID: 40444029

Mullin, D. S. (2023). Motoric Cognitive Risk: epidemiology of a walking speed-based syndrome to predict dementia.

Munk, P., Brinch, C., Synnott, A., & Hendriksen, R. S. (2022). Global genomic surveillance of antimicrobial resistance: A One Health approach. *Nature Microbiology, 7*(9), 1291–1304. DOI: 10.1038/s41564-022-01149-4

Muro, F. J., Lyamuya, F. S., Kwobah, C., Bollinger, J., Bodinayake, C. K., Nagahawatte, A., Piyasiri, B., Kurukulasooriya, R., Ali, S., Mallya, R., Rolfe, R., Ruwanpathirana, A., Sheng, T., Østbye, T., Drew, R., Kussin, P., Woods, C. W., Anderson, D. J., Mmbaga, B. T., & Tillekeratne, L. G. (2022). Opportunities for Improving Antimicrobial Stewardship: Findings From a Prospective, Multi-Center Study in Three Low- or Middle-Income Countries. *Frontiers in Public Health, 10*, 848802. DOI: 10.3389/FPUBH.2022.848802/BIBTEX PMID: 35548085

Murray, C. J. L., Ikuta, K. S., Sharara, F., Swetschinski, L. R., Aguilar, G. R., Gray, A., Han, C., Bisignano, C., Rao, P., Wool, E., Johnson, S. C., Browne, A. J., Chipeta, M. G., Fell, F., Hackett, S., Haines-Woodhouse, G., Hamadani, B. H. K., Kumaran, E. A. P., McManigal, B., & Naghavi, M. (2022). Global burden of bacterial antimicrobial resistance in 2019: A systematic analysis. *Lancet, 399*(10325), 629–655. PMID: 35065702

Muteeb, G.. (2023). Origin of antibiotics and antibiotic resistance, and their impacts on drug development: A narrative review. *Pharmaceuticals, 16*(11), 1615.

Naas, T.. (2017). Beta-lactamase database (BLDB)–structure and function. *Journal of Enzyme Inhibition and Medicinal Chemistry, 32*(1), 917–919.

Naeem, M. I., Aziz, S., Akhtar, T., Asghar, M., Tanveer, K., Rehman, A., Zahid, R., Tehseen, U., Arbab, Z., & Ahmad, H. M. (2023). Use of nanotechnology to mitigate antimicrobial resistance.

Nasirian, H. (2017). Infestation of cockroaches (Insecta: Blattaria) in the human dwelling environments: A systematic review and meta-analysis. *Acta Tropica, 167*, 86–98. DOI: 10.1016/j.actatropica.2016.12.019 PMID: 28012906

Naylor, N. R., Hasso-Agopsowicz, M., Kim, C., Ma, Y., Frost, I., Abbas, K., Aguilar, G., Fuller, N., Robotham, J. V., & Jit, M. (2025). The global economic burden of antibiotic-resistant infections and the potential impact of bacterial vaccines: A modelling study. *BMJ Global Health*, *10*(6). Advance online publication. DOI: 10.1136/BMJGH-2024-016249 PMID: 40537271

Nazir, A.. (2025). The Global Challenge of Antimicrobial Resistance: Mechanisms, Case Studies, and Mitigation Approaches. *Health Science Reports*, *8*(7), e71077.

Ndung'u, M. H., Gachara, G., Ontweka, L., Menza, N., Musyoki, A., & Muturi, M. (2023). Review of Rapid Diagnostic Methods for Vibrio Cholerae Detection in the Last Decade (2011–2022). *The East African Health Research Journal*, *7*(2), 131. PMID: 39219657

Nekahiwot, S. (2024). "Multi-drug resistant gonorrhea: an emerging global threat." Multi-Drug Resistant Gonorrhea: An Emerging Global Threat.

Ng, E., Tay, J. R. H., Boey, S. K., Laine, M. L., Ivanovski, S., & Seneviratne, C. J. (2024). Antibiotic resistance in the microbiota of periodontitis patients: An update of current findings. *Critical Reviews in Microbiology*, *50*(2), 329–340. DOI: 10.1080/1040841X.2023.2201411 PMID: 37140235

Nickerson, R., Thornton, C. S., Johnston, B., Lee, A. H. Y., & Cheng, Z. (2024). Pseudomonas aeruginosa in chronic lung disease: Untangling the dysregulated host immune response. *Frontiers in Immunology*, *15*, 1405376. DOI: 10.3389/FIMMU.2024.1405376/XML/NLM PMID: 39015565

Nikaido, H. (2003). Molecular basis of bacterial outer membrane permeability revisited. *Microbiology and Molecular Biology Reviews : MMBR*, *67*(4), 593–656. DOI: 10.1128/MMBR.67.4.593-656.2003 PMID: 14665678

Nikaido, H. (2018). RND transporters in the living world. *Research in Microbiology*, *169*(7-8), 363–371.

Nordmann, P., Naas, T., & Poirel, L. (2012). Global spread of carbapenemase-producing Enterobacteriaceae. *Emerging Infectious Diseases*, *17*(10), 1791–1798. DOI: 10.3201/eid1710.110655

Nowak, J.. (2021). Inactivation of the gene encoding the cationic antimicrobial peptide resistance factor MprF increases biofilm formation but reduces invasiveness of Listeria monocytogenes. *Journal of Applied Microbiology*, *130*(2), 464–477.

O'Neill, J. (2016). *Tackling drug-resistant infections globally: Final report and recommendations*. Review on Antimicrobial Resistance.

O'Neill, J. (2016). Tackling drug-resistant infections globally: Final report and recommendations. Review on Antimicrobial Resistance. https://amr-review.org

O'Neill, J. (2020). *Tackling drug-resistant infections globally: Final report and recommendations*. UK Government.

OECD. (2022). *Stemming the Superbug Tide: Just a Few Dollars More*. OECD Publishing., DOI: 10.1787/9789264307599-

Ogunsola, F. T., & Mehtar, S. (2020). Challenges regarding the control of environmental sources of contamination in healthcare settings in low-and middle-income countries - a narrative review. *Antimicrobial Resistance & Infection Control 2020 9:1, 9*(1), 81-. https://doi.org/DOI: 10.1186/S13756-020-00747-0

Okesanya, O. J., Ahmed, M. M., Ogaya, J. B., Amisu, B. O., Ukoaka, B. M., Adigun, O. A., Manirambona, E., Adebusuyi, O., Othman, Z. K., & Oluwakemi, O. G. (2025). Reinvigorating AMR resilience: Leveraging CRISPR–Cas technology potentials to combat the 2024 WHO bacterial priority pathogens for enhanced global health security—a systematic review. *Tropical Medicine and Health, 53*(1), 43. PMID: 40176174

Olaitan, M. O.. (2025). Prevalence of ESBL-producing Escherichia coli in sub-Saharan Africa: A meta-analysis using a One Health approach. *One Health, 20*, 101090.

Olalekan, A., Bader, B. K., Iwalokun, B., Wolf, S., Lalremruata, A., Dike, A., Mannie-Udoh, M., Lo Presti, L., Liese, J., Guther, J., D'alvise, P., & Peter, S. (2023). High incidence of carbapenemase-producing Pseudomonas aeruginosa clinical isolates from Lagos, Nigeria. *JAC-Antimicrobial Resistance, 5*(2). Advance online publication. DOI: 10.1093/JACAMR/DLAD038 PMID: 37051191

Olatunji, A. O., Olaboye, J. A., Maha, C. C., Kolawole, T. O., & Abdul, S. (2024). Next-Generation strategies to combat antimicrobial resistance: Integrating genomics, CRISPR, and novel therapeutics for effective treatment. *Engineering Science & Technology Journal, 5*(7), 2284–2303.

Olawade, D. B., Fapohunda, O., Egbon, E., Ebiesuwa, O. A., Usman, S. O., Faronbi, A. O., & Fidelis, S. C. (2024). Phage therapy: A targeted approach to overcoming antibiotic resistance. *Microbial Pathogenesis, 197*, 107088. DOI: 10.1016/J.MICPATH.2024.107088 PMID: 39477033

Onyeyili, I. N., Ogbozor, F. I., Kehinde, A. B., & Chiemerie, C. (2025). Phage-based CRISPR delivery systems for targeted eradication of drug-resistant bacterial infections.

Oppenheimer-Shaanan, Y., Steinberg, N., & Kolodkin-Gal, I. (2013). Small molecules are natural triggers for the disassembly of biofilms. *Trends in Microbiology, 21*(11), 594–601. DOI: 10.1016/j.tim.2013.08.005 PMID: 24080023

Organization, W. H. (2024). *WHO Strategic and Technical Advisory Group for Antimicrobial Resistance (STAG-AMR): report of the fourth meeting 11-13 June 2024*. World Health Organization.

Organization, W. H. (2022). *Global antimicrobial resistance and use surveillance system (GLASS) report 2022*. World Health Organization.

Organization, W. H. (2024). *WHO bacterial priority pathogens list, 2024: bacterial pathogens of public health importance, to guide research, development, and strategies to prevent and control antimicrobial resistance*. World Health Organization.

Ortega, M. A., Guzmán Merino, A., Fraile-Martínez, O., Recio-Ruiz, J., Pekarek, L., Guijarro, L. G., García-Honduvilla, N., Álvarez-Mon, M., Buján, J., & García-Gallego, S. (2020). Dendrimers and dendritic materials: From laboratory to medical practice in infectious diseases. *Pharmaceutics, 12*(9), 874. DOI: 10.3390/pharmaceutics12090874 PMID: 32937793

Osman, A.-H.. (2023). The potential of bacteriophage-antibiotic combination therapy in treating infections with multidrug-resistant bacteria. *Antibiotics (Basel, Switzerland), 12*(8), 1329.

Oubekka, S. D., Briandet, R., Fontaine-Aupart, M.-P., & Steenkeste, K. (2012). Correlative time-resolved fluorescence microscopy to assess antibiotic diffusion-reaction in biofilms. *Antimicrobial Agents and Chemotherapy, 56*(6), 3349–3358. DOI: 10.1128/AAC.00216-12 PMID: 22450986

Ouwehand, A. C., Salminen, S., & Isolauri, E. (2002). Probiotics: An overview of beneficial effects. *Antonie van Leeuwenhoek, 82*(1), 279–289. DOI: 10.1023/A:1020620607611 PMID: 12369194

Overman, P. R. (2007). Biofilm: A new view of plaque. *The Journal of Contemporary Dental Practice, 1*(3), 18–29. DOI: 10.5005/jcdp-1-3-18 PMID: 12167880

Oyeyemi, O. T., Agbaje, M. O., & Okelue, U. B. (2016). Food-borne human parasitic pathogens associated with household cockroaches and houseflies in Nigeria. *Parasite Epidemiology and Control, 1*(1), 10–13. DOI: 10.1016/j.parepi.2015.12.001

Ozma, M. A., Abbasi, A., Asgharzadeh, M., Pagliano, P., Guarino, A., Köse, S., & Kafil, H. S. (2022). Antibiotic therapy for pan-drug-resistant infections. *Le Infezioni in Medicina, 30*(4), 525. DOI: 10.53854/LIIM-3004-6 PMID: 36482958

Pachón-Ibáñez, M. E., Smani, Y., Pachón, J., & Sánchez-Céspedes, J. (2017). Perspectives for clinical use of engineered human host defense antimicrobial peptides. *FEMS Microbiology Reviews, 41*(3), 323–342. DOI: 10.1093/femsre/fux012 PMID: 28521337

Paharik, A. E., & Horswill, A. R. (2016). The staphylococcal biofilm: Adhesins, regulation, and host response. *Microbiology Spectrum, 4*(2). Advance online publication. DOI: 10.1128/microbiolspec.VMBF-0022-2015 PMID: 27227309

Pai, H.-H. (2013). Multidrug resistant bacteria isolated from cockroaches in long-term care facilities and nursing homes. *Acta Tropica, 125*(1), 18–22. DOI: 10.1016/j.actatropica.2012.08.016 PMID: 22960645

Pai, H.-H., Chen, W.-C., & Peng, C.-F. (2005). Isolation of bacteria with antibiotic resistance from household cockroaches (Periplaneta americana and Blattella germanica). *Acta Tropica, 93*(3), 259–265. DOI: 10.1016/j.actatropica.2004.11.005 PMID: 15716054

Pai, M., Schumacher, S. G., & Abimbola, S. (2018). Surrogate endpoints in global health research: Still searching for killer apps and silver bullets? *BMJ Global Health, 3*(2), e000755. DOI: 10.1136/bmjgh-2018-000755

Pal, C., Bengtsson-Palme, J., Kristiansson, E., & Larsson, D. G. J. (2015). Co-occurrence of resistance genes to antibiotics, biocides, and metals reveals novel insights into their co-selection potential. *BMC Genomics, 16*(1), 964. DOI: 10.1186/s12864-015-2153-5

Pallares, C. J., Porras, J., De La Cadena, E., García-Betancur, J. C., Restrepo-Arbeláez, N., Viveros, S. M. C., Cornistein, W., Castañeda-Méndez, P., Cuellar, L., Boldim-Ferreira, D., Chaverri-Murillo, J., Labarca, J. A., & Villegas, M. V. (2023). Antimicrobial stewardship programs in seven Latin American countries: facing the challenges. *BMC Infectious Diseases 2023 23:1, 23*(1), 463-. https://doi.org/DOI: 10.1186/S12879-023-08398-3

Panchpuri, M., Painuli, R., & Kumar, C. (2025). Artificial intelligence in smart drug delivery systems: A step toward personalized medicine. *RSC Pharmaceutics.*

Pandey, S.. (2024). Antibiotic resistance in livestock, environment and humans: One Health perspective. *Journal of Animal Science and Technology, 66*(2), 266.

Pandrangi, S. L., ... (2025). Omics Approaches in Diagnosis of Polymicrobial Biofilms and Identification of Novel Therapeutic Drugs. Omics Approaches in Biofilm Research: Perspectives and Applications, Springer: 369-389.

Pang, Z., Raudonis, R., Glick, B. R., Lin, T. J., & Cheng, Z. (2019). Antibiotic resistance in Pseudomonas aeruginosa: Mechanisms and alternative therapeutic strategies. *Biotechnology Advances, 37*(1), 177–192. DOI: 10.1016/J.BIOTECHADV.2018.11.013 PMID: 30500353

Parcell, B. J. (2021). *Whole genome sequencing service: investigating healthcare associated infections*. University of St Andrews.

Park, A. R., Kim, S. B., Jung, S. W., Chun, J. W., Kim, J. H., Kim, J., Lazarte, Y. R., Jang, J. M. S., Jang, H. B., Thompson, K. D., Jung, T. S., & Cha, I. S. (2022). Membrane vesicles from antibiotic-resistant Staphylococcus aureus transfer antibiotic resistance to antibiotic-susceptible Escherichia coli. *Journal of Applied Microbiology, 132*(4), 2746–2759. PMID: 35019198

Partridge, S. R., Kwong, S. M., Firth, N., & Jensen, S. O. (2018). Mobile genetic elements associated with antimicrobial resistance. *Clinical Microbiology Reviews, 31*(4), e00088–e17.

Patel, R. (2015). MALDI-TOF MS for the diagnosis of infectious diseases. *Clinical Chemistry, 61*(1), 100–111. DOI: 10.1373/clinchem.2014.221770 PMID: 25278500

Paulson, D., & Johnson, A. (2025). Integrating Artificial Intelligence with Genomic and Biomarker Data for the Advancement of Personalized Therapeutics in a Human-Centric Framework.

Pauly, B., Revai, T., Marcellus, L., Martin, W., Easton, K., & MacDonald, M. (2021). "The health equity curse": Ethical tensions in promoting health equity. *BMC Public Health, 21*(1), 1567. PMID: 34407781

Pei, Y., Hamar, P., & Pei, D. S. (2025). Deciphering Multidrug-Resistant Pseudomonas aeruginosa: Mechanistic Insights and Environmental Risks. *Toxics 2025, Vol. 13, Page 303, 13*(4), 303. https://doi.org/DOI: 10.3390/TOXICS13040303

Peiffer-Smadja, N., Rawson, T. M., Ahmad, R., Buchard, A., Georgiou, P., Lescure, F.-X., Birgand, G., & Holmes, A. H. (2020). Machine learning for clinical decision support in infectious diseases: A narrative review of current applications. *Clinical Microbiology and Infection, 26*(5), 584–595. DOI: 10.1016/j.cmi.2019.09.009 PMID: 31539636

Peñil Celis, A. (2025). Inclusión del pangenoma para la vigilancia genómica de los serovares Typhi y Hadar de Salmonella enterica.

Pennisi, F., Pinto, A., Ricciardi, G. E., Signorelli, C., & Gianfredi, V. (2025). The role of artificial intelligence and machine learning models in antimicrobial stewardship in public health: A narrative review. *Antibiotics (Basel, Switzerland)*, *14*(2), 134. PMID: 40001378

Pentland, D. R., ... (2020). "CO2 enhances the ability of Candida albicans to form biofilms, overcome nutritional immunity and resist antifungal treatment." bioRxiv: 2020.2003. 2031.018200.

Pepi, M., Focardi, S., Area, M., & Int, J. E. (2021). Antibiotic-Resistant Bacteria in Aquaculture and Climate Change: A Challenge for Health in the Mediterranean Area. *International Journal of Environmental Research and Public Health 2021, Vol. 18, Page 5723, 18*(11), 5723. https://doi.org/DOI: 10.3390/IJERPH18115723

Pérez Maldonado, M., Ofori-Darko, D., Nichols, V., French, J., Spence, K., Reid-Smith, R. J., & Parmley, E. J. (2025). Investigating the occurrence of antimicrobial resistance in the environment in Canada: A scoping review. *Canadian Journal of Microbiology*, *71*, 1–13. PMID: 40279669

Pérez-Varela, M.. (2019). Roles of efflux pumps from different superfamilies in the surface-associated motility and virulence of Acinetobacter baumannii ATCC 17978. *Antimicrobial Agents and Chemotherapy*, *63*(3), 02190–02118. DOI: 10.1128/aac

Pérez-Varela, M., Tierney, A. R., Dawson, E., Hutcheson, A. R., Tipton, K. A., Anderson, S. E., Haldopoulos, M. E., Song, S., Tomlinson, B. R., & Shaw, L. N. (2022). Stochastic activation of a family of TetR-type transcriptional regulators controls phenotypic heterogeneity in *Acinetobacter baumannii*. *PNAS Nexus*, *1*(5), pgac231. Advance online publication. DOI: 10.1093/pnasnexus/pgac231

Peri, A. M.. (2024). Rapid diagnostic tests and antimicrobial stewardship programs for the management of bloodstream infection: What is their relative contribution to improving clinical outcomes? A systematic review and network meta-analysis. *Clinical Infectious Diseases*, *79*(2), 502–515.

Perry, J. A., & Wright, G. D. (2013). The antibiotic resistance "mobilome": Searching for the link between environment and clinic. *Frontiers in Microbiology*, *4*, 138. DOI: 10.3389/fmicb.2013.00138 PMID: 23755047

Pervez, M. T., Hasnain, M. J. U., Abbas, S. H., Moustafa, M. F., Aslam, N., & Shah, S. S. M. (2022). [Retracted] A Comprehensive Review of Performance of Next-Generation Sequencing Platforms. *BioMed Research International*, *2022*(1), 3457806. PMID: 36212714

Petronio, D. G. P. Study of fluoroquinolone resistance in Lactobacillus spp.

Pettorelli, N., Graham, N. A., Seddon, N., Maria da Cunha Bustamante, M., Lowton, M. J., Sutherland, W. J., Koldewey, H. J., Prentice, H. C., & Barlow, J. (2021). Time to integrate global climate change and biodiversity science-policy agendas. *Journal of Applied Ecology*, *58*(11), 2384–2393.

Pfeifer, N. M.. (2025). Escherichia coli resistant to the highest priority critically important fluoroquinolone or 3rd and 4th generation cephalosporin antibiotics persist in pigsties. *Applied and Environmental Microbiology*, •••, 01386–01324.

Phan, S., Feng, C. H., Huang, R., Lee, Z. X., Moua, Y., Phung, O. J., & Lenhard, J. R. (2023). Relative Abundance and Detection of Pseudomonas aeruginosa from Chronic Wound Infections Globally. *Microorganisms*, *11*(5), 1210. DOI: 10.3390/MICROORGANISMS11051210 PMID: 37317184

Pierce, J. D.. (2022). Post-COVID-19 syndrome. *Nursing Research*, *71*(2), 164–174.

Pilar, R.-G.. (2025). New Drugs, Old Problems: A Narrative Review of Antibiotic Stewardship Program in the era of novel Gram-negative antibiotics. *Clinical Microbiology and Infection*.

Pinheiro, L., Brito, C. I., Pereira, V. C., Oliveira, A., Camargo, C. H., & Cunha, M. L. R. S. (2014). Reduced susceptibility to vancomycin and biofilm formation in methicillin-resistant *Staphylococcus epidermidis* isolated from blood cultures. *Memorias do Instituto Oswaldo Cruz*, *109*(7), 871–878. DOI: 10.1590/0074-0276140128 PMID: 25410990

Pirnay, J. (2020). Phage therapy in the year 2035. *Frontiers in Microbiology*, *11*, 1171.

Pirnay, J. P., Verbeken, G., Rose, T., Jennes, S., Zizi, M., Huys, I., & Merabishvili, M. (2022). Introducing phage therapy to Western medicine. *Emerging Infectious Diseases*, *28*(1), 16–23. DOI: 10.3201/eid2801.210157

Piscaglia, M.. (2025). Exploring human use of monoclonal antibodies against critical bacteria: A scoping review of clinical trials. *Infectious Diseases and Therapy*, •••, 1–29.

Plackett, B. (2020). Why big pharma has abandoned antibiotics. *Nature*, *586*, S50–S52.

Pliakos, E. E., Andreatos, N., Shehadeh, F., Ziakas, P. D., & Mylonakis, E. (2018). The Cost-Effectiveness of Rapid Diagnostic Testing for the Diagnosis of Bloodstream Infections with or without Antimicrobial Stewardship. *Clinical Microbiology Reviews*, *31*(3). Advance online publication. https://doi.org/10.1128/CMR.00095-17

Polemis, M., Theofili, E., & Tryfinopoulou, K. (2024). Rapid increase of multi-drug resistant Pseudomonas aeruginosa in Greece - WHONET-Greece (2020-2023). *European Journal of Public Health, 34*(Supplement_3). Advance online publication. DOI: 10.1093/EURPUB/CKAE144.2154

Poole, K. (2007). Efflux pumps as antimicrobial resistance mechanisms. *Annals of Medicine*, *39*(3), 162–176. DOI: 10.1080/07853890701195262

Prestinaci, F., Pezzotti, P., & Pantosti, A. (2015). Antimicrobial resistance: A global multifaceted phenomenon. *Pathogens and Global Health*, *109*(7), 309–318. https://doi.org/10.1179/2047773215Y.0000000030

Pulcini, C., Binda, F., Lamkang, A. S., Trett, A., Charani, E., Goff, D. A., Harbarth, S., Hinrichsen, S. L., Levy-Hara, G., Mendelson, M., Nathwani, D., Gunturu, R., Singh, S., Srinivasan, A., Thamlikitkul, V., Thursky, K., Vlieghe, E., Wertheim, H., Zeng, M., & Gandra, S. (2019). Developing core elements and checklist items for global hospital antimicrobial stewardship programmes: A consensus approach. *Clinical Microbiology and Infection*, *25*(1), 20–25. https://doi.org/10.1016/j.cmi.2018.03.033

Pungartnik, P. C., Abreu, A., Dos Santos, C. V. B., Cavalcante, J. R., Faerstein, E., & Werneck, G. L. (2023). The interfaces between One Health and Global Health: A scoping review. *One Health*, *16*, 100573. PMID: 37363235

Puraswani, M., Ashita, A., Kumari Ambashta, N., Aggrawal, R., Soni, K. D., Kumar, S., Sagar, S., Gupta, A., Farooque, K., & Mathur, P. (2025). Transmission dynamics of multidrug resistant Klebsiella pneumoniae from an Indian hospital. *Indian Journal of Medical Microbiology*, *55*, 100848. https://doi.org/10.1016/j.ijmmb.2025.100848

Pursey, E., Sünderhauf, D., Gaze, W. H., Westra, E. R., & van Houte, S. (2018). CRISPR-Cas antimicrobials: Challenges and future prospects. *PLoS Pathogens*, *14*(6), e1006990. DOI: 10.1371/journal.ppat.1006990 PMID: 29902258

Qin, S.. (2022). Pseudomonas aeruginosa: Pathogenesis, virulence factors, antibiotic resistance, interaction with host, technology advances and emerging therapeutics. *Signal Transduction and Targeted Therapy*, *7*(1), 199.

Qiu, J. (2024). Innovations in combating antimicrobial resistance: Unveiling nanotechnology, gene technology, and molecular diagnostics. *Theoretical and Natural Science*, *44*, 203–208.

Qudrat-Ullah, H. (2024). Future Prospects and Emerging Technologies. *Sustainable Energy: A Myth or Reality*, 185-202.

Rabaan, A. A., Alhumaid, S., Mutair, A. A., Garout, M., Abulhamayel, Y., Halwani, M. A., Alestad, J. H., Bshabshe, A. A., Sulaiman, T., & AlFonaisan, M. K. (2022). Application of artificial intelligence in combating high antimicrobial resistance rates. *Antibiotics (Basel, Switzerland), 11*(6), 784. PMID: 35740190

Rafiq, M. K., Kamran, H., Sultan, B., Khan, Y. A., Wadud, F., Ayub, M., Ali, S., & Ali, A. (2022). Outcome of the Choice of Wound Closure Technique in Emergency Laparotomy. *Journal of Ayub Medical College, Abbottabad, 34*(1), 164–168. DOI: 10.55519/JAMC-01-8797 PMID: 35466646

Rahman, M. M., Alam Tumpa, M. A., Zehravi, M., Sarker, M. T., Yamin, M., Islam, M. R., Harun-Or-Rashid, M., Ahmed, M., Ramproshad, S., Mondal, B., Dey, A., Damiri, F., Berrada, M., Rahman, M. H., & Cavalu, S. (2022). An overview of antimicrobial stewardship optimization: The use of antibiotics in humans and animals to prevent resistance. *Antibiotics (Basel, Switzerland), 11*(5), 667. PMID: 35625311

Rajakumari, K.. (2024). Comprehensive review of DNA gyrase as enzymatic target for drug discovery and development. *European Journal of Medicinal Chemistry Reports, 12*, 100233.

Ramatla, T., Nkhebenyane, J., Lekota, K. E., Thekisoe, O., Monyama, M., Achilonu, C. C., & Khasapane, G. (2025). Global prevalence and antibiotic resistance profiles of carbapenem-resistant Pseudomonas aeruginosa reported from 2014 to 2024: A systematic review and meta-analysis. *Frontiers in Microbiology, 16*, 1599070. DOI: 10.3389/FMICB.2025.1599070/BIBTEX PMID: 40761277

Ramirez, M. S., & Tolmasky, M. E. (2010). Aminoglycoside modifying enzymes. *Drug Resistance Updates, 13*(6), 151–171.

Rao, H.. (2021). Approaches for mitigating microbial biofilm-related drug resistance: A focus on micro-and nanotechnologies. *Molecules (Basel, Switzerland), 26*(7), 1870.

Ratiner, K., Ciocan, D., Abdeen, S. K., & Elinav, E. (2024). Utilization of the microbiome in personalized medicine. *Nature Reviews. Microbiology, 22*(5), 291–308. PMID: 38110694

Raven, K. E., Reuter, S., Reynolds, R., Brodrick, H. J., Russell, J. E., Török, M. E., Parkhill, J., & Peacock, S. J. (2016). A decade of genomic history for healthcare-associated *Enterococcus faecium* in the United Kingdom and Ireland. *Genome Research, 26*(10), 1388–1396. https://doi.org/10.1101/gr.204024.116

Rawson, T. M., Moore, L. S. P., Hernandez, B., Charani, E., Castro-Sanchez, E., Herrero, P., Hayhoe, B., Hope, W., Georgiou, P., & Holmes, A. H. (2017). A systematic review of clinical decision support systems for antimicrobial management: Are we failing to investigate these interventions appropriately? *Clinical Microbiology and Infection, 23*(8), 524–532. https://doi.org/10.1016/j.cmi.2017.02.028

Razzaque, M. S. (2021). Implementation of antimicrobial stewardship to reduce antimicrobial drug resistance. *Expert Review of Anti-Infective Therapy, 19*(5), 559–562. DOI: 10.1080/14787210.2021.1858802 PMID: 33084432

Rees, T. W., Ho, P. Y., & Hess, J. (2023). Recent advances in metal complexes for antimicrobial photodynamic therapy. *ChemBioChem, 24*(16), e202200797. DOI: 10.1002/cbic.202200797 PMID: 36917084

Rehman, S. (2024). Ethical Implications of Genetic Engineering: Balancing Innovation and Responsibility. *Frontiers in Biotechnology and Genetics, 1*(1), 37–55.

Rehm, Z. J., Gonzaga, C., Merakou, A., DiGiandomenico, G. P., & Priebe, B. H. A. (2021). A Pseudomonas aeruginosa-Derived Particulate Vaccine Protects against P. aeruginosa Infection. *Vaccines, 9*(7), 803. DOI: 10.3390/vaccines9070803 PMID: 34358220

Reighard, K. P. (2015). Antibacterial action of nitric oxide-releasing chitosan oligosaccharides against *Pseudomonas aeruginosa* under aerobic and anaerobic conditions. *Antimicrobial Agents and Chemotherapy, 59*(10), 6506–6513. DOI: 10.1128/AAC.01208-15 PMID: 26239983

Reig, S., Le Gouellec, A., & Bleves, S. (2022). What Is New in the Anti–Pseudomonas aeruginosa Clinical Development Pipeline Since the 2017 WHO Alert? *Frontiers in Cellular and Infection Microbiology, 12*, 909731. DOI: 10.3389/FCIMB.2022.909731/TEXT PMID: 35880080

Reygaert, W. C. (2018). An overview of the antimicrobial resistance mechanisms of bacteria. *AIMS Microbiology, 4*(3), 482–501. DOI: 10.3934/microbiol.2018.3.482 PMID: 31294229

Reynolds, D., & Kollef, M. (2021). The Epidemiology and Pathogenesis and Treatment of Pseudomonas aeruginosa Infections: An Update. *Drugs 2021 81:18, 81*(18), 2117–2131. https://doi.org/DOI: 10.1007/S40265-021-01635-6

Ribeiro, Á. C. da S., Crozatti, M. T. L., da Silva, A. A., Macedo, R. S., Machado, A. M. de O., & Silva, A. T. de A. (2019). Pseudomonas aeruginosa in the ICU: Prevalence, resistance profile, and antimicrobial consumption. *Revista da Sociedade Brasileira de Medicina Tropical*, *53*, e20180498. DOI: 10.1590/0037-8682-0498-2018 PMID: 31859938

Rice, L. B. (2008). Federal funding for the study of antimicrobial resistance in nosocomial pathogens: No ESKAPE. *The Journal of Infectious Diseases*, *197*(8), 1079–1081. DOI: 10.1086/533452 PMID: 18419525

Rice, L. B. (2010). Progress and challenges in implementing the research on ESKAPE pathogens. *Infection Control and Hospital Epidemiology*, *31*(S1), S7–S10. PMID: 20929376

Riddle, M. S., Kaminski, R. W., Di Paolo, C., Porter, C. K., Gutierrez, R. L., Clarkson, K. A., Weerts, H. E., Duplessis, C., Castellano, A., Alaimo, C., Paolino, K. M., Gormley, R., & Gambillara Fonck, V. (2016). Safety and immunogenicity of a candidate bioconjugate vaccine against Shigella flexneri 2a administered to healthy adults: A single-blind, randomized phase I study. *Clinical and Vaccine Immunology; CVI*, *23*(12), 908–917. DOI: 10.1128/CVI.00224-16 PMID: 27581434

Ridha, D. M., Al-Awady, M. J., Abd Al-Zwaid, A. J., Balakit, A. A., Al-Dahmoshi, H. O. M., Alotaibi, M. H., & El-Hiti, G. A. (2024). Antibacterial and antibiofilm activities of selenium nanoparticles-antibiotic conjugates against anti-multidrug-resistant bacteria. *International Journal of Pharmaceutics*, *658*, 124–214. DOI: 10.1016/j.ijpharm.2024.124214

Ridyard, K. E., & Overhage, J. (2021). The potential of human peptide LL-37 as an antimicrobial and anti-biofilm agent. *Antibiotics (Basel, Switzerland)*, *10*(6), 650. DOI: 10.3390/antibiotics10060650

Riwu, K. H. P., Effendi, M. H., & Rantam, F. A. (2020). A Review of Extended Spectrum β-Lactamase (ESBL) Producing Klebsiella pneumoniae and Multidrug Resistant (MDR) on Companion Animals. *Systematic Reviews in Pharmacy*, *11*(7).

Robinson, T. P., Bu, D. P., & Carrique-Mas, J.. (2016). Antibiotic resistance is the quintessential One Health issue. *Transactions of the Royal Society of Tropical Medicine and Hygiene*, *110*(7), 377–380. DOI: 10.1093/trstmh/trw048

Rodrigues, G., Santos, L. S., & Franco, O. L. (2022). Antimicrobial peptides controlling resistant bacteria in animal production. *Frontiers in Microbiology*, *13*, 874–153. DOI: 10.3389/fmicb.2022.874153

Rodrigues, S. H., Nunes, G. D., Soares, G. G., Ferreira, R. L., Damas, M. S. F., Laprega, P. M., Shilling, R. E., Campos, L. C., da Costa, A. S., & Malavazi, I. (2024). First report of coexistence of blaKPC-2 and blaNDM-1 in carbapenem-resistant clinical isolates of Klebsiella aerogenes in Brazil. *Frontiers in Microbiology*, *15*, 1352851. PMID: 38426065

Rodríguez-Baño, J., Rossolini, G. M., Schultsz, C., Tacconelli, E., Murthy, S., Ohmagari, N., Holmes, A., Bachmann, T., Goossens, H., Canton, R., Roberts, A. P., Henriques-Normark, B., Clancy, C. J., Huttner, B., Fagerstedt, P., Lahiri, S., Kaushic, C., Hoffman, S. J., Warren, M., & Zoubiane, G. (2021). Antimicrobial resistance research in a post-pandemic world: Insights on antimicrobial resistance research in the COVID-19 pandemic. *Journal of Global Antimicrobial Resistance*, *25*, 5–7. https://doi.org/10.1016/j.jgar.2021.02.013

Rodríguez-Guerrero, E., Callejas-Rodelas, J. C., Navarro-Marí, J. M., & Gutiérrez-Fernández, J. (2022). Systematic review of plasmid AmpC type resistances in Escherichia coli and Klebsiella pneumoniae and preliminary proposal of a simplified screening method for AmpC. *Microorganisms*, *10*(3), 611. PMID: 35336186

Román Hurtado, F. (2022). Genome mining of the strain Streptomyces sp. CA-170360: Identification and heterologous expression of secondary metabolite biosynthetic gene clusters [Doctoral dissertation, University of Granada].

Rugarabamu, S., & Mwanyika, G. (2025). Biotechnological Innovations to Combat Antimicrobial Resistance and Advance Global Health Equity. *Bacteria*, *4*(3), 46.

Rush, L.. (2019). Communicating antimicrobial resistance and stewardship in the national press: Lessons from sepsis awareness campaigns. *The Journal of Infection*, *78*(2), 88–94.

Rushton, J. (2015). Anti-microbial use in animals: How to assess the trade-offs. *Zoonoses and Public Health*, *62*(Suppl. 1), 10–21. DOI: 10.1111/zph.12126

Saeidi, N.. (2011). Engineering microbes to sense and eradicate Pseudomonas aeruginosa, a human pathogen. *Molecular Systems Biology*, *7*(1), 521.

Saffari Natanzi, A.. (2025). Innovative approaches to combat antibiotic resistance: Integrating CRISPR/Cas9 and nanoparticles against biofilm-driven infections. *BMC Medicine*, *23*(1), 486.

Saha, M., & Sarkar, A. (2021). Review on multiple facets of drug resistance: A rising challenge in the 21st century. *Journal of Xenobiotics*, *11*(4), 197–214. DOI: 10.3390/jox11040013 PMID: 34940513

Sahli, C., Moya, S. E., Lomas, J. S., Gravier-Pelletier, C., Briandet, R., & Hémadi, M. (2022). Recent advances in nanotechnology for eradicating bacterial biofilm. *Theranostics, 12*(5), 2383–2405. PMID: 35265216

Saidi, B., Mafirakureva, P., & Mbanga, J. (2013). Antimicrobial resistance of Escherichia coli isolated from chickens with colibacillosis in and around Harare, Zimbabwe. *Avian Diseases, 57*(1), 152–154. DOI: 10.1637/10268-060412-ResNote.1 PMID: 23678746

Sainz-Mejías, M., Jurado-Martín, I., & McClean, S. (2020). Understanding Pseudomonas aeruginosa–Host Interactions: The Ongoing Quest for an Efficacious Vaccine. *Cells 2020, Vol. 9, Page 2617, 9*(12), 2617. https://doi.org/DOI: 10.3390/CELLS9122617

Sakagianni, A., Koufopoulou, C., Feretzakis, G., Kalles, D., Verykios, V. S., & Myrianthefs, P. (2023). Using machine learning to predict antimicrobial resistance—A literature review. *Antibiotics (Basel, Switzerland), 12*(3), 452. PMID: 36978319

Sakagianni, A., Koufopoulou, C., Koufopoulos, P., Kalantzi, S., Theodorakis, N., Nikolaou, M., Paxinou, E., Kalles, D., Verykios, V. S., & Myrianthefs, P. (2024). Data-driven approaches in antimicrobial resistance: Machine learning solutions. *Antibiotics (Basel, Switzerland), 13*(12), 1052. DOI: 10.3390/antibiotics13121052 PMID: 39596745

Sakib, M. A. N., Mitro, P., Oishee, F. Y., Talukdar, P. R., Mazumder, Z., Islam, R., Khaiat, S. B., Hossain, M. Z., & Hossain, M. M. (2025). Assessing knowledge, attitudes, and preventive practices of smallholder livestock farmers toward antimicrobial use, resistance, and sources in Bangladesh. *IJID One Health, 2025*, 100101.

Saliba, R., Zahar, J. R., Dabar, G., Riachy, M., Karam-Sarkis, D., & Husni, R. (2023). Limiting the Spread of Multidrug-Resistant Bacteria in Low-to-Middle-Income Countries: One Size Does Not Fit All. *Pathogens 2023, Vol. 12, Page 144, 12*(1), 144. https://doi.org/DOI: 10.3390/PATHOGENS12010144

Sandgren, A., Strong, M., Muthukrishnan, P., Weiner, B. K., Church, G. M., & Murray, M. B. (2009). Tuberculosis drug resistance mutation database. *PLoS Medicine, 6*(2), e1000002. DOI: 10.1371/journal.pmed.1000002

Sangeetha Vijayan, P.. (2024). A review of immune modulators and immunotherapy in infectious diseases. *Molecular and Cellular Biochemistry, 479*(8), 1937–1955.

Sani, R. A., Rachmawati, A., Sunandar, S., Pertela, G., Jahja, E. J., Suandy, I., van den Broek, J., de Wit, S. J., Wagenaar, J. A., Speksnijder, D. C., & Velkers, F. C. (2025). Longitudinal evaluation of interventions on antimicrobial use and antimicrobial resistance on broiler farms in West Java, Indonesia. *Poultry Science, 104*(12), 106010. PMID: 41274108

Santamarina-Fernández, R., Fuentes-Valverde, V., Silva-Rodríguez, A., García, P., Moscoso, M., & Bou, G. (2025). Pseudomonas aeruginosa Vaccine Development: Lessons, Challenges, and Future Innovations. *International Journal of Molecular Sciences, 26*(5), 2012. DOI: 10.3390/IJMS26052012/S1 PMID: 40076637

Sanya, D. R. A., Onésime, D., Vizzarro, G., & Jacquier, N. (2023). Recent advances in therapeutic targets identification and development of treatment strategies towards Pseudomonas aeruginosa infections. *BMC Microbiology 2023 23:1, 23*(1), 1–18. https://doi.org/DOI: 10.1186/S12866-023-02832-X

Sao, P., Vats, S., & Singh, S. (2022). *Porphyromonas gingivalis* resistance and virulence: An integrated functional network analysis. *Gene, 839*, 146734. DOI: 10.1016/j.gene.2022.146734 PMID: 35835406

Saranraj, P., Singh, S., Manigandan, M., Nisha, R., Lokeshwari, B., & Gayathri, K. (2025). Pharmacological Effects of Medicinal Herbs: Recent Development and Progress. In Pharmacology of Plants and Plant Derived Biologically Active Molecules (pp. 30-45). CRC Press.

Saranraj, P., & Manigandan, M. (2025). Antibacterial Efficacy of Moringa oleifera Leaf Extract against Salmonella typhimurium in a Rat Model: An Experimental Study on Infection Treatment. *Al-Anbar Journal of Veterinary Sciences, 18*(1), 19–23.

Saranraj, P., Sayyed, R. Z., Kokila, M., Salomi, V., Sivasakthivelan, P., Manigandan, M., & Mawar, R. (2023). Evolving concepts of biocontrol of phytopathogens by endophytic Pseudomonas fluorescence. In *Plant growth promoting microorganisms of arid region* (pp. 365–388). Springer Nature Singapore.

Sassi, A.. (2025). The Role of the Environment (Water, Air, Soil) in the Emergence and Dissemination of Antimicrobial Resistance: A One Health Perspective. *Antibiotics (Basel, Switzerland), 14*(8), 764.

Sastalla, I.. (2025). *NIAID workshop report: systematic approaches for ESKAPE bacteria antigen discovery*. MDPI.

Sathe, N., Beech, P., Croft, L., Suphioglu, C., Kapat, A., & Athan, E. (2023). Pseudomonas aeruginosa: Infections and novel approaches to treatment "Knowing the enemy" the threat of Pseudomonas aeruginosa and exploring novel approaches to treatment. *Infectious Medicine*, *2*(3), 178–194. DOI: 10.1016/J.IMJ.2023.05.003 PMID: 38073886

Sati, H., et al. (2025). "The WHO Bacterial Priority Pathogens List 2024: a prioritisation study to guide research, development, and public health strategies against antimicrobial resistance." The Lancet infectious diseases.

Sattari-Maraji, A., Nikchi, M., Shahmiri, M., Ahadi, E. M., Firoozpour, L., Moazeni, E., Jabalameli, F., Pourmand, M. R., & Kharrazi, S. (2024). Jellein-I-conjugated gold nanoparticles: Insights into the antibacterial, antibiofilm activities against MRSA, and anticancer properties. *Journal of Drug Delivery Science and Technology*, *101*, 106–218. DOI: 10.1016/j.jddst.2024.106218

Schuts, E. C., Hulscher, M. E. J. L., Mouton, J. W., Verduin, C. M., Stuart, J. W. T. C., Overdiek, H. W. P. M., van der Linden, P. D., Natsch, S., Hertogh, C. M. P. M., Wolfs, T. F. W., Schouten, J. A., Kullberg, B. J., & Prins, J. M. (2016). Current evidence on hospital antimicrobial stewardship objectives: A systematic review and meta-analysis. *The Lancet. Infectious Diseases*, *16*(7), 847–856. https://doi.org/10.1016/s1473-3099(16)00065-7

Schwartz, D. C., Ritchie, A., & Smith, M. A. (2023). AI-driven diagnostic models for predicting antimicrobial resistance. *Nature Biotechnology*, *41*(2), 254–266. DOI: 10.1038/s41587-023-01750-5

Scoffone, V. C.. (2025). The evolution of antimicrobial resistance in Acinetobacter baumannii and new strategies to fight it. *Antibiotics (Basel, Switzerland)*, *14*(1), 85.

Sema, T.. (2025). Global Prevalence and Risk Factors of Multidrug Resistance Escherichia Coli in Human and Animal Samples (2015-2023): A Systematic Review and Meta-Analysis. *J Gastro Endosc*, *3*(2), 1–10.

Sendra, E., Fernández-Muñoz, A., Zamorano, L., Oliver, A., Horcajada, J. P., Juan, C., & Gómez-Zorrilla, S. (2024). Impact of multidrug resistance on the virulence and fitness of Pseudomonas aeruginosa: a microbiological and clinical perspective. *Infection 2024 52:4*, *52*(4), 1235–1268. https://doi.org/DOI: 10.1007/S15010-024-02313-X

Servetas, S. L., Daschner, P. J., Guyard, C., Thomas, V., Affagard, H., Sergaki, C., Sokol, H., Wargo, J. A., Wu, G. D., & Sabot, P. (2022). Evolution of FMT–From early clinical to standardized treatments. *Biologicals*, *76*, 31–35. PMID: 35086768

Shabbir, M. A. B., Shabbir, M. Z., Wu, Q., Mahmood, S., Sajid, A., Maan, M. K., Ahmed, S., Naveed, U., Hao, H., & Yuan, Z. (2019). CRISPR-cas system: Biological function in microbes and its use to treat antimicrobial resistant pathogens. *Annals of Clinical Microbiology and Antimicrobials*, *18*, 21. Advance online publication. DOI: 10.1186/s12941-019-0317-x PMID: 31277669

Shabi, Y., & Algarni, A., Al bshabshe, A., Alazraqi, T., Patriquin, G., Bawazeer, A. O. S., Mohammed, S. A., Habbash, S., Somily, A., Alqahtani, A. J., & Alhamhhum, S. M. S. (2025). A decade of antimicrobial resistance trends in Pseudomonas aeruginosa: Insights from a tertiary care hospital in Saudi Arabia (2013–2022). *Frontiers in Microbiology*, *16*, 1617522. DOI: 10.3389/FMICB.2025.1617522/BIBTEX PMID: 40693146

Shah, C., Baral, R., Bartaula, B., & Shrestha, L. B. (2019). Virulence factors of uropathogenic *Escherichia coli* (UPEC) and correlation with antimicrobial resistance. *BMC Microbiology*, *19*(1), 204. DOI: 10.1186/s12866-019-1587-3 PMID: 31477018

Shah, M., Nawaz, S., Jan, H., Uddin, N., Ali, A., Anjum, S., Giglioli-Guivarc'h, N., Hano, C., & Abbasi, B. H. (2020). Synthesis of bio-mediated silver nanoparticles from Silybum marianum and their biological and clinical activities. *Materials Science and Engineering C*, *112*, 110889. DOI: 10.1016/j.msec.2020.110889

Shahsavand, A., Golestani, A., Akbarpour, S., Salehi, M., Seifi, A., Mohammadi, K., & Shafaati, M. (2025). Burden of antimicrobial resistance and estimated economic impact of Klebsiella pneumoniae in Iran—A 2000 to 2021 analysis. *New Microbes and New Infections*, *68*, 101675. PMID: 41377034

Sharma, V. ETHICAL AND SAFETY CONSIDERATIONS: MICROBIAL GENETIC RESEARCH. *MICROBIAL GENETICS*, 85.

Sharma, D., Misba, L., & Khan, A. U. (2019). Antibiotics versus biofilm: An emerging battleground in microbial communities. *Antimicrobial Resistance and Infection Control*, *8*, 76. DOI: 10.1186/s13756-019-0533-3 PMID: 31131107

Sheng, J.. (2025). Global geographic and genomic epidemiology analysis of carbapenem-resistant Escherichia coli carrying bla NDM-9. *MSphere*, •••, 00704–00725.

Shortridge, D., Pfaller, M. A., Castanheira, M., & Flamm, R. K. (2018). Antimicrobial activity of ceftolozane-tazobactam tested against Enterobacteriaceae and Pseudomonas aeruginosa collected from patients with bloodstream infections isolated in United States hospitals (2013–2015) as part of the Program to Assess Ceftolozane-Tazobactam Susceptibility (PACTS) surveillance program. *Diagnostic Microbiology and Infectious Disease*, *92*(2), 158–163. DOI: 10.1016/J.DIAGMICROBIO.2018.05.011 PMID: 29891184

Shree, P., Singh, C. K., Sodhi, K. K., Surya, J. N., & Singh, D. K. (2023). Biofilms: Understanding the structure and contribution towards bacterial resistance in antibiotics. *Medicine in Microecology*, *16*, 100084. DOI: 10.1016/j.medmic.2023.100084

Shrestha, P., Cooper, B. S., Coast, J., Oppong, R., Do Thi Thuy, N., Phodha, T., Celhay, O., Guerin, P. J., Wertheim, H., & Lubell, Y. (2018). Enumerating the economic cost of Antimicrobial Resistance per antibiotic consumed to inform the evaluation of interventions affecting their use. *Antimicrobial Resistance and Infection Control*, *7*, 98. Advance online publication. DOI: 10.1186/s13756-018-0384-3 PMID: 30116525

Shukla, V., Singh, S., Verma, S., Verma, S., Rizvi, A. A., & Abbas, M. (2024). Targeting the microbiome to improve human health with the approach of personalized medicine: Latest aspects and current updates. *Clinical Nutrition ESPEN*, *63*, 813–820. PMID: 39178987

Simon, B. O., Nnaji, N. D., Anumudu, C. K., Aleke, J. C., Ekwueme, C. T., Uhegwu, C. C., Ihenetu, F. C., Obioha, P., Ifedinezi, O. V., & Ezechukwu, P. S. (2025). Microbiome-based interventions for food safety and environmental health. *Applied Sciences (Basel, Switzerland)*, *15*(9), 5219.

Sindeldecker, D., & Stoodley, P. (2021). The many antibiotic resistance and tolerance strategies of Pseudomonas aeruginosa. *Biofilm*, *3*, 100056. DOI: 10.1016/J.BIOFLM.2021.100056 PMID: 34471871

Singh, S., Kumar, M., Sarma, D. K., Kumawat, M., Verma, V., kriti, M., & Tiwari, R. (2025). Advancing AMR Surveillance: Confluence of One Health and Big Data Integration: S. Singh, et al. *EcoHealth*, 1-12.

Singha, B., Singh, V., & Soni, V. (2024). Alternative therapeutics to control antimicrobial resistance: A general perspective. *Frontiers in Drug Discovery*, *4*, 1385460. DOI: 10.3389/FDDSV.2024.1385460/XML

Singhal, L., Gupta, P., & Gupta, V. (2025). Diagnostic stewardship in clinical microbiology: An indispensable component of patient care. *Infectious Disorders Drug Targets*, *25*(2), E030724231543. PMID: 38963103

Singh, P. K., Schaefer, A. L., Parsek, M. R., Moninger, T. O., Welsh, M. J., & Greenberg, E. P. (2007). Quorum-sensing signals indicate that cystic fibrosis lungs are infected with bacterial biofilms. *Nature*, *407*(6805), 762–764. DOI: 10.1038/35037627 PMID: 11048725

Singh, R. K., Prasad, A., Maurya, J., & Prasad, M. (2022). Regulation of small RNA-mediated high temperature stress responses in crop plants. *Plant Cell Reports*, *41*(4), 765–773. DOI: 10.1007/s00299-021-02829-3

Singh, S. B., Young, K., & Silver, L. L. (2017). What is an "ideal" antibiotic? Discovery challenges and path forward. *Biochemical Pharmacology*, *133*, 63–73. DOI: 10.1016/j.bcp.2017.01.003 PMID: 28087253

Sivalingam, P.. (2025). Microplastics, Nanoplastics and Nanoparticles: Emerging Dynamic Carriers of Extracellular DNA Antibiotic Resistance Genes in the Environment. *BioNanoScience*, *15*(1), 198.

Sivamani, Y., Chakraborty, A., Kounin, A. P., & Elayaperumal, S. (2025). Microbiome Engineering and its Applications. In *Microbiome Engineering* (pp. 13–34). CRC Press.

Slawomirski, L., Kelly, D., de Bienassis, K., Kallas, K.-A., & Klazinga, N. (2025). *The economics of diagnostic safety*.

Smith, W. D., Bardin, E., Cameron, L., Edmondson, C. L., Farrant, K. V., Martin, I., Murphy, R. A., Soren, O., Turnbull, A. R., Wierre-Gore, N., Alton, E. W., Bundy, J. G., Bush, A., Connett, G. J., Faust, S. N., Filloux, A., Freemont, P. S., Jones, A. L., Takats, Z., & Davies, J. C. (2017). Current and future therapies for Pseudomonas aeruginosa infection in patients with cystic fibrosis. *FEMS Microbiology Letters*, *364*(14), 121. DOI: 10.1093/FEMSLE/FNX121 PMID: 28854668

Sole, E., Trinchera, M., Gaetano, S. De, Midiri, A., Piccolo, G., Mancuso, G., Schepici, G., & Biondo, C. (2025). The Paradox of Healthcare in the 'Superbugs' Era: Current Challenges and Future Directions. *Pathogens 2025, Vol. 14, Page 1199*, *14*(12), 1199. https://doi.org/DOI: 10.3390/PATHOGENS14121199

Sonderholm, M., Bjarnsholt, T., Alhede, M., Kolpen, M., Jensen, P. Ø., Kuhl, M., & Kragh, K. N. (2017). The consequences of being in an infectious biofilm: Microenvironmental conditions governing antibiotic tolerance. *International Journal of Molecular Sciences*, *18*(12), 2688. DOI: 10.3390/ijms18122688 PMID: 29231866

Souza, S. S., Piper, K. R., Ikhimiukor, O. O., Marcovici, M. M., Zac Soligno, N. I., Harmon, A. J., Eckhardt, E. M., Carreiro, N., Workman, A. A., & Martin, I. W. (2025). Variants of β-lactamase-encoding genes are disseminated by multiple genetically distinct lineages of bloodstream Escherichia coli. *Communications Medicine*, *5*(1), 260. PMID: 40595425

Spagnolo, A. M., Sartini, M., & Cristina, M. L. (2021). Pseudomonas aeruginosa in the healthcare facility setting. *Reviews in Medical Microbiology : a Journal of the Pathological Society of Great Britain and Ireland*, *32*(3), 169–175. DOI: 10.1097/mrm.0000000000000271

Spellberg, B., Guidos, R., Gilbert, D., Bradley, J., Boucher, H. W., Scheld, W. M., Bartlett, J. G., & Edwards, J. (2008). The epidemic of antibiotic-resistant infections: A call to action for the medical community from the Infectious Diseases Society of America. *Clinical Infectious Diseases*, *46*(2), 155–164. PMID: 18171244

Srivastav, A. K., Das, P., & Srivastava, A. K. (2024). Future trends, innovations, and global collaboration. In *Biotech and IoT: an introduction using cloud-driven labs* (pp. 309–398). Springer.

Standyło, A.. (2022). The correlation between second-hand tobacco smoke exposure and biofilm formation in chronic rhinosinusitis. *Journal of Education, Health and Sport*, *12*(6), 268–275.

Stark, Z., Glazer, D., Hofmann, O., Rendon, A., Marshall, C. R., Ginsburg, G. S., Lunt, C., Allen, N., Effingham, M., & Hastings Ward, J. (2025). A call to action to scale up research and clinical genomic data sharing. *Nature Reviews. Genetics*, *26*(2), 141–147. PMID: 39375561

Stoitsova, S.. (2022). The concept for the antivirulence therapeutics approach as alternative to antibiotics: Hope or still a fiction? *Biotechnology, Biotechnological Equipment*, *36*(1), 697–705.

Strathdee, S. A., Hatfull, G. F., Mutalik, V. K., & Schooley, R. T. (2023). Phage therapy: From biological mechanisms to future directions. *Cell*, *186*(1), 17–31. PMID: 36608652

Struelens, M. J., Ludden, C., Werner, G., Sintchenko, V., Jokelainen, P., & Ip, M. (2024). Real-time genomic surveillance for enhanced control of infectious diseases and antimicrobial resistance. *Frontiers in Science*, *2*, 1298248.

Suay-García, B., & Pérez-Gracia, M. T. (2019). Present and future of carbapenem-resistant Enterobacteriaceae (CRE) infections. *Antibiotics (Basel, Switzerland)*, *8*(3), 122. DOI: 10.3390/antibiotics8030122 PMID: 31430964

Subramaniam, G., & Girish, M. (2020). Antibiotic resistance: A cause for re-emergence of infections. *Indian Journal of Pediatrics, 87*(11), 937–944. PMID: 32026301

Suessmuth, R. D.. (2025). Fighting antimicrobial resistance: Innovative drugs in antibacterial research. *Angewandte Chemie International Edition, 64*(10), e202414325.

Sukhum, K. V., Diorio-Toth, L., & Dantas, G. (2019). Genomic and metagenomic approaches for predictive surveillance of emerging pathogens and antibiotic resistance. *Clinical Pharmacology and Therapeutics, 106*(3), 512–524. PMID: 31172511

Sultana, A., Zare, M., Thomas, V., Kumar, T. S., & Ramakrishna, S. (2022). Nano-based drug delivery systems: Conventional drug delivery routes, recent developments and future prospects. *Medicine in Drug Discovery, 15*, 100134.

Sunderland, K. S., Yang, M., & Mao, C. (2017). Phage-enabled nanomedicine: From probes to therapeutics in precision medicine. *Angewandte Chemie International Edition, 56*(8), 1964–1992. PMID: 27491926

Tacconelli, E., Carrara, E., & Savoldi, A.. (2018). Discovery, research, and development of new antibiotics: The WHO priority list of antibiotic-resistant bacteria and tuberculosis. *The Lancet. Infectious Diseases, 18*(3), 318–327. DOI: 10.1016/S1473-3099(17)30753-3

Tagini, F., & Greub, G. (2020). Bacterial genome sequencing in clinical microbiology: A pathogen-oriented review. *European Journal of Clinical Microbiology & Infectious Diseases, 39*(5), 785–802.

Taheri, M., Arabestani, M. R., Kalhori, F., Soleimani Asl, S., Asgari, M., & Hosseini, S. M. (2024). Antibiotics-encapsulated nanoparticles as an antimicrobial agent in the treatment of wound infection. *Frontiers in Immunology, 15*, 1435151. DOI: 10.3389/fimmu.2024.1435151

Talat, A., Blake, K. S., Dantas, G., & Khan, A. U. (2023). Metagenomic insight into microbiome and antibiotic resistance genes of high clinical concern in urban and rural hospital wastewater of northern India origin: A major reservoir of antimicrobial resistance. *Microbiology Spectrum, 11*(2), e04102–e04122. PMID: 36786639

Tamma, P. D., Avdic, E., & Li, D. X. (2022). Association of adverse events with antibiotic use in hospitalized patients. *JAMA Internal Medicine, 177*(9), 1308–1315. DOI: 10.1001/jamainternmed.2017.1938 PMID: 28604925

Tamma, P. D., & Cosgrove, S. E. (2011). Antimicrobial stewardship. *Infectious Disease Clinics of North America, 25*(1), 245–260. PMID: 21316003

Tang, X. (2024). Conifer Genome Sequencing and Functional Study of Disease Resistance Genes. *Tree Genetics and Molecular Breeding, 14.*

Tang, K. W. K., Millar, B. C., & Moore, J. E. (2023). Antimicrobial resistance (AMR). *British Journal of Biomedical Science*, *80*, 11387. PMID: 37448857

Tavares-Carreon, F.. (2023). Serratia marcescens antibiotic resistance mechanisms of an opportunistic pathogen: A literature review. *PeerJ*, *11*, e14399.

Tehrani, K. H., & Martin, N. I. (2018). β-lactam/β-lactamase inhibitor combinations: An update. *MedChemComm*, *9*(9), 1439–1456.

Tesema, M. Y., & Birhanu, A. G. (2024). One Health initiative to mitigate the challenge of antimicrobial resistance in the perspectives of developing countries. *Bulletin of the National Research Center*, *48*(1), 14.

Thai, P. K., Ky, L. X., Binh, V. N., Nhung, P. H., Nhan, P. T., Hieu, N. Q., Dang, N. T. T., Tam, N. K. B., & Anh, N. T. K. (2018). Occurrence of antibiotic residues and antibiotic-resistant bacteria in effluents of pharmaceutical manufacturers and other sources around Hanoi, Vietnam. *The Science of the Total Environment*, *645*, 393–400. DOI: 10.1016/j.scitotenv.2018.07.126 PMID: 30029118

Thanush, D., Basavaraj, H., & Gowrav, M. (2023). Current regulation and initial considerations for successful development and commercialization of microbiome therapies. *Advanced Gut & Microbiome Research*, *2023*(1), 6657515.

Theivendren, P., Kunjiappan, S., Pavadai, P., Ravi, K., Murugavel, A., Dayalan, A., & Santhana Krishna Kumar, A. (2024). Revolutionizing cancer immunotherapy: Emerging nanotechnology-driven drug delivery systems for enhanced therapeutic efficacy. *ACS Measurement Science Au*, *5*(1), 31–55. PMID: 39991031

Theuretzbacher, U. (2009). Accelerating resistance, inadequate antibacterial drug pipelines and international responses. *International Journal of Antimicrobial Agents*, *33*(3), 195–199. PMID: 22341298

Thompson, L. (2024). The Impact of Antimicrobial Resistance on Public Health: Challenges and Strategic Responses. *Insight into Epidemiology, 1*(1).

Tiwari, G., Tiwari, R., & Srivastava, P. (2023). Nanocarrier-assisted delivery of antimicrobial peptides: A frontier in combating multidrug resistance. *Drug Delivery and Translational Research*, *13*(2), 234–248. DOI: 10.1007/s13346-023-01198-z

Tosas Auguet, O., et al. (2025). "Global antibiotic resistance surveillance report 2025."

Tracanna, V., de Jong, A., Medema, M. H., & Kuipers, O. P. (2017). Mining prokaryotes for antimicrobial compounds: From diversity to function. *FEMS Microbiology Reviews, 41*(3), 417–429. DOI: 10.1093/femsre/fux014 PMID: 28402441

Treffon, J., Heppner, B., Eismann, J., Bothe, J., Omengo, B., & Mellmann, A. (2022). Single nucleotide polymorphism-based real-time PCR screening assay for rapid tracking of bacterial infection clusters to complement whole-genome sequencing efforts during outbreak investigations. *Microbiology Spectrum, 10*(6), e03036–e03022. PMID: 36250868

Tsalidou, M., Stergiopoulou, T., Bostanitis, I., Nikaki, C., Skoumpa, K., Koutsoukou, T., & Papaioannidou, P. (2023). Surveillance of antimicrobial resistance and multidrug resistance prevalence of clinical isolates in a regional hospital in Northern Greece. *Antibiotics (Basel, Switzerland), 12*(11), 1595. PMID: 37998797

Tseng, Y. S., Wu, D. C., Chang, C. Y., Kuo, C. H., Yang, Y. C., Jan, C. M., Su, Y. C., Kuo, F. C., & Chang, L. L. (2009). Amoxicillin resistance with beta-lactamase production in *Helicobacter pylori. European Journal of Clinical Investigation, 39*(9), 807–812. DOI: 10.1111/j.1365-2362.2009.02166.x PMID: 19614952

Tsere, B. (2023). Assessing Antibiotic-Resistance Patterns and Clinical outcomes among People-Living with Hiv/Aids with Features of Sepsis. In *Northern Tanzania.* NM-AIST.

Tumbarello, M., Repetto, E., Trecarichi, E. M., Bernardini, C., De Pascale, G., Parisini, A., Rossi, M., Molinari, M. P., Spanu, T., Viscoli, C., Cauda, R., & Bassetti, M. (2011). Multidrug-resistant Pseudomonas aeruginosa bloodstream infections: Risk factors and mortality. *Epidemiology and Infection, 139*(11), 1740–1749. DOI: 10.1017/S0950268810003055 PMID: 21226988

Turner, N. A., Sharma-Kuinkel, B. K., Maskarinec, S. A., Eichenberger, E. M., Shah, P. P., Carugati, M., Holland, T. L., & Fowler, V. G. (2019). Methicillin-resistant Staphylococcus aureus: An overview of basic and clinical research. *Nature Reviews. Microbiology, 17*(4), 203–218. https://doi.org/10.1038/s41579-018-0147-4

Uddin, T. M., Chakraborty, A. J., Khusro, A., Zidan, B. R. M., Mitra, S., Emran, T. B., Dhama, K., Ripon, M. K. H., Gajdács, M., Sahibzada, M. U. K., Hossain, M. J., & Koirala, N. (2021). Antibiotic resistance in microbes: History, mechanisms, therapeutic strategies and future prospects. *Journal of Infection and Public Health, 14*(12), 1750–1766. DOI: 10.1016/j.jiph.2021.10.020 PMID: 34756812

Umansky, A. A., & Fortier, L. C. (2023). The long and sinuous road to phage-based therapy of Clostridioides difficile infections. *Frontiers in Medicine, 10*, 1259427. PMID: 37680620

United Nations Interagency Coordination Group on Antimicrobial Resistance. (2019). *No time to wait: Securing the future from drug-resistant infections.*

Urban-Chmiel, R.. (2022). Antibiotic resistance in bacteria—A review. *Antibiotics (Basel, Switzerland), 11*(8), 1079.

Uwitonze, A. M., Ojeh, N., Murererehe, J., Atfi, A., & Razzaque, M. S. (2020). Zinc adequacy is essential for the maintenance of optimal oral health. *Nutrients, 12*(4), 949. DOI: 10.3390/nu12040949 PMID: 32235426

Valentin, J. D. P., Straub, H., Pietsch, F., Lemare, M., Ahrens, C. H., & Schreiber, F. (2022). Role of the flagellar hook in the structural development and antibiotic tolerance of *Pseudomonas aeruginosa* biofilms. *The ISME Journal, 16*(5), 1176–1186. DOI: 10.1038/s41396-021-01157-9

Valiakos, G., & Kapna, I. (2021). Colistin resistant mcr genes prevalence in livestock animals (swine, bovine, poultry) from a multinational perspective. A systematic review. *Veterinary Sciences, 8*(11), 265. PMID: 34822638

van Belkum, A., Bachmann, T. T., Lüdke, G., Lisby, J. G., Kahlmeter, G., Mohess, A., Becker, K., Hays, J. P., Woodford, N., Mitsakakis, K., Moran-Gilad, J., & Consortium, T. D. (2019). Developmental roadmap for antimicrobial susceptibility testing systems. *Nature Reviews. Microbiology, 17*(1), 51–62. DOI: 10.1038/s41579-018-0098-9 PMID: 30333569

Van Boeckel, T. P., Glennon, E. E., Chen, D., Gilbert, M., Robinson, T. P., Grenfell, B. T., Levin, S. A., Bonhoeffer, S., & Laxminarayan, R. (2017). Reducing antimicrobial use in food animals. *Science, 357*(6358), 1350–1352. PMID: 28963240

van der Meij, A., Worsley, S. F., Hutchings, M. I., & van Wezel, G. P. (2017). Chemical ecology of antibiotic production by Actinomycetes. *FEMS Microbiology Reviews, 41*(3), 392–416. DOI: 10.1093/femsre/fux005 PMID: 28521336

van Duin, D., & Doi, Y. (2017). The global epidemiology of carbapenemase-producing Enterobacteriaceae. *Virulence, 8*(4), 460–469. DOI: 10.1080/21505594.2016.1222343

Vasala, A., Hytönen, V. P., & Laitinen, O. H. (2020). Modern tools for rapid diagnostics of antimicrobial resistance. *Frontiers in Cellular and Infection Microbiology, 10*, 308. PMID: 32760676

Vatansever, C.. (2025). Evaluating the Antibiofilm Effects of Antibiotics on Staphylococcus Species from Pediatric Hematology–Oncology Patients. *Microbial Drug Resistance (Larchmont, N.Y.), 31*(6), 178–188.

Veerachamy, S., Yarlagadda, T., Manivasagam, G., & Yarlagadda, P. K. (2014). Bacterial adherence and biofilm formation on medical implants: A review. *Proceedings of the Institution of Mechanical Engineers. Part H, Journal of Engineering in Medicine*, *228*(10), 1083–1099. DOI: 10.1177/0954411914556137 PMID: 25406229

Ventola, C. L. (2015). The antibiotic resistance crisis: Part 1: Causes and threats. *P&T : a Peer-Reviewed Journal for Formulary Management*, *40*(4), 277–283. PMID: 25859123

Ventola, C. L. (2015). The antibiotic resistance crisis: Part 1—Causes and threats. *P&T : a Peer-Reviewed Journal for Formulary Management*, *40*(4), 277–283. PMID: 25859123

Verderosa, A. D., Totsika, M., & Fairfull-Smith, K. E. (2019). Bacterial biofilm eradication agents: A current review. *Frontiers in Chemistry*, *7*, 824. DOI: 10.3389/fchem.2019.00824 PMID: 31850313

Verma, A., Vishwakarma, A., Singh, R., & Yadav, P. MICROBIOME-TARGETED THERAPIES: UNLOCKING THE GUT MICROBIOME FOR DISEASE TREATMENT.

Verraes, C., Van Boxstael, S., Van Meervenne, E., Van Coillie, E., Butaye, P., Catry, B., de Schaetzen, M. A., Van Huffel, X., Imberechts, H., Dierick, K., Daube, G., Saegerman, C., De Block, J., Dewulf, J., & Herman, L. (2013). Antimicrobial resistance in the food chain: A review. *International Journal of Environmental Research and Public Health*, *10*(7), 2643–2669. DOI: 10.3390/ijerph10072643

Viasus, D., Puerta-Alcalde, P., Cardozo, C., Suárez-Lledó, M., Rodríguez-Núñez, O., Morata, L., Fehér, C., Marco, F., Chumbita, M., Moreno-García, E., Fernández-Avilés, F., Gutiérrez-Garcia, G., Martínez, J. A., Mensa, J., Rovira, M., Esteve, J., Soriano, A., & Garcia-Vidal, C. (2020). Predictors of multidrug-resistant Pseudomonas aeruginosa in neutropenic patients with bloodstream infection. *Clinical Microbiology and Infection*, *26*(3), 345–350. DOI: 10.1016/J.CMI.2019.07.002 PMID: 31295551

Vidyadhari, A. and A. K. Singh Immunogenicity of Cell-Based Therapy. Nano-erythrocytes in Cancer Therapy, CRC Press: 192-222.

Visan, A. I., & Negut, I. (2024). Coatings based on essential oils for combating antibiotic resistance. *Antibiotics (Basel, Switzerland)*, *13*(7), 625.

Vliex, L. M. M. (2024). The gut microbiome and metabolic health in humans: Individualised impact of antibiotic and prebiotic use.

Vrancianu, C. O.. (2020). Antibiotic resistance profiles, molecular mechanisms and innovative treatment strategies of Acinetobacter baumannii. *Microorganisms, 8*(6), 935.

Vuong, C., Voyich, J. M., Fischer, E. R., Braughton, K. R., Whitney, A. R., DeLeo, F. R., & Otto, M. (2004). Polysaccharide intercellular adhesin (PIA) protects *Staphylococcus epidermidis* against major components of the human innate immune system. *Cellular Microbiology, 6*(3), 269–275. DOI: 10.1046/j.1462-5822.2004.00367.x PMID: 14764110

Waddington, C., Carey, M. E., Boinett, C. J., Higginson, E., Veeraraghavan, B., & Baker, S. (2022). Exploiting genomics to mitigate the public health impact of antimicrobial resistance. *Genome Medicine, 14*(1), 15. PMID: 35172877

Walsh, C. (2000). Molecular mechanisms that confer antibacterial drug resistance. *Nature, 406*(6797), 775–781. DOI: 10.1038/35021219 PMID: 10963607

Walsh, C., & Collyns, T. (2017). The pathophysiology of urinary tract infections. *Surgery (Oxford), 35*(6), 293–298. DOI: 10.1016/j.mpsur.2017.03.007

Wan, C., Gao, C., Xie, Q., Wang, Y., Cheng, X., Fang, Y., Liu, Z., Zhang, W., Zou, Q., Lu, G., & Gu, J. (2021). Flagella hook protein FlgE is a novel vaccine candidate of Pseudomonas aeruginosa identified by a genomic approach. *Vaccine, 39*(17), 2386–2395. DOI: 10.1016/J.VACCINE.2021.03.051 PMID: 33775439

Wang, G., Yang, H., Olczak, A. A., Maier, S. E., & Maier, R. J. (2006). Dual roles of *Helicobacter pylori* NapA in inducing and combating oxidative stress. *Infection and Immunity, 74*(12), 6839–6846. DOI: 10.1128/IAI.00991-06 PMID: 17030577

Wang, H., Ren, L., Yu, X., Hu, J., Chen, Y., He, G., & Jiang, Q. (2017). Antibiotic residues in meat, milk and aquatic products in Shanghai and human exposure assessment. *Food Control, 80*, 217–225. DOI: 10.1016/j.foodcont.2017.04.034

Wang, H., Wang, D., Huangfu, H., Lv, H., Qin, Q., Ren, S., Zhang, Y., Wang, L., & Zhou, Y. (2022). Branched AuAg nanoparticles coated by metal–phenolic networks for treating bacteria-induced periodontitis via photothermal antibacterial and immunotherapy. *Materials & Design, 224*, 111401.

Wang, L.. (2017). The antimicrobial activity of nanoparticles: Present situation and prospects for the future. *International Journal of Nanomedicine*, •••, 1227–1249.

Wang, R.. (2025). Research Progress on the Influence Factors of the Quorum Sensing System Regulating the Growth of Wastewater Treatment Biofilm. *Water (Basel), 17*(13), 1944.

Wang, Z., Li, S., You, R., Zhu, S., Zhou, X. J., & Sun, F. (2021). ARG-SHINE: Improve antibiotic resistance class prediction by integrating sequence homology, functional information and deep convolutional neural network. *NAR Genomics and Bioinformatics*, *3*(3), lqab066. PMID: 34377977

Warnes, S. L., Highmore, C. J., & Keevil, C. W. (2012). Horizontal transfer of antibiotic resistance genes on abiotic touch surfaces: Implications for public health. *mBio*, *3*(6), e00489–e12. DOI: 10.1128/mBio.00489-12 PMID: 23188508

Wassmann, T., Kreis, S., Behr, M., & Buergers, R. (2017). The influence of surface texture and wettability on initial bacterial adhesion on titanium and zirconium oxide dental implants. *International Journal of Implant Dentistry*, *3*(1), 32. DOI: 10.1186/s40729-017-0093-3 PMID: 28714053

Watts, N.. (2021). The 2020 report of The Lancet Countdown on health and climate change: Responding to converging crises. *Lancet*, *397*(10269), 129–170.

Weber, D. J., Anderson, D., & Rutala, W. A. (2013). The role of the surface environment in healthcare-associated infections. *Current Opinion in Infectious Diseases*, *26*(4), 338–344. https://doi.org/10.1097/qco.0b013e3283630f04

Wei, X. C., Zhao, M. F., & Xiao, X. (2024). Evaluating omadacycline dosing regimens against drug-resistant pathogens including Staphylococcus aureus, Streptococcus pneumoniae and Haemophilus influenzae in adults: A pharmacokinetic/pharmacodynamic analysis using Monte Carlo simulation. *Journal of Chemotherapy (Florence, Italy)*, *36*(7), 532–539. DOI: 10.1080/1120009X.2024.2339706 PMID: 38591989

Welch, K. T., Virga, K. G., Whittemore, N. A., Ozen, C., Wright, E., Brown, C. L., Lee, R. E., & Serpersu, E. H. (2005). Discovery of non-carbohydrate inhibitors of aminoglycoside-modifying enzymes. *Bioorganic & Medicinal Chemistry*, *13*(22), 6252–6263. DOI: 10.1016/j.bmc.2005.06.059 PMID: 16140014

Wensel, C. R., Pluznick, J. L., Salzberg, S. L., & Sears, C. L. (2022). Next-generation sequencing: Insights to advance clinical investigations of the microbiome. *The Journal of Clinical Investigation*, *132*(7). PMID: 35362479

Werner, G., Couto, N., Feil, E. J., Novais, A., Hegstad, K., Howden, B. P., Friedrich, A. W., & Reuter, S. (2023). Taking hospital pathogen surveillance to the next level. *Microbial Genomics*, *9*(4), 1. DOI: 10.1099/mgen.0.001008 PMID: 37099616

WHO. (2022). *Global Tuberculosis Report 2022*. World Health Organization.

WHO. (2023). *Global antimicrobial resistance and use surveillance system (GLASS) report 2023*. World Health Organization.

WHO. (2024). *Global action plan on antimicrobial resistance: Progress report.* World Health Organization.

Wiens, J., & Shenoy, E. S. (2017). Machine Learning for Healthcare: On the Verge of a Major Shift in Healthcare Epidemiology. *Clinical Infectious Diseases, 66*(1), 149–153. https://doi.org/10.1093/cid/cix731

Winter, S. E.. (2010). Gut inflammation provides a respiratory electron acceptor for Salmonella. *Nature, 467*(7314), 426–429.

Wong, J. L.. (2022). Recurrent emergence of Klebsiella pneumoniae carbapenem resistance mediated by an inhibitory ompK36 mRNA secondary structure. *Proceedings of the National Academy of Sciences of the United States of America, 119*(38), e2203593119.

Wood, T. K., Knabel, S. J., & Kwan, B. W. (2013). Bacterial persister cell formation and dormancy. *Applied and Environmental Microbiology, 79*(23), 7116–7121. DOI: 10.1128/AEM.02636-13 PMID: 24038684

World Bank. (2023). *Pulling together to beat superbugs: Knowledge and implementation gaps in addressing antimicrobial resistance.* Washington, DC.

World Health Organization (WHO). (2020). *Antimicrobial resistance: A global threat.* https://www.who.int/antimicrobial-resistance/en/

World Health Organization. (2015). Global action plan on antimicrobial resistance.

World Health Organization. (2020). *Global antimicrobial resistance and use surveillance system (GLASS) report 2020.* https://www.who.int/glass

World Health Organization. (2023). *One Health Joint Plan of Action 2022–2026.* WHO Press.

World Health Organization. (2024). *Global Antimicrobial Resistance and Use Surveillance System (GLASS) Report 2024.* WHO.

Wu, P., & Grainger, D. W. (2006). Drug/device combinations for local drug therapies and infection prophylaxis. *Biomaterials, 27*(11), 2450–2467. DOI: 10.1016/j.biomaterials.2005.09.032

Yakout, M. A., & Ali, G. H. (2022). A novel parC mutation potentiating fluoroquinolone resistance in Klebsiella pneumoniae and Escherichia coli clinical isolates. *Journal of Infection in Developing Countries, 16*(02), 314–319. PMID: 35298427

Yamasaki, S.. (2023). Drug resistance and physiological roles of RND multidrug efflux pumps in Salmonella enterica, Escherichia coli and Pseudomonas aeruginosa. *Microbiology*, *169*(6), 001322.

Yang, H., Li, Y., Zhang, Y., Dong, B., Duan, B., Guo, L., Wang, T., Lv, X., Zheng, M., & Cui, X. (2023). Prevalence, drug resistance spectrum and virulence gene analysis of Campylobacter jejuni in broiler farms in central Shanxi, China. *Poultry Science*, *102*(3), 102419. PMID: 36599220

Yan, X.. (2023). Applications of synthetic biology in medical and pharmaceutical fields. *Signal Transduction and Targeted Therapy*, *8*(1), 199.

Yayan, J., Ghebremedhin, B., & Rasche, K. (2015). Antibiotic Resistance of Pseudomonas aeruginosa in Pneumonia at a Single University Hospital Center in Germany over a 10-Year Period. *PLoS One*, *10*(10), e0139836. DOI: 10.1371/JOURNAL.PONE.0139836 PMID: 26430738

Yin, C., Alam, M. Z., Fallon, J. T., & Huang, W. (2024). Advances in Development of Novel Therapeutic Strategies against Multi-Drug Resistant Pseudomonas aeruginosa. *Antibiotics 2024, Vol. 13, Page 119, 13*(2), 119. https://doi.org/DOI: 10.3390/ANTIBIOTICS13020119

Yin, L., Zhang, Y., Azi, F., Zhou, J., Liu, X., Dai, Y., Wang, Z., Dong, M., & Xia, X. (2022). Inhibition of biofilm formation and quorum sensing by soy isoflavones in Pseudomonas aeruginosa. *Food Control*, *133*, 108629. DOI: 10.1016/J.FOODCONT.2021.108629

Yosef, I., Manor, M., Kiro, R., & Qimron, U. (2015). Temperate and lytic bacteriophages programmed to sensitize and kill antibiotic-resistant bacteria. *Proceedings of the National Academy of Sciences of the United States of America*, *112*(23), 7267–7272. DOI: 10.1073/pnas.1500107112 PMID: 26060300

Youf, R.. (2021). Antimicrobial photodynamic therapy: Latest developments with a focus on combinatory strategies. *Pharmaceutics*, *13*(12), 1995.

Youssef, R. A., Sakr, M. M., Shebl, R. I., Saad, B. T., & Aboshanab, K. M. (2024). Genomic characterization, in vitro, and preclinical evaluation of two microencapsulated lytic phages VB_ST_E15 and VB_ST_SPNIS2 against clinical multidrug-resistant Salmonella serovars. *Annals of Clinical Microbiology and Antimicrobials*, *23*(1), 1–17. PMID: 38360595

Yu, V. L. (2011). Guidelines for hospital-acquired pneumonia and health-care-associated pneumonia: A vulnerability, a pitfall, and a fatal flaw. *The Lancet. Infectious Diseases*, *11*(3), 248–252. DOI: 10.1016/S1473-3099(10)70306-5 PMID: 21371658

Yu, Y., Xue, J., Lin, F., Liu, D., Zhang, W., Ru, S., & Jiang, F. (2024). Global primary antibiotic resistance rate of *Helicobacter pylori* in recent 10 years: A systematic review and meta-analysis. *Helicobacter, 29*(1), e13103. DOI: 10.1111/hel.13103 PMID: 38898622

Zakaria, N. F. S.. (2023). Multiple bacterial strategies to survive antibiotic pressure. *RE:view*.

Zaman, S. B., Hussain, M. A., Nye, R., Mehta, V., Mamun, K. T., & Hossain, N. (2017). A review on antibiotic resistance: Alarm bells are ringing. *Cureus, 9*(6), e1403. DOI: 10.7759/cureus.1403 PMID: 28852600

Zangirolami, A. C., Dias, L. D., Blanco, K. C., Vinagreiro, C. S., Inada, N. M., Arnaut, L. G., Pereira, M. M., & Bagnato, V. S. (2020). Avoiding ventilator-associated pneumonia: Curcumin-functionalized endotracheal tube and photodynamic action. *Proceedings of the National Academy of Sciences of the United States of America, 117*(37), 22967–22973. DOI: 10.1073/pnas.2006759117 PMID: 32868444

Zhang, D., Zhang, J., Kalimuthu, S., Liu, J., Song, Z.-M., He, B.-b., Cai, P., Zhong, Z., Feng, C., & Neelakantan, P. (2023). A systematically biosynthetic investigation of lactic acid bacteria reveals diverse antagonistic bacteriocins that potentially shape the human microbiome. *Microbiome, 11*(1), 91. PMID: 37101246

Zhang, J., Chu, A., Yang, P., Ouyang, X., Li, B., Mao, W., Wu, X., Zhong, C., Gou, S., Zhang, Y., Liu, H., & Ni, J. (2025). De novo design of mirror-image dimeric antimicrobial peptides with low drug resistance and in vivo efficacy. *Journal of Medicinal Chemistry, 68*(19), 20304–20323. PMID: 41023587

Zhang, L., Gowardman, J., Morrison, M., Runnegar, N., & Rickard, C. M. (2016). Microbial biofilms associated with intravascular catheter-related bloodstream infections in adult intensive care patients. *European Journal of Clinical Microbiology & Infectious Diseases, 35*(2), 201–205. DOI: 10.1007/s10096-015-2532-5 PMID: 26610337

Zhang, L., & Webster, T. J. (2009). Nanotechnology and nanomaterials: Promises for improved tissue regeneration. *Nano Today, 4*(1), 66–80. DOI: 10.1016/j.nantod.2008.10.014

Zhang, Y., Yew, W. W., & Barer, M. R. (2012). Targeting persisters for tuberculosis control. *Antimicrobial Agents and Chemotherapy, 56*(5), 2223–2230. DOI: 10.1128/AAC.06288-11

Zhao, F., Liu, J., Shi, W., Huang, F., Liu, L., Zhao, S., & Zhang, J. (2019). Antimicrobial susceptibility and genotyping of Mycoplasma pneumoniae isolates in Beijing, China, from 2014 to 2016. *Antimicrobial Resistance and Infection Control*, *8*, 18. Advance online publication. DOI: 10.1186/s13756-019-0470-1 PMID: 30697421

Zhao, W.. (2024). Increased risk of antibiotic resistance in surface water due to global warming. *Environmental Research*, *263*, 120149.

Zhao, X., Chen, Z., Yang, T., Jiang, M., Wang, J., Cheng, Z., Yang, M., Zhu, J., Zhang, T., Li, H., Li, A., Chen, H., & Wang, H. (2021). Glutamine promotes antibiotic uptake to kill multidrug-resistant uropathogenic bacteria. *Science Translational Medicine*, *13*(625), eabj0716. Advance online publication. DOI: 10.1126/scitranslmed.abj0716 PMID: 34936385

Zhou, M., Xu, B., Guo, Z., Zeng, Y., Lei, J., Kritsotakis, E. I., & Wang, J. (2024). Clinical burden of community-associated infections caused by multidrug-resistant Pseudomonas aeruginosa: A propensity-matched longitudinal cohort study in Southern China. *GMS Hygiene and Infection Control*, *19*, Doc51. DOI: 10.3205/DGKH000506 PMID: 39553304

Zhou, S., Zhao, X., & Meng, F. (2025). Method development and clinical validation of LAMP-CRISPR/Cas12a for rapid detection of respiratory pathogens in children. *Frontiers in Pediatrics*, *13*, 1533100. PMID: 40292114

Zhou, Y., Zhong, Z., Hu, S., Wang, J., Deng, Y., Li, X., Chen, X., Li, X., Tang, Y., Li, X., Zheng, Z., & Li, B. (2022). A survey of *Helicobacter pylori* antibiotic-resistant genotypes and strain lineages by whole-genome sequencing in China. *Antimicrobial Agents and Chemotherapy*, *66*(4), e02188–e21. DOI: 10.1128/aac.02188-21 PMID: 35652644

Zimmermann, S., Klinger-Strobel, M., Bohnert, J. A., Wendler, S., Rödel, J., Pletz, M. W., & Löffler, B. (2019). Clinically approved drugs inhibit the *Staphylococcus aureus* multidrug NorA efflux pump and reduce biofilm formation. *Frontiers in Microbiology*, *10*, 2762. DOI: 10.3389/fmicb.2019.02762 PMID: 31849901

Ziran, B. H. (2007). Osteomyelitis. *The Journal of Trauma and Acute Care Surgery*, *62*(6), S59. DOI: 10.1097/TA.0b013e318065abb6 PMID: 17556977

Zurek, L., & Ghosh, A. (2014). Insects represent a link between food animal farms and the urban environment for antibiotic resistance traits. *Applied and Environmental Microbiology*, *80*(12), 3562–3567. DOI: 10.1128/AEM.00600-14 PMID: 24705326

About the Contributors

Syed Sohail Ahmad is an emerging leader in medical microbiology and scientific publishing, recognized for his editorial expertise and research contributions in antimicrobial resistance and medical diagnostics. He currently lectures in Medical Laboratory Technology at Rehman Medical Institute, Peshawar, and has previously served as Head of Department and Assistant Professor at the Khyber Pakhtunkhwa Institute of Medical Sciences. His research portfolio spans biofilm disruption, antimicrobial resistance mechanisms, and innovative diagnostic strategies, with publications in respected journals including Molecules and the International Journal of Pathology. He has presented at international conferences and facilitated workshops on research fundamentals, proposal development, and academic publishing, reflecting his commitment to advancing biomedical sciences. Syed Sohail is the Chief Editor of the Dinkum Journal of Medical Innovations, where he oversees peer review, editorial workflows, and scientific quality assurance. He also serves as International Book Editor for Combatting Antimicrobial Resistance Through Medical Microbiology (IGI Global, USA), collaborating with global scholars to curate cutting-edge research addressing one of the most urgent challenges in healthcare. Beyond editorial leadership, he mentors undergraduate and postgraduate researchers through the NOVA Research Program, guiding them in study design, data analysis, and manuscript preparation for publication. His dual MPhil degrees in Medical Microbiology and Medical Laboratory Sciences, combined with a BS in Medical Laboratory Technology, underpin his academic rigor and editorial vision. Honored by the Higher Education Commission of Pakistan for academic excellence, and recognized for his leadership as president of the Society for Peace and Conflict Management, Syed Sohail continues to shape the future of medical microbiology and scientific publishing. His career reflects a rare blend of editorial precision, research innovation, and international collaboration, positioning him as a dynamic voice in the global fight against antimicrobial resistance.

Aman Ullah is the Principal of Rehman College of Allied Health Sciences at Rehman Medical Institute, Peshawar, Pakistan. He holds a PhD in Microbiology and has completed postdoctoral research in advanced biomedical sciences. With extensive academic and administrative experience, he has played a pivotal role in strengthening medical education and research culture in Pakistan. His research interests span medical microbiology, infectious diseases, antimicrobial resistance, and translational therapeutics. Prof. Ullah has contributed to numerous peer-reviewed publications, book chapters, and collaborative projects, with a focus on bridging laboratory findings to clinical applications. He has co-edited volumes on antimicrobial resistance and continues to mentor students and early-career researchers in microbiology and allied health sciences. As an academic leader, Prof. Ullah has been instrumental in curriculum development, faculty training, and fostering international collaborations. His vision emphasizes innovation, interdisciplinary research, and the integration of modern diagnostic and therapeutic approaches to address global health challenges.

***

Maria Nazir is an MPhil Scholar in Microbiology at the Cholistan University of Veterinary and Animal Sciences (CUVAS), Bahawalpur, Pakistan. She is part of an NRPU-funded project focusing on the molecular characterization of Corynebacterium pseudotuberculosis and its implications for animal and human health. Her research interests include genetics, molecular biology, and bioinformatics.

Farman Alam is a BS Biotechnology student at Bahauddin Zakariya University, Multan, with interests in climate change, sustainability, biodiversity, and health biotechnology. He has worked on projects related to antimicrobial resistance, public health stigmatization, and species extinction. He is currently seeking research and internship opportunities to expand his scientific experience.

B. Ramya holds a Doctorate in Biochemistry and has 22 years of extensive teaching and research experience. A total of 32 research publications and 2 book chapters have been authored. Active participation, presentation, and organization of conferences, seminars, and workshops have been undertaken. Three life memberships in recognized professional bodies are held. Guidance has been successfully provided to 32 M.Phil. scholars, mentorship extended to 105 postgraduate students, and supervision carried out for 10 undergraduate group projects. Active involvement as a member in various co-curricular and extracurricular activities has been maintained. At present, the position of Assistant Professor in the PG and Research Department of Biochemistry at Auxilium College, Vellore, is being held.

Lara Donaldson is a principal investigator at the International Centre for Genetic Engineering and Biotechnology (ICGEB), Cape Town. Her research interest lies in understanding how plants and their microbiomes sense, signal, respond, and adapt to their environments and promote growth. She has studied plant hormones like plant natriuretic peptides, second messengers such as Ca2+ and cyclic nucleotides (cGMP), proteins that produce these second messenger signals, including adenylyl and guanylyl cyclases, and cyclic nucleotide binding proteins that help plants respond to differing environmental challenges, whether caused by living or non-living factors.

Huzaif Khan is an MS in Microbiology and Immunology, with expertise in microbial mechanisms and immune responses. His research focuses on infectious diseases and immunotherapy, aiming to contribute impactful insights.

Ayoigbala Monioluwa Lawal is a lecturer in the department of Microbiology, Federal University Oye-Ekiti, Nigeria. Her research focuses on probiotics, functional foods, food preservation, safety, and processing innovations.

Lovleen Marwaha, Professor, Department of Zoology, School of Bioscience and Bioengineering, Lovely Professional University, Punjab, India Mail ID: lovleenmarwaha@gmail.com Mobile no: 6283587688 Dr. Lovleen Marwaha, Ph.D., is a Professor at the Department of Zoology, School of Bioengineering and Biosciences, Lovely Professional University, Phagwara, India. She has completed her M.S. and Ph.D. in Cytogenetics from the Department of Zoology, Punjab University, Chandigarh. She has worked on the evaluation of pesticide genotoxicity using insect genomes, specifically on different mosquito species and Drosophila melanogaster. She has carried out an intensive study on the correlation between pesticide exposure limit and inductive genotoxic consequences on Dipteran larval salivary polytene chromosomes. Furthermore, she has studied chromosomal and gene mutations in mosquito and fruit fly genomes due to pesticide exposure. Currently, she is working on Apiculture and Sericulture-related topics. She has many research papers published in National and International Journals of repute. Presently, she is working on insecticide resistance in mosquitoes, pesticide genotoxicity evaluation, honey bee development, honey processing, silk fiber, and pearl quality improvement. She has published three authored books on Apiculture and on Mobile Genetic Elements. Forthcoming books include Worker Honey Bees, Apiculture Products, Basic Concepts of Genetics, and Introduction to Sericulture.

Busayo Olowe is a lecturer and researcher in the Department of Biological Sciences, Bamidele Olumilua University of Education Science and Technology, Ikere Ekiti. Her research areas include water, environmental microbiology, and metagenomics.

Kehinde Adewole Oyeniran is a lecturer in the Department of Biological Sciences, Bamidele Olumilua University of Education Science and Technology, Ikere-Ekiti, and presently a postdoctoral fellow with the plant systems biology group, ICGEB Cape Town, South Africa. His multidisciplinary research combines bioinformatics and gold-standard wet-lab approaches to gain insights into the molecular mechanisms underlying pathogen emergence.

Olubukola Helen Oyeniran is a lecturer in the Department of Biochemistry, Federal University Oye-Ekti. Her research focus is on the use of plants as functional foods for management of degenerative diseases, using Drosophila melanogaster and Rattus norvegicus as study models.

P. Saranraj holds a Ph.D. in Microbiology from Annamalai University, Chidambaram, India, and is NET (ASRB–ICAR) qualified in Microbiology. He is currently serving as Assistant Professor and Head, Department of Microbiology, at Sacred Heart College (Autonomous), Tirupattur, Tamil Nadu, India. In addition, he is the Proprietor and Managing Director of JPS Scientific Publications, contributing actively to academic publishing and research dissemination. Dr. Saranraj has over 15 years of research experience and 10 years of teaching experience in the fields of Environmental Microbiology, Agricultural Microbiology, Industrial Microbiology, Bioremediation, Microbial Biotechnology, and Sustainable Ecosystem Management. His research work has focused on Microbial degradation of pollutants, Effluent treatment, Soil health improvement, Plant–microbe interactions, and Applied environmental sustainability. He has an extensive publication record, with more than 240 international research articles, over 90 books (international and national), and 70+ book chapters published with reputed academic publishers.

Gautam Palshikar is currently working as an Assistant Professor in the Department of Pharmacognosy, with 17 years of teaching experience and 7 years of research experience. He has been actively involved in academic activities, contributing to the advancement of pharmacy field through research, publications, and book chapters in national and international forums. His expertise bridges both educational and practical healthcare settings, providing a unique perspective on herbal applications. He is also an active member of professional organizations in his field.

P. Parthiban is an accomplished researcher in Biochemistry, Environmental Biotechnology, and Microbial Technology, with over ten years of experience in interdisciplinary research, innovation management, and analytical instrumentation. His work spans bioprocess development, wastewater and sludge valorization, microbial degradation pathways, nano-bioformulations, and phytochemical-based therapeutics. He has contributed to major DST and DRDO-funded projects exceeding 10 crore and has published 30+ peer-reviewed SCI/Scopus articles, reflecting a strong commitment to high-impact research. Dr. Parthiban is also an active innovator, holding 4 utility patents and 7 design patents, and his additional role as a Patent Analyst has strengthened his expertise in prior art search, patent drafting, and technology evaluation. His research aims to develop sustainable, scalable bioprocesses while bridging scientific discovery with societal and industrial applications.

R Swadhi. working as Coordinator, Academic and Examination Cell, Saraswathi Institute of Medical Sciences, Hapur. She Completed Ph.D. in the Department of Physics, AMET University, Chennai Specialized in Nano Bio materials. Served as Assistant Professor in Nirmala College, Coimbatore, Lecturers & Exam coordinator in DMI-St.Eugene University Zambia published 20+ articles in peer reviewed journals and edited book chapters.

R. Ramya is a seasoned healthcare administrator dedicated to enhancing public health systems and empowering communities through outreach programs. With extensive experience and academic qualifications in Public Administration and Hospital Management, she serves as Vice Chairperson at Saraswathi Institute of Medical Sciences, Hapur driving excellence in healthcare delivery and education. Through her leadership and initiatives via charitable trusts, she addresses healthcare disparities and promotes community welfare, embodying a commitment to social impact and public health advancement.

Zahid Ahmad Thoker Research Scholar, Department of Zoology, School of Bioscience and Bioengineering, Lovely Professional University, Punjab, India Mail ID: za7710917@gmail.com, Orcid id: 0009-0002-6897-5835 Mobile No: 9906499012 Mr. Zahid Ahmad Thoker is a serious research Scholar at Lovely Professional University who is working on Insects (Entomology), specifically on Honey Bees. He graduated with his Master's degree in Zoology from Chandigarh University, Gharuan, Mohali, where he developed a very solid academic grounding in life sciences. Zahid has already contributed greatly to academia; one of his research papers was published, one review paper, and over 25 book chapters in reputable national and international volumes. His academic publication is an indication of the desire to promote science, especially in the biological sciences. As a visionary who desires to make a difference in the research world and in society, Zahid hopes to broaden his academic and professional experiences with integrity and excellence. He is also strongly driven by the goal of benefiting society with his research work and making his parents proud by leaving his mark on the field of science and scholarship.

Sivaranjani Varadharajan is currently working as an Assistant Professor in the Department of Biochemistry, with 4 years of teaching experience and 12 years of research and hospital-based professional experience. She has been actively involved in clinical and academic activities, contributing to the advancement of biochemistry through research, publications, and book chapters in national and international forums. Her expertise bridges both educational and practical healthcare settings, providing a unique perspective on translational biochemistry applications. She is also an active member of professional organizations in her field.

Index

Symbols

A

B

C

D

E

G

H

I

M

N

www.ingramcontent.com/pod-product-compliance
Lightning Source LLC
LaVergne TN
LVHW062336300926
849161LV00007B/1717